Sustainable Housing in a Circular Economy

This book relates circular economy principles to housing design and construction and highlights how those principles can result in both monetary savings, positive environmental impact, and socio-ecological change.

Chapters focus on three key circular economy principles and apply them to architectural construction and design, namely rethinking of the end-of-use phase of a building and the potential of design-for-disassembly; the role of digitization and data standardization in fostering evidence-based circular economy design decision-making; and presenting space as a resource to conserve, via exploration of the sharing economy and flexibility principles. Beyond waste management and material cycles, this book provides a holistic understanding of the opportunities across the building life cycle that can allow for sustainable and affordable circular housing. With case studies from 13 different countries, including but not limited to the Hammarby Sjöstad district in Sweden, the Circle House in Denmark, Benny Farm in Canada, VMD Prefabricated House in Mexico, and the Deep Performance Dwelling in China, authors pair theoretical frameworks with real-world examples.

This will be a useful resource for upper-level students and academics of architecture, construction, and planning, especially those studying and researching housing design, building technology, green project management, and environmental design.

Naomi Keena is an Assistant Professor at McGill University's Peter Guo-hua Fu School of Architecture. Keena's research aims to rethink our built environment as an untapped material resource in a continuous cycle of reuse.

Avi Friedman is a Full Professor at McGill's Peter Guo-hua Fu School of Architecture where he directs the Affordable Homes Research Group. Friedman researches and develops innovative housing prototypes and is known for the Grow and Next Homes designs.

Sustainable Housing in a Circular Economy

Naomi Keena and Avi Friedman

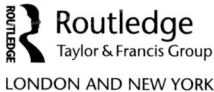

Routledge
Taylor & Francis Group

LONDON AND NEW YORK

Cover design by Naomi Keena, Avi Friedman, Martha Milagros Pomasonco Alvis and Daniel R. Rondinel-Oviedo. Image credit: mycola.

First published 2024
by Routledge
4 Park Square, Milton Park, Abingdon, Oxon OX14 4RN

and by Routledge
605 Third Avenue, New York, NY 10158

Routledge is an imprint of the Taylor & Francis Group, an informa business

British Library Cataloguing-in-Publication Data
A catalogue record for this book is available from the British Library

Library of Congress Cataloging-in-Publication Data
Names: Keena, Naomi, author. | Friedman, Avi, 1952- author.
Title: Sustainable housing in a circular economy / Naomi Keena and Avi Friedman.
Description: Abingdon, Oxon ; New York, NY : Routledge, 2024. | Includes bibliographical references and index. |
Identifiers: LCCN 2023042176 | ISBN 9781032368221 (hbk) | ISBN 9781032368214 (pbk) | ISBN 9781003333975 (ebk)
Subjects: LCSH: Ecological houses. | Sustainable architecture. | Circular economy. | Housing--Environmental aspects. | Dwellings--Design and construction--Case studies.
Classification: LCC TH880 .K44 2024 | DDC 690/.80286--dc23/eng/20231227
LC record available at https://lccn.loc.gov/2023042176

ISBN: 978-1-032-36822-1 (hbk)
ISBN: 978-1-032-36821-4 (pbk)
ISBN: 978-1-003-33397-5 (ebk)

DOI: 10.4324/9781003333975

Typeset in Helvetica
by KnowledgeWorks Global Ltd.

Contents

Preface

Current residential design and construction practices, with their many far-reaching negative implications, necessitate a fundamental rethinking. When an attempt is made to diagnose the root cause that led to poor practices in the homebuilding sector, ignorance of the inner workings of three pivotal issues, environment, economy, and society, can arguably be one of the reasons. Mainstream developments are often regarded as a *product*, rather than a *process*, which this book interrogates through outlining the promise of whole-building life cycle thinking. Such mainstream developments rely on a linear paradigm of *take, make, waste* in the construction of housing. However, although housing construction has negative environmental impacts, globally, there is a housing crisis and a need to provide shelters and homes for a growing population. To disrupt this negative cycle, it's necessary to revisit how we build. Through this book we question, is it possible to provide affordable housing that can benefit our environment? This question is explored through the concept of a *circular economy* which offers a promising approach to tackle housing supply.

A circular economy envisions a sustainable future where waste is eliminated in the built environment and materials and buildings are kept in use for as long as possible. Circular economy aims to rethink the built environment as an untapped material resource in a continuous cycle of reuse. Such an approach encourages a paradigm shift away from the current status quo that facilitates a culture of take-make-waste, toward resilient built environments which aim to benefit human health, economic growth, and the environment. The intention is to put in place effective measures and guidelines for achieving waste recovery to support an effort to significantly curb global greenhouse gas emissions. Therefore, a circular economy approach can offer solutions to challenges of housing supply at the end of a building cycle, revealing its materials as a bank of resources rather than waste. However, such an approach to housing can go beyond solely waste recovery by keeping buildings in use for as long as possible, by promoting flexibility and design-for-disassembly in the early design phases, and by reducing waste and costs of new housing construction. This book outlines a new thought process on how data-driven approaches to circular design decision-making can facilitate sustainable, affordable, and circular housing design. We presented and illustrated this new thought process through systematically exploring, considering, and implementing a series of concepts and theories regarding the environmental, social, and economic aspects of a circular approach as described below.

On the environmental front, the causes of phenomena such as global warming, depletion of natural resources, and waste generation can be blamed on several sectors. Yet, close examination of the data shows that residential follows the industrial and transportation sectors in energy consumption. This data comes as no surprise. From the middle of the 20th century, the size of an average home underwent constant expansion, with significant environmental ramifications. Most low-density, low-rise homes are constructed of solid-sawn lumber. Considered to be an inexpensive renewable resource with low embodied energy, wood has become the material of choice over light gauge steel, for example, in house buildings consuming vast amounts of forested land. The building process is also responsible for a large amount of waste generated all of which is shipped to landfills.

Along with the expansion in house size, the energy consumed grew. Since most of the energy used in the residential sector is for space heating and cooling, the increase can be attributed to a rise in the home's area, the number of windows installed, a lack of bioclimatic design, and poor construction practices. Since cooling is more energy-intensive than heating, the increase can also be due to a rise in the use of air conditioners in the modern home. The need to rethink residential design and construction from material and energy consumption standpoints is critical in the fight to combat climate change and is one of the tenets of this book.

In the social domain, a significant demographic change is affecting residential design. In general, society's demographic composition is much more diverse than in previous decades to include groups such as singles, and single-parent families that in the past were considered marginal by homebuilders. Concurrently, the proportion of seniors is also rising rapidly in many nations. By some accounts, the elderly homeowners are trading a large, costly-to-maintain home for a smaller dwelling unit. There is a growing interest in adaptable living arrangements that accommodate Aging in Place, multi-generational homes, and assisted living. The need to develop housing prototypes that simplify interior adaptability while avoiding waste generation is rapidly becoming a priority and is also addressed in this book.

The change in the economic landscape and its effect on the residential sector calls for attention as well. An affordability gap has emerged, where the rate of increase of house prices has far surpassed the growth of household incomes putting dwellings beyond the reach of a growing number of first-time home buyers, increasing the demand for less expensive, smaller units. This widening gulf in affordability can be explained by higher land, materials, and infrastructure costs, offering another argument for a need to save resources and make dwelling adaptable.

Transformations are also visible on the technological front. Contemporary advancements in technology have provided designers and builders with not only more efficient mechanisms to design and construct but also to reach and accommodate customers' space needs. The digital revolution has had a significant effect on design. These methods and technologies allow for simple integration of innovative designs and products contributing to the cost reduction of design and construction, making homes affordable and cost-efficient as well as reducing their carbon footprint. Among recent innovations, a renewed attention to prefabricated homes as a way of solving some of these above-mentioned challenges has emerged. Fully automated production where panels are produced using robotics for all aspects of fabrication, including cutting, nailing, and installing insulation. These advanced cost- and resource-saving production methods are explored in this book.

When looking for an overarching term to coin the contemporary negative practices in residential development, the word *unsustainable* comes to mind. Present consumption of natural resources at the expense of future needs is the practice's mark. The proliferation of the term *sustainable development* and the background that brought it about can be traced to the 1970s and 1980s. In a report, *Our Common Future* the World Commission on Environment and Development (WCED) defined sustainable development as "development that meets present needs without compromising the ability of future generations to meet their own needs". The definition puts in place a conceptual approach to development whereby every action has to be taken while considering its future effect.

Environmental sustainability relates to the ecological burden that the construction and upkeep of development, including the residential sector, creates. A *cradle-to-cradle* whole-building life cycle assessment is necessary when the planning of a development is pursued. It regards not only the initial effect of choice of materials, for example, but also the construction ecology, the impact of sourcing and producing the materials, their long-term performance, and their reusability and recyclability once their use is ended.

This book explores and outlines housing in a circular economy and is divided into four parts, the first, Housing and the Circular Economy sets the stage for the ones that follow. It includes chapters on the housing supply challenge and sustainability, offers historical background and definition of circular economy, and looks into circular business models and financing methods as well as introducing policy considerations and their contributions to the United Nations Sustainable Development Goals.

Part 2, Applications of Circular Economy Principles to Housing, lays the ground for design methods using circular economy. The part introduces housing passports, explores cost-reduction methods using circular economy principles, and outlines flexibility in housing design.

Part 3, Designing Low Carbon Circular Housing, moves into the implementation phase of a project. It investigates methods for the design of low-carbon and low-energy homes, relates construction practices for the circular economy to digitalization, and discusses the concept of clean operational energy in buildings.

Part 4, Fostering Circularity, Implementation Strategies and Tools, examines the building's end of use and investigates opportunities for upcycling. It then studies and lists the key stakeholders that are involved in the residential process and articulates their redefined roles in a circular marketplace and their capacity to enable change.

As societal pressures call for an urgent new direction in residential design, we do hope that this book will serve as a guide to members of homebuilding sector to regard circular economy practices as an integral part of the design and the construction process.

Naomi Keena and Avi Friedman

Acknowledgments

Researching and writing on circular economy as it relates to materials and their use, energy consumption, construction practices, and sustainable and affordable housing design were subjects of our work and practice for a long time. It included collaboration with and contribution by numerous colleagues, assistants, and students who directly and indirectly inspired this work. Our apologies if we have mistakenly omitted someone's name and we will do our best to correct it in future editions.

This book could not have been written without background research, compiling data, writing, and assembling case studies material by our former students Ava Klein, Claire Troyer, and Ciara Wade. Special thanks to Ava Klein for organizing the manuscript for publication, to Rachel O for generating the illustrations and laying out the sample chapters, and to Martha Milagros Pomasonco Alvis and Daniel R. Rondinel-Oviedo for the cover design. The team's hard work, talent, dedication, and punctuality are most appreciated.

Inspiring the writing of this book and its content was a two-phase research project called Data Homebase that was funded by Canada Mortgage and Housing Corporation (CMHC) as part of the national Housing Supply Challenge program. Phase one participants were Prof. Michael Jemtrud from McGill University, McGill research team members Sahil Adnan, Nadia Antoniadis, Liliane Bamdadian, Hermine Demael, Fabrice Grenier Arellano, Arielle Lasry, Jonah Rappaport, Maria Teleman, and Frédéric Verrier-Paquette. Phase two's team included postdoctoral researcher and project manager Dr. Mojtaba Parsaee, students Emma Brice, Finn Clements, Kareem Hammami, Prasoon Jain, Jihoon Jeon, Ajwad Kabir, Felicity Li, Maria Lederer, Madeline Mussio, Daniel R. Rondinel-Oviedo, Alexa Sharp, Teagan Vincent, and Osman Warsi. Special thanks to our collaborators Prof. Alica Beth Rod (McGill Library), Prof. Anna Dyson and Dr. Mohamed Aly Etman (Yale Center for Ecosystems and Architecture), Dr. Marco Raugei (Oxford Brookes University), and Dr. Paulo Pinheiro (Rensselaer Polytechnic Institute). We thank them all.

Many thanks to the design firms and organizations who made material about their projects available to feature in our case studies. These exemplary projects showcase the implementation of a circular approach.

Thanks goes to our colleagues at McGill's Peter Guo-hua Fu School of Architecture.

To Francesca Ford, Senior Publisher, Lydia Kessell, Commissioning Editor, and Jake Millicheap, Editorial Assistant, Architecture at Routledge, many thanks for the guidance and support.

Finally, our heartfelt thanks and appreciation to our families for their love and support.

Naomi Keena and Avi Friedman

PART 1

Housing and the Circular Economy

Chapter 1

Contemporary Housing Challenges and Sustainability

1.1 Setting the Stage: Contemporary Urban Issues

With a rapidly growing and continually changing urban population, an unstable housing market, and a norm of overconsumption and waste generation, the global need for sustainable urban development is more pressing than ever. The UN Intergovernmental Panel on Climate Change (IPCC) stresses the imminent threat of global warming reaching 1.5°C, which would cause irreversible harm to our ecosystems and human populations (IPCC, 2022). Coupled with the threat of climate change, Wetzstein (2017) states that cities are facing a global urban affordability crisis. In 2021, the price to buy a home in the United States was on average 4.4 times the average income of prospective buyers, the highest price-to-income ratio since 2006 (Joint Center for Housing Studies, 2021). An examination of the built environment and the residential sector can help explain why and how housing affordability and environmental challenges are inextricably linked. This chapter sets the stage for a new paradigm shift, detailing some of the challenges that cities throughout the world face today and stressing the need to adopt a new approach to construction and building practices. Environmental challenges, such as urban sprawl and energy overconsumption; economic challenges that lead to housing unaffordability; aging construction methods; and a changing sociodemographic makeup will be examined, as well as an explanation as to why a sustainable developmental approach is the necessary solution. The circular economy is a suitable response to many of these urban issues and fulfills key sustainable development principles. While the term has been defined in a multitude of ways, the circular economy is a reconceptualization of the current economic system, with the goal of minimizing the disposal of construction materials and components as much as possible. The current economic model that underpins contemporary urban design and housing is linear, meaning that it relies on a "take-make-waste" model. Extracted raw material is used for a period of time and then disposed of as the stock grows old or the use of the dwelling, for instance, ends. In a circular economy, however, the end-of-life idea that defines linearity is replaced with revitalization, through the use of renewable resources, impeccable design of products to maintain quality, and the eventual reuse of material at the end of a product's useful life (see Figure 1.1) (Hobson, 2016; Moreau et al., 2017). In this sense, the circular economy aims to remove waste from the building process, which has significant implications for ecosystems, the economy, and society at large.

DOI: 10.4324/9781003333975-2

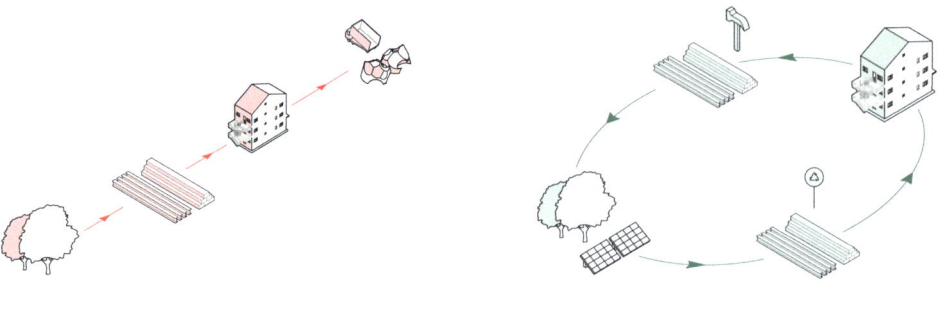

LINEAR ECONOMY   **CIRCULAR ECONOMY**

Figure 1.1 Linear Economy Compared to Circular Economy.

The linear approach to housing and urban design has created or worsened many environmental, economic, and societal issues, producing unsustainable cities. To understand why sustainable development, and specifically the circular economy, is essential for cities to adopt, it is pertinent to understand some of the current obstacles that cities are facing.

1.1.1 Construction, Sprawl, and Overconsumption: Environmental Challenges

Urban design and contemporary housing practices are environmentally detrimental. From construction methods to the sprawled layout of cities to cultural norms of overconsumption, the linear sentiment that cities extract resources and then discard them is engrained in the urban fabric.

Indeed, the building sector accounts for about 50 percent of total raw material use and 36 percent of global final energy use (Norouzi et al., 2021). In the European Union, construction and demolition waste accounts for one-third of total generated waste, with most ending up in landfills (Norouzi et al., 2021). Similarly, in Canada, construction and demolition waste makes up 27 percent of the total municipal solid waste disposal in landfills despite 75 percent of that waste having a residual value (Yeheyis et al., 2013). In 2010, Canada produced about 4 million metric tons of construction and demolition waste with residential construction, demolition, and renovation accounting for over 60 percent (Light House, 2021; Yeheyis et al., 2013). The US Environmental Protection Agency (USEPA) also found that in 2018 the United States generated more than 544 million metric tons (600 million US tons) of construction and demolition waste with demolition accounting for 90 percent of the total debris produced. This waste generation has increased in the United States by 342 percent since 1990 (United States Environmental Protection Agency, 2020). This, in part, comes down to poor management, as well as insufficient material choices, such as non-renewable resources, that are difficult to recycle.

Urban sprawl is another major concern for the environment. Zoning policies in the United States, for instance, are designed to designate space to function, denying a more natural flow between uses and prolonging trip distance between locations (Rosni et al., 2018). Single-family zoning may force industry and jobs farther away from the home, leading residents to rely on automobiles as their primary form of transportation, which further enables low-density development and contributes to greenhouse gas emissions (Friedman, 2021).

Moreover, the low density that comes from urban sprawl incentivizes the construction of larger, often detached, homes. As the floor and surface area of a home increases with more facades exposed, as is the case in detached homes, more heating and cooling technology is required to regulate the temperature of the dwelling (Wahlström & Hårsman, 2015). This has significant environmental costs and contributes to the energy consumption of a household. In the United States, the average residential energy consumption in 2021 was about 10,632 kilowatt-hours (kWh), comparatively higher than many countries in the world (US Energy Information Administration, 2022). The average person in China consumes one-third of the electricity of an average American (International Energy Agency, 2018). In Canada, the average annual electrical consumption per capita is about 15,000 kWh, the highest energy use per person globally (Canadian Energy Regulator, 2022). As will be discussed in Chapter 9, poor construction practices that hinder passive heating and cooling of a dwelling force residents to rely on energy-consumptive mechanical systems, such as heating, ventilation, and air conditioning (HVAC) systems. About 30 percent of households globally own an air conditioner, contributing to the share of residential electricity demand growing from 54 percent between 2000 and 2017 to a projected 70 percent between 2025 and 2040 (International Energy Agency, 2018). In advanced economies, such as the United States and Japan, about 90 percent of households have an air conditioner (International Energy Agency, 2018). According to the World Energy Outlook report, the fast growth in household appliance ownership, particularly air conditioners, accounts for 65 percent of the increase in the building sector's electricity demand (International Energy Agency, 2018). With rising global average temperatures, the current overreliance on HVAC systems to regulate household temperatures will only worsen. Hence, urban sprawl reinforces the construction of detached and semi-detached low-density housing that, due to exposed surface area, typically increases the need for mechanical systems.

In these examples, the linear economy perspective is foundational. When constructing homes, a lack of consideration for waste management leads to enormous disposal and an overloaded system of construction waste. Sprawled-out city planning similarly treats the land as disposable, choosing to build far apart and larger in area, thus infiltrating on precious ecological green space. Lastly, as a result of poor building design, residents rely on wasteful energy consumption habits to regulate the temperature in their home. This could be avoided by proper planning of the home where temperature regulation is designed into the building (see Chapter 9). The wasteful design of space has, therefore, effects both on energy use and on building materials. Treating space as a *resource* to conserve can allow for a new design paradigm that transitions from a linear economy to a circular one. Circular design can close the loop on material waste (at the building and urban scale) and promote designs that use energy resourcefully.

1.1.2 Too Many People, Not Enough Housing: A Global Affordability Crisis

Factors such as zoning and urban sprawl do not only affect the environment but also contribute to the growing housing affordability crisis that has emerged in almost every major city worldwide. The global urban housing affordability crisis is defined as a situation in which the expenses required to buy and maintain a house are rising faster than salaries and wages, making it difficult for first-time buyers to afford a home (Wetzstein, 2017). This leads to a myriad of negative outcomes: overcrowding, a decrease of financial security, evictions, and displacement from the urban center. This trend is expected to worsen, with the McKinsey Global Institute predicting that about half a billion households globally will live in overcrowded, poor dwelling conditions by 2025 (Woetzel et al., 2014).

A range of factors contribute to the housing affordability crisis, but one major factor is that the population rate of cities continues to grow and the number of dwelling units becomes scarce, inflating prices. A report by the Canada Mortgage and Housing Corporation argues that a solution to the housing supply issue is not only to create more housing but also to expand housing diversity, providing a range of choices in housing types for different household compositions (CMHC et al., 2022). This includes decreasing the number of single-detached homes and building more small-scale units. Contemporary zoning policies in many North American cities prevent any dwelling unit except for single-detached family homes from being built, which makes it difficult for smaller, denser, and more affordable dwelling units to be constructed. Therefore, while a range of policy changes must be put in place, one necessary change to aid in the housing supply challenge and affordability crisis is to build denser and smaller. The rigidity of housing construction is similarly reflective of this linear perspective on the economy. In this system, value is based on making new housing that can be sold at a higher price, incentivizing larger homes, and rigid construction practices that force people to move as their life circumstances change. In a circular economy, by contrast, value comes from lengthening the useful lifespan of a product, such as housing, through high-quality materials, renewable resources, reuse of materials, and reconfigurable housing designs that enable expansion and contraction over time. In this respect, housing is viewed as adaptable to the needs of the buyer.

1.1.3 Changing Sociodemographic Conditions

There are also changes that are occurring in the sociodemographic composition of our cities that the current built environment does not support. The percentage of citizens aged 55 or older has been increasing at a rapid pace in the Global North. A 2019 UN report calls aging a "global phenomenon," as almost every country in the world is seeing a rise in their older populations. In 2019, there were about 703 million persons aged 65 or older in the world, and this number is expected to double by 2050 to about 1.5 billion (United Nations, 2019). The old-age dependency ratio, which is the ratio of the number of persons aged 65 or older compared to those aged 20–64 years, is projected to increase, doubling in many countries of the Global South (United Nations, 2019). The aging population is expected to put pressure on old-age support systems, making it difficult for cities to sustain their current approach to elderly support. Vanleerberghe et al. (2017) suggest that for the quality of life of older persons, policies and services must prioritize "aging in place", a concept that stresses the importance and right for a person to grow old in their stable home environment rather than a specialized institution.

Moreover, there has been a global fall in household composition sizes, presenting another change in the size requirements for a house. In France, for instance, household size went from 3.1 persons per household to 2.3 between 1968 and 2011 (United Nations, 2017). Similarly, in Canada, the average household size fell from 4.3 persons per household to 2.5 from 1941 to 2011 (Statistics Canada, 2018). Consistently, there seem to be important sociodemographic trends – there are more people living today than ever before, yet the number of people living within a household is shrinking; as well, the number of older persons is rapidly increasing, warranting the need for adaptable housing to accommodate aging in place. This requires building more diverse dwelling units, including smaller dwelling units that can easily and efficiently adapt to the needs of the population.

An examination of some of the most pertinent urban problems underscores how environmental, economic, and sociodemographic issues are inextricably linked in the housing sector. A solution must touch on all three issues to be successful. Sustainable development is thus the necessary solution.

1.2 A New Approach to Housing

Sustainable development is a term that encompasses many facets of society, not only the environment but the economy, society, culture, and governance as well.

1.2.1 Contemporary History of Sustainability and Its Relevance to Housing

The origin of sustainable development comes from the 1972 United Nations Conference on the Human Environment in Stockholm. This was the first international conference that discussed how to move forward with the knowledge of environmental damage and climate change, setting the precedent for development practices that considered future environmental effects (United Nations, 1972). A 1987 report, *Our Common Future*, written by the World Commission on Environment and Development (WCED) introduced the term "sustainable development" as a process that "meets the needs of the present without compromising the ability of future generations to meet their own needs" (Brundtland, 1987). In this report, three

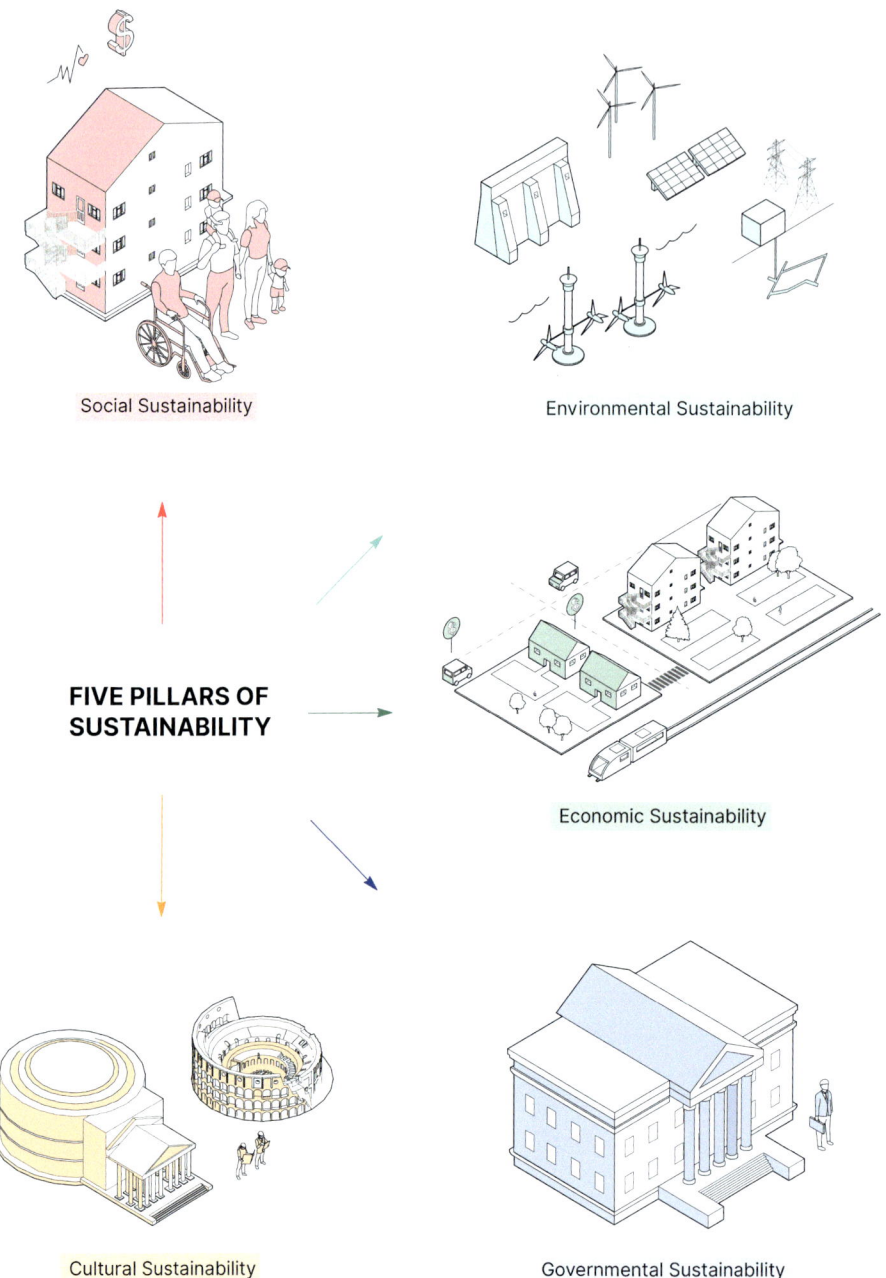

Social Sustainability

Environmental Sustainability

FIVE PILLARS OF SUSTAINABILITY

Economic Sustainability

Cultural Sustainability

Governmental Sustainability

Figure 1.2 Five Pillars of Sustainability.

pillars of sustainable development are presented as follows: social, economic, and environmental (Brundtland, 1987). Stephen Wheeler (2004) calls this the "Three Es" – environment, economy, and equity. In recent years, however, culture and governance were integrated as the fourth and fifth pillars of sustainability (see Figure 1.2). This idea of "sustainable development" has been on the top of the mind

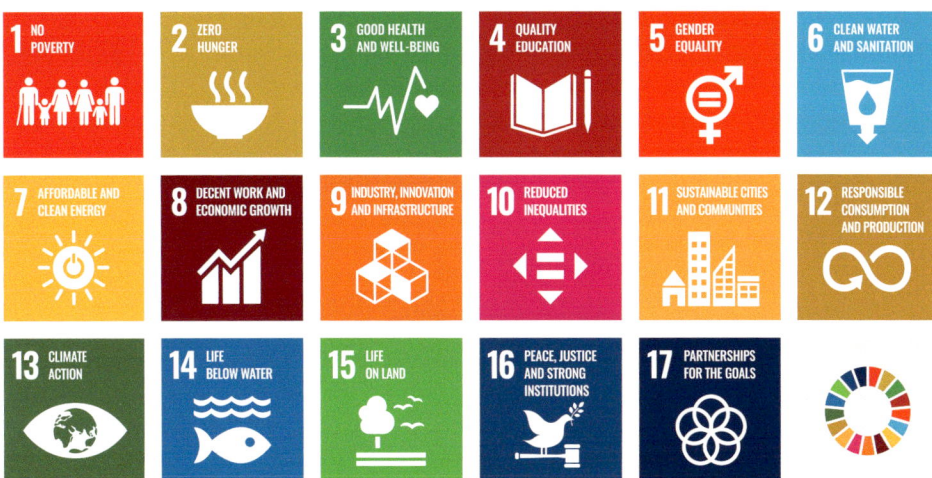

Figure 1.3 United Nations Sustainability Goals.

of major global conferences, namely the United Nations, which has produced their Sustainable Development Goals (SDGs) in 2015, with a timeline of 15 years (see Figure 1.3) (UN General Assembly, 2015). The 17 goals outlined in this report touch on the three pillars of the 1987 report, including social and economic goals, such as Goal 1 – no poverty, 4 – quality education, and 3 – ensure health and well-being for all ages. Environmental goals are featured prominently, from protecting terrestrial ecosystems (Goal 15), conserving marine life (Goal 14), and most notably, Goal 13 – "Take urgent action to combat climate change and its impacts" (UN General Assembly, 2015).

Goal 11 of the UN report is especially relevant – "Make cities and human settlements inclusive, safe, resilient and sustainable" (UN General Assembly, 2015). By 2030, the United Nations aims to ensure that safe and affordable housing be available to all, reduce per capita environmental impact of cities, and foster healthy economic, social, and environmental connections between urban, peri-urban, and rural areas (UN General Assembly, 2015). The weight of the 2030 UN Sustainable Development Goals rests on the global scale of its ambitions and it has become evident as cities around the world start adopting "Green City Thinking" perspectives to planning. The 2016 UN Habitat Conference on Housing and Sustainable Urban Development (Habitat III) narrowed in on concepts outlined in Goal 11 (United Nations General Assembly, 2017). This conference established the New Urban Agenda, a plan for building more sustainable cities and urban developments, pointing to a paradigm shift in planners' and local officials' approaches to the construction, design, waste management, and development of cities (United Nations General Assembly, 2017). A "Green City" is defined by the Asian Development Bank as cities that are moving toward or have achieved long-term environmental sustainability (OECD, 2013). Other relevant definitions include the Organisation for Economic Co-operation and Development (OECD), which defines green growth as promoting economic development while reducing environmentally damaging activity, such as greenhouse gas emission, inefficient resource usage, depletion of biodiversity, and overproduction of waste (OECD, 2013). Cohen's definition of "Sustainable Cities" requires cities to use renewable resources, efficiently use water and energy sources, and reduce and recycle construction waste (Cohen, 2018). Green cities can adopt some key urban design features, such as transit-oriented development, livable density, green technology, and green space.

1.2.2 Environmental Sustainability

An environmentally sustainable development is one that fulfills present needs while being attentive to the needs of the environment and ecosystem, presenting no future harm to the environment (see Figure 1.4) (Kaswan et al., 2018). The Paris Agreement aims to lower emissions to 30 percent below 2005 levels by 2050 (United Nations, 2015). One of the central ways to achieve this goal and foster environmental sustainability is to opt for renewable energy resources over non-renewable. Renewable resources are those that can be replenished through natural cycles, such as water, sun, or air (Friedman, 2007). Solar energy is one example of a renewable resource and can come in the form of solar panels on roofs or through proper orientation of the house and its windows to retain heat from the sun. Geothermal energy taps into natural ground temperature to use as a power source; hydroelectric power relies on the flow of water against turbines to create energy; and biomass uses the burning of waste and wood to create energy. The switch from non-renewable resources, such as fossil fuels, to renewable resources, significantly decreases greenhouse gas emissions. For instance, Skaftkärr is an energy-efficient neighborhood in Finland, relying on renewable heating and distributed energy generation (Finnish Innovation Fund Sitra, VTT Technical Research Centre of Finland, Tekes, 2011). This is done by tapping into biopower and solar energy, raising the share of renewable energy to 90 percent (Finnish Innovation Fund Sitra, VTT Technical Research Centre of Finland, Tekes, 2011).

Some regions, such as the province of Quebec in Canada, already rely mainly on renewable energy (hydroelectric power). In this case, the proper choice of building materials is another important way to decrease waste production and result in more environmentally sustainable construction. The key is to choose materials with low embodied carbon, meaning the amount of carbon dioxide emitted by producing the material is low, factoring in the extraction process, transportation process, and manufacturing process. In Quebec, Canada, for instance, solid saw

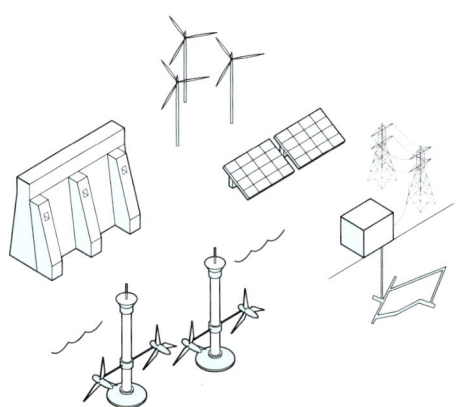

Figure 1.4 Environmental Sustainability.

lumber has low embodied carbon as well as being an inexpensive and renewable resource. As a result, lumber is often chosen over materials such as light gauge steel for home construction. However, this requires careful maintenance so as not to over-exploit forests. Nonetheless, timber's potential to be recycled and reused, its proximity to construction sites, and its relative energy efficiency would lessen long-term environmental impacts than other building materials in the province. However, the recycling process for lumber is not as straightforward and often requires much energy and materials to remanufacture the product into a new structural member. To make recycled lumber structural, an engineered board is typically produced as an output of the remanufacturing process. In this case the embodied carbon can be increased by recycling as opposed to landfilling (Keena et al., 2023). Hence, from an environmental sustainability approach, it's crucial to consider low-carbon materials during the design phase but to also consider the end-of-life phase during the design process. During the building's end-of-life how can greenhouse gas emissions be mitigated? Can the specified building materials be reused? If not, can they be recycled? What are the greenhouse gas emissions associated with reusing and recycling the chosen materials? The whole life cycle of a material must be considered when designing a building if an environmentally sustainable and circular logic is to be practiced. Avoiding the use of virgin materials is the first key principle, followed by designing out waste across the building life cycle. Chapter 7, "Low Carbon Footprints and Material Efficiency", delves deep into the topic of material choice, use, and low-carbon approaches.

Environmentally sustainable solutions require large-scale assessments to ensure that a choice is environmentally neutral in both the short- and long term. One way this can be done is through a "cradle-to-cradle" whole building life cycle assessment (LCA), where planning of a development considers not only the immediate effects of material choice or construction methods but also their long-term performance and ability for reuse once its current use has ended (see Figure 1.5) (Friedman, 2007;

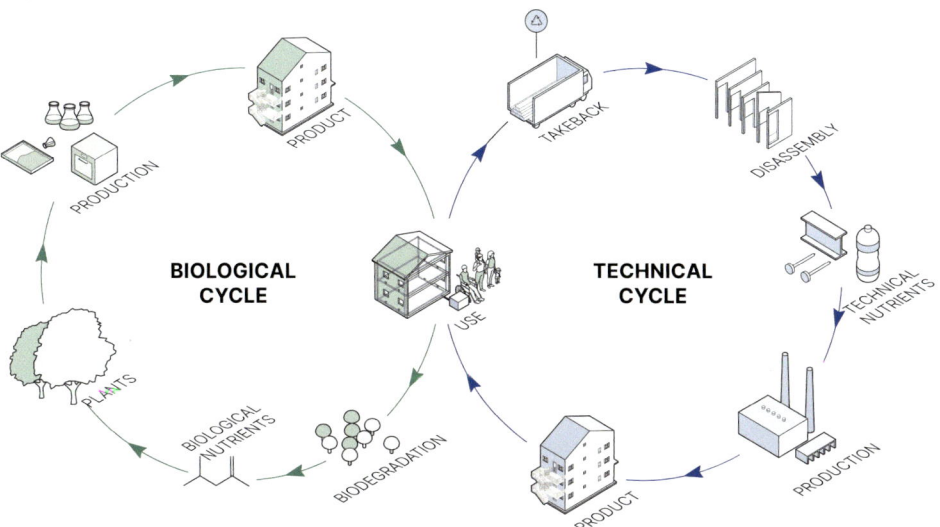

Figure 1.5 Taking a Cradle-to-Cradle Life Cycle Approach in the Built Environment.

Keena & Dyson, 2017; Keena et al., 2022). Environmental sustainability, thus, values long-term resource use which extends the life of the material, followed by reuse, and recyclability.

1.2.3 Social Sustainability

Building cities that are socially sustainable entails building adaptable environments that accommodate and support major shifts in lifestyles (see Figure 1.6). This involves developing communities that have social capital, are resilient, and feature social supports, human rights, public health, and labor rights (Friedman, 2021). Social sustainability becomes relevant, for instance, when low-income families seek housing. Often, lower income families must rent over purchasing a home, denying them the benefit of accumulating capital. Not only are lower income families likely to segment a large portion of their monthly income to housing expenses, but the lack of ownership over their home may lead to extreme monetary need as they age. Without proper social support, such as affordable housing options, low-income families are in a more vulnerable situation. In this example, social support presented at present can mitigate social vulnerability in the long term. Moreover, with an aging population it is important that housing ensures "aging in place". Latham et al. (2015) found that the environment in which older adults live, and their ability to remain in their long-term residence, has psychosocial effects that influence their ability to adapt to health concerns, retirement, and other changes in their lifestyle. Since older adults primarily occupy their home and neighborhood, these environments have a large impact on their health and well-being. While maintaining affordable housing is one central component to ensuring residential stability, as older adults have reduced mobility, modifications to the home as they age must be available and accessible as well. This could include building a ramp at the entrance for wheelchairs, widening doorways, or installing handrails. The idea that one's dwelling is supportive to the resident as the resident grows and evolves in their lifetime is key to long-term social support. Another way that the built environment can support social sustainability is by offering a range of services for the community. Setting a sharing or service economy, as depicted in Figure 1.6, where buildings function as sites of multiple activities, can be a helpful way to support and meet the needs of a community. For instance, designing homes that also have office spaces supports the needs of people professionally while functioning as a place of rest outside of work hours. This kind of design ensures the social needs of people while saving space and money.

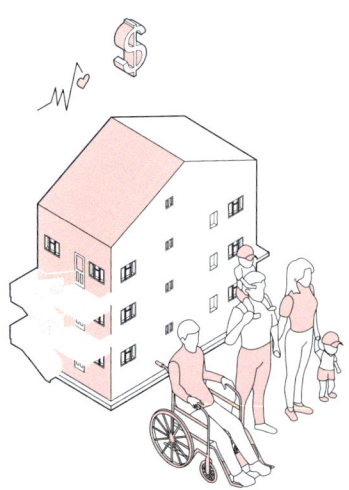

Figure 1.6 Social Sustainability.

1.2.4 Economic Sustainability

Economic sustainably aims to avoid poor present decisions and transfer of costs for future generations (Friedman, 2007). As Wheeler (2004) explains, the current economic structure is unsustainable for a few key reasons. For instance, it is difficult to monetarily quantify environmental and social goods or make economic decisions for public goods, such as roads and public space (Wheeler, 2004). As well, there is an incentive in our society to prioritize short-term profit over long-term costs, contradicting the core philosophy of sustainable development (Wheeler, 2004). Therefore, for cities to produce economically sustainable conditions, they must lessen their environmental impact, factor in the financial security of citizens, and consider future challenges. For instance, some cities have implemented "polluter pays" principles, which considers the social and environmental cost of typically polluting activities and factors in funding for cleanup. This can be found in such policies as "eco-taxes", where people who choose to engage in environmentally harmful activities are responsible to fund the long-term environmental cleanup (see Figure 1.7). In 2007, for instance, Canada implemented an excise tax on fuel-inefficient vehicles, requiring one to pay a fee when buying environmentally harmful cars (Canada Revenue Agency, 2022). In terms of housing, an economically unsustainable practice is featured when developers prioritize single-family dwellings, which has a high cost of service provision compared to smaller, denser dwelling units. Not only would a development such as this be environmentally harmful, contributing to energy overconsumption, automobile reliance, and sprawl, but it would also put a strain on home-buyers' financial security (Friedman, 2021). Economic sustainability is helpful in combining ecological and social goals of sustainability through an economic lens.

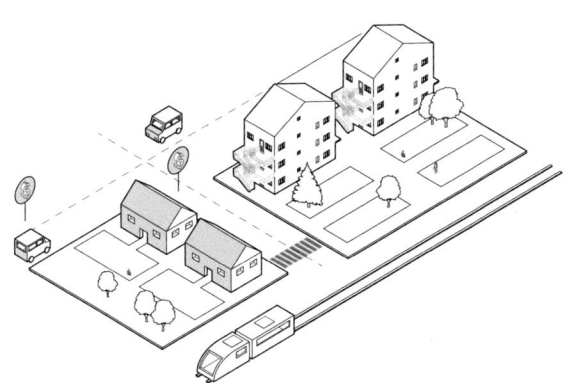

Figure 1.7 Economic Sustainability.

1.2.5 Cultural Sustainability

Appreciation for cultural sustainability is becoming more commonplace and it is often grouped with social sustainability goals. While overlapping, Hawkes (2001) defines cultural vitality as an environment that provides a sense of belonging, shared identity and meaning, and respect for its society, creativity, and education. In this way, cultural sustainability goes beyond social sustainability, to focus specifically on fostering culture and tradition in a place. The UNESCO Decade of Culture and Development (1988–1997) focuses on this relationship between culture and development, and the subsequent "Our Creative Diversity Report", by the World Commission on Culture and Development (WCCD), cemented culture within the realm of development (World Commission on Culture and Development, 1995). One way to promote cultural sustainability is by supporting vernacular culture and traditions (Friedman, 2021). This can come in the form of historic heritage buildings. While building denser development is key to affordability, older buildings are important reminders of a city's past. By maintaining important heritage sites, planners and architects can

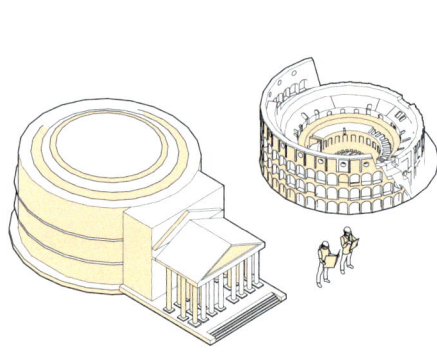

Figure 1.8 Cultural Sustainability.

improve upon the quality, undergoing retrofits of the buildings to avoid demolition, and working to diminish overuse of natural resources coming from new construction (see Figure 1.8) (Friedman, 2021). Another way to promote cultural sustainability is by using buildings as sites to offer cultural services in an easy and accessible way (Soini & Birkeland, 2014). In both instances, there is an effort to conserve cultural capital for future generations.

1.2.6 Governmental Sustainability

A sustainable government can adopt and support long-term sustainability plans (see Figure 1.9) (Schraad-Tischler & Seelkopf, 2015). To achieve the aforementioned four pillars of sustainability, governments must structure policy and decision-making on a longer term scale. Most governments act in the short term, focusing on the short-term economic gain and immediate political praise that may lead to resource exploitation and accumulation of public debt, resulting in detrimental long-term consequences (Schraad-Tischler & Seelkopf, 2015). This is in part due to the short electoral terms of politicians – it is common for new politicians to come in and discard the ongoing plans made by their predecessor. Examining the level of economic, social, and environmental policies being implemented, to what extent local officials are being held accountable for long-term policy decisions, and to what degree citizens are actively and democratically participating in politics, are all important indicators of sustainable governance.

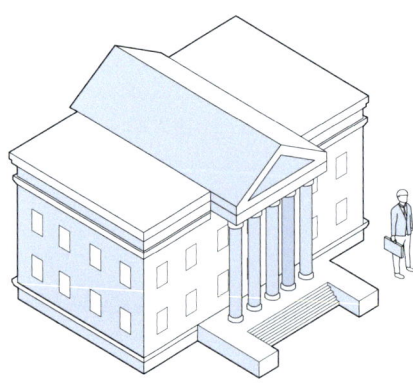

Figure 1.9 Governmental Sustainability.

Employing new data technology can help governments achieve long-term sustainability goals since they can help plan for the distant future, creating complex strategies that involve multiple stakeholders.

While each pillar holds importance on its own, effective solutions to urban problems, particularly when it comes to construction and building, must acknowledge the symbiotic relationship between these five pillars and design accordingly.

1.3 Principles of Sustainable Systems

In the urban design realm specifically, there are four principles of sustainability that can help planners and decision makers practically approach urban development projects. Following these principles allows sustainable urban development to flourish.

1.3.1 The Path of Least Negative Impact

This first principle requires decision makers and planners to choose the development process that leads to the least unsustainable effect. At the beginning of a building project, decision makers must assess potential short- and long-term consequences on the environment, society, economy, culture, and government (Friedman, 2007). For example, plans to build a luxury condominium development in a lower income neighborhood may result in short-term economic gain. However, an assessment at the outset would reveal the serious risk of displacement for low-income residents through gentrification and rising rents in both the short- and long term, leading to economic and social inequality and unsustainability. Furthermore, a development that is planned to be constructed rapidly and cheaply is likely to lead to environmentally harmful construction practices, an overconsumption of household heating and cooling due to poor thermal regulation, and fast turnover of materials, which all have environmentally harmful effects. An initial assessment may lead to more upfront costs and time but will mitigate the long-term negative effects. Governmentally, this may look like relying less on heavy polluting industries that could lead to long-term health problems for the population.

This idea of designing for the least negative impact goes hand-in-hand with the core concept of "closed cycles thinking" that Korhonen et al. (2018) describe in the circular economy. Unlike a traditional recycling concept, which focuses on converting waste to reusable material, circular economy factors in value maintenance at each point of the material's lifespan. Recycling and reusing materials are viewed as some of the last steps of a circular economy's material life cycle (the last being disposal to landfills). In the meantime, the central goal should be to maintain a product (e.g., a dwelling) to its highest possible quality for as long as possible (Korhonen et al., 2018). This is done by constructing a dwelling to its highest quality and design at the outset, designing for flexibility to allow adaptive reuse later in a building life, and ensuring

15

maintenance and repairs throughout its lifespan. This sustains both the material value of a building and the economic value of the dwelling as well as people's comfort levels within that dwelling. In this sense, a circular economy's focus on value maintenance through a closed-cycle perspective touches on a multitude of sustainability goals.

1.3.2 Self-Sustaining Process

Not only should urban design mitigate future harm, but also a sustainable built environment can act as a self-sustaining generator of resources by designing renewable energy features into the development (Friedman, 2007). Photovoltaic panels or solar panels on the rooftops of houses actively collect solar energy that can help fuel homes, such as heating water (Friedman, 2007). This approach designs the home to be a generator of resources, decreasing its reliance on public utilities. However, this is not the only way that the built environment can design self-sustenance. Relating to the social and economic branches of sustainability, offering a mix of dwelling units of different sizes and configurations is another useful example of self-sustaining social networks. If a development designs units for young families as well as sustainable accommodations for older adults, key intergenerational bonds can form within the dwelling, building reciprocal relationships of aid and support (Friedman, 2007).

The concept of the resilient city is another relevant example of a self-sustaining process. Resilient cities are cities that can withstand shocks, be they environmental, social, economic, or other, and recover quickly (Kesik, 2017). Particularly in the current time period, when climate change has increased the risk of extreme weather events, buildings must incorporate robust enclosure design, energy efficiency, and secure construction techniques to withstand extreme weather events and allow their occupants to be safe and comfortable (Kesik, 2017). What resilient planning calls for is design that allows the built environment and the home to protect itself and its inhabitants from extreme disaster scenarios to the best of its ability. This requires decision makers to engage seriously in disaster planning as a way for the built environment to consistently sustain itself and its inhabitants. This concept is not necessarily new. Before cities relied on energy grids, the home itself was designed to regulate temperature effectively and conform to weather conditions (see Chapter 9). The porch functioned as a cooling system, providing natural ventilation, windows provided sun and heating depending on where they were located, and dwellings were heated by wood (Kesik, 2017). Furthermore, residents grew their own food and built ties with community members that led to natural self-sufficiency instead of an overreliance on external energy sources, fossil fuels, and outsourced labor. Indeed, community resilience occurs when individuals harness local expertise and resources to protect themselves in cases of emergency (UK Cabinet Office, 2011). Like formal architectural resilience, community resilience can be fostered through good urban design, such as incorporating livable density, which is healthy density that allows for walkability, social capital, and small businesses to flourish (Sim & Gehl, 2019).

Therefore, planning the built environment to withstand extreme events – be they environmental, economic, political, or social – allows the city to be self-sustaining. Circular economy's emphasis on high-quality design and reusability of products relates strongly to this self-sustaining process principle. Kennedy and Linnenluecke (2022) offer the global medical supply chain crisis as a useful example of the circular economy's potential for resilience planning – if medical supplies were designed to be repurposed or used for a long period of time at high quality, this would have increased the resilience of cities against the imminent supply chain crisis. This can similarly relate to housing. To create long-term high-quality dwellings, it is pertinent that dwellings are designed to be resilient against a myriad of situations and act as a self-sustaining process.

1.3.3 Supporting Relations

This chapter has continued to stress the interlocking relationship between the five pillars of sustainability, and it is this understanding that decision makers and planners must factor into development plans (see Figure 1.10). By acknowledging the

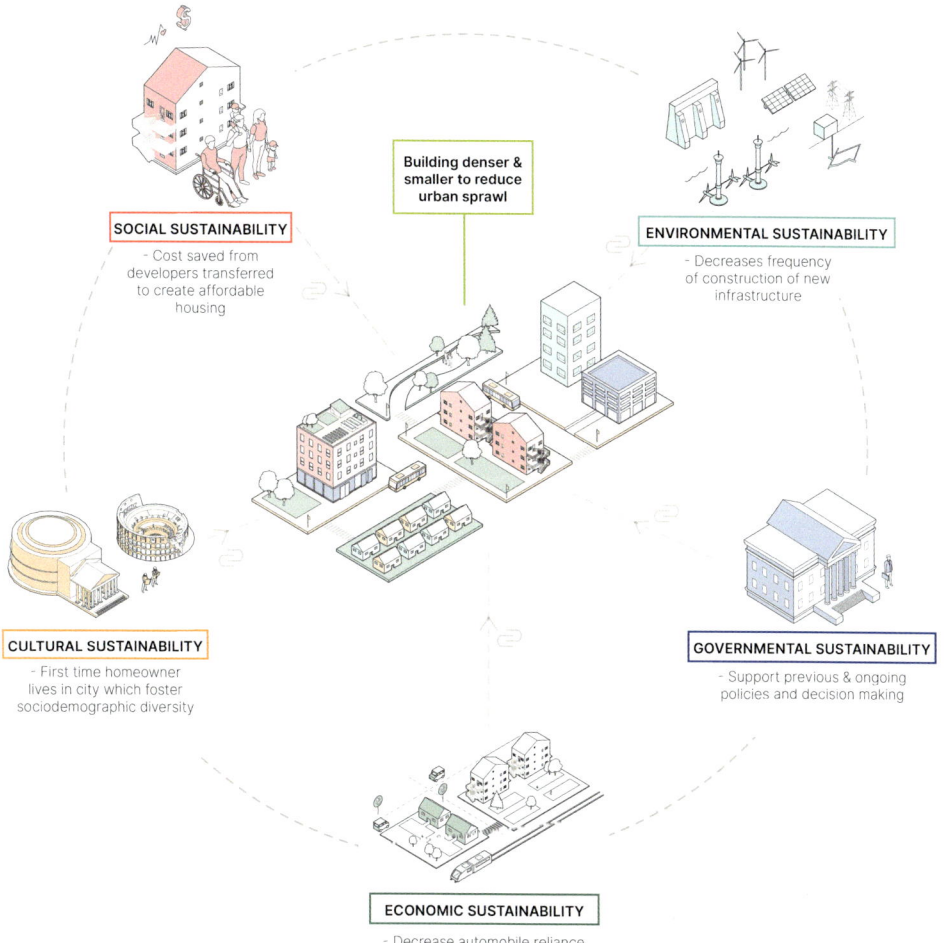

Figure 1.10 The Interlocking Relationship of the Five Pillars of Sustainability to Improve Urban Conditions.

symbiosis between these five pillars, planners and decision makers can use features from one component as a catalyst for activity in another. For example, building denser and smaller dwelling units reduces urban sprawl, which will decrease automobile reliance and thus decrease infrastructure costs for parking and road expansions. This will save costs for developers which can be transferred to the end user in the form of affordable housing. In this capacity, an environmental decision for construction triggers an economic advantage as well. Furthermore, building denser cities contributes to much-needed housing supply, ensuring that young, first-time homeowners continue to live in the city, fostering sociodemographic diversity and supporting the aging population. Making an environmental decision contributes to social and cultural sustainability as well. This is in line with another major element of circular economy – systems thinking. Like an ecosystem, every actor is interconnected to each other, and every action influences another action (Robinson, 2022). Understanding circular economy as a system allows decision makers to visualize the immediate effects as well as long-term effects of construction decisions, creating supporting relations as a result.

1.3.4 Life Cycle Approach

Adopting a life cycle approach means a project is able to sustain itself throughout its life cycle. As climate change shapes cities, sociodemographic conditions morph, and economic conditions continue to shift, it is crucial that cities adapt and accommodate for a long-term and ongoing evolution to achieve sustainability. Dwellings must be made with good quality construction materials despite the higher upfront cost. If a project is well-constructed, homeowners are likely to maintain this quality, replacing windows when needed for proper insulation, and thus save on energy consumption in the long run. Moreover, a building must be elastic and adaptable. For instance, as sociodemographic conditions shift and the size of a household changes, their dwelling should be able to shift as well, avoiding potential demolition and extending the dwelling's useful life. This approach can also be applied to governance. Too often, when political power shifts in municipal government, old objectives and goals are discarded for new ones. This political structure does not support the long-term goals of a city. Instead, a continuity between policies must be established for sustainable governance. Codes and bylaws must also be open to adaptation or amendment as the city requires. For instance, single-family-exclusively-zoned areas have negative effects on sprawl and affordability. A more flexible zoning code could allow different configurations of dwelling units to be built that better meet the needs of the public.

These examples emphasize the demand for cities to evolve and adapt over time according to their needs. In terms of housing, for instance, designing flexibility at the onset will extend the useful life of the dwelling and prevent demolition, which is the main objective of the circular economy. In a linear economy, emphasis is made on the end-of-life phase of a product through end-of-life waste treatment. In other words, resources are extracted, used, and then a reactionary approach is done when the product's use is "over". These end-of-life treatments are waste management systems that process waste before dumping it into a landfill. In a circular economy, paying attention to the entire life cycle or supply chain is more important than reacting to the end step of a product's life. Gheewala and Silalertruksa (2021) provide a good example of the difference between a linear end-of-life approach and a circular life cycle approach. In the case of car design, replacing a steel-framed car with a composite carbon fiber car will lead to lighter vehicles, which will minimize the fuel usage needed to drive a car and reduce damage to asphalt on roads. In terms of the useful phase of a vehicle's life, it appears that this shift in automobile's material is an environmentally sustainable solution. However, steel is almost completely recyclable, while carbon fiber is not, creating environmentally harmful conditions for the end-of-life phase of a vehicle. By focusing on one specific part of a vehicle's environmental impact instead of its entire life cycle, a manufacturer may be wrongly convinced that this material change would be environmentally beneficial. Therefore, when selecting environmentally sustainable building materials for houses, for instance, it is important to factor in the entire process of extraction, transportation, longevity, etc., to assess its environmental impact accurately. Using a life cycle approach avoids these mistakes, forcing decision makers to plan the entire life cycle of a product instead of focusing on one stage of a product's life (see Figure 1.11).

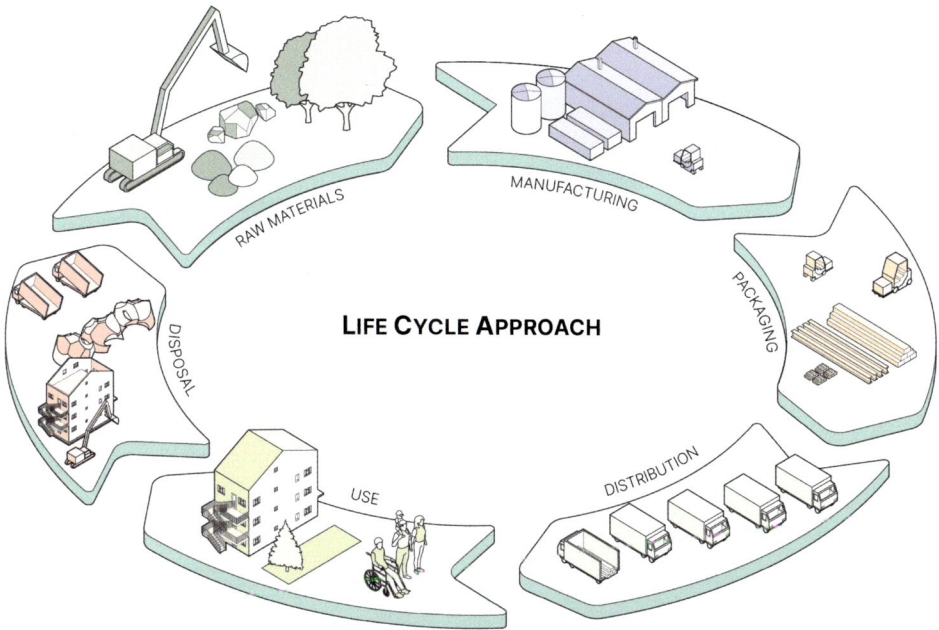

Figure 1.11 A Life Cycle Approach to the Design and Construction Process.

1.4 Supporting a Call for Circular Economy

The city and housing sector are crucial actors in implementing a circular economy. Two-thirds of the population is projected to live in urban areas by 2050, and by 2030 the middle class is projected to grow from 2 billion to over 4 billion, stressing the need to build larger and denser (Norouzi et al., 2021). With no change to the construction and planning practices, this urbanization is likely to increase annual resource requirements to 90 billion metric tons by 2050 – 60 billion metric tons more than the annual resource consumption in 2010. This, coupled with the current environmental, social, and economic junctures affecting the urban environments, calls for a fundamental shift in how cities are planned and constructed. Just as urban design and architectural issues are interrelated, so are their solutions. The term "sustainability", thus, relates appropriately, encompassing the interconnectedness between environmental, economic, social, cultural, and governmental action. Concepts, such as the path of least negative impact, self-sustaining process, supporting relations, and a life cycle approach, are all helpful for bringing these tenets of sustainability into the built environment. These concepts are already being explored and enacted in cities around the world with great success. For instance, Hammarby Sjöstad, a borough of Stockholm, Sweden, uses an urban symbiosis approach that designs pillars of circular economy and sustainability into the foundation of the city, rather than relying on a surface-level behavioral change by its residents.

Circular economy offers a promising approach to housing that considers the symbiotic relationships within sustainability and touches on each of these sustainability principles. The fundamental issue that leads to unsustainable housing is the "take-make-waste" approach to construction. In this linear approach, material and energy are taken for construction of dwelling units, used for a period, and then discarded into a landfill as construction waste. If the take-make-waste approach is the foundation of unsustainable development, the circular economy offers the alternative – closing this linear approach for a "reduce, reuse, repair, and recycle" perspective. In a circular housing economy, the goal is not to produce and sell as many dwelling units as possible, but to adapt, accommodate, and conserve current construction to reduce waste and lengthen the functional use of a dwelling unit for as long as possible. This flexible approach to housing not only aids in environmental conditions, but also touches on sociodemographic change, and reorients housing as a tool to evolve with the residents rather than get discarded. In this sense, the circular economy has the potential to touch on the key aspects of sustainable development. The next chapter will go in-depth on what circular economy entails exactly, its origins, and its design focus.

1A

Project:
Hammarby Sjöstad

Locations:
Hammarby Sjöstad, Sweden

Year:
2017

Team:
The City of Stockholm

**Mapping to Circular
Economy Framework:**

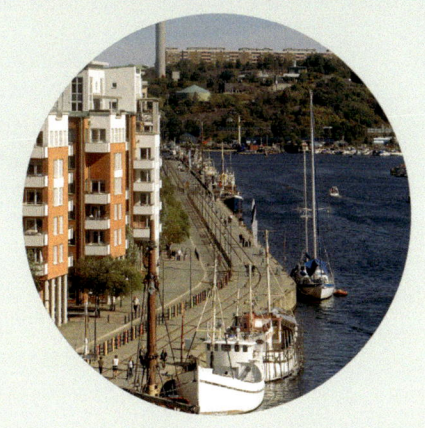

CIRCULAR ECONOMY PRACTICES

LIFE CYCLE PHASES

	Recovery	Life Extension	Sharing Platforms	Service Models	Regenerate	Virtualize
Work of Geobiosphere						
Sourcing						
Manufacturing						
Design & Construction						
Use						
End-of-Use						

LAYERS + LIFESPAN
Structural Layers | Long Life
Skin, MEP Layers | Medium Life
Interior Layers | Short Life

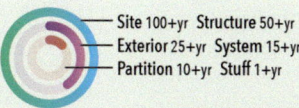

Site 100+yr   Structure 50+yr
Exterior 25+yr   System 15+yr
Partition 10+yr   Stuff 1+yr

Hammarby Sjöstad is a borough in a formerly industrial zone and brownfield of Stockholm, Sweden, and surrounds lake Hammarby Sjö on both sides (see Figures 1.12 and 1.13). Construction that follows ambitious and broad environmental goals, dating back to 1990, was finalized in 2017 and exemplifies this necessary shift to a life cycle and circular economic approach to construction.

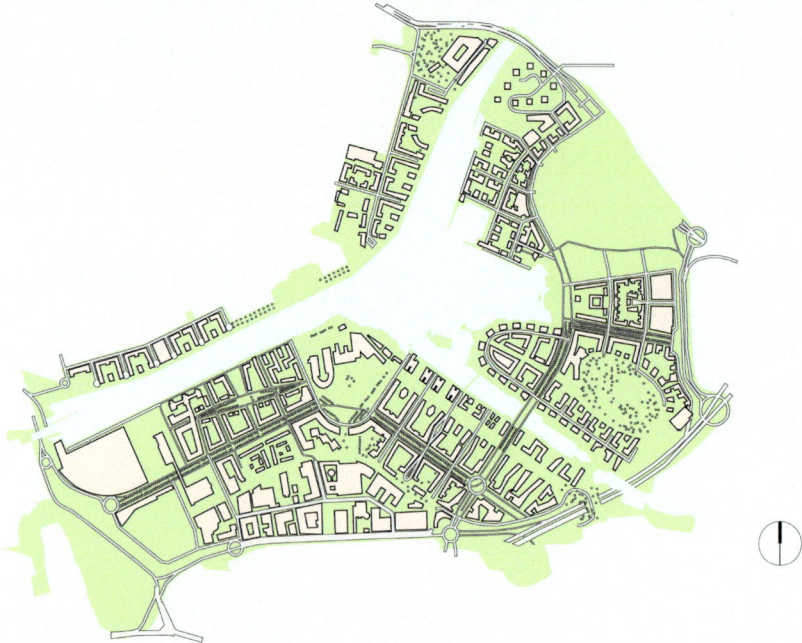

Figure 1.12 Map of Hammarby Sjöstad, Sweden.

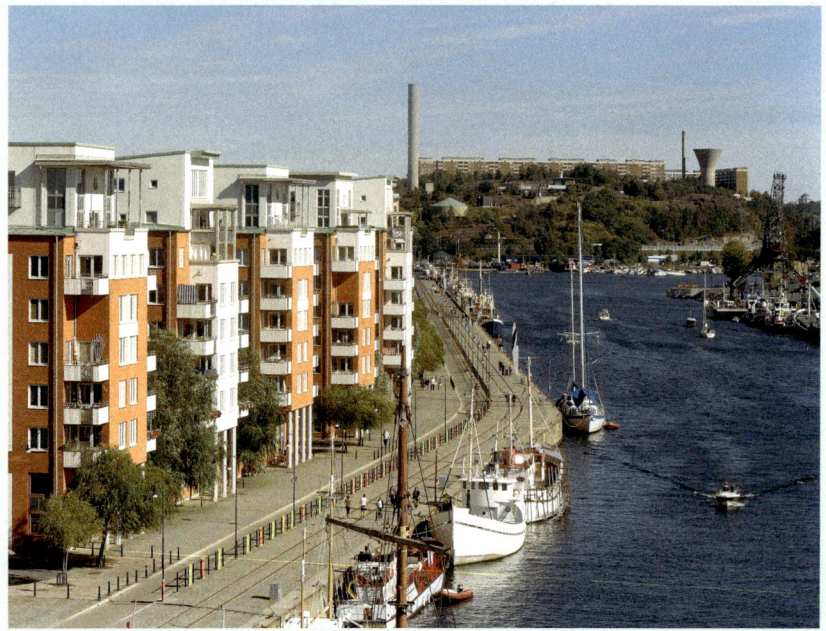

Figure 1.13 Hammarby Docks.

22

The city was developed based on seven key intentions: soil remediation, dense and diverse urban form, walkability and integrated public transport, green buildings, energy efficiency and recovery, responsible waste management, and water efficiency (Bernard et al., 2019). These principles were approached through an integrated resource management system referred to as the Hammarby Model, which prioritized the reuse of resources in a circular process. The urban area is now home to roughly 25,000 residents and 10,000 additional workers, as a blend of residential, commercial, waterfront, and green spaces, with a common modern architectural style featuring flat roofs, large windows, and colorful façades.

The borough utilizes a sustainable development strategy to increase **recovery and recycling** that focuses on technical solutions and urban symbiosis instead of putting the burden on the occupants to change their behavior (Iveroth, 2014). Urban symbiosis, in this case, refers to the integration of infrastructural systems, including energy, waste collection, water, and transportation, to achieve high environmental performance of the system at large, circulating resources and limiting waste. An example of this symbiotic system is the treatment of wastewater sludge to be used as fertilizer, and the use of biogas produced from this treatment as fuel for transit vehicles.

The intentionally designed urban form facilitates the time-tested **sharing platform** of public transportation to reduce emissions and pressure on road infrastructure associated with automobile reliance. A centralized network of pedestrian and bike paths, efficient bus and tram routes, free ferry service, as well as carpooling and car-sharing programs, have reduced car ownership when compared to the rest of Stockholm (see Figures 1.14–1.16). Close to 80 percent of all daily journeys of both residents and

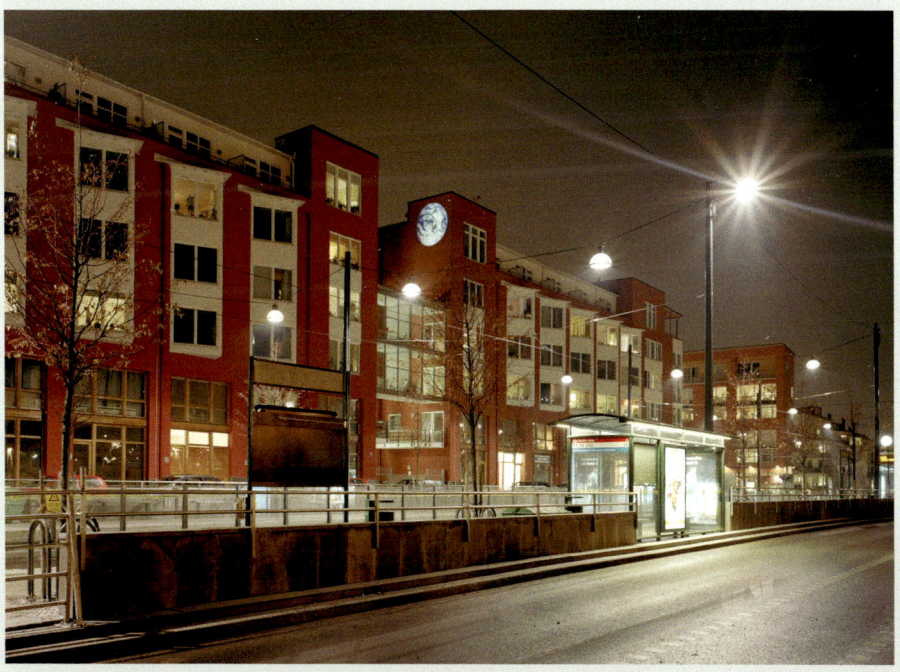

Figure 1.14 A Night Bus Stop in Hammarby Sjöstad.

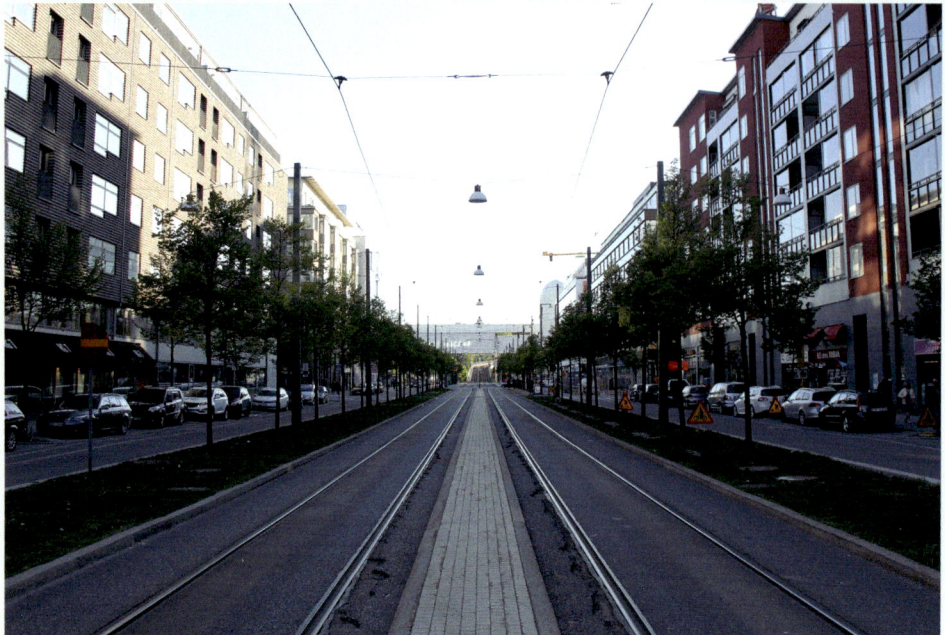

Figure 1.15 Tram Lines in Hammarby Sjöstad.

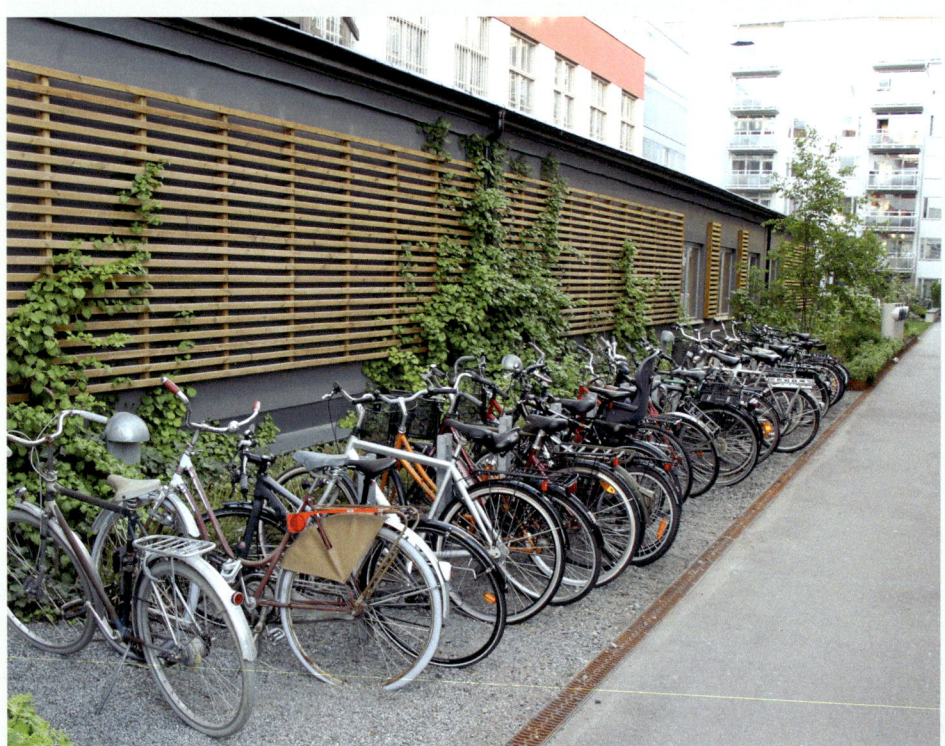

Figure 1.16 Bicycle Parking in Hammarby Sjöstad.

workers are completed by using public transportation, walking, or cycling, due to this focus on walkability and density (Bernard et al., 2019).

Regeneration of this site, which was generally unsafe and polluted prior to the development, was another one of the original intentions of the project. The former industrial zone required sanitization of contaminated soil to ensure public health, and this responsibility was shared between The City of Stockholm and private developers (Jonas Jernberg & Huang, 2015). Developers were given the option to buy contaminated land at a reduced price under the condition that they must finance soil treatment. All land was sold under this condition, showing the potential of shared financial burden between public and private sources to achieve environmental goals. Hammarby Sjöstad is a fine example of future urban planning in a time of increased demand and limited resources. The development shows the value that sustainable practices can add to an area, how environmentally sustainable goals can address multiple sustainability pillars, and how designing for sustainability from the beginning can lead to a self-sustaining process.

References

Bernard, C., Eleazar, A., & Huddlestun, R. M. (2019). *Hammarby Sjöstad: Planning precedent. Precedents, 8.* https://digitalcommons.calpoly.edu/paradise_pr/8

Brundtland, G. (1987). *Report of the World Commission on Environment and Development: Our common future.* United Nations General Assembly document A/42/427.

Canada Revenue Agency. (2022). *Excise taxes and other levies notices.* Retrieved January 23 from https://www.canada.ca/en/revenue-agency/services/tax/technical-information/excise-taxes-special-levies/excise-taxes-special-levies-notices.html

Canadian Energy Regulator. (2022). *Provincial and territorial energy profiles – Canada.* Canadian Energy Regulator. https://www.cer-rec.gc.ca/en/data-analysis/energy-markets/provincial-territorial-energy-profiles/provincial-territorial-energy-profiles-canada.html

CMHC, Bond, E., & Cortellino, F. (2022). *Housing supply report.* https://assets.cmhc-schl.gc.ca/sites/cmhc/professional/housing-markets-data-and-research/market-reports/housing-supply-report/housing-supply-report-2022-05-en.pdf?rev=e66a4117-594f-4b3e-8477-c33fbe1e7766

Cohen, S. (2018). *The sustainable city.* Columbia University Press.

Finnish Innovation Fund Sitra, VTT Technical Research Centre of Finland, Tekes. (2011). *World-class sustainable solutions from Finland*(Outlook No. 48). Helsinki.

Friedman, A. (2007). *Sustainable residential development: Planning and design for green neighborhoods.* McGraw-Hill.

Friedman, A. (2021). *Fundamentals of sustainable urban design.* Springer. https://doi.org/10.1007/978-3-030-60865-1

Gheewala, S. H., & Silalertruksa, T. (2021). Life cycle thinking in a circular economy. In L. Liu & S. Ramakrishna (Eds.), *An introduction to circular economy* (pp. 35–53). Springer Singapore. https://doi.org/10.1007/978-981-15-8510-4_3

Hawkes, J. (2001). *The fourth pillar of sustainability: Culture's essential role in public planning.* Common Ground.

Hobson, K. (2016). Closing the loop or squaring the circle? Locating generative spaces for the circular economy. *Progress in Human Geography, 40*(1), 88–104. https://doi.org/10.1177/0309132514566342

International Energy Agency. (2018). *World energy outlook 2018.* IEA, Paris. https://www.iea.org/reports/world-energy-outlook-2018

IPCC. (2022). Summary for policymakers. In H.-O. Pörtner, D. C. Roberts, E. S. Poloczanska, K. Mintenbeck, M. Tignor, A. Alegría, M. Craig, S. Langsdorf, S. Löschke, V. Möller, & A. Okem (Eds.), *Climate change 2022: Impacts, adaptation and vulnerability* (pp. 3–33). Cambridge University Press.

Iveroth, S. P. (2014). *Industrial ecology for sustainable urban development – The case of Hammarby Sjöstad* [Doctoral dissertation, KTH Royal Institute of Technology]. https://www.diva-portal.org/smash/get/diva2:716823/FULLTEXT01.pdf

Joint Center for Housing Studies. (2021). *The State of the nation's housing.* https://www.jchs.harvard.edu/sites/default/files/reports/files/Harvard_JCHS_State_Nations_Housing_2021.pdf

Jernberg, J., Hedenskog, S., & Huang, C. C. (2015). *China Development Bank Capital.* 2015_https://energyinnovation.org/wp-content/uploads/2015/12/Hammarby-Sjostad.pdf

Kaswan, V., Choudhary, M., Kumar, P., Kaswan, S., & Bajya, P. (2018). *Green production strategies.* https://doi.org/10.1016/B978-0-08-100596-5.22292-0

Keena, N., & Dyson, A. (2017). Qualifying the quantitative in the construction of built ecologies. In D. Benjamin (Ed.), *Embodied energy and design: Making architecture between metrics and narratives.* Columbia University GSAPP Lars Müller.

Keena, N., Raugei, M., Lokko, M.-l, Aly Etman, M., Achnani, V., Reck, B. K., & Dyson, A. (2022). A life-cycle approach to investigate the potential of novel biobased construction materials toward a circular built environment. *Energies, 15*(19), 7239. https://doi.org/10.3390/en15197239

Keena, N., Rondinel-Oviedo, D. R., De-los-Ríos, A. A., Sarmiento-Pastor, J., Lira-Chirif, A., Raugei, M., & Dyson, A. (2023). Implications of circular strategies on energy, water, and GHG emissions in housing of the Global North and Global South. *Cleaner Engineering and Technology*. https://doi.org/10.1016/j.clet.2023.100684

Kennedy, S., & Linnenluecke, M. K. (2022). Circular economy and resilience: A research agenda. *Business Strategy and the Environment*. https://doi.org/10.1002/bse.3004

Kesik, T. (2017). *Resilience planning guide* (Version 1). University of Toronto.

Korhonen, J., Nuur, C., Feldmann, A., & Birkie, S. E. (2018). Circular economy as an essentially contested concept. *Journal of Cleaner Production, 175*, 544–552. https://doi.org/10.1016/j.jclepro.2017.12.111

Latham, K., Clarke, P. J., & Pavela, G. (2015). Social relationships, gender, and recovery from mobility limitation among older Americans. *Journals of Gerontology, Series B: Psychological and Social Sciences, 70*(5), 769–781. https://doi.org/10.1093/geronb/gbu181

Light House. (2021). *Residential construction waste analysis*. https://www.light-house.org/wp-content/uploads/2021/05/Residential-Construction-Waste-Analysis-May-27-2021.pdf

Moreau, V., Sahakian, M., Van Griethuysen, P., & Vuille, F. (2017). Coming full circle: Why social and institutional dimensions matter for the circular economy. *Journal of Industrial Ecology, 21*(3), 497–506. https://doi.org/10.1111/jiec.12598

Norouzi, M., Chàfer, M., Cabeza, L. F., Jiménez, L., & Boer, D. (2021). Circular economy in the building and construction sector: A scientific evolution analysis. *Journal of Building Engineering, 44*, 102704. https://doi.org/10.1016/j.jobe.2021.102704

OECD. (2013). *Green growth in cities*. In *OECD green growth studies*. OECD Publishing.

Robinson, S. (2022). Chapter 3—A systems thinking perspective for the circular economy. In *Circular economy and sustainability* (Vol. 1: Management and Policy, pp. 35–52). Elsevier. https://doi.org/10.1016/b978-0-12-819817-9.00034-x

Rosni, N. A., Ponrahono, Z., & Mohd Noor, N. (2018). Segregated land use sprawl: TOD approach for mixed-use housing development in Kuala Lumpur. *Planning Malaysia Journal, 16*. https://doi.org/10.21837/pmjournal.v16.i5.418

Schraad-Tischler, D., & Seelkopf, L. (2015). *Concept and methodology—Sustainable governance indicators 2015*. Dollacker & Waldik GbR.

Sim, D., & Gehl, J. (2019). *Soft city: Building density for everyday life*. Island Press. http://ebookcentral.proquest.com/lib/mcgill/detail.action?docID=6317985

Soini, K., & Birkeland, I. (2014). Exploring the scientific discourse on cultural sustainability. *Geoforum, 51*, 213–223. https://dx.doi.org/10.1016/j.geoforum.2013.12.001

Statistics Canada. (2018). The shift to smaller households over the past century. https://www150.statcan.gc.ca/n1/pub/11-630-x/11-630-x2015008-eng.htm

UK Cabinet Office. (2011). *Strategic national framework on community resilience*. https://www2.oxfordshire.gov.uk/cms/sites/default/files/folders/documents/fireandpublicsafety/emergency/StrategicNationalFramework.pdf

UN General Assembly. (2015). *Transforming our world: The 2030 agenda for sustainable development*. United Nations. https://sdgs.un.org/publications/transforming-our-world-2030-agenda-sustainable-development-17981

United Nations. (1972). *Report of the United Nations conference on the human environment*. https://digitallibrary.un.org/record/523249?ln=en

United Nations. (2015). *Paris agreement*. https://unfccc.int/sites/default/files/english_paris_agreement.pdf

United Nations. (2017). *Household size and composition around the world 2017*. https://www.un.org/en/development/desa/population/publications/pdf/ageing/household_size_and_composition_around_the_world_2017_data_booklet.pdf

United Nations. (2019). *World population ageing 2019: Highlights*. https://www.un.org/en/development/desa/population/publications/pdf/ageing/WorldPopulationAgeing2019-Highlights.pdf

United Nations General Assembly. (2017, January 25). Resolution adopted by the General Assembly on 23 December 2016: 71/256, "New Urban Agenda." United Nations.

United States Environmental Protection Agency. (2020). *Advancing sustainable materials management: 2018 fact sheet*. https://www.epa.gov/sites/default/files/2021-01/documents/2018_ff_fact_sheet_dec_2020_fnl_508.pdf

US Energy Information Administration. (2022). *How much energy does a person use in a year?* https://www.eia.gov/tools/faqs/faq.php?id=85&t=1

Vanleerberghe, P., De Witte, N., Claes, C., Schalock, R. L., & Verté, D. (2017). The quality of life of older people aging in place: A literature review. *Quality of Life Research*, *26*(11), 2899–2907. https://doi.org/10.1007/s11136-017-1651-0

Wahlström, M. H., & Hårsman, B. (2015). Residential energy consumption and conservation. *Energy and Buildings*, *102*, 58–66. https://doi.org/10.1016/j.enbuild.2015.05.008

Wetzstein, S. (2017). The global urban housing affordability crisis. *Urban Studies*, *54*(14), 3159–3177. https://doi.org/10.1177/0042098017711649

Wheeler, S. (2004). *Planning for sustainability: Creating livable, equitable and ecological communities* (1st ed.). Routledge. https://doi.org/10.4324/9780203300565

Woetzel, J., Ram, S., Mischke, J., Garemo, N., & Sankhe, S. (2014). *A blueprint for addressing the global affordable housing challenge*. https://www.mckinsey.com/~/media/mckinsey/featured%20insights/urbanization/tackling%20the%20worlds%20affordable%20housing%20challenge/mgi_affordable_housing_full%20report_october%202014.ashx

World Commission on Culture and Development. (1995). *Our creative diversity: Report of the World Commission on Culture and Development* (Publication No. 14). https://unesdoc.unesco.org/ark:/48223/pf0000101651

Yeheyis, M., Hewage, K., Alam, M. S., Eskicioglu, C., & Sadiq, R. (2013). An overview of construction and demolition waste management in Canada: A lifecycle analysis approach to sustainability. *Clean Technologies and Environmental Policy*, *15*(1), 81–91. https://doi.org/10.1007/s10098-012-0481-6

Chapter 2

Circular Economy

Definition and Historical Overview

2.1 Sustainability and Circular Economy

Chapter 1 traced the history and origins of sustainability and sustainable development, and how it relates to circular economy. In this chapter, the emphasis will be on the circular economy itself, and how it can be specifically applied to the built environment as illustrated in Figure 2.1. The circular economy is a regenerative model that aims at reducing waste and emissions through maintenance, long-lasting design, repair, and reuse. This model has important implications for the built environment, a sector, as discussed in the previous chapter, that struggles with waste management and enormous pollution and emission rates. To rethink how architects structure design criteria first requires an understanding of existing knowledge and assessment methods. The first section outlines key energy theories to understand different ways of assessing the environmental impact of architecture and the built environment. This sets a foundation for understanding exactly what entails a "sustainable" circular economic approach – it must be assessed through the lens of multiple energy theories and seen as environmentally sustainable in all. This chapter then explores the origins and conceptual underpinnings of the circular economy model itself, including ecological economics, environmental economics, industrial ecology, bioeconomy, and green economy. One can think of a circular economy in terms of its treatment of flows and stock. In a linear economy, emphasis is on the quick flow of material to its point of sale, creating enormous waste. Loop economy, lake economy, and performance economy are three ways to conceptualize a circular economy's framing of stock value, which shifts from a strong emphasis on flows to a maintenance of stock value for a long period of time. The circular economy is first and foremost a design strategy, and thus, the last section explores core design goals for a circular built environment and recommendations to achieve said goals, including adjusting building size, sourcing materials appropriately, and incorporating data and technological innovations into the construction sector. The aim of this chapter is to provide a comprehensive introduction to the central concept this book rests upon – circular economy – going through its origin and conceptual underpinnings.

DOI: 10.4324/9781003333975-3

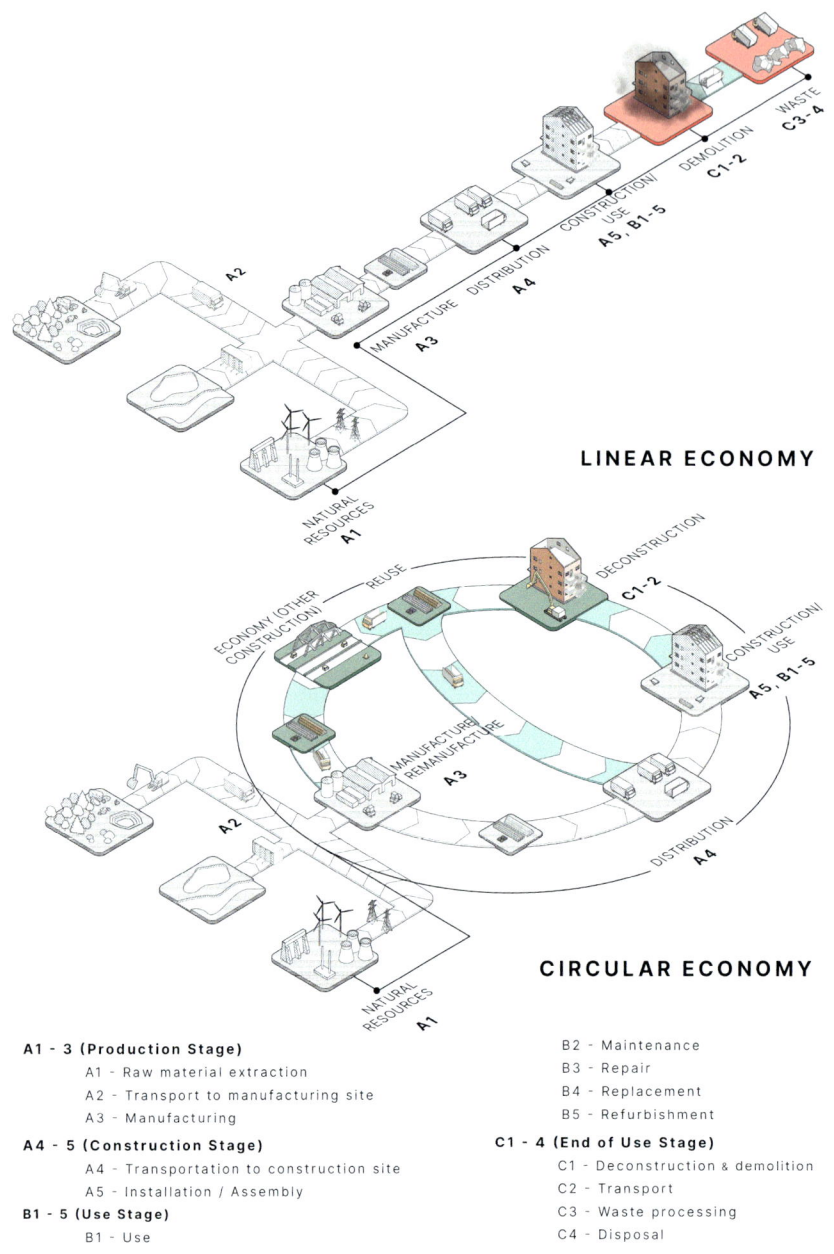

LINEAR ECONOMY

CIRCULAR ECONOMY

A1 - 3 (Production Stage)
    A1 - Raw material extraction
    A2 - Transport to manufacturing site
    A3 - Manufacturing
A4 - 5 (Construction Stage)
    A4 - Transportation to construction site
    A5 - Installation / Assembly
B1 - 5 (Use Stage)
    B1 - Use

    B2 - Maintenance
    B3 - Repair
    B4 - Replacement
    B5 - Refurbishment
C1 - 4 (End of Use Stage)
    C1 - Deconstruction & demolition
    C2 - Transport
    C3 - Waste processing
    C4 - Disposal

Figure 2.1 Lifespan of the Built Environment Process.

2.2 Historical Developments and Differences in Energy Theories: From Bullard and Herendeen's Embodied Energy to Odum's Emergy

How one conceptualizes energy and material can affect building and assessment decisions in construction. There are three major energy theories – embodied energy, life cycle assessment, and emergy analysis – that will be discussed further, as well

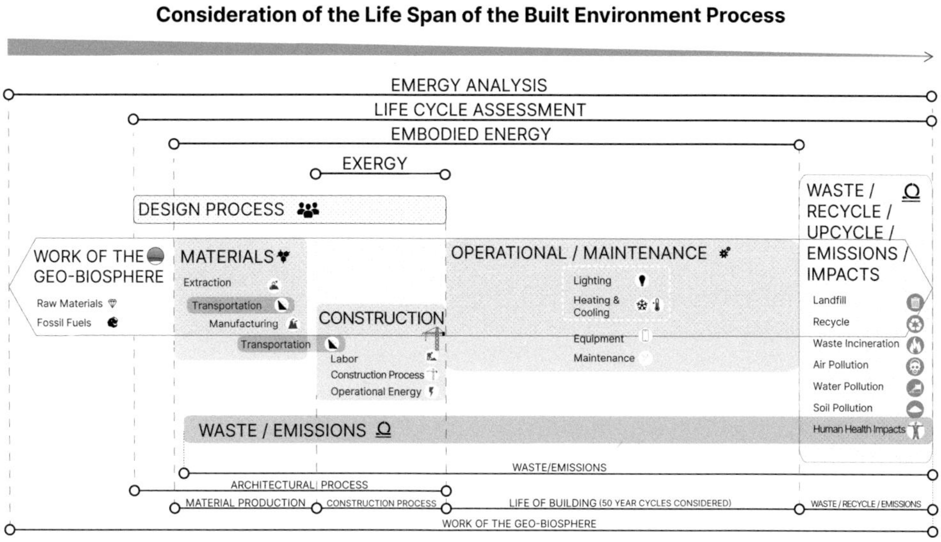

Consideration of the Life Span of the Built Environment Process

Figure 2.2 Lifespan of the Built Environment Process.

as their respective strengths and weaknesses. Each theory considers direct and indirect outputs differently, painting a different picture of the extent to which an activity is environmentally detrimental (see Figure 2.2). These theories are helpful in setting the theoretical foundation on which builders and architects implement a circular economic model.

2.2.1 Embodied Energy Analysis

Embodied energy analysis considers all the exergy needed to produce a good or service (see Figure 2.3). Exergy is a term used in thermodynamics to define the potential to do work when it is brought into thermodynamic equilibrium with its environment (Benjamin et al., 2017). Embodied energy can be helpful when considering the true environmental benefit of certain building decisions. For instance, rather than merely calculating the amount of greenhouse gas emissions saved by building energy-efficient dwellings, an embodied energy analysis will factor in the emissions caused by transporting goods, constructing the energy-saving features, extracting necessary materials, etc., to paint a comprehensive image of the genuine environmental benefit of such a decision. This approach thus looks at a product or service with a life cycle view, factoring in all energy inputs and outputs before, during, and after a product's life.

There are three approaches to measuring embodied energy: process analysis, input-output analysis (I-O analysis), and hybrid models (Bullard et al., 1978). Theoretically, these approaches will factor in the same data, but the extent to which each factor is measured differs. Process analysis uses an iterative process of identifying energy inputs to a target product until the input amount is negligible to the total energy use of a product. As a result, process analysis accounts almost solely for

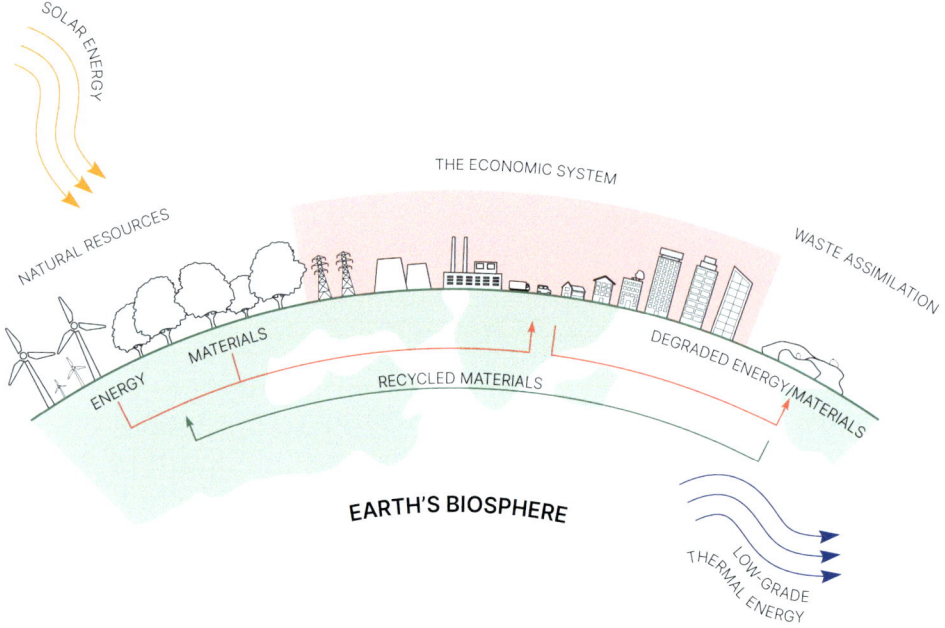

Figure 2.3 The Work of the Geo-Biosphere and the Overall Ecological System that Enables Access to the Energy and Material Resources Used in the Built Environment.

direct energy that has the clearest impact on a building. This approach risks neglecting the myriad of indirect energy inputs that are nearly negligent on their own but may accumulate to a substantial effect when summed together. I-O analysis, by contrast, accounts for the direct and indirect energy to produce a good or service in the economy, factoring in labor, land, and capital (Costanza, 1980). Direct energy would be energy that is directly used by a product, such as cement used in a building, or electricity to heat a dwelling. Indirect energy would be energy that is used outside of the product, but to produce goods and services that then become direct energy inputs to the building. Labor to extract raw materials that then turn into cement would be an indirect energy input (Bullard et al., 1978). The main difference between Process and I-O analysis is their view on the relationship between factors of economic production (e.g., labor, land, government services, and raw material extraction). In the former approach, many of these primary factors of production are considered independent and thus irrelevant to the calculation of embodied energy of a product; however, the I-O approach draws its boundary of consideration to include many of these net inputs, or primary factors of production, viewing many industries that go into producing a good or service as being *inter*dependent. Comprehensive matrix tables are made for I-O analysis to account for direct inputs (e.g., the direct resources used to build a dwelling), indirect inputs (e.g., labor required to extract resources), and induced inputs (e.g., resources to allow workers to extract material). By using national averages of energy and economic data, I-O models are able to turn purchases from energy sectors to financial terms; however, using national averages makes analysis on energy consumption of individual products somewhat inaccurate (Treloar et al., 2001).

Therefore, to accurately assess a building's embodied energy, a hybrid model of Process and I-O techniques is suggested (Keena & Dyson, 2017).

2.2.2 Life Cycle Assessment (LCA)

A life cycle assessment of energy and material flows examines each stage of a product or service's life (see Figure 2.4a). This is typically conceptualized as a "cradle-to-grave" logic, meaning that a good or service's environmental impact is assessed from the conception of the good (e.g., extracting raw materials), to material consumption, manufacturing, and then to the eventual demolition and waste (grave). This allows a cumulative and comprehensive assessment of a product's impact on the environment. There is a range of other interpretations of life cycle analysis. "Cradle-to-gate" entails assessing a product's life from its extraction to production, omitting the use and demolition phase. LCA can also be framed as "cradle-to-cradle", in which a product's environmental impact is assessed from its conception to its reuse in another sector. In a circular economy there are often suggestions to use a life cycle assessment to help understand if a building process is becoming circular. While the embodied energy analysis assesses the sum of energy needed to extract and produce a good or service, life cycle assessment has a more temporal and multifaceted lens, factoring in numerous environmental and human health impacts from a product's inception to after the product is built, as well as its demolition.

LCA is governed by standards which support consistency across analyses, such as the ISO standards 14040 and 14044 (ISO, 2006). It is noteworthy that life cycle analyses of the same material or process can differ greatly over time and from region to region. This can be due to transportation factors, the grid-mix composition for regional electricity production, or the technological processes used. Therefore, employing local specific data which expresses regional conditions and processes that are used (or are assumed to be used) throughout a building's life cycle is preferable. Where local data is unobtainable, data is typically acquired from similar projects outlined in the literature. Data is captured in the life cycle inventory (LCI) model. The life cycle impact assessment (LCIA) stage is used to evaluate the magnitude and significance of the life cycle flows for each phase of the life cycle or to compare different design options with respect to their human health and environmental impacts, such as climate change, human toxicity, and biodiversity. Hence, an LCA goes beyond solely measuring global warming potential (GWP) or embodied carbon and energy, by including impact assessment methods which help to characterize the potential consequences a building design in a particular region may have on human health and the environment.

To understand the three central pillars of sustainability (environment, economy, and social needs) from a life cycle perspective, two other life cycle assessment methods are important to discuss, namely Life Cycle Cost Assessment (LCCA), and Social-LCA (S-LCA), which, respectively, aim to measure the economic, and social impacts associated with a product or service life cycle (see Figure 2.4).

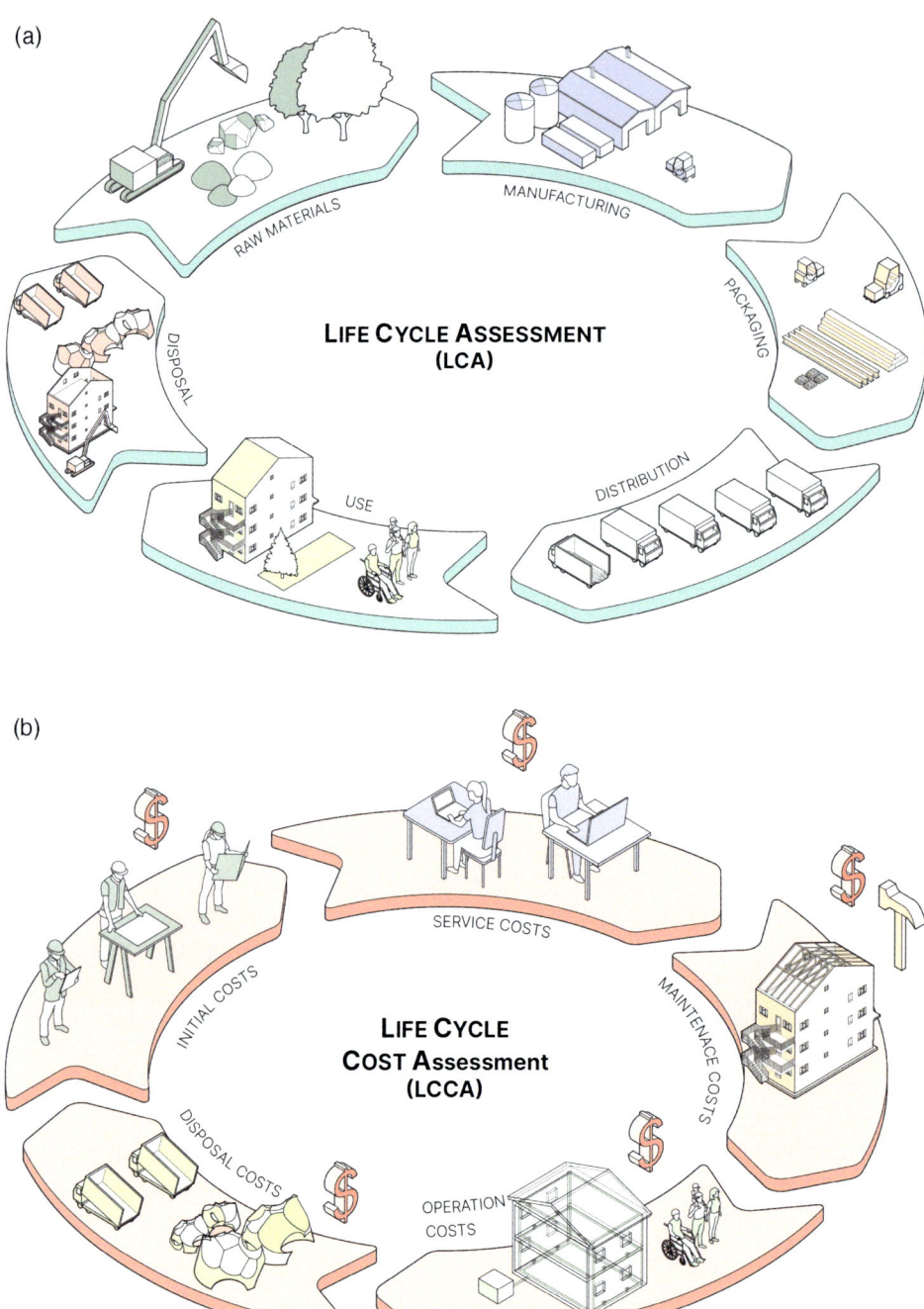

Figure 2.4 Holistic Life Cycle Design Thinking in the Built Environment: (a) Life Cycle Assessment, (b) Life Cycle Cost Assessment. (*Continued*)

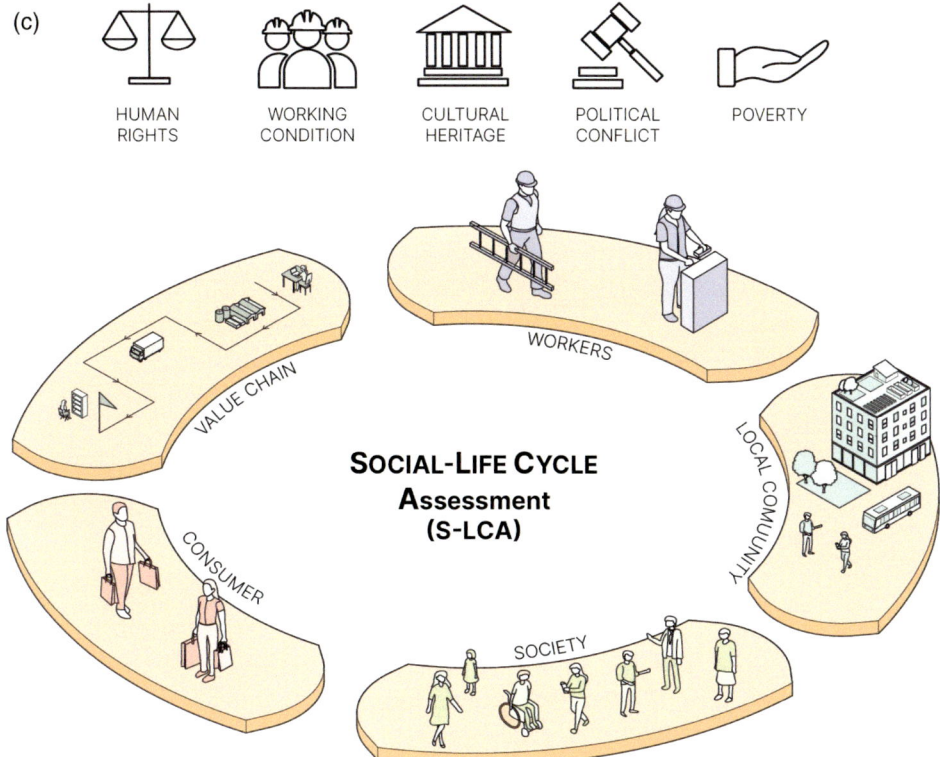

(c)

HUMAN RIGHTS   WORKING CONDITION   CULTURAL HERITAGE   POLITICAL CONFLICT   POVERTY

Figure 2.4 (*Continued*) Holistic Life Cycle Design Thinking in the Built Environment: (c) Social Life Cycle Assessment.

Life Cycle Cost Assessment (LCCA)

Similar to how an environmentally focused LCA will measure the cumulative environmental impact of each phase of a building's life, an LCCA calculates the most cost-effective route to, in this case, construction, factoring in costs from creation, operation, and disposal (Liu & Qian, 2019). As discussed in Chapter 1, the core of sustainability is a consideration of long-term effects of human decisions. An LCCA similarly factors in long-term service costs and maintenance costs of construction decisions and, as a result, an option that has a higher upfront cost but better quality and durability may present the economic benefits of a more circular approach in an LCCA over an option with a short linear, lifespan but cheaper upfront costs.

Social-Life Cycle Assessment (S-LCA)

S-LCA is used to measure a range of potential social impacts likely to be experienced by a range of stakeholders at each phase of the building life cycle. An S-LCA will compare the different socio-economic impacts of material decisions throughout a building's life cycle. Some factors accounted for in an S-LCA would be those that directly impact a company's stakeholders, including human rights, cultural heritage, poverty, working conditions, labor, and political conflict that may result from a building project (Hosseinijou et al., 2014). Social impact assessment is done to five categories of stakeholders: workers, the local community, society, consumers, and value chain actors (Liu & Qian, 2019). The conversation on how to measure qualitative social impacts is complicated, but the UNEP has created guidelines and a methodology for conducting S-LCA, which divides social impact into two categories: stakeholders and impacts (United Nations Environment Programme, 2009). While the S-LCA is less firmly established as the environmental or economic LCA, long-term scrutiny of a production process helps clarify the dynamic social impact that production decisions have on multiple stakeholders.

2.2.3 Emergy Analysis and a Regenerative Approach

Emergy is the amount of an individual source's energy that is needed, either directly or indirectly, to produce and/or support a particular good or service. Figure 2.5 depicts an energy circuit diagram that illustrates the differences between emergy from other energy evaluation methods. All energy sources are measured by "unit emergy values" (UEVs), which is the total exergy used from the source's formation (Raugei et al., 2014). Unlike an embodied energy or LCA, which was conceived to assess human-made systems, emergy was conceived by Howard T. Odum (1988) to measure energy required to fuel natural ecosystems. As a result, this approach to energy analysis is the most macro of the four, viewing all processes of production from the perspective of the geo-biosphere. While embodied energy and LCA use economic approaches, such as giving a monetary value to energy to measure environmental impact, emergy analysis believes economies can be measured by energy units. While both are valuable perspectives, embodied energy and LCA analysis omit "free" ecological resources, which become difficult to translate into a monetary value (Benjamin et al., 2017). By converting natural capital to UEVs, emergy analysis can account for both human-applied and environmental resources.

The four energy analysis methods differ in terms of their respective scopes of consideration. A combination of each energy method allows each to complement different aspects of a building development and help determine whether a building fulfills core requirements of circularity. The Ellen MacArthur Foundation provides three pillars of circular economy: (1) eliminate waste and pollution, (2) circulate products and materials at their highest values, and (3) regenerate nature (1996). Emergy analysis is the only energy theory to properly measure how regenerative a project is because it factors in the ecological geo-biosphere. According to Mark Brown and Herendeen (1996), emergy analysis can be described as "donor"-based, in that a product's value comes from how much goes into it rather than how much one is willing to pay for it. With this

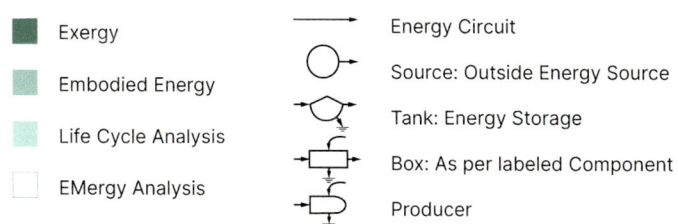

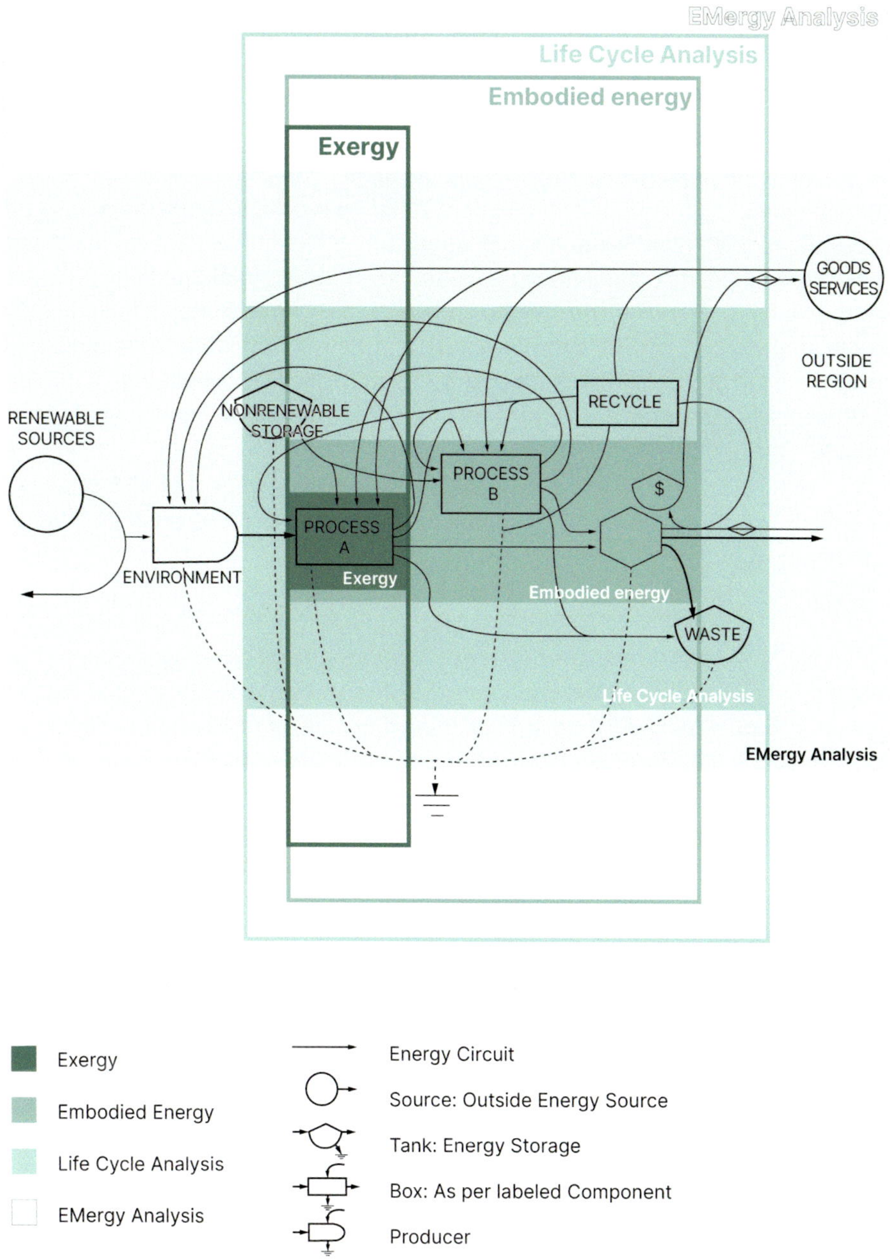

Figure 2.5 Energy Circuit Diagram.

logic, embodied energy and LCA, in contrast, are "receiver"-based. They derive a product's environmental impact by taking into account only those resources which are paid for. If we take sand as an example, in embodied energy and LCA calculations, sand is considered a raw material input. In emergy analysis sand is considered a raw material input, but the natural bio-geophysical processes such as sedimentary cycles that make sand over millions of years are also considered. Assessing goods and services with both a human-based lens and a purely environmental lens, or ideally a *socio-ecological* lens, allows for a deeper understanding of human's effect on the environment.

Section 2.2 outlined energetic theories that have been applied to architectural considerations to gain an understanding of the energy, material, and information flows of a building's life cycle. All of these approaches rely on systems thinking and taking a life cycle view when considering buildings and their designs. The scope of the defined lifespan is different depending on the methodology used, but all three theories outlined aim to go beyond the idea of a building in abstraction, fixed solely in the operational phase, but rather a building as a system that acknowledges the broad scope and terrestrial scale at which the built environment operates. Circular economy builds on such systems thinking and life cycle approach, as is explained in the next section.

2.3 Introducing the Idea of a Circular Economy

Geissdoerfer et al. (2017) describe a circular economy as a regenerative system that minimizes energy waste and emissions by closing or lessening energy loops. This is done by designing high quality from a product's inception, and maintaining that quality throughout a product's life, through repairs and refurbishments. This approach to development maintains the value of a product for as long as possible, eliminating waste and elongating the lifespan of both the dwelling and its composed-of parts. The current approach to manufacturing is linear, resting on a "take-make-waste" attitude toward construction. Goods are produced through a process of raw material extraction, then undergoes a single use for a period of time. After its usefulness ends, either due to wear-and-tear or contextual conditions, the product is disposed of, creating enormous waste. As the Ellen MacArthur Foundation (2013) writes, this framework is inherently inequitable. Most consumers are in Western nations, but industries acquire material resources in abundance across the globe. The notably inexpensive material cost compared to the cost of human labor incentivizes industries to disregard the need for recycling and reuse, emphasizing quick turnover of materials for maximum profit (Sariatli, 2017). The Ellen MacArthur Foundation (2013) cites the Sustainable Europe Research Institute's (SERI) study that 21 billion metric tons of production materials are wasted in the production process due to inefficient practices. As well, they cite that 2.7 billion metric tons (2.45 billion metric tons) of material inputs were discarded as waste, with only 40 percent recycled or reused. In a circular economy, the end-of-life perspective that a linear economy is contingent upon is replaced with revitalization, through the use of renewable resources, quality design of products, and the eventual reuse of material at the end of a product's useful life (Hobson, 2016; Moreau et al., 2017). The central aim of a circular economic approach is to remove waste from the building process, which has implications for the ecosystem, the economy, and society. As mentioned previously, there are three principles to achieve circularity in a system. First, a system must use design to eliminate waste; second, to maintain the usefulness of materials for as long as possible; and lastly, to regenerate the natural systems (Foundation, 2020). These components can be viewed as a "closed cycle" perspective, which looks at material cycles like an ecosystem, in which every residual component is reused. In a closed cycle, renewable energy is thus prioritized and does away with toxic substances that cannot be reused and regenerated. This allows for every product to extend its own useful life and be upcycled. Moreover, the idea of "systems thinking" is also crucial in all three aspects of this definition, which underscores the idea that every actor, industry, and material is connected in a system. As a result, every action influences another action.

This systemic perspective is reiterated by Haas et al. (2015), who stress that a circular economy requires a macro-view of environmental sustainability, resulting in an overhaul of our basic economic and industrial structure. Instead of a virtually ineffective eco-efficiency perspective, a circular economy values eco-effectiveness. In other words, in a linear economy, an environmentally conscious aim may be to lessen the relative environmental impact of a product to get the same result as before. Although a system being less ecologically detrimental than previously is beneficial, a relative approach does not ensure improvements to the ecology. Eco-effectiveness, by contrast, focuses not on minimizing harmful impacts of systems, but on rethinking systems to be environmentally, economically, and socially beneficial. Rather than downcycling, which relies on breaking down a product (e.g., concrete), into smaller parts to be used in a different setting (e.g., asphalt in the road), the circular economy relies on upcycling, which turns "end-of-life" material into a product of higher quality. Some benefits from a circular economy include self-evident environmental benefits – increased use of renewable resources, a decrease in emission rates, a reduction of residual material waste, and less input of natural resources (Antikainen et al., 2018). This construction reform also comes with significant economic benefits. A reduction of waste accumulation means that companies and municipalities save on costly waste management problems (Antikainen et al., 2018). Furthermore, labor is valued over cheap raw materials because efforts are put in place to upcycle used materials, resulting in a growth in jobs. The Ellen McArthur Foundation (2015) estimates that an incorporation of a circular economy would result in a 3 percent growth annually of resource productivity and a 7 percent rise in gross domestic product (GDP) in Europe.

2.4 Origins and Conceptual Underpinnings of a Circular Economy

The idea of using waste as a resource for economic activity is not a new concept. Before the Industrial Revolution, material waste management facilities were known as material recovery facilities, and they used manual sorting to create secondary raw materials in Western Europe (Velis et al., 2009). As will be expanded on in the following case study, repurposing building waste into new sculptures, columns, or monuments was also a common practice in the late antiquity, known as "spolia". The Arch of Constantine in Rome is a prime example of upcycling previous construction materials into a secondary life. Rather than framing the circular economy as a completely new concept, Antikainen et al. (2018) suggest that it is more accurate to view the circular economy as another step in an evolution of waste management systems. Nonetheless, the term "CE" started to gain traction in the late 1970s, influenced by Boulding's seminal text "The Economics of the coming Spaceship Earth" (Boulding & Jarrett, 1966). He describes the earth as a closed, circular system that has a limited capacity. As a result, the economy and environment should rest at an equilibrium for long-term sustainability. Stahel (1982) then introduces the idea of the closed loop (spiral-loop) to establish cyclical ecological systems instead of a linear model. The term "circular economy" was officially coined by Pearce and Turner (1990) who wrote about how natural resources affect the economy and described a system in which waste is reintegrated into a closed system as useful inputs. In 1994, Germany was one of the first countries to establish a Closed Substance Cycle and Waste Management Act (Kreislaufwirtschafts und Abfallgesetz), with the goal of conserving natural resources by promoting a closed cycle of waste management. Japan is another pioneer of sustainable waste management policies, enacting the Basic Law for Establishing a Recycling-Based Society, in 2002, which set a legal framework for environmentally friendly material cycles.

While circular economy itself was coined officially in the end of the 20th century, there are key concepts that set the foundation for a circular economic model. These include ecological economics, environmental economics, industrial ecology, bioeconomy, and green economy.

2.4.1 Ecological Economics

An ecological economic perspective is somewhat a response to the more mainstream neoclassical economic vision. The neoclassical perspective views economics as a relationship between firms and households, in which each has a mutual reliance on the other for goods and services. However, in neoclassical economics, the environment is excluded from conversations of the economy. While firms and households are important in fostering the economy, these entities are encompassed by the ecology – firms supply households and demand labor, households supply workers and demand goods, but the firm-household dynamic demands environmental resources and supplies waste to the environment. As well, the environment, through ecological processes such as the carbon cycle, is somewhat able to replenish itself, thus creating an everlasting circular system of ecological supply for the economy. Ecological economics stems from Boulding's 1966 ideas of closed earth and closed human sphere of activity and the attempt to have the ecological and economic fields interact in a meaningful way (Antikainen et al., 2018). This framework believes that

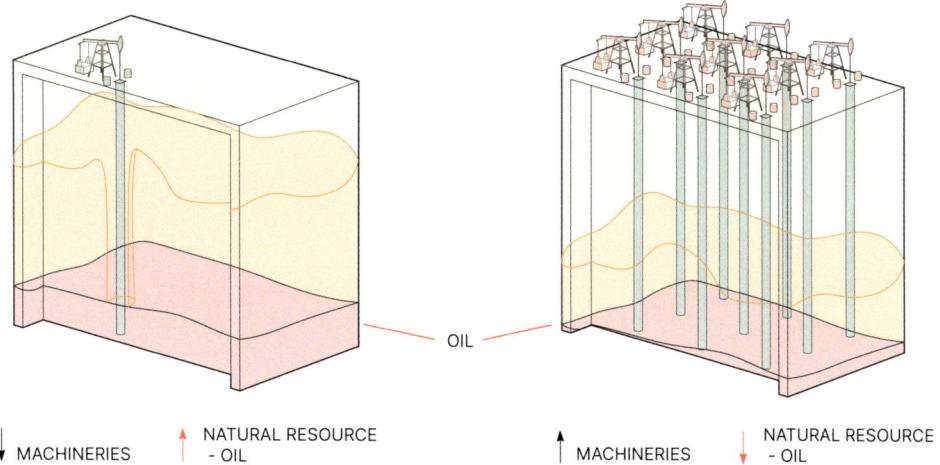

OIL

↓ MACHINERIES   ↑ NATURAL RESOURCE - OIL   ↑ MACHINERIES   ↓ NATURAL RESOURCE - OIL

Figure 2.6 Boulding's Closed Cycle System Can Be Demonstrated in the Economic System's Relationship with Crude Oil. When the Economy Is So Reliant on This Natural Resource, It Becomes Inextricably Linked to This Environmental Resource in a Way Where the Economy Becomes a Subset of the Natural Resource.

the economy is a subset of the environment, meaning that not only is the economy a factor in affecting the environment, through its scale or process, but the economy is also a reflection of the environment, and can be measured on a biological scale (see Figure 2.6). In a circular economy framework, this idea that the environment is a significant driver of the economy is key.

2.4.2 Environmental Economics

While ecological economics is fundamentally the notion that the economy is a subsystem within the larger ecosystem, environmental economics promotes the idea of minimizing negative externalities from environmental policy. In an open-ended system, price is determined by supply and demand – to determine an appropriate price for a good, a company must hit the equilibrium. In other words, a good must be sold high enough to make up the lost money of production but low enough to be attractive to buyers. However, environmental economics pushes this idea forward, factoring in externalities that are required to produce such a good. Environmental externalities are indirect costs that affect a third party, in this case the environment, but are not included in the market price of a good (see Figure 2.7). For instance, when buying an automobile, the price of the car may be determined by the cost of manufacturing, production, and transportation that the automobile company had to spend to construct the car. However, the long-term cost of carbon emissions from motor vehicle engines can be viewed as an externality that, despite leading to a large environmental and monetary cost for society in terms of public health issues, is not factored into the price of the automobile. circular economy's emphasis on interdisciplinary analysis is in line with environmental economic thinking. Through

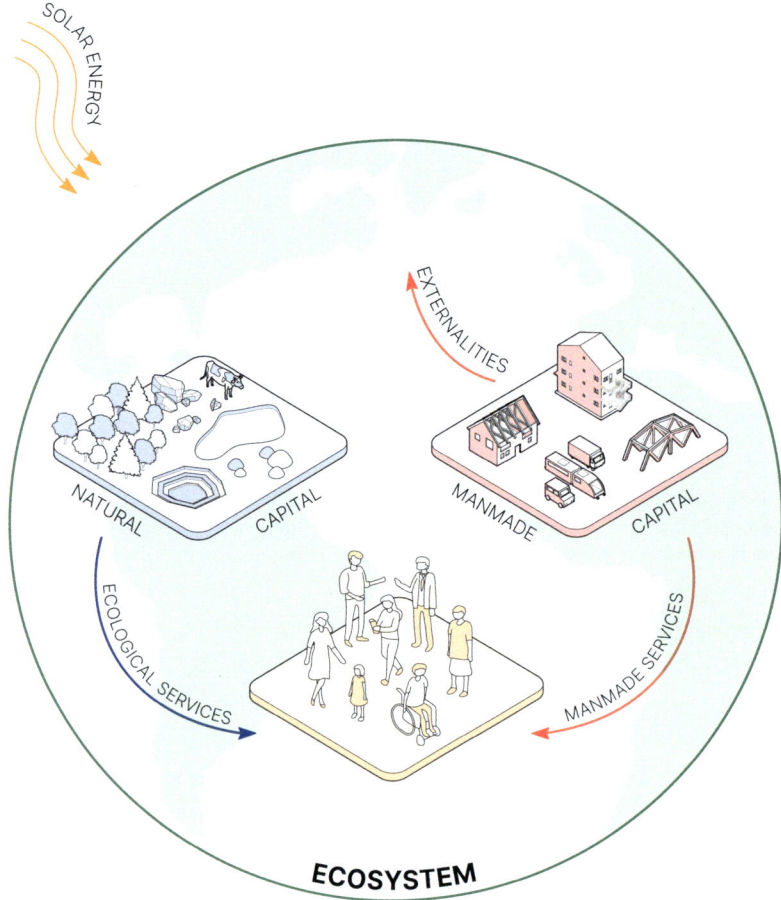

Figure 2.7 Visual Illustration of the Disregard for Externalities when Determining the Value of a Good or Service.

interdisciplinary analysis that accounts for environmental consequences, negative externalities can be accounted for in environmental policy (Andersen, 2007).

2.4.3 Industrial Ecology

Unlike the previous two conceptual underpinnings, whose respective focuses were on the relationship between the environment and economy, industrial ecology looks at the relationship between the environment and industrial systems, looking through the lens of a systems-based approach. Like the circular economy, industrial ecology uses a life cycle assessment as a means to achieve energy efficiency in the industrial sector. The principal idea of this concept is, as the name implies, that industrial economics can be viewed as an extension of the natural ecosystem. This overlap in the industrial and natural realm is fundamental in a circular economy. If the industrial sector is an extension of the natural ecosystem, which replenishes itself circularly, industrial frameworks can also act as a sort of ecosystem, replenishing itself through developing closed cycles. This concept is called biomimicry – where human-made systems emulate natural systems. This idea rests upon the assumption that natural systems are the model for sustainable design and that industrial systems can be viewed as a reflection of natural systems. Industrial ecology's primary aim is to improve the metabolic pathways of industrial processes, design for a closed-loop industrial ecosystem, and dematerialize industrial outputs (Antikainen et al., 2018).

2.4.4 Bioeconomy

Bioeconomy is another concept connected to the circular economy and refers to the portion of the economy based on biological resources, such as plants and microorganisms (Gallo, 2022). The United Nations Food and Agriculture Organization (FAO) defines this as:

> The production, use and conservation of biological resources, including related knowledge, science, technology, and innovation to provide information, products, processes and services to all economic sectors with the aim of moving towards a sustainable economy.
>
> (Trigo et al., 2021)

One of the aims of bioeconomy is to foster circularity, namely reuse, repair, and recycle. A bioeconomy grows bio-based resources, converts these resources into bio-based products, and uses bio-based waste to upcycle products (Gallo, 2022; see Figure 2.8). Instead of a take-make-waste model, the bioeconomy's emphasis on using bio-based resources throughout the life cycle of a product is circular in concept. A crop can be grown to feed an animal but can also be converted to a food product for the market, such as barley and beer. The "waste" of the barley, which was not incorporated in the bio-based product, can then be converted to a bio-based energy source to power homes, thus using every part of a biological substance to foster circularity and sustainability.

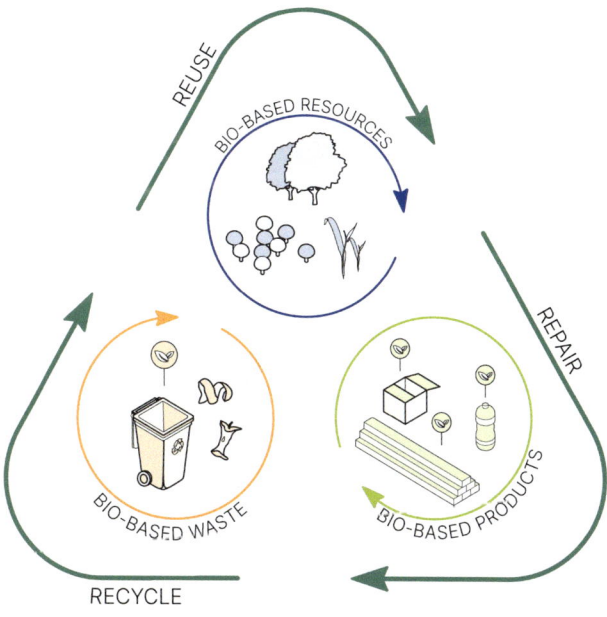

Figure 2.8 Bioeconomy.

2.4.5 Green Economy

The green economy is a broader concept to describe an economy that significantly reduces "environmental risks and ecological scarcities" (United Nations Environment Programme, 2011). In a green economy, social inclusion, carbon reduction, and resource efficiency are prioritized. The green economy runs in relation with UN Sustainability Goals, recognizing that economic reform is a crucial tool in achieving sustainable development. Like sustainable development goals discussed in Chapter 1, a green economy values social and environmental sustainability and sees these realms as interconnected. The circular economy is one component of a green economy that is crucial to ensuring that homes are built for long-term usefulness and products do not conform to a throwaway culture of waste.

2.5 Three Interpretations of CE

The basis of circular economy, in the simplest sense, is a rejection of linear economy, which rests on a once-through industrial economy of stock and material flows. A linear economy treats capital stock and flows as something to accumulate and thus the industrial economy's measure of success is the sum of all the flows (GDP). The focus is on management of such material flows until its point of sale, where the responsibility is then lifted from the manufacturer and put onto the consumer to decide to what extent they will maintain the product and eventually dispose of it (Stahel & Clift, 2016). Circular economy rejects this notion of linear maintenance, emphasizing value preservation over value added. Yet, models for understanding exactly how a circular economy handles capital stock and material flows differ. Stahel and Clift (2016) outline three interpretations of circular economy to help understand how this framework functions: loop economy, lake economy, and performance economy.

2.5.1 Loop Economy

A loop economy, also known as a cradle-to-cradle concept, focuses on the flow of materials whereby materials for products are recycled for the same use as before in a loop format (see Figure 2.9) (Stahel & Clift, 2016). These loops include reuse, repair, remanufacturing, and repossession of material, in the local, regional, and global economies and supply chains (Antikainen et al., 2018). In a reuse loop, second-hand markets, such as garage sales, and private reuse, such as refilling empty bottles, are local ways to reuse stock. Remanufacturing can be local or regional in scale, entailing repairing or upgrading a good to meet new technological standards (Stahel & Clift, 2016). Recycling does not repair a product but reprocesses it to secondary material with the aim that it returns to the same use. Reprocessing is typically on the regional or global scale, as Stahel and Clift (2016) describe, and tries to recycle or downcycle materials. In the simplest sense, a loop economy perspective views the circular

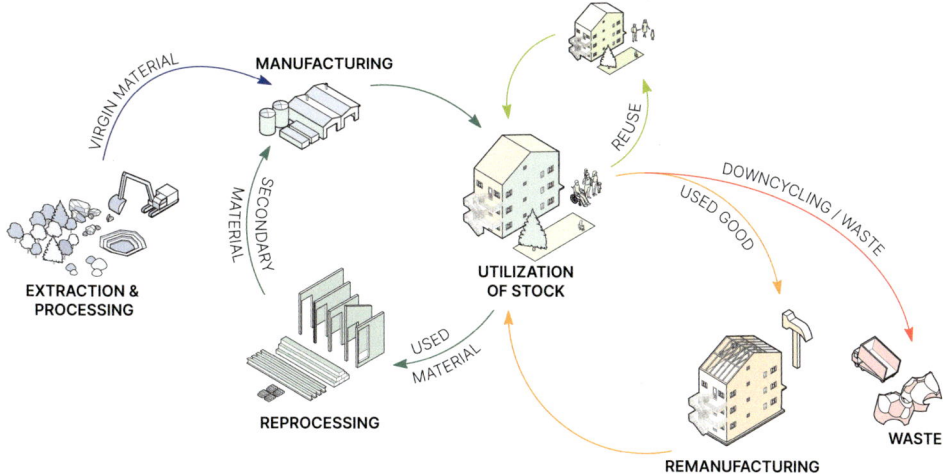

LOOP ECONOMY

Figure 2.9 Loop Economy.

economy as a tool to recycle production materials to return to the same use so as not to discard waste (Stahel & Clift, 2016). Stahel (1982) suggests that a loop economy that prioritizes waste prevention and material reuse entails an emphasis on utilization over ownership of goods, meaning that industries can profit off sustainability without enduring external costs and risks of waste management. This is how China interprets circular economy, defining the term as "the activities of decrement, recycling and resource recovery in production, circulation, and consumption" (Jintao, 2009).

2.5.2 Lake Economy

One disadvantage of a loop economy is that it is arguably the least profitable interpretation of circular economy, as it disregards ways to optimize economic performance of stock. A loop economy focuses mainly on good waste management, but the useful lifespan of a product may be the same as in a linear industrial economy. Another way to interpret circular economy is as a lake economy, which has the central goal of preventing waste rather than managing waste in a sustainable fashion. It focuses on optimizing the stock and preserving value without switching ownership (Stahel & Clift, 2016). Fleet managers, as they are called, are the central economic actors of a lake economy, responsible for overseeing a range of operations. Ownership stays on the fleet manager, who is responsible for having their fleet of stock repaired and remanufactured when necessary (see Figure 2.10). In this model, management of stock trumps management of flow to maintain value. This model is more economically advantageous than a simple loop economy because the fleet manager can make a profit from reuse and remanufacturing.

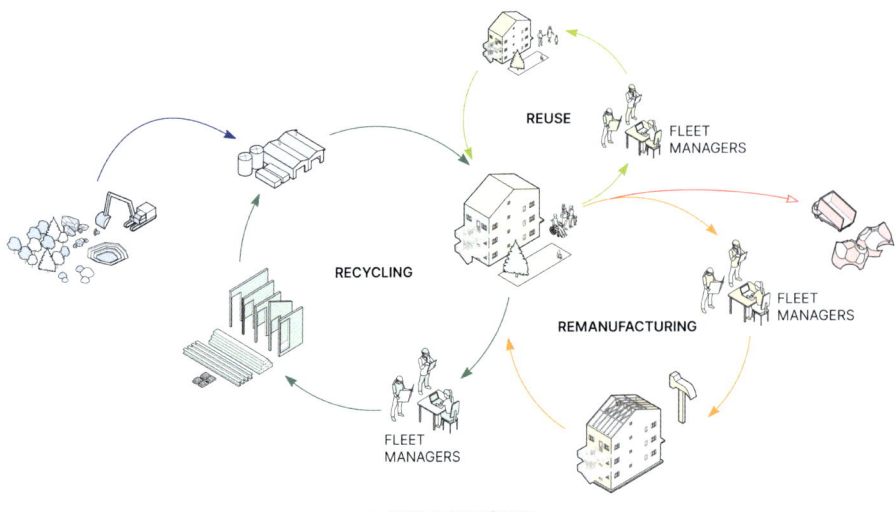

LAKE ECONOMY

Figure 2.10 Lake Economy.

2.5.3 *Performance Economy*

Performance economy pushes this idea forward, in which value of a good is optimized through business models that present goods as services (Stahel & Clift, 2016). This model disincentivizes the production (and subsequent waste) of many goods and instead rewards goods that serve the highest use value for the longest period. An example of this could be selling tires by the kilometer instead of by quantity, which would incentivize tire companies to produce the longest lasting tire instead of the highest quantity of tires. In this model, reuse and remanufacturing are key to maintaining stock of high quality for as long as possible. This approach also contributes to social sustainability, as it subverts the current low-labor and high-resource cost. Reuse and remanufacturing are labor intensive, leading to more jobs (see Figure 2.11). Businesses can afford to hire more workers from the capital saved

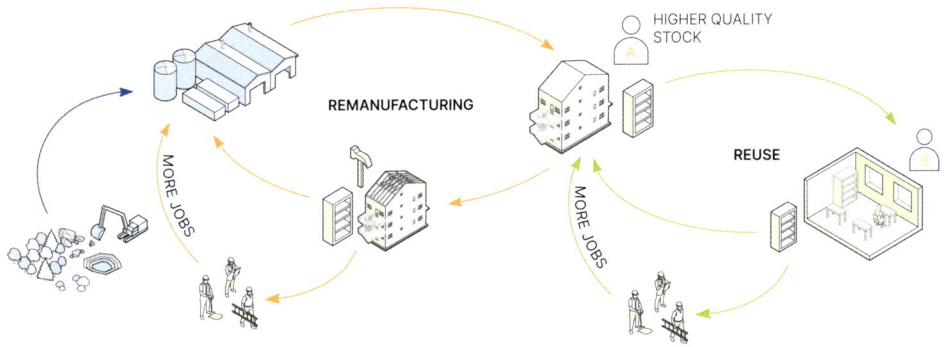

PERFORMANCE ECONOMY

Figure 2.11 Performance Economy.

on reducing virgin material production and primary manufacturing (Stahel & Clift, 2016). In the current industrial economy, capital is accumulated by value added, contributing to the overall GDP of a country. This does not reward quality and long-term value maintenance of products. In a performance economy, profit comes from maintaining stock, not from flows.

These interpretations fundamentally differ in terms of where value comes from and how ownership is viewed. In a loop economy, value still comes from flow and management of flows, while in the lake and performance economy, value shifts to stock and stock maintenance. As resource prices continue to increase and resource scarcity is expected to become a major political point of contention, a paradigm shift in how resources are valued is necessary. Managing existing stock, rather than burning through and depleting stock, will give nations resource security. If a stock value is maintained, ownership does not often shift the way it would in a linear economy. This allows owners to maintain resources at previously lower prices and contribute to its future resource supply.

2.6 Circular Economy: A Design Focus

This chapter has outlined key foundational concepts that influence and shape the circular economy. The key difference between circular economy and these conceptual underpinnings is that circular economy is first and foremost a design strategy, focused on redesigning the way things are done. In the context of architecture, circular economy seeks to redesign the built environment process – that is, the pre-building, building, and post-building lifespan of a built environment (Keena & Dyson, 2020). The built environment process encompasses the extraction of materials, the manufacturing of construction products, the construction of the building, the operation of the building, and the end of the building's useful life – all aspects that a circular economy lens would address (see Figure 2.1). One component of this circular built environment is decreasing negative externalities, which include water, noise, air, and soil pollution (Zimmerman et al., 2016). Transitioning to a circular built environment requires the efforts of multiple stakeholders who are involved in the entire life cycle of a building. Policies must support cross-industry collaboration. Technology and Big Data can aid in the flow of materials and set collaborative networks between sectors (Keena & Dyson, 2020). In the above discussion on energy theories, there is an emphasis on the need to design buildings to be both ecologically beneficial as well as economically sustainable. Evidently, this is crucial in the context of a circular built environment, in which both the ecology, but also multiple stakeholders, including municipalities, companies, and residents, are affected by building choices. Therefore, what differentiates circular economy and makes it appealing to stakeholders, over other economic models discussed, is its pragmatic nature. Multiple institutions and organizations have provided design criteria and business models to achieve circularity in the built environment, which benefits ecology, economics, and the social sphere. This next section details the design goals of the circular economy and proposed strategies for reaching said goals.

2.6.1 Design Goals for Circular Economy

Multiple institutions have come out with sustainable building targets. As discussed in Chapter 1, the UN SDGs are large-scale development goals that touch on the five pillars of sustainability (environmental, economic, social, cultural, and governmental). The American Institute of Architects' (AIA) Design Excellence Goals, the Leadership in Energy and Environmental Design (LEED) program, the Building Research Establishment Environmental Assessment Method (BREEAM), and the WELL Building Standard are other frameworks specific to architecture. Standards such as BREEAM and LEED provide assessments and certifications to designate a building as sustainable. The AIA proposes ten measures for "design excellence" (AIA, 2020). These measures seek to achieve a "zero-carbon, equitable, resilient, and healthy built environment" (AIA, 2020). In terms of circularity, there are three general goals that many of the standards encourage and relate directly to the built environment: building smaller and building less, choosing the right materials, and incorporating data and technology for waste management.

2.6.2 Building Smaller and Building Less

Choosing the right size for one's building can conserve space and promote economic design (Keena & Dyson, 2020). Bigger area size requires more energy consumption and costs more money to heat and cool. Not only is this environmentally detrimental (see Chapter 1) but also economically draining. A building efficiency ratio calculation (net square footage divided by gross square footage) can help builders determine the available conserved space in their dwelling. When budget cuts come, reducing space in an efficient manner is far more economically and environmentally sustainable than reducing material quality (Keena & Dyson, 2020).

While some net zero energy goals and green certification rating systems reward reducing the amount of energy an individual building uses, Miflin (2019) argues against this measurement, pushing for space to be used more often and by more people. The goal should be not only to build more compactly but to build less in general, so as to save on costly, timely, and environmentally draining construction projects. This can be done by assigning spaces to multiple functions, such as "gymnatoriums" in schools, which combine a gymnasium and auditorium to reduce the number of large area spaces in schools and conserve energy and costs (Miflin, 2019). While this may lead to more energy an individual building uses, the overall energy saved by reducing construction will be substantial.

Moreover, making efforts to modify existing buildings for reuse instead of building new can save on money and environmental cost. Changing single-family-zoned areas to allow for multifamily developments and accessory dwelling units can densify areas near core transit hubs, reducing the need for parking lots and the overall reliance on automobiles. This saves money for municipalities, developers, business owners, and individuals (Keena & Dyson, 2020). Regional Plan Association's Fourth Regional Plan finds that affordable housing in the New York-New Jersey-Connecticut Metropolitan Area can be achieved without building new, through modifying zoning laws (Regional Plan Association, 2019).

The emphasis of this first goal is to effectively use space to reduce overall costs. This can be done by building smaller, leading to less energy consumption costs. However, creating spaces that are multifunctional is another way to use area effectively, preventing people from building outward to perform their duties. The United Kingdom's 2013 HM Treasury Infrastructure Carbon Review suggests that in the planning stage of development, it is pertinent to ask whether the desired outcome of a development can be achieved without building more and instead using the existing built environment more efficiently (Macdonald et al., 2013).

2.6.3 Material Choice and End-Of-Life Design

Use of material is another "best practice" guiding economic and environmental building design. What materials builders choose determines economic success, safety and resilience, and environmental impact.

The AIA guidelines recommend reducing excess or unneeded construction materials to reduce the overall cost per square foot. Like with the previous recommendation, the AIA recommends choosing materials that serve more than one function, such as structural shear walls. This material is impact resistant as well as sound and fireproof (AIA, n.d.). A life cycle assessment can guide builders on the long-term efficiency of material choices, creating a resilient building. When natural disaster strikes, it is vital that materials can recover and sustain disaster for economic viability and waste reduction (see Section 1.3.2). While a material may have more upfront costs, when a long-term LCA is performed, this can highlight valuable long-term pay-back of materials in terms of energy saving, environmental impact, and durability (Keena & Dyson, 2020). Another way to promote safety and environmental protection via material choice is by rejecting "chemicals of concern" from the building process (Keena & Dyson, 2020). The AIA has a measure that sets goals in terms of the material selection so that the contractor is aware of any health concerns regarding material selection.

Material sourcing is another important aspect to achieve sustainable building practices, such as choosing materials that can replenish natural air, water, and biological cycles. Using material impact tracking throughout the construction process via Environmental Product Declarations EPDs, for instance, can help builders ensure that extraction and material sourcing are done in an environmentally respectful way (Keena & Dyson, 2020). Builders should choose materials that are reclaimed, such as reclaimed brick, that has high potential for reuse and recycling at its end-of-use phase. As well, through a life cycle assessment, builders should make a concerted effort to choose materials with low embodied carbon, such as wood and bio-based products. This includes choosing materials that are locally sourced, which has the added benefit of supporting the local economy and building community links.

This second goal highlights the need for architects and builders to pay attention to the economic and environmental implications of their material choice. Using non-toxic, renewable, and reclaimed material leads to long-term benefits.

2.6.4 Using Data and Technology to Reduce Waste Generation

Data and technology should be utilized by builders to properly assess the long-term and interconnected impact that building choices have on the environment and economy. The construction sector is one of the least digitized in the world, often seeing timely and costly projects with low labor-productivity growth compared to other sectors (McKinsey Global Institute, 2017). One method of improving productivity is by digitizing supply-chain management to allow for better planning and more transparency between contractors and suppliers (McKinsey Global Institute, 2017). For instance, Katerra, a US-based construction company, has created a data-enhanced global sourcing model that tracks supply chains and predicts potential market dynamics and replenishment of supplies (McKinsey Global Institute, 2017). Other techniques such as integrating a "Last Planner System" (LPR) and using key performance indicators (KPS) to assess productivity and ensure building plans are communicated between actors. One way to do this is by designing a building information modeling (BIM) system within construction companies which will enact transparency in the design, cost, and progress visualization of a project (McKinsey Global Institute, 2017). Moreover, the Waste Calculator, created by the AIA in their zero-waste guidelines uses data to approximate how much waste a building is expected to produce depending on the operating scenario (Miflin et al., 2017). The BREEAM standard emphasizes the need for better disclosure and reporting techniques. Using data and technology and third-party assurance throughout the entire life cycle of a building, stakeholders are able to understand important insights into their construction impact and affect decisions to align with sustainability goals (BREEAM, n.d.). Using advanced predictive data and technology to visualize the life cycle of the building post-construction allows planners and architects to plan for waste prevention and management before the building is made.

McKinsey (2017) underscores the need to move to a more holistic operating system to reduce construction waste. By adopting new data and technology techniques, the building sector has the potential to add about $1.6 trillion to the total economy, increasing the global economy by about 2 percent (McKinsey Global Institute, 2017). Many of the data and technological advancements promoted by McKinsey's comprehensive report adopt the idea of systems thinking into the construction project – a core tenet of the circular economy. By improvement construction efficiency, collaboration between partners, and transparency of cost and building materials, builders can design out waste. Chapters 10 and 11 expand on this idea, stressing how virtualization can improve construction efficiency and communication between stakeholders.

2A

Arch of Constantine

Location:
Rome, Italy –

Year:
312 AD (materials from 98 to 180 AD)

Team:
Ancient Romans

Mapping to Circular Economy Framework:

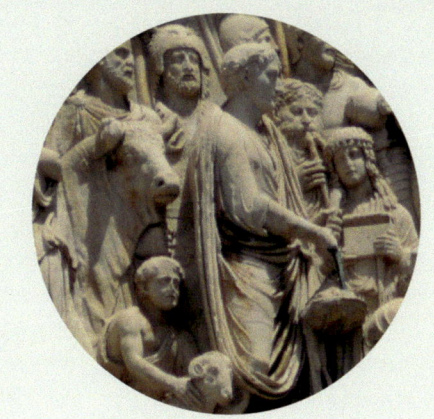

CIRCULAR ECONOMY PRACTICES

LIFE CYCLE PHASES	Recovery	Life Extension	Sharing Platforms	Service Models	Regenerate	Virtualize
Work of Geobiosphere	●	●	○	○	○	○
Sourcing	●	●	○	○	○	○
Manufacturing	●	●	○	○	○	○
Design & Construction	●	●	○	○	○	○
Use	●	●	○	○	○	○
End-of-Use	◐	○	○	○	○	○

LAYERS + LIFESPAN
Structural Layers | Long Life
Skin, MEP Layers | Medium Life
Interior Layers | Short Life

Site 100+yr Structure 50+yr
Exterior 25+yr System 15+yr
Partition 10+yr Stuff 1+yr

A circular approach to construction is not a new concept. Circular material sourcing techniques were at one point the norm in some ancient cultures, effectively reducing labor, limiting raw material extraction, and preserving ideological and aesthetic heritage. In ancient Greece and Rome, a recycling and material reuse method later named "spolia" repurposed building materials, primarily stone, for new construction. This ancient and widespread practice enabled stone and masonry that had been quarried, cut, and used in a built structure to be salvaged and used elsewhere, generating unique, ad-hoc, and wonderfully textured building façades and interiors. This reuse practice was first used extensively during the era of Constantine, with columns, architraves, and ornamental components of demolished buildings given new lives across the empire (Brenk, 1987). Although not a dwelling, the Arch of Constantine is an excellent example of the use of spolia where much of the construction materials are repurposed from earlier monuments (see Figures 2.12–2.15).

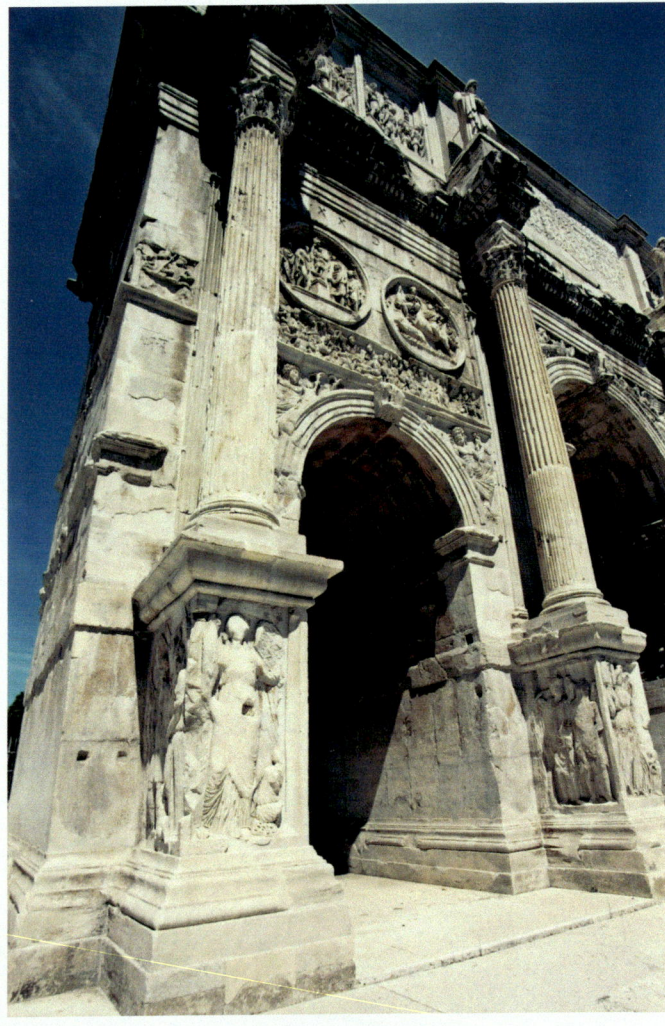

Figure 2.12 Ground Eye View of the Arch of Constantine.

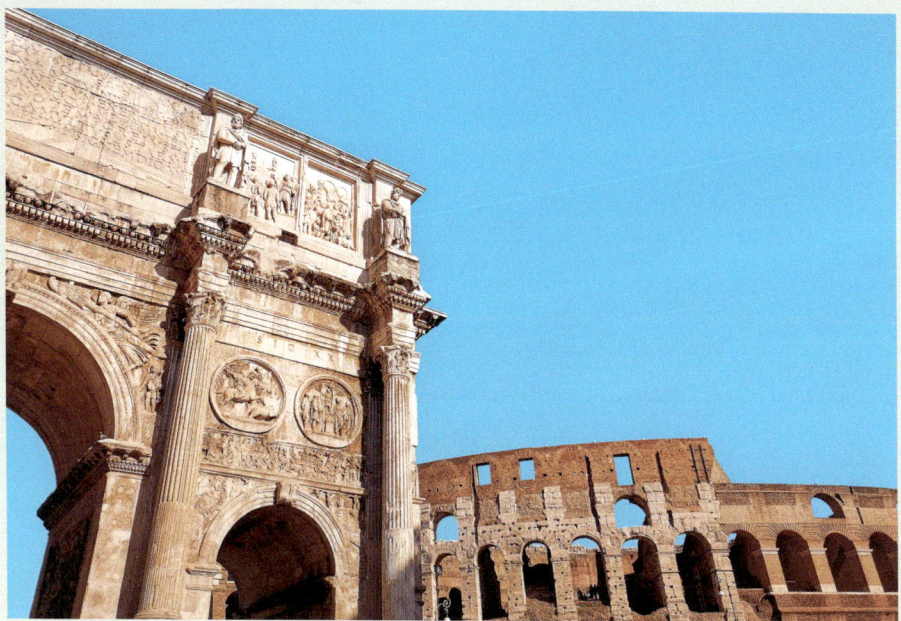

Figure 2.13 Arch of Constantine and Colosseum.

The historical landmark was erected in 312 AD and stands at almost 21 meters (70 ft) high as a dedication to Constantine the Great, who ruled Rome as emperor between 306 and 337 AD. The Arch of Constantine remains today as a cultural relic and is popular among travelers and historians alike. One reason why the arch has

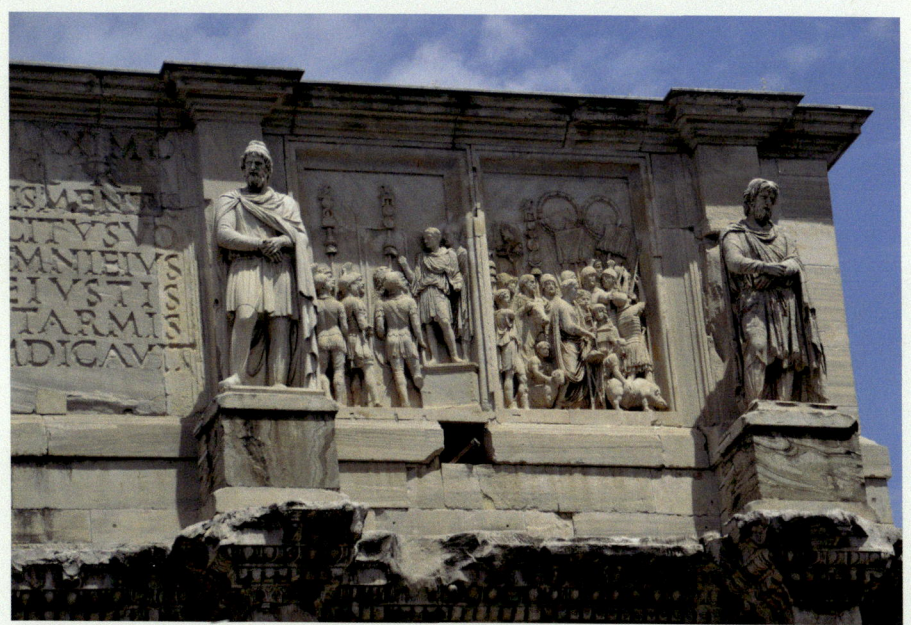

Figure 2.14 Detail of the Arch of Constantine.

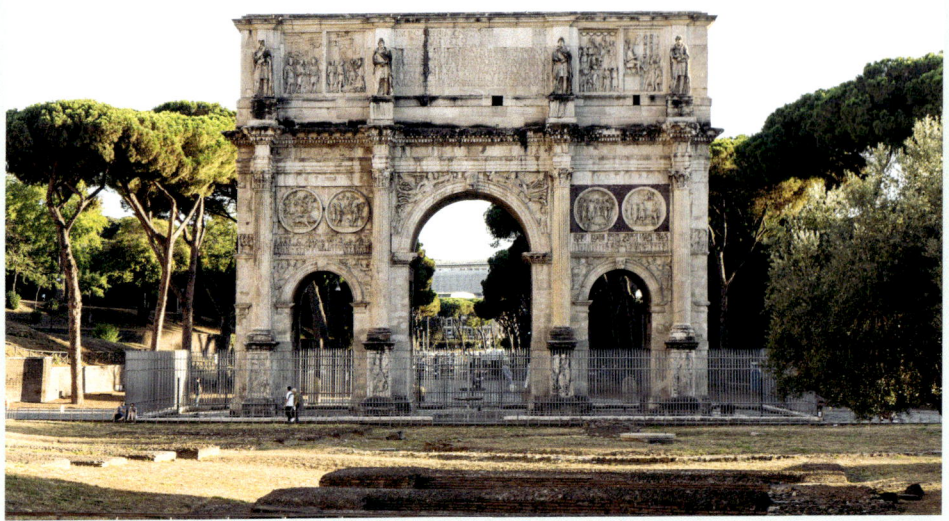

Figure 2.15 Arch of Constantine Today.

remained a topic of interest for many today is its incorporation of spolias, decorative reliefs, and statues from monuments spanning from the Trajan (98–117 AD) to the Marcus Aurelius Era (161–180 AD). Eight Dacian prisoners stand atop the arch's Corinthian columns on the structure's long façades, and these statues are thought to be derived from Trajan's forum of the Trajan era (Prusac, 2012). Constantine mounted these recognizable sculptures, along with other instances of reuse in the same structure, to reference Rome's previous victories and present himself as rightful and heroic caretaker of the empire.

Although the reasoning for material reuse in ancient times was largely political, the benefits of this practice represented by the Arch of Constantine are far-reaching. The incorporation of culturally significant, previously used stone carvings and blocks encourages **recovery and recycling** within construction practices. This circular principle prolongs the life of materials and, in ancient Rome's case, keeps stone in a cycle of use thus reducing the need for raw material extraction from the geo-biosphere. The repurposing of carvings and materials by Constantine and many rulers proceeding him allowed for the preservation of aesthetic and cultural heritage under a new context within the empire (Prusac, 2012). The widespread adoption of this tradition in late antiquity meant the development of required skills for stone extraction and reconstruction within the workforce, allowing for efficient **product life extension** of stone. The Arch of Constantine gave new life to materials and artwork in a new political environment, providing an excellent example of the power of circular construction techniques that are often associated with modernity. Circularity within the built environment is not new, and there is much to be learned from previous cultures to achieve it in our future.

2.7 Conclusion

This chapter has outlined important foundational concepts related to sustainability and circular economy. Embodied energy, life cycle assessment, and emergy analysis are interconnected concepts that describe how energy moves through space and time and has important implications to energy conservation practices involved in a circular economy. Outlining the origins and conceptual underpinnings of circular economy reveals how circular economy is not an entirely new concept, but an extension of waste management systems of environmental and ecological concepts already in place. While ecological economics, environmental economics, industrial ecology, bioeconomy, and green economy are helpful concepts, they differ distinctly from circular economy in terms of their respective pragmatism. The literature for these frameworks is focused on theory, while circular economy's central concern is to redesign the current linear framework to design out waste, unsustainable production methods, and incorporate renewable and resource-efficient sources practically. The relationship between the ecological and economic view of sustainability is especially relevant in a circular built environment, which is partly why businesses have found a particular interest in a circular economy framework, as will be discussed in the next chapter. Therefore, the examination of a loop, lake, and performance economy becomes helpful in understanding where profit rests when moving away from a take-make-waste production model. Incorporating circular economy into the built environment is fundamentally a design shift, and thus outlining different goals and recommendations for design excellence is pertinent in the discussion on practical architectural techniques. Focusing on three general categories of design targets in a circular economy also points to circular economy's connection with the five pillars of sustainability – environment, economy, society, culture, and government. Building smaller, choosing appropriate materials, and incorporating data and technology, all have clear environmentally beneficial impacts. However, as a life cycle assessment would find, these design targets also provide economic benefits for stakeholders, by saving money on building new dwellings, for instance, and decreasing waste management costs through reuse. Streamlining construction and planning phases by utilizing data and technology methods provides governmental efficiency as well. Furthermore, providing multifunctional space, as mentioned in Chapter 1, allows for cultural vibrancy and social accessibility. The next chapter will continue this discussion, examining specific circular business models and design drivers to achieve the UN sustainable development goals in residential development.

References

AIA. (n.d.). *Design for economy*. American Institute of Architects. Retrieved January 24 from https://www.aia.org/showcases/6082495-design-for-economy

AIA (2020). *AIA framework for design excellence*. American Institute of Architects.

Andersen, M. S. (2007). An introductory note on the environmental economics of the circular economy. *Sustainability Science*, 2(1), 133–140. https://doi.org/10.1007/s11625-006-0013-6

Antikainen, R., Lazarevic, D., & Seppälä, J. (2018). *Circular economy: Origins and future orientations*. In (pp. 115–129). Springer International Publishing. https://doi.org/10.1007/978-3-319-50079-9_7

Benjamin, D., Addington, M., Andraos, A., Barber, D. A., Bayer, E., Brownell, B., Carlisle, S., Dent, A., Dyson, A., & Hebel, D. E. (2017). *Embodied energy and design: Making architecture between metrics and narratives*. Columbia University Press.

Boulding, K. E., & Jarrett, H. (1966). *Environmental quality in a growing economy: Essays from the sixth RFF forum*. Published for Resources for the Future, Inc. by the Johns Hopkins Press.

BREEAM. (n.d.). *Disclosures and reporting: Making disclosures and reporting easier with BREEAM*. Retrieved January 24, 2023 from https://bregroup.com/products/breeam/breeam-solutions/breeam-disclosures-and-reporting/

Brenk, B. (1987). Spolia from Constantine to Charlemagne: Aesthetics versus ideology. *Dumbarton Oaks Papers*, *41*, 103–109.

Brown, M. T., & Herendeen, R. A. (1996). Embodied energy analysis and EMERGY analysis: A comparative view. *Ecological Economics*, *19*(3), 219–235. https://doi.org/10.1016/S0921-8009(96)00046-8

Bullard, C. W., Penner, P. S., & Pilati, D. A. (1978). Net energy analysis: Handbook for combining process and input-output analysis. *Resources and Energy*, *1*(3), 267–313. https://doi.org/10.1016/0165-0572(78)90008-7

Costanza, R. (1980). Embodied energy and economic valuation. *Science*, *210*(4475), 1219–1224. https://doi.org/10.1126/science.210.4475.1219

Ellen MacArthur Foundation. (2013). Towards a circular economy. *Journal of Industrial Ecology*, *2*(1), 23–44.

Ellen MacArthur Foundation. (2020). Circular economy introduction: What is a Circular Economy? https://www.ellenmacarthurfoundation.org/topics/circular-economy-introduction/overview

Ellen MacArthur Foundation, SUN, & McKinsey Center for Business and Environment. (2015). *Growth within: a circular economy vision for a competitive Europe*. https://www.ellenmacarthurfoundation.org/assets/downloads/publications/EllenMacArthurFoundation_Growth-Within_July15.pdf

Gallo, M. E. (2022). The bioeconomy: A primer. Congressional Research Service. https://crsreports.congress.gov/product/pdf/R/R46881

Geissdoerfer, M., Savaget, P., Bocken, N. M. P., & Hultink, E. J. (2017). The circular economy – A new sustainability paradigm? *Journal of Cleaner Production*, *143*, 757–768. https://doi.org/10.1016/j.jclepro.2016.12.048

Hobson, K. (2016). Closing the loop or squaring the circle? Locating generative spaces for the circular economy. *Progress in Human Geography*, *40*(1), 88–104. https://doi.org/10.1177/0309132514566342

Hosseinijou, S. A., Mansour, S., & Shirazi, M. A. (2014). Social life cycle assessment for material selection: A case study of building materials. *The International Journal of Life Cycle Assessment*, *19*(3), 620–645. https://doi.org/10.1007/s11367-013-0658-1

ISO. (2006). ISO 14044:2006 Environmental management – Life cycle assessment – Requirements and guidelines (1st ed.). ISO.

Jintao, H. (2009). *Circular Economy Promotion Law*. S. C. O. E. I. S. Platform. https://www.greengrowthknowledge.org/sites/default/files/downloads/policy-database/CHINA%29%20Circular%20Economy%20Promotion%20Law%20%282008%29.pdf

Keena, N., & Dyson, A. (2017). Qualifying the quantitative in the construction of built ecologies. In D. Benjamin (Ed.), *Embodied energy and design: Making architecture between metrics and narratives*. Columbia University GSAPP Lars Müller.

Keena, N., & Dyson, A. (2020). *State of play for circular built environment in North America. A report compiling the regional state of play for circularity in the built environment in North America across the United States of America*. Yale Center for Ecosystems in Architecture, Yale University and United Nations One Planet Network Sustainable Buildings and Construction Programme.

Liu, S., & Qian, S. (2019). Towards sustainability-oriented decision making: Model development and its validation via a comparative case study on building construction methods. *Sustainable Development*, *27*(5), 860–872. https://doi.org/10.1002/sd.1946

MacDonald, M., Enzer, M., Manidaki, M., Radford, J., & Ellis, T. (2013). *Infrastructure carbon review*. HM Treasury.

McKinsey Global Institute. (2017). *Reinventing construction: A route to higher productivity*. https://www.mckinsey.com/business-functions/operations/our-insights/reinventing-construction-through-a-productivity-revolution

Miflin, C. (2019, January 24). Build Less. For More People. Design Circular. *AIA KnowledgeNet*. https://network.aia.org/blogs/clare-j-miflin-aia1/2019/10/15/build-less-for-more-people-design-circular

Miflin, C., Spertus, J., Miller, B., & Grace, C. (2017). *Zero waste design guidelines*. American Institute of Architects.

Moreau, V., Sahakian, M., Van Griethuysen, P., & Vuille, F. (2017). Coming full circle: Why social and institutional dimensions matter for the circular economy. *Journal of Industrial Ecology*, *21*(3), 497–506. https://doi.org/10.1111/jiec.12598

Odum, H. T. (1988). Self-organization, transformity, and information. *Science*, *242*(4882), 1132–1139. https://doi.org/10.1126/science.242.4882.1132

Pearce, D. W. T. R. K. (1990). *Economics of natural resources and the environment*. Johns Hopkins University Press.

Prusac, M. (2012). The arch of Constantine: Continuity and commemoration through reuse. *Acta ad archaeologiam et artium historiam pertinentia*, *25*, 127–157.

Raugei, M., Rugani, B., Benetto, E., & Ingwersen, W. W. (2014). Integrating emergy into LCA: Potential added value and lingering obstacles, *Ecological Modelling*, *271*, 4–9, http://www.sciencedirect.com/science/article/pii/S0304380012005637

Regional Plan Association. (2019). *The fourth regional plan for the New York-New Jersey-Connecticut metropolitan area: Making the region work for all of us*. Regional Plan Association.

Sariatli, F. (2017). Linear economy versus circular economy: A comparative and analyzer study for optimization of economy for sustainability. *Visegrad Journal on Bioeconomy and Sustainable Development*, *6*(1), 31–34. https://doi.org/doi:10.1515/vjbsd-2017-0005

Stahel, W. R. (1982). The product life factor. *An inquiry into the nature of sustainable societies: The role of the private sector (Series: 1982 Mitchell Prize Papers), NARC*, 74-96.

Stahel, W. R., & Clift, R. (2016). *Stocks and flows in the performance economy*. In R. Clift & A. Druckman (Eds.), *Taking stock of industrial ecology* (pp. 101–112). Springer. https://doi.org/10.1007/978-3-319-20571-7_7

Treloar, G. J., Love, P. E. D., & Holt, G. D. (2001). Using national input/output data for embodied energy analysis of individual residential buildings. *Construction Management and Economics*, *19*(1), 49–61. https://doi.org/10.1080/014461901452076

Trigo, E., Chavarria, H., Pray, C., Smyth, S. J., Torroba, A., Wesseler, J., Zilberman, D., & Martinez, J. F. (2021). *The bioeconomy and food systems transformation*. https://sc-fss2021.org/wp-content/uploads/2021/03/FSS_Brief_Bioeconomy_and_Food_Systems_Transformation.pdf

United Nations Environment Programme. (2009). *Guidelines for social life cycle assessment of products*. https://wedocs.unep.org/bitstream/handle/20.500.11822/7912/-Guidelines%20for%20Social%20Life%20Cycle%20Assessment%20of%20Products-20094102.pdf?sequence=3&%3BisAllowed=

United Nations Environment Programme. (2011). *Towards a green economy: Pathways to sustainable development and poverty eradication – A synthesis for policy makers* [Report]. United Nations Environment Programme, Nairobi. https://www.unep.org/resources/report/towards-green-economy-pathways-sustainable-development-and-poverty-eradication-10

Velis, C. A., Wilson, D. C., & Cheeseman, C. R. (2009). *19th century London dust-yards: A case study in closed-loop resource efficiency*. https://doi.org/10.1016/j.wasman.2008.10.018

Zimmerman, R., O'Brien, H., Hargrave, J., & Morrell, M. (2016). *The circular economy in the built environment*. Arup. https://www.arup.com/perspectives/publications/research/section/circular-economy-in-the-built-environment

Chapter 3

Circular Business Models and UN SDGs as Design Drivers in Residential Developments

3.1 Introduction

Circular economy is unique in presenting a practical approach to creating waste-free and resilient economies. It is evident from previous chapters that sustainability principles must be incorporated into the built environment and circular economy is an effective way to do so. This chapter tackles the next step – how to practically implement circularity into the building sector. This chapter is divided into five parts. First, a discussion on six dimensions that must be addressed when implementing a circular economic framework into a built environment. All six must be touched on for circular economy principles to be successfully adopted in all aspects of the built environment, including production, operation, and end-of-life. Second, a review of five business models is described in detail by Lacy and Rutqvist (2015) in their book *Waste to Wealth*. The five business models underscore how implementing circular economy principles is not only beneficial for the environment but also acts as a smart business strategy for many companies and consumers. These business models provide a helpful touchstone for companies to follow when implementing circularity. The third section reiterates the importance of the United Nations (UN) Sustainable Development Goals (SDGs) (UN SDGs) discussed in Chapter 1. Just as the five business models are a helpful reference points for implementing a circular economy, the UN SDGs are an integral reference point that all circularity assessments must consider. This leads to the fourth section, in which several existing sustainable certification systems for design and construction within the building sector are compared. While these certification systems serve different and important functions of assessment, none provide entirely sufficient criteria for building design professionals to follow if they want to implement circularity principles specifically. As a result, the last section provides a new circular economy framework that incorporates the ReSOLVE circular economy framework by the Ellen MacArthur Foundation, the five business models of Lacy and Rutqvist, the 17 UN SDGs, and applicable aspects of existing certification systems. This circular economy framework hopes to help architects better implement circularity into new building design and assess circularity of existing buildings.

DOI: 10.4324/9781003333975-4

3.2 Six Dimensions for Implementing Circular Economy in the Built Environment

As discussed in Chapter 2, there are a number of core conceptual underpinnings supporting the emergence of a circular economic framework. While the concept of circular economy is broad and encompasses many of these ideas, this section explores what dimensions are required to get a circular economic framework successfully implemented, including a focus on the meso-scale, governmental policy influence, behavioral shifts, social collaboration, economic reframing, and technological incorporation.

Circular economy literature tends to focus either on the macro- or the micro-scale, such as the neighborhood or material parts, respectively. The meso-scale, or the scale of an individual building, therefore, is often ignored (Pomponi & Moncaster, 2017). However, as Pomponi and Moncaster (2017) stress, all three scales are crucial in a proper circular economy (see Figure 3.1). Buildings are unique in that they encompass both small-scale manufactured products on the micro-scale but, when assembled, represent a complex long-term product that makes up a large-scale neighborhood or city (Keena et al., 2023).

In order to build "circular buildings", or buildings designed, operated, and maintained following principles of circular economy, multiple disciplines must coordinate with one another (Pomponi & Moncaster, 2017). Indeed, buildings are a result of material production, governmental policy, and an economic framework and have impacts on multiple sectors of society. For instance, policy that makes the market price for steel low disincentives builders to reuse steel (Corbey et al., 2016). Alternatively, Adams (2016) writes that governments providing tax breaks for buildings that use reclaimed materials can aid in applying a circular economy to the built environment.

Just as governmental policy can influence the success of a circular built environment, so do people's general attitudes toward these circular economy principles. People must be on board for actions like recycling and energy and carbon reduction to be adopted. Roy Fishwick notes that this is one of the biggest obstacles for the implementation of a circular economy in the built environment – people are more attracted to new versus old (Corbey et al., 2016). Adams (2016) finds, however, that this is not a hard-and-fast rule. In the case of reclaimed wood, for instance, people will choose reclaimed over new wood for the aesthetic appeal (see Figure 3.2), meaning that people's perception of the aesthetic quality of materials can change. A similar trend

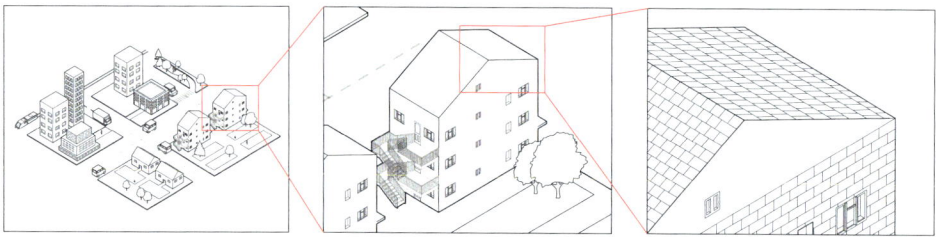

Figure 3.1 The Meso-Scale of a Building.

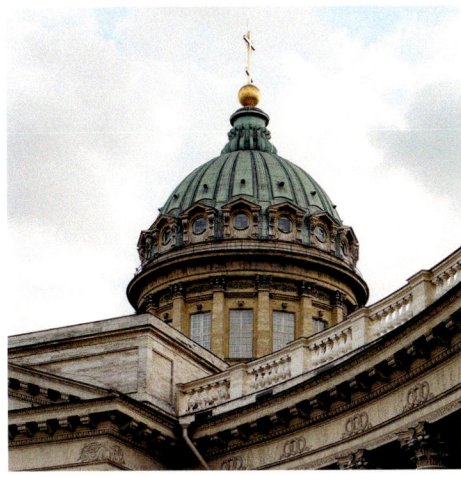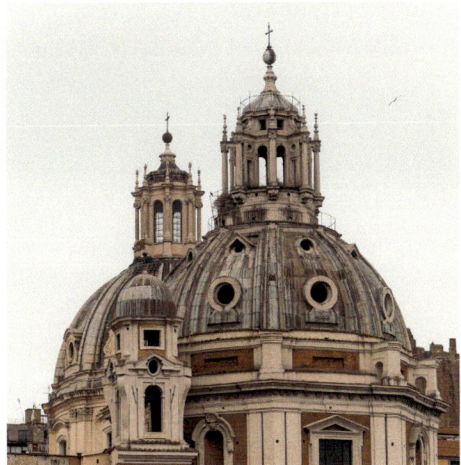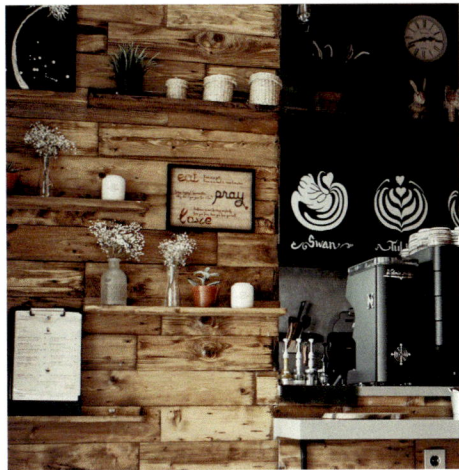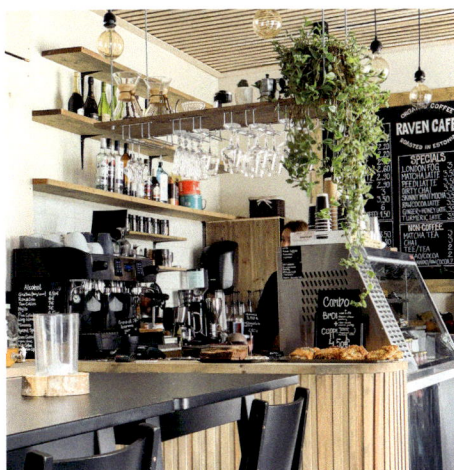

Figure 3.2 Examples of the Popularization of Reused and Aged Materials in Architecture.

is seen with the patina effect of copper that is often sought after but only achievable after the copper is exposed to natural weathering over several years (see Figure 3.2).

Implementing a circular economy also requires a social dimension, collaborating with multiple stakeholders, partnerships, and networks for resource sharing. Circular economy is, as the name suggests, fundamentally an economic model, which requires a change in the ownership models taken for granted in a linear economy. Shifting economic profit from quantity of goods produced, which leads to enormous waste, to longevity and quality performance is key.

Lastly, a technological dimension is a central part of a circular approach, to connect supply and demand and aid in management of data that reduces inefficiency and waste in the circular economy production stream. For instance, Khoo (2015) discusses online platforms for resource sharing, making it easy for collaboration to occur and information to disperse among stakeholders (see Chapter 10).

An examination of the built environment in relation to circular economy underscores the unique issue of scale in relation to framing a circular built environment. The next section expands on these six dimensions of a circular economy, outlining five different business models for circular economy implementation.

3.3 Circular Business Models

Circular economy is a pragmatic approach to sustainable development that comes from an economic perspective, ensuring profit from environmentally beneficial shifts. This attention to the economy makes a circular economy particularly attractive for business owners as well as any stakeholder concerned with profit. As a result, Lacy and Rutqvist (2015) came up with five business models for circular economy, which outline how developers and manufacturers can create value and profit while minimizing negative environmental and social impact. The ReSOLVE framework by the Ellen MacArthur Foundation similarly covers how to transition to a circular economy. In this framework, each tenet is reflected in one of these circular business models: Regenerate (Circular Supply-Chain business model), Loop (Recovery and Recycling business model), Share (using the Sharing Platform business model), Optimize (the Product Life Extension business model), Exchange (Product as a Service [PaaS] business model), and Virtualize (incorporating Technological Innovation into the Building Process). The included case study on the Circular Building, a 2016 prototype dwelling designed by Arup, covers how this framework can practically look in an architectural setting. As Zimmerman et al. (2016) explain, like the actions of the ReSOLVE framework, these five business models can be applied to buildings, neighborhoods, and cities.

3.3.1 Circular Supply-Chain Model

In a linear economic approach, manufacturers are incentivized to extract virgin resources to produce their goods, which are often toxic and nonrecyclable (Lacy & Rutqvist, 2015). In a linear model, this is often the cheapest method of acquiring resources, giving the largest profit margin, despite having enormous environmental costs. With a circular supply chain, by contrast, value is made while reducing the consumption of raw materials, excluding toxic materials from the manufacturing process, using high-quality materials that can be reused and recycled, and using renewable materials that are bio-based and biodegradable (Thelen et al., 2018). In this business model, every aspect of a product is capable of reuse and disassembly, meaning that the circularity of the model is only complete when a product's initial use is complete, and it enters a new cycle (see Figure 3.3). This

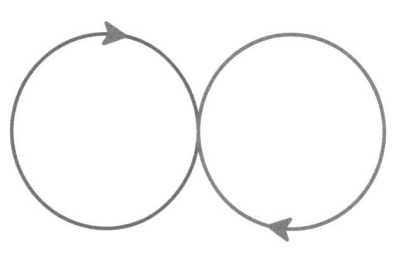

Source: Adapted from Accenture Strategy Circular Advantage

Figure 3.3 Simple Circular Supply-Chain Model.

can be done in two ways: either by getting turned into a new product within a company's manufacturing process, or through reselling the product to another company (GXN & Assets, 2018).

There are two major characteristics of this business model according to the World Business Council for Sustainable Development (WBCSD) (2018). First, in a circular supply-chain model, there is a minimization of material use, meaning that lightweight and compact construction is prioritized. At the beginning of a building process, two questions must be asked – first, can refurbishment of existing buildings be done to avoid new construction? If not, building design from its onset should try to minimize virgin material usage through compact design. Each part of a building should be planned for renewal and disassembly so that refurbishment can be easily and cost-effectively done in the future. In line with building compact space, space must be designed for multiple functions, touching not only on environmental impacts but social impacts as well (WBCSD, 2018). Second, applying life cycle thinking to materials minimizes waste generated during resource extraction (WBCSD, 2018).

Advantages and Obstacles

Minimization of material use and life cycle thinking have been discussed in previous chapters as methods for environmentally sound construction, but how does this model economically benefit a manufacturer or business owner? First, by distancing a reliance on non-renewable, and/or toxic resources, manufacturers will use more long-term and predictable materials in production, which are less likely to get affected by volatile resource depletion (Lacy & Rutqvist, 2015). Second, this approach gives manufacturers a competitive edge – a customer who wants to reduce risk and ensure long-term pricing and supply are more likely to become stable partners since one's materials are not subject to volatile price fluctuations and depletion (Lacy & Rutqvist, 2015).

Global supply chains experienced such volatility during the Covid-19 pandemic where logistical supply chain issues. Moreover, if the price is equal to that of an unsustainable alternative, most consumers will likely choose the more sustainable option (Lacy & Rutqvist, 2015). Ikea is a good example of a company that has economically succeeded through a circular supply chain. Peter Agnefjall, the CEO of Ikea, established at the UN Climate Summit in 2014 that the company will only use renewable and recycled plastics in its home furnishing products by 2020. This has secured the company of having a consistent supply of plastic as well as saving about 700,000 metric tons of carbon dioxide emissions per year (IKEA, 2014). The energy, chemical, mining and metals sectors have all seen adoption of this model as well.

Nonetheless, there are logistical challenges to implementing such a model. Lengthy and costly research and development processes are required before implementation, companies and consumers must be willing to work in collaboration with one another, substantial initial capital investment is required, and suppliers must understand the specific environmental conditions across the product life cycle to choose products that can show their full environmental potential.

Relevance to the Built Environment

Regenerating and restoring natural capital are the closest ReSOLVE actions to the circular supply-chain business model. This model leads to building performance that is both efficient and circular, since negative externalities are reduced and primary resource consumption and waste are diminished (Zimmerman et al., 2016). Negative externalities are indirect social costs, such as pollution or environmental degradation. By reducing such externalities, the built environment is able to foster more resilience, tapping into environmental and social sustainability as discussed in Chapter 1. For instance, applying net zero strategies to cities leads to low-impact building design that helps reduce environmental, social, and economic consequences to the built environment by lowering emission rates and waste costs (Zimmerman et al., 2016). For companies, avoiding waste-to-landfill streams, improving air quality, and employing material efficiency not only make the built environment more sustainable but also improve the reputation of companies and industries, underscoring how this first business model can apply to the built environment successfully (see Figure 3.4) (Zimmerman et al., 2016).

3.3.2 Recovery and Recycling

When waste management systems first emerged, the focus was on removing waste from cities to improve population health. This focus eventually shifted to creating landfills for waste. Now, landfills are unable to handle the amount of waste disposed of. This next business model, Recovery and Recycling, comes from a similar lens of trying to remove waste, but rather than dumping it in another location, this model seeks to eliminate the concept of waste all together. Unlike recycling, in which waste is seen as an entity to be dealt with through waste management, in this model, businesses view "waste" as a valuable commodity, trying to recapture the sources they would have lost in a linear process by making new raw materials or products and reselling. What in a linear model would be considered waste and subsequently discarded, in the Recovery and Recycling model, would be upcycled to create additional revenue streams for the producer, thus benefiting the environment

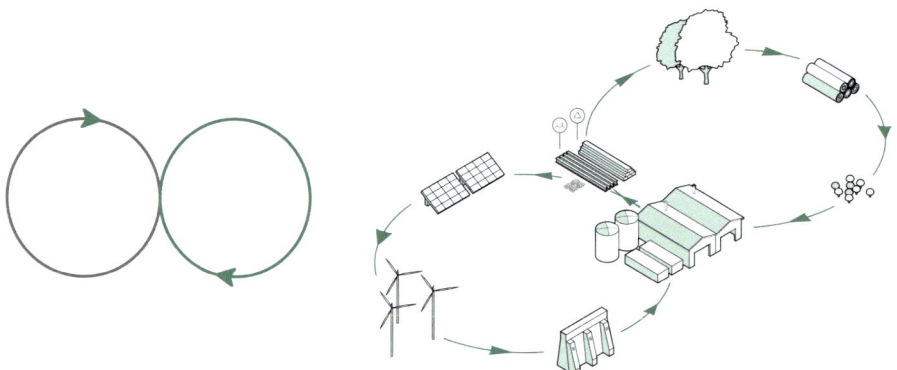

Figure 3.4 How the Circular Supply-Chain Model Applies to the Built Environment.

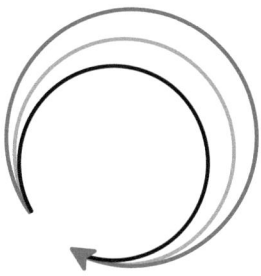

while making a larger profit for manufacturers (see Figure 3.5). Recycling and recovery do not only have to occur within a single company. Rather, industrial symbiosis can be an effective way for multiple companies to benefit financially from recycling and recovery – companies can share by-product resources, integrating closed-loop recycling and cradle-to-cradle design so that products disposed of in one industry can be taken up and reprocessed in another (Lacy & Rutqvist, 2015).

Source: Adapted from Accenture Strategy Circular Advantage

Figure 3.5 Recovery and Recycling Model.

Advantages and Obstacles

There is a range of benefits to adopting such a model, including reducing the cost of waste management, gaining revenue from selling one's disposed-of products to other industries, gaining deeper knowledge on how products are disposed of (which allows product developers to design for recyclability), dealing with a lower material bill between primary and secondary resources, and, of course, reducing harmful environmental impacts from waste (Lacy & Rutqvist, 2015).

However, companies need to figure out how to maintain ownership of high-quality materials and return flows to benefit from the product's post-life value. Also, when companies have recovered resources, infrastructure must be in place to maximize the quality of such resources through sorting, reprocessing, and refining technology (Lacy & Rutqvist, 2015).

Relevance to the Built Environment

Keeping materials in loop makes a significant impact on the built environment. Within construction, repurposing materials for circularity reduces the need to build with virgin resources (see Figure 3.6). Remanufacturing reduces waste by keeping

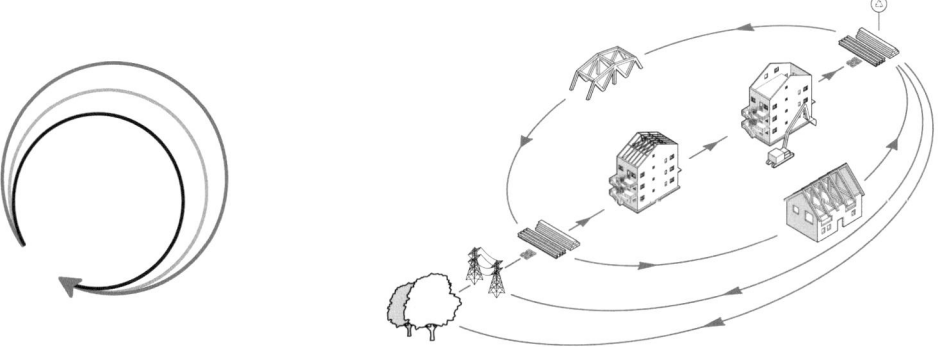

Figure 3.6 How the Recovery and Recycling Model Applies to the Built Environment.

buildings and materials in use for longer. Caterpillar is a company that remanufactures building parts to reduce, reuse, recycle, and reclaim materials, returning materials to same-as-new conditions for a small cost in comparison to producing new. By employing the Recycling & Reuse business model, Caterpillar saves a significant cost for its own operations, namely through labor costs, and its customers save as well. Through this technique, the company has saved over 500,000 metric tons (550,000,000 kg) of materials (Zimmerman et al., 2016). Moreover, buildings should be designed to be easily disassembled for reuse and recycling. Creating material passports to understand and standardize components can similarly help maximize the number of recycled materials from a building. Maersk, for instance, uses a cradle-to-cradle passport to identify recycled steel from the shipping industry. The saved embodied environmental impact of using recycled and reused steel is 2–10 percent for a whole building, according to Zimmerman et al. (2016). This also saves the builder up to 16 percent per metric ton of recycled steel compared to conventional building material (Zimmerman et al., 2016).

3.3.3 Product Life Extension

Within a linear approach, increasing flow of products, or throughput, is prioritized as an efficient way to accumulate capital; however, this approach exacerbates material waste and degrades the environment. The Product Life Extension model extends the useful life of a product, relying on revenue through longevity of a product's service rather than product accumulation (see Figure 3.7). Durability, functionality, and quality are valued as the source of revenue for the company. There are three ways that companies can embody this model. First, and most self-evident, the manufacturer can build products of high quality with a long lifespan. In this method, manufacturers must design with upgrades, add-ons, and long-life cycle planning in mind (Lacy & Rutqvist, 2015). Second, a company can act as a channel player, which means that a company can work to find consumers to buy underused products to extend its useful life (Lacy & Rutqvist, 2015). Third, a field service company can repair and upgrade products to maintain their useful life.

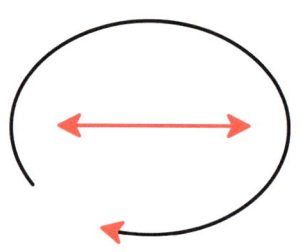

Source: Adapted from Accenture Strategy Circular Advantage

Figure 3.7 Product Life Extension Model.

Advantages and Obstacles

While an obvious barrier to adopting such a model could be the potential for higher upfront costs, this is not necessarily required. Some digital "freemium" models allow products to be sold for free while upgrades and add-ons generate the bulk of revenue, just as Amazon does with Kindle (Lacy & Rutqvist, 2015). One central challenge, however, is for companies to choose which products should have their life extended. For instance, when products are influenced by changing consumer tastes, implementing this business model may not be profitable for companies. High-value equipment found in construction sectors is likely to benefit from this model, however, as it can be used between businesses.

Relevance to the Built Environment

"Optimize" is the third action of the ReSOLVE framework and parallels the goals of the Product Life Extension business model. In the built environment, maintaining high-quality materials throughout the design and construction process, while maximizing efficiency, eliminating waste, and promoting reuse, can extend the life of a building to the environment and economy's benefit (see Figure 3.8) (Zimmerman et al., 2016). Establishing durable materials and construction standards can ensure a building's longevity and reduce maintenance costs. Standardization of quality controls can also minimize structural errors and building degradation. Designing for flexibility is another key method for the built environment to implement the Product Life Extension model. For instance, if an area's zoning laws change from commercial to residential, instead of tearing commercial buildings to build residential, buildings should be able to easily convert, thus saving costs of demolition and construction, and reducing enormous waste and building-related carbon emissions. For example, Derwent London's White Collar Factory on Old Street, London, features commercial, residential, and public space. Allford Hall Monaghan Morris, the architecture firm in charge of this project, designed exposed services and flexible floor plates for subdivision, flexibility, and interactivity as time goes on (Allford Hall Monaghan Morris Architects, 2016).

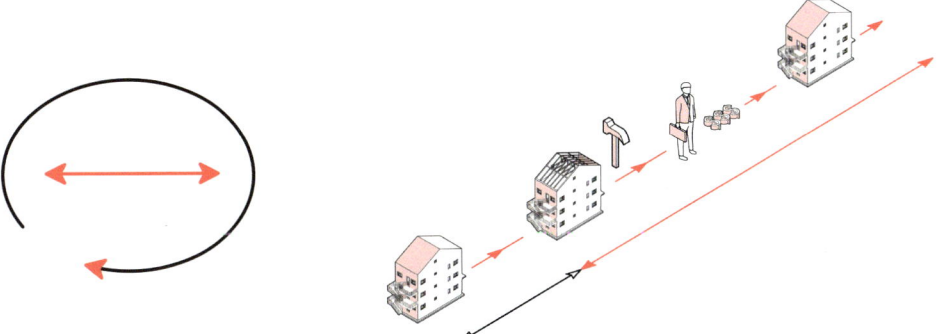

Figure 3.8 How the Product Life Extension Model Applies to the Built Environment.

3.3.4 *Sharing Platform*

The Sharing Platform business model connects owners of products to organizations and individuals that would like to use them (see Figure 3.9) (Lacy & Rutqvist, 2015). A co-ownership platform allows a product to continually be in use, which reduces the demand for more production. This business model has parallels to circular economy and sharing economy. A product's life is extended as it serves multiple uses and customers at the same time. In a sharing economy, resource utilization and long-life cycles are prioritized, tapping into core tenets of circular economy.

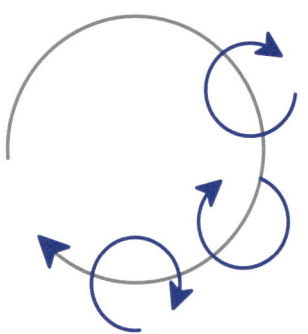

Source: Adapted from Accenture Strategy Circular Advantage

Figure 3.9 Sharing Platform Model.

Advantages and Obstacles

There are three main reasons to adopt a Sharing Platform model (Lacy & Rutqvist, 2015). First, this model is more convenient for the consumer, who has a more varied range of resources available to them (Lacy & Rutqvist, 2015). Second, without full ownership of a product, customers can benefit from lower prices, allowing individuals to take advantage of multiple platforms and services to suit their needs without the burden or commitment of full ownership. Third, sharing platforms are often found online, meaning that better service quality is vital for a successful business (Lacy & Rutqvist, 2015).

While a sharing platform should be based on a motivation for community-building capitalism, sharing economy companies are mainly motivated by profit seeking, which is one challenge faced by this platform. Furthermore, as found in services like Uber, a lack of protection to citizens engaging in sharing platforms has the potential to create poor working conditions with insecure incomes and benefits (Lacy & Rutqvist, 2015). Lastly, sharing platforms often avoid taxes and regulations which threaten companies operating in the formal economy.

Relevance to the Built Environment

In a built environment setting, sharing space, or designing for multifunctional space, is an effective example of the sharing platform. By allowing multiple people to use a space or building for different functions, the building is constantly in use and thus the need to build more, which leads to a strain on the environment, is reduced (see Chapter 2) (Zimmerman et al., 2016). In the built environment, asset owners can rent or share space that is underused. An example of this that has become popular in dense cities is shared working space, in which people of different careers share one building and conduct their respective business, thus minimizing the amount of time the space is unused. When Lloyds Banking Group implemented flexible working

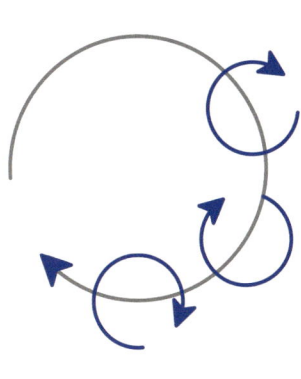

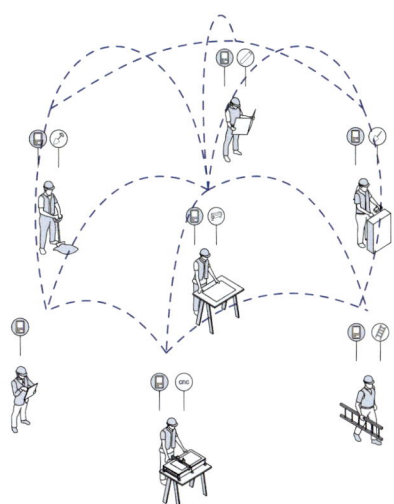

Figure 3.10 How the Sharing Platform Model Applies to the Built Environment.

space for 20 percent of its office, it saved 10 million UK Pounds (about 12.25 million USD) because less desks and office space were required (Zimmerman et al., 2016). Furthermore, The Collective and Common both provide co-living spaces, where multiple people live in a space with communal areas like kitchens and dining rooms, which can convert to other functions. This can become an effective strategy for saving space, reducing cost of living, and reducing the environmental damage that building new dwellings entails. Moreover, sharing built environment materials helps foster collaboration between owners, operators, technology companies, and other industries (see Figure 3.10) (Bhatia & Steinmuller, 2018). Globechain matches businesses that have unwanted stock and equipment to other businesses or individuals that are looking for said materials (globechain.com, n.d.). Not only does a platform like this share supplies and materials, foster reuse, and elongate the life of a material, but Telefonica, who used Globechain to donate unused office furniture, saves a substantial amount in landfill costs (3,675 USD).

3.3.5 *Product as a Service*

Similar to the sharing model, the Product as a Service (PaaS) model offers services to multiple people (see Figure 3.11). The difference is that while in a sharing platform there can be models of shared ownership between companies and customers, in a PaaS model, the companies retain ownership but offer it out to customers (Lacy & Rutqvist, 2015). As well, in a sharing model, a product itself is being used by multiple consumers, while in a PaaS model, it is the service that is the object of value, not the product.

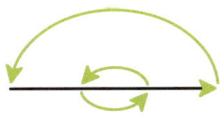

Figure 3.11 Product as a Service Model.

69

Advantages and Obstacles

For the customer, this is an advantageous model since the ownership remains on the provider, meaning that they continue to bear responsibility for the quality of the product throughout its lifespan (Lacy & Rutqvist, 2015). In terms of housing, this would avoid poor housing construction that degrades fast, where the burden goes on the homeowner, or the landlord who may neglect quality checks for their tenants. An alignment of interests between the consumer and producer is a central component of this model – the better and longer a product performs, the more a consumer will use it, thus driving revenue for the producer.

The main obstacle for this approach is the need for producers to always keep current information on the quality and performance of their products, which is timely and difficult. As well, companies need to maintain a relationship with customers to listen to feedback and concerns. This all requires regulatory infrastructure to be built, which takes time and technological innovation.

Relevance to the Built Environment

In the built environment, a PaaS model would look like replacing existing energy sources with buildings that generate energy and heat through closed-loop anaer-

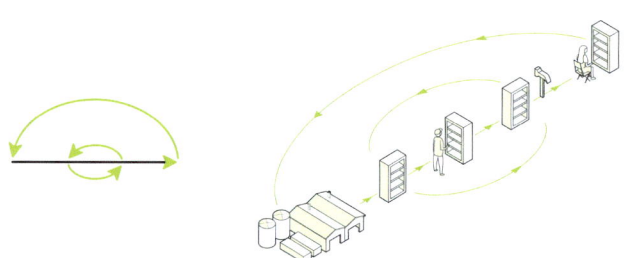

obic digestion systems (see Figure 3.12) (Zimmerman et al., 2016). In this way, the building's service of providing energy is the focal point of the construction. Furthermore, incorporating advanced technology into the built environment can extend the life cycle of a building, help with repairs, and allow for flexible upgrades and easy disassembly (McKinsey Global

Figure 3.12 How the Product as a Service Model Applies to the Built Environment.

Institute, 2017; Zimmerman et al., 2016). This is connected to the exchange pillar of the ReSOLVE framework, which emphasizes replacing and upgrading old systems for new, more sustainable options.

3.4 UN Sustainable Development Goals and Their Relationship to Circular Economy

While a successful circular built environment must be financially profitable for businesses and consumers, a circular built environment must also fulfill key sustainability pillars outlined by the UN SDGs (see Figure 3.13). Created in 2015 and composed of

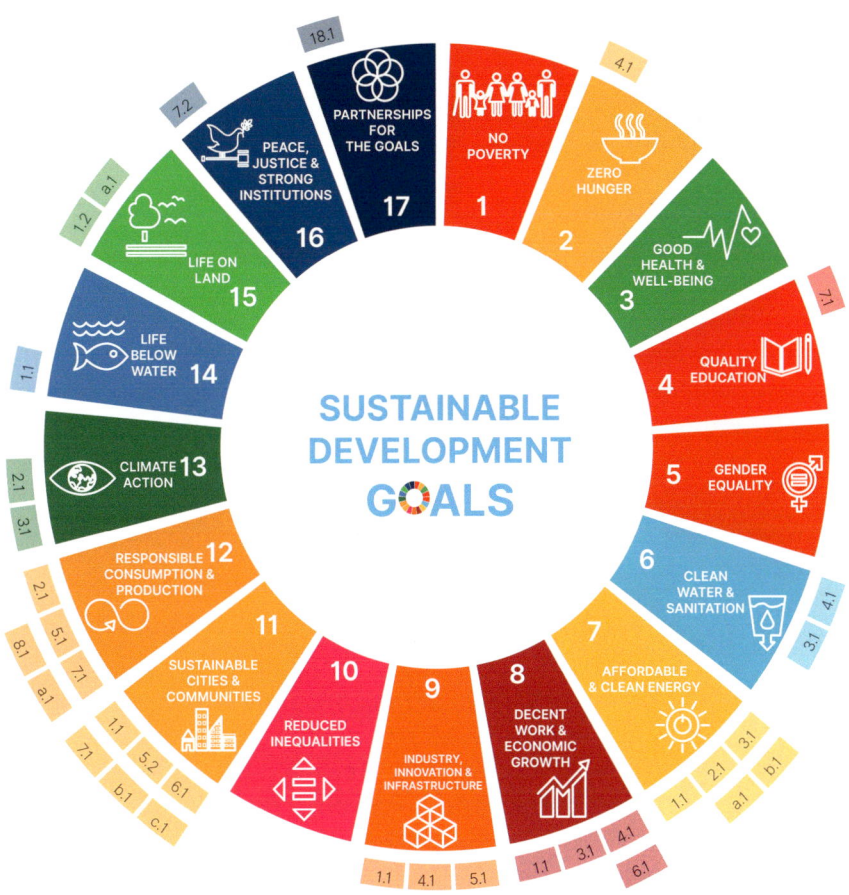

Figure 3.13 Circular UN Sustainable Development Goals. Source: Created by Iyer-Raniga and Huovila (2020).

17 goals, this report aims at global change in environmental, economic, and social sustainability, with a timeline of 15 years (UN General Assembly, 2015). Like the three main pillars of sustainability (environment, economy, and equity) (Wheeler, 2004), circular economy touches on these pillars in its quest for a sustainable built environment (see Chapter 1).

Goal 11: *Sustainable Cities and Communities* is especially relevant, aiming to "make cities and human settlements inclusive, safe, resilient and sustainable" (UN General Assembly, 2015). Within this report, safe and affordable housing is outlined as a central goal and reducing per capita environmental impact of cities, as well as fostering healthy economic, social, and environmental connections between urban, peri-urban, and rural areas (UN General Assembly, 2015). Goal 3 wants to establish good health and well-being globally, Goal 7 aims to foster affordable and clean energy, Goals 8 and 9 focus on economic growth and industrial innovation, respectively, and Goal 13 targets climate action – all goals that are in line with circularity principles. The Ecological Living Module (ELM), for example, is a demonstration housing project that seeks to address the UN SDGs in its architecture through a circular systems-based approach (Dyson et al., 2020). As is detailed in the following case study, the ELM is a rich example of the natural overlap between the UN SDGs and circular economy.

Iyer-Raniga and Huovila (2020) measure the SDGs and indicators in relation to the underpinnings of a circular built environment sector. They found that 12 of the 17 SDGs have particular relevance to circularity (1, 3, 4, 6, 7, 8, 9, 11, 12, 13, 15, 17). Iyer-Raniga and Huovila (2020) also examined how regions compared in terms of their respective emphases on certain SDG goals. In general, in the Global North, much of the urban fabric has already been built, so in terms of circular economy, refurbishment and the reuse of materials is emphasized. In the Global South, however, the focus is more on new construction and ways to design out waste in the development phase. With a growth in urbanization and population density expected in the coming years, it is especially pertinent that cities going forward shape their built environment in line with the UN SDG 2030 targets.

3.5 An Overview of Sustainable Certification Programs

Along these lines, a number of institutions and organizations have created standards, goals, and certification programs to help architects assess and design for sustainability. Leadership in Energy and Environmental Design (LEED), WELL Building Standard, the Living Building Challenge (LBC), Building Research Establishment Environmental Assessment Method (BREEAM) (BRE Group, n.d.), EDGE certification (IFC, n.d.), and the American Institute of Architects Design Goals are all examples of these standards (AIA, 2020). These programs have grown in popularity since the 1990s as a way to support a sustainable built environment but differ in their weight given to different realms of sustainability and the scope of sustainability (e.g., whole life cycle or only the operational phase) (Nguyen & Altan, 2011). A comparative analysis of the different certification programs reveals the gaps in the current sustainability assessment frameworks and how a new set of guidelines can build off of and improve these conventions.

BREEAM and LEED certification programs are known worldwide for sustainable building assessments. The respective building certifications have gained traction in different parts of the world. BREEAM is European-based and most used in the UK/ Continental European context, LEED is more common in North America, and EDGE is popular in the Global South.

LEED's conceptual underpinnings are management, policy, and economics, outlining how the construction sector can combat environmental degradation and, in turn, the architectural design process (Keena, 2017; USGBC, 2009). For LEED and BREEAM, construction is the focal point, not design, and eco-efficiency is prioritized over eco-effectiveness. In other words, while a system like LBC aims to add a positive impact on the earth's ecosystem, other certification systems aim to "do no harm" to the ecosystems. For instance, LEED's Platinum certification, and EDGE's highest certification, both represent when a building achieves net zero energy, meaning that it produces enough energy through renewable sources without relying on an external utility source (Keena, 2017). The Living Building Challenge, by contrast, assumes net zero energy as the minimum and builds from there to achieve regenerative design, or a design that benefits ecology (International Living Future Institute, 2019, n.d.; Keena, 2017; Thomas, 2016). Moreover, while LEED and BREEAM list criteria and benchmarks for architects to check off, the Living Building Challenge and WELL use holistic language to describe a philosophical goal to shift architects' minds on the purpose and function of design (International Well Building Institute, 2016; Keena, 2017). Interestingly, each certification system, or standard, prides itself on providing a holistic approach to sustainable building assessment; however, the scope differs between the different assessments. WELL, AIA, EDGE, and BREEAM fail to consider the environmental impacts of demolition, giving sustainable certification without consideration of a sustainable demolition plan. LEED and EDGE do not review refurbishment projects, which discourages building owners from improving existing buildings over building new.

Furthermore, while a standard lexicon for sustainability principles is easy to follow, the generality can be ultimately ineffective. For instance, LEED uses a points system to determine what ranking a building gets. Incorporating certain design principles into a building can accumulate more points. However, this certification system is not entirely climate specific, so the impact a design choice will make is not accurately measured within its respective context (Swanson, 2018). As well, a points system allows builders to accumulate many points from so-called low-hanging fruit measures, such as putting up educational displays in their building, without making significant changes like incorporating renewable resources into construction (Schnaars & Morgan, 2012).

These different sustainability certification systems emphasize different definitions of sustainability. LEED and BREEAM speak mainly of environmental sustainability, WELL and Living Building Challenge have a strong focus on human health and well-being, and EDGE centers around economic sustainability. While these certification systems are useful, none display a fully comprehensive set of criteria for a circular building to follow.

3.6 A New Circular Economy Framework Targeted at Housing Design and Construction

Throughout this chapter, several sustainability certification systems were outlined, as well as core business models for successfully incorporating circularity into the production process. The ReSOLVE framework was outlined with the tenets of *Regenerate*, *Optimize*, *Loop*, *Virtualize*, and *Exchange*. Each business model appears to reflect these core tenets, respectively, with the Circular Supply-Chain model, the Sharing Platform, the Product Life Extension, Recovery and Recycling, and PaaS business model. The aims of these business models and the Ellen MacArthur ReSOLVE framework reflect many of the goals and indicators of the 17 UN SDGs, which similarly discuss the role of data and technology, collaboration, climate action, economic growth, and health and well-being. From the previous discussion on existing sustainable building certification systems, gaps exist in the current frameworks. LEED and BREEAM come from a mainly environmental lens, applying generic sustainability criteria on a points system for buildings to achieve certification. Other models, like WELL and the Living Building Challenge, come from a health and well-being perspective, concerned for the practical impacts that buildings have on the residents who occupy them, and the ecology they are situated in. EDGE takes a more economic focus, assessing efficiency and strategic ways for buildings to score green funding opportunities. Upon reflection of the ReSOLVE framework, the Five New Business Models for Circular Growth, and the UN SDGs, and building off existing building certification systems, we have proposed a comprehensive circular economy framework to assess the circularity of building design and construction projects and move away from the linear building process depicted in Figure 3.14.

1. ***Circular Supply Chain*** – Adopting similar ideas from the Circular Supply-Chain business model, this criterion stresses the importance of the material phase and extracting material responsibly and sustainably (see Figure 3.15).

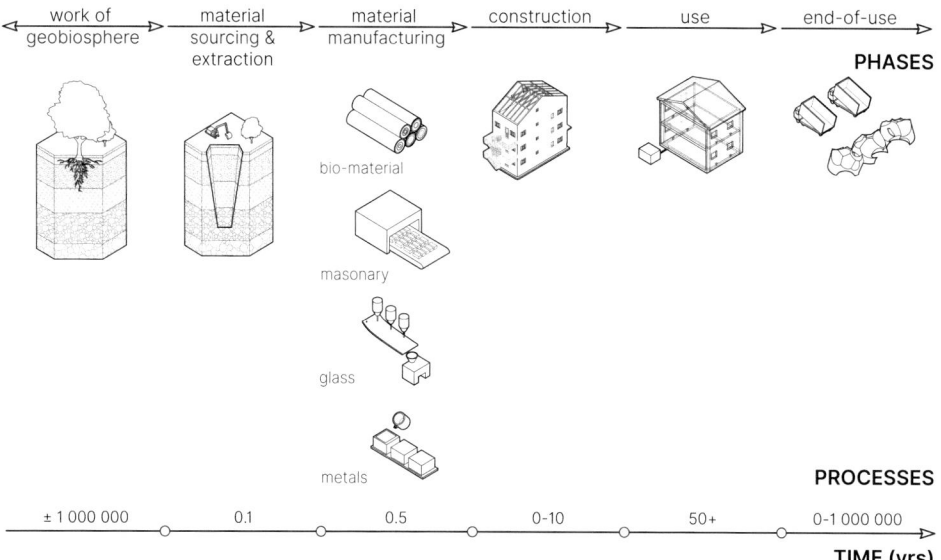

Figure 3.14 **The Linear Building Process.**

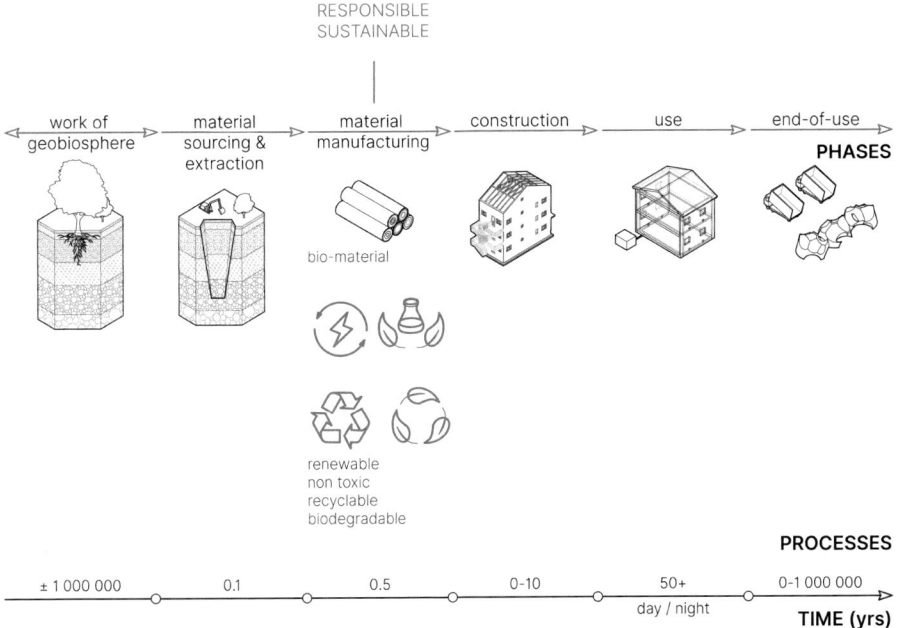

Figure 3.15 How the Circular Supply-Chain Influences the Building Process.

2. **_Recovery and Recycling_** – This criterion encourages products and materials to remain in useful cycles for as long as possible, prioritizing inner loops – remanufacturing, refurbishing products and components, and recycling materials. Building projects can incorporate this in the end-of-use, construction, and renovation phases (see Figure 3.16).

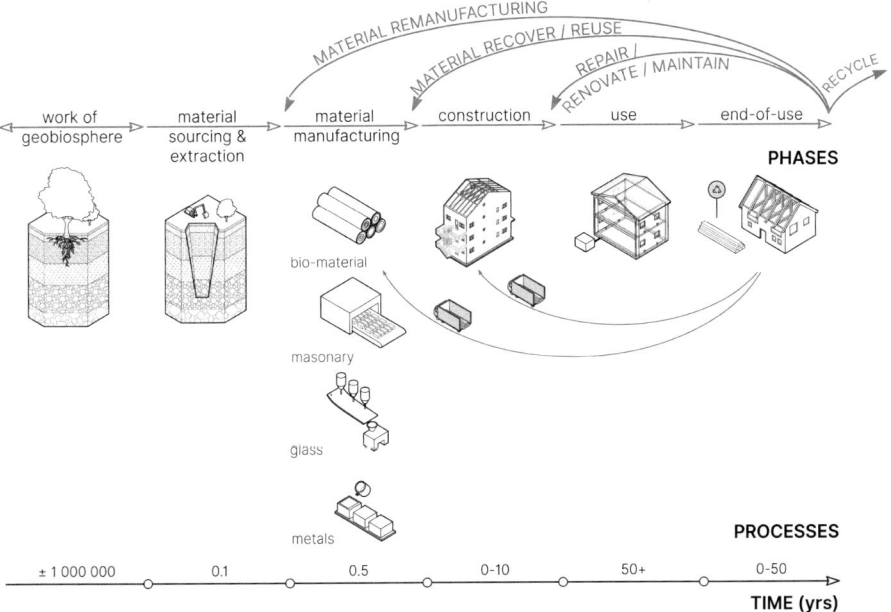

Figure 3.16 How Recovery and Recycling Influences the Building Process.

75

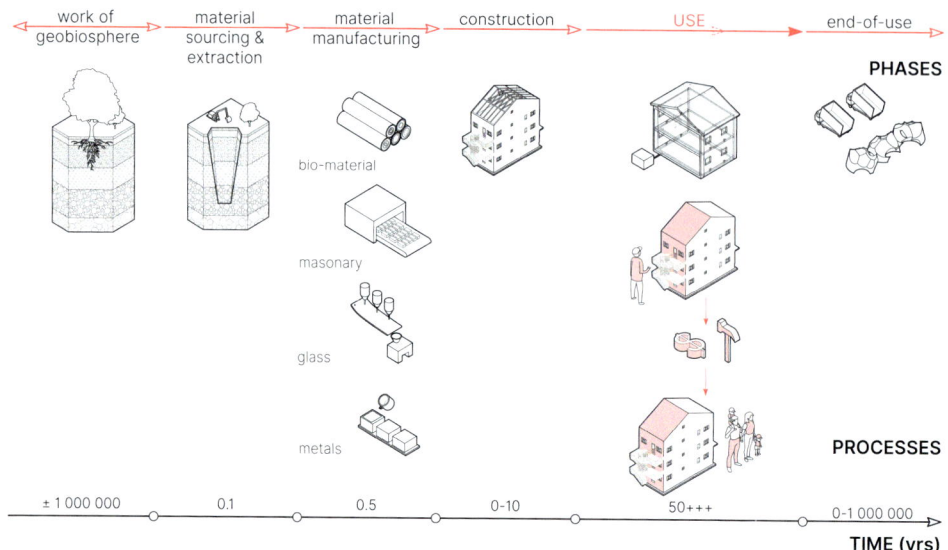

Figure 3.17 How Product Life Extension Influences the Building Process.

3. ***Product Life Extension*** – Similar to the previous principle and the corresponding business model, this tenet focuses on the design phase and end-of-use phase, prioritizing adaptability, and design-for-disassembly in order to extend the lifespan of a building (see Figure 3.17).

4. ***Sharing Platform*** – In an architectural setting, the sharing platform principle focuses on sharing of space for a more efficient and socially sustainable built environment. This principle applies for the operational use phase of a building, treating space as a resource to conserve. For instance, converting a cafe to a restaurant at night, office during the day facilitated via technology, and co-living spaces. The construction phase can help design off-site construction (fabrication) facilities and equipment that can be shared to elevate costs among smaller contractor companies (see Figure 3.18).

5. ***Service Model*** – In the built environment context, the service model requires selecting resources and technology wisely. For instance, using renewable energies, using alternative material inputs (e.g., biomaterials), using advanced technology (e.g., digitalization), and service-centric delivery models as opposed to product-centric ones. This model applies to the material and use phases. For instance, material rental, space rental, and shared space are all ways for the service model to be applied to an architectural setting (see Figure 3.19).

6. ***Regenerate*** – The regenerate model focuses on restoring natural capital such as returning valuable biological nutrients safely to the biosphere and reducing environmental overloading. An understanding of a socio-ecological approach to the built environment is necessary to justify this tenet. As described by Keena (2017), the built environment process (BEP) houses the Technosphere, or the sphere of health management systems, socio-cultural systems, and economic systems. The Technosphere

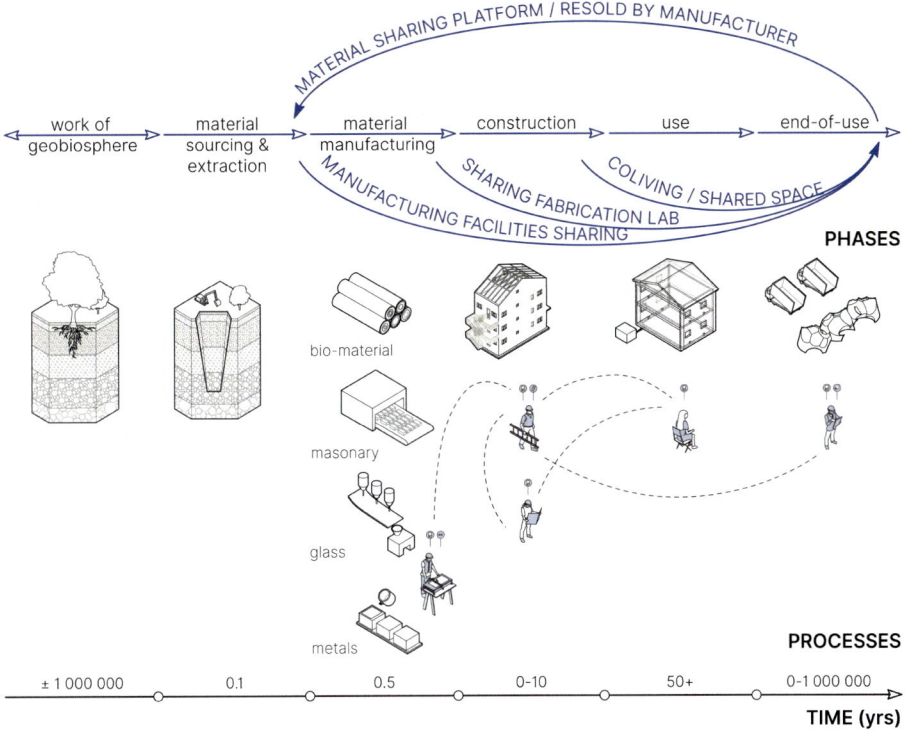

Figure 3.18 How Sharing Platform Influences the Building Process.

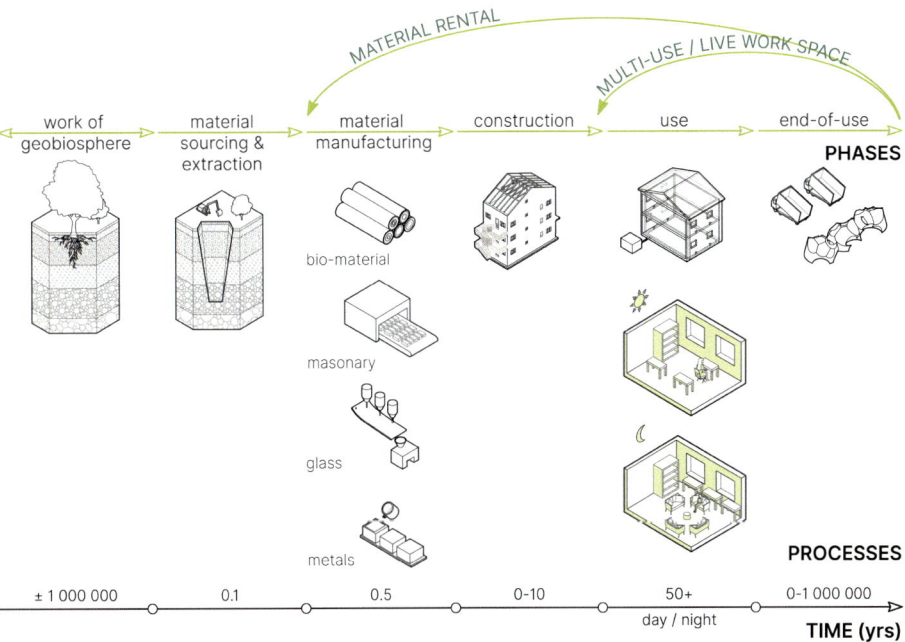

Figure 3.19 How Service Model Influences the Building Process.

77

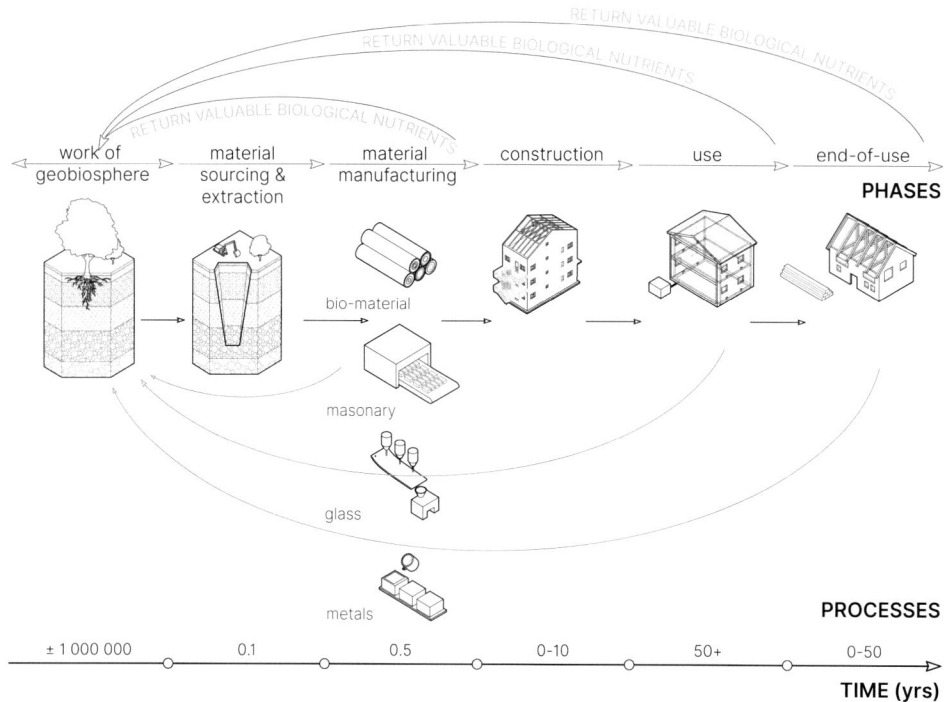

Figure 3.20 How Regenerate Influences the Building Process.

and BEP use aspects of the geo-biosphere, such as clean air, water, and raw materials, constantly, throughout the lifespan of a building. This risks environmental overloading that, in turn, leads to adverse effects to the Technosphere (e.g., poor health due to pollution). This tenet applies in the manufacturing phase by avoiding harmful extraction methods, applies to the operational phase by avoiding environmental overloading through energy consumption, and applies to the design phase by considering biomaterials which can sequester carbon and consider how they can be safely returned to the biosphere. Circular thinking is required for this model by factoring in the end-of-use phase in the design phase. Ultimately, understanding the consequences of climate change globally involves studying the interconnections between the natural, built, and social systems people rely on and their vulnerability to cascading impacts. The regenerate model aims to highlight this broader mindset during the design process (see Figure 3.20).

7. ***Virtualize*** – Virtualization and the incorporation of data and technological innovation is useful in the manufacturing, design, and construction phases. Virtualizing the construction phase can help avoid waste at the outset via using technology in fabrication of buildings which occurs off-site in a controlled facility. It can also be useful at the end-of-use phase to monitor the number of materials and/or components being sent for reuse or recycling thereby providing advanced notice to recycling and reuse companies and suppliers, which allows them to plan for incoming stock accordingly (see Figure 3.21).

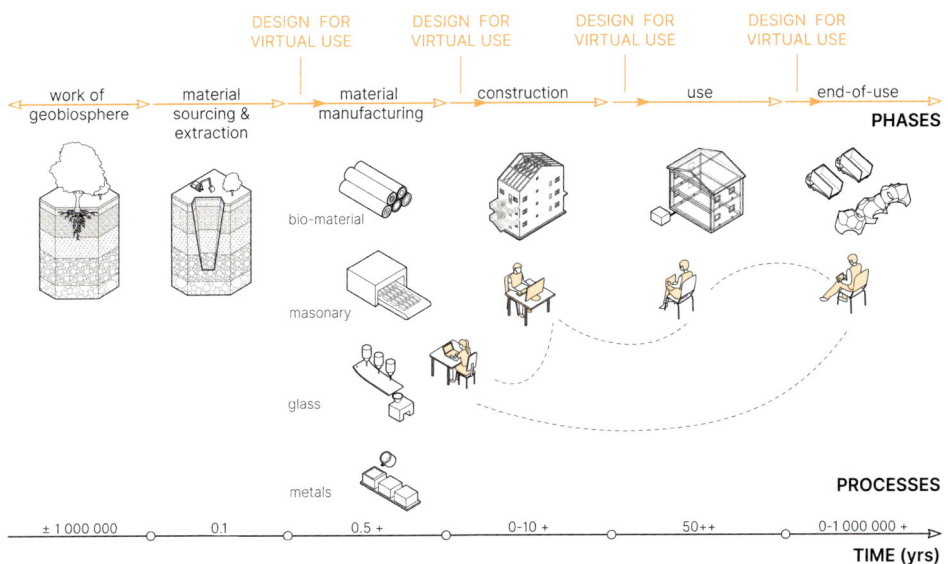

Figure 3.21 How Virtualize Influences the Building Process.

3.6.1 How the Circular Economy for Housing Design Framework Relates to the Built Environment

Understanding how this circular economy for Housing Design framework can apply to the built environment can help visualize how changes in both the architectural design phases, and throughout the building's entire life cycle, can continuously reinforce circularity (Keena et al., 2023). The principles outlined in our circular economy framework are not mutually exclusive but should work together at different stages of a product's life cycle to create a well-rounded circular building (Carra & Magdani, 2017). As Carol Lemmens explains, the built environment is a complex system that requires a rethinking of every aspect of its production system to successfully integrate circularity (Carra & Magdani, 2017). Take a co-living environment, which prioritizes the sharing of spaces and amenities to reduce cost for tenants. In Germany, the Baugruppen, or "building groups", are shared living quarters that feature the sharing platform (Bhatia & Steinmuller, 2018). Space is designed for shared amenities and social interaction – by having multiple people share a space, the amount of time the space is not in use decreases. The Product Life Extension model is also employed, as many units in the Baugruppen are "blank", meaning that the units have the flexibility to be built out to accommodate for each individual owner's preferences and needs throughout their lifetime (Bhatia & Steinmuller, 2018). This extends the usefulness and relevance of a unit. The Circular Supply-Chain model also applies to a co-living environment, as more people living in dwellings lead to more compact construction and less construction in general, reducing material usage and waste. It also includes the Recovery and Recycling model as the design

79

of new shared spaces can incorporate the use of secondary materials where possible to avoid primary material extraction and manufacturing. Share House, a co-living space in Asia for youth aged 5–15, exemplifies how this housing model employs the PaaS model as well. In this space, the dwelling is designed for the service of temporary residents who are likely students and need a space that accommodates their studying schedule and low income (Bhatia & Steinmuller, 2018). The rental or leasing form of the service model would be used. Moreover, Virtualize is gaining prominence in this model as well, with sites such as coliving.com, that help people find co-living space to move into. Functionally, it is evident that multiple pillars of the circular economy framework can be employed simultaneously to ensure circularity in a building's lifespan.

If this co-living space's building life cycle is thus paired with a circular architectural process, such as planning for disassembly in the pre-design phase, choosing materials that are renewable and recyclable, and incorporating data and technology to improve construction efficiency, pillars of our circular economy framework will also be employed in the pre-operational phase to ensure circularity in the construction itself. Planning to design out harmful extraction methods and incorporate biomaterials, which can be returned to the biosphere after use, is aspects that the architectural design phase can include in the design of the actual building to ensure circularity.

What this example stresses is that circularity is not only done through the materials used in the building itself – although this is an impactful aspect – but through the role the building plays, its function, and its capability to adapt and change over time. When a professional considers these seven tenets in architectural design, choices such as building material and construction assembly design aspects must be considered, as well as the function of the building, its relationship to its occupants, its relationship with the larger built environment, and how its function changes over time.

The consideration of multiple functions and aspects of the building, which this co-living case study provides, enables the achievement of the UN SDGs. Environmentally, co-living is beneficial in that it increases densification and shared amenities, which decreases superfluous construction and energy consumption. Circular architectural design choices will ensure that the construction of the building is also environmentally sound. Economically, co-living is one solution to housing affordability issues. Not only is rent cheaper as amenities are shared, but co-living rents are often all-inclusive in terms of utilities and Wi-Fi (CBRE+Streetsense, 2020). Socially, the sharing platform and service model featured in this co-living example allow for dynamic social formations (Bhatia & Steinmuller, 2018). These circular economy framework pillars, when incorporated in a built environment context, should be incorporated at multiple different phases of a building's life cycle to service different aspects of sustainability.

3A

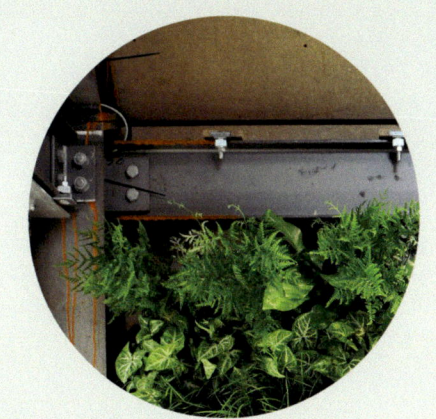

Project:
The Circular Building

Location:
London, United Kingdom

Year:
2016

Team:
Arup, Frener & Reifer facades,
BAM Construction, and the Built
Environment Trust

**Mapping to Circular
Economy Framework:**

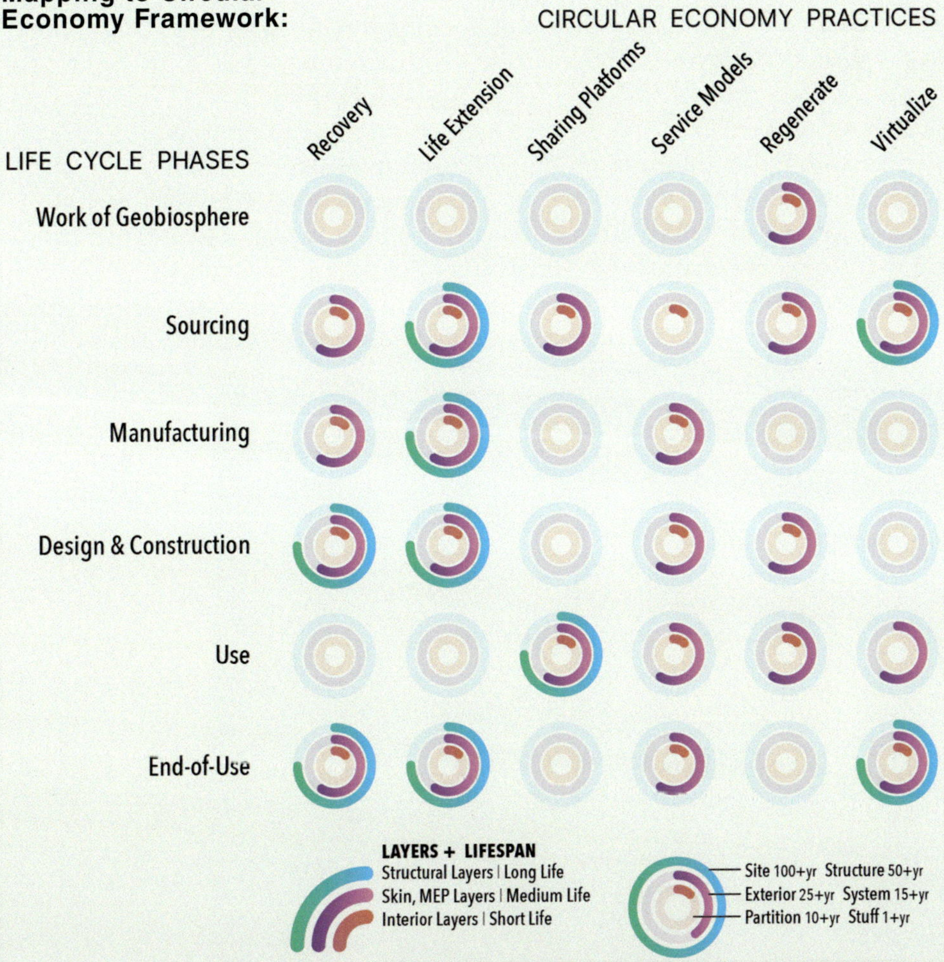

CIRCULAR ECONOMY PRACTICES

LIFE CYCLE PHASES	Recovery	Life Extension	Sharing Platforms	Service Models	Regenerate	Virtualize
Work of Geobiosphere						
Sourcing						
Manufacturing						
Design & Construction						
Use						
End-of-Use						

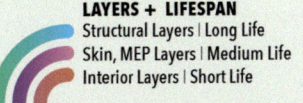

LAYERS + LIFESPAN
Structural Layers | Long Life
Skin, MEP Layers | Medium Life
Interior Layers | Short Life

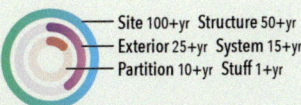

Site 100+yr Structure 50+yr
Exterior 25+yr System 15+yr
Partition 10+yr Stuff 1+yr

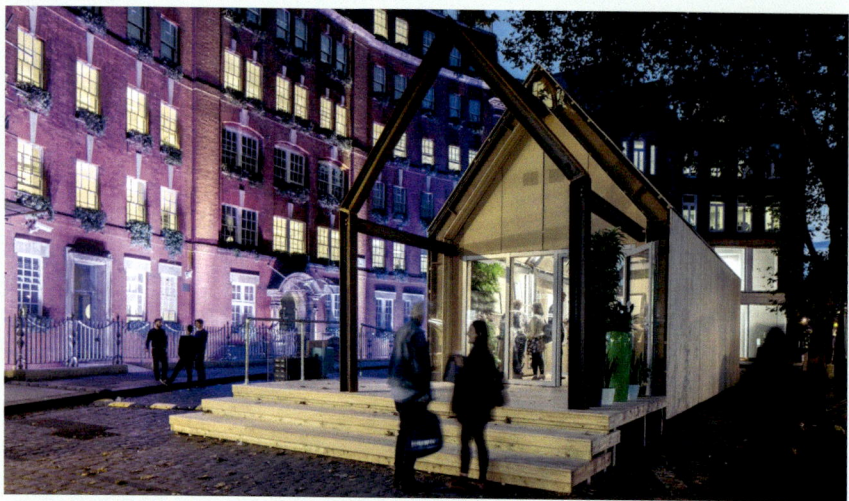

Figure 3.22 The Circular Building Prototype Was Demonstrated at the 2016 London Design Festival.

The Circular Building is a prototype dwelling designed by Arup for the 2016 London Design Festival as illustrated in Figure 3.22. The showcase was a collaboration between global architecture firm Arup, Frener & Reifer facades, BAM Construction, and the Built Environment Trust, to demonstrate the potential of circular principles across the construction industry to create waste-free housing. To test the feasibility of circularity at a larger scale, Arup has applied collaboration and digitalization to produce a completely reusable building. The building utilizes the principles of circular models – Recovery and Recycling, Product Life Extension, Service models, and Virtualization – in the design concept and overall construction value chain. Figure 3.23 gives a peak of the interior of the Circular Building.

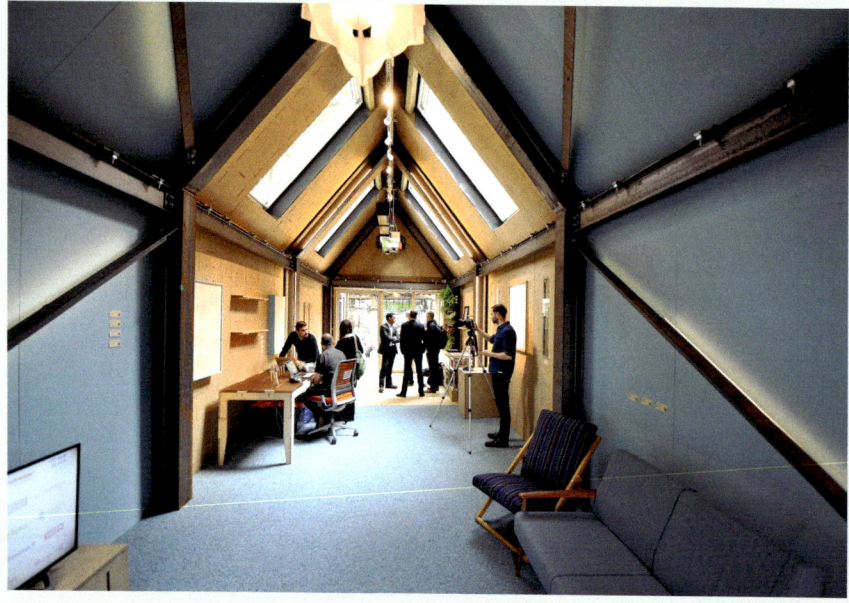

Figure 3.23 Interior View of the Circular Building.

Through considering the housing prototype as a series of layers – including façade, structure, systems, and "things" – Arup aimed to maximize the life span of these elements to come together in an example of comfortable and beautiful circular housing (Fernandez, 2016). The potential of the circular economy model, **Product Life Extension**, is explored through a design that facilitates a minimally damaging deconstruction process at the end of a building's useful life. The operational phase is also considered such as the inclusion of a greenwall to enhance indoor air quality as seen in Figure 3.24. This *design-for-disassembly* is achieved through dry construction techniques, such as mechanical push-fit connections and structural joints visible to the interior, to simplify the separation of building layers and promote the reuse of construction materials at the end-of-use phase. Arup used prefabrication construction, with its inherent precision and efficiency, to design these state-of-the-art building components that fit together effortlessly on-site and retain their value post-use (Archello, 2016).

Every part of the building can be disassembled with minimum damage, facilitating recovery and therefore reuse, remanufacturing, and recycling of its materials and components. The circular principle of **recovery and recycling** is also investigated through the material sourcing phase, as Arup sought to integrate recycled components, materials that had already served another use in another life. The steelwork that composes the building's structure is made from off-cuts from local construction

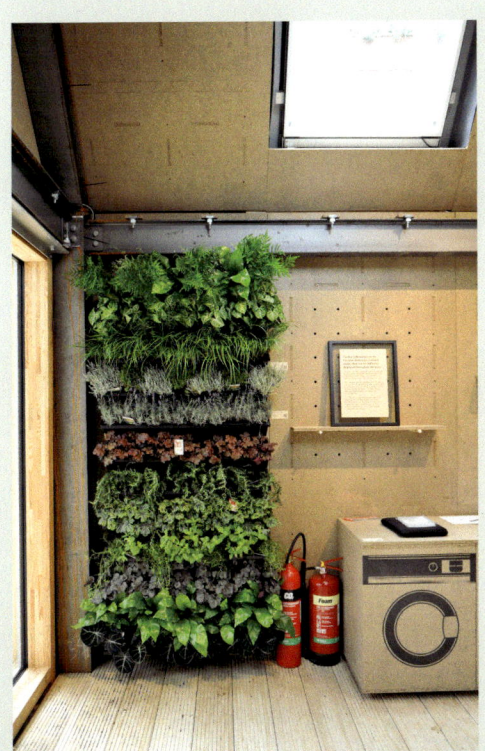

Figure 3.24 View of the Greenwall Which Supports Indoor Air Quality within the Circular Building.

sites (Antonini et al., 2020). The very dimensions of the dwelling were influenced by the lengths of steel available, illustrating the need for circular thinking across a building's life stages, from design to construction to end-of-use, in order to minimize waste. Boards of compressed agricultural waste make up the building's façade, exemplifying another recycled material. The sourcing of different recycled materials limits the need for raw material extraction while keeping these materials out of landfills. In the material sourcing phase, Arup also put **service models** to the test, with the interior carpeting being leased from its manufacturer. Desso supplied the carpet on a 'takeback' scheme, collecting and replacing the carpeting when worn out, and refurbishing and reusing the materials (Archello, 2016). This leasing method ensures high-quality products that are made to last, as it is in the manufacturer's best interest to replace and remanufacture products infrequently.

Virtualization was a crucial technique in the Circular Building to eliminate waste in multiple approaches (see Figure 3.25). The internal environment was monitored using integrated sensors which fed information to a cloud system which then controlled skylights, blinds, and lighting (Archello, 2016). This data-driven system ensured minimal use of energy to achieve comfortable lighting, temperature, and ventilation. A virtual building information model (BIM), now a commonly used tool in the industry to produce architectural and system drawings, collected and displayed internal environment data as well as a *Material Database* (Zimmerman et al., 2016). All building components and items within the prototype are 'tagged' with unique QR codes that, when scanned, provide users, construction professionals, or demolition experts with a product's information. This information, which is also stored in the BIM model, assists maintenance and reuse efforts to eliminate unnecessary trash. This prototypical dwelling, completely designed for reuse, illustrates the possibility within our construction industry to work toward a healthier future free of waste.

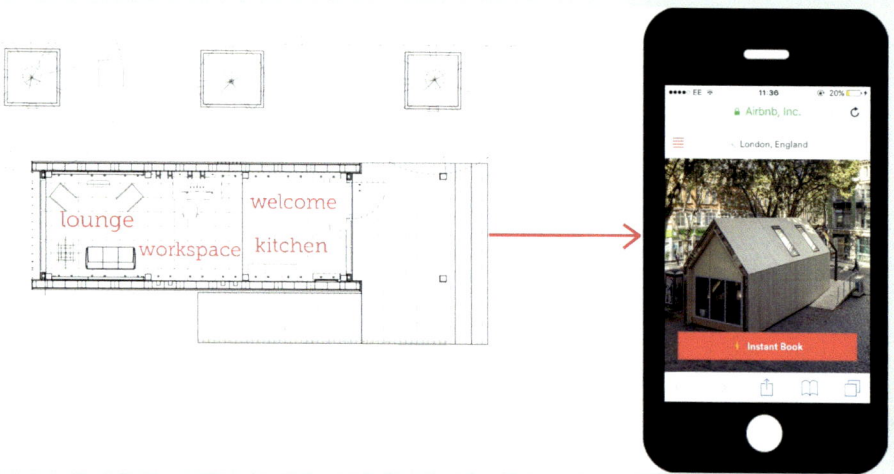

Figure 3.25 Virtualization in the Circular Building Design Enhanced Its Ability to Engage in a Circular Economy.

3B

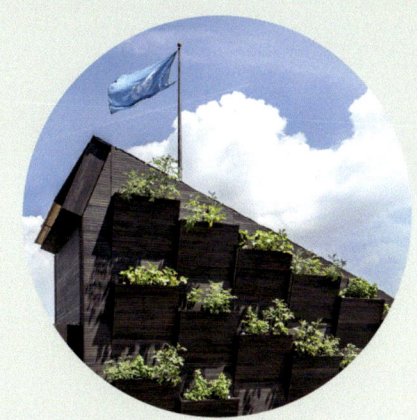

Project:
Ecological Living Module

Location:
New York City, USA

Year:
2018

Team:
Yale Center for Ecosystems +
Architecture and Gray Organschi
Architecture in collaboration with
UN Environment Programme and
UN-Habitat

**Mapping to Circular
Economy Framework:**

CIRCULAR ECONOMY PRACTICES

LIFE CYCLE PHASES

	Recovery	Life Extension	Sharing Platforms	Service Models	Regenerate	Virtualize
Work of Geobiosphere						
Sourcing						
Manufacturing						
Design & Construction						
Use						
End-of-Use						

LAYERS + LIFESPAN

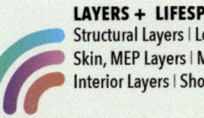

Structural Layers | Long Life
Skin, MEP Layers | Medium Life
Interior Layers | Short Life

Site 100+yr   Structure 50+yr
Exterior 25+yr   System 15+yr
Partition 10+yr   Stuff 1+yr

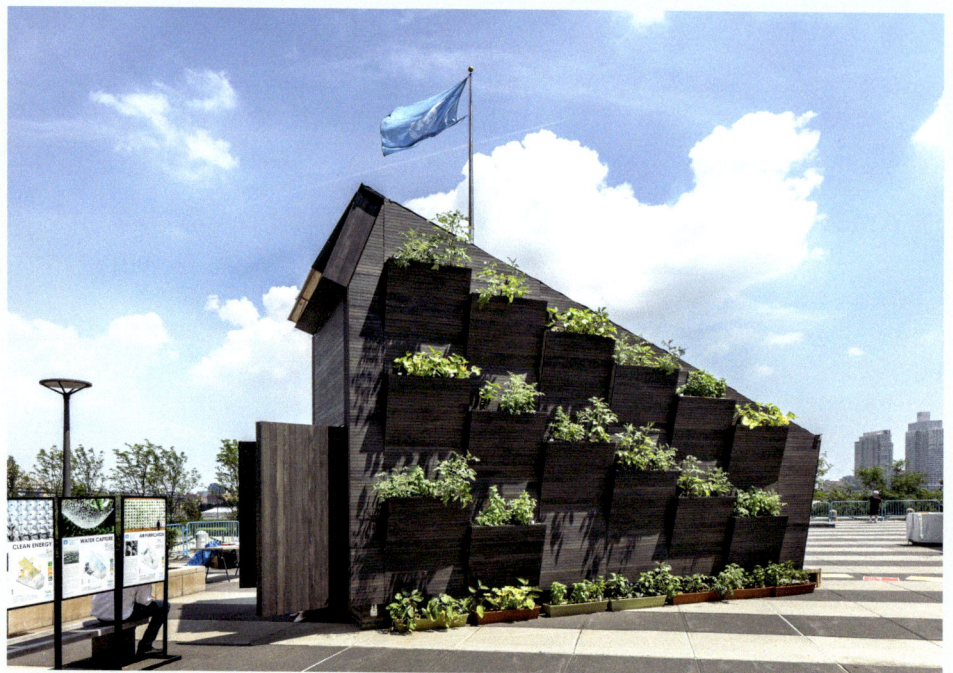

Figure 3.26 Demonstration of the Ecological Living Module on the UN Plaza, New York City July to August 2018. © David Sundberg/Esto.

The ELM is a 22 m² housing module designed for a family of four as a collaboration between Yale Center for Ecosystems and Architecture (Yale CEA), Gray Organschi Architecture, UN Environment Programme, and UN-Habitat. The self-sufficient home was demonstrated on the UN Plaza in New York City during the High-Level Political Forum, 2018 (see Figure 3.26). The home's modular, prefabricated structure, and environmental systems were developed off-site in controlled environments before being assembled on-site within a three-day period with no need for industrial equipment. The demonstration project was designed as a joint effort between architects, engineers, data scientists, and policy experts to explore the potential of a built ecologies approach to housing to achieve social and environmental goals set out by the UN 2030 agenda (UN General Assembly, 2015). As is illustrated in Figure 3.27, ELM strives to achieve the UN SDGs through circular practices and a systems-thinking approach considering the relationships across five main areas: food, air, solar, water, and materials (Dyson et al., 2020).

ELM's integrated approach to food production strives to meet SDG 2 which outlines the goal to *End hunger, achieve food security and improved nutrition, and promote sustainable agriculture.* The project features a micro-farming exterior wall (see Figure 3.28), located on the western-facing façade to achieve optimal sunlight for fruit and vegetable growth. The micro-farm includes fruits and vegetables native to New York, which are irrigated with harvested rainwater collected on the ELM roof and distributed via channels in the walls to each planter. This system provides 65 percent of the recommended nutrient-dense fruit and vegetable servings for a family of

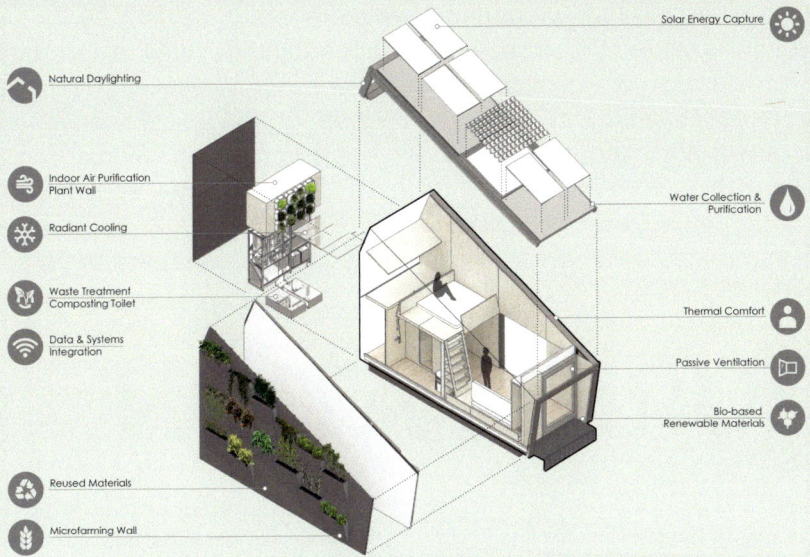

Figure 3.27 ELM's Toolkit for Sustainable On-Site Self-Sufficiency. Source: Gray Organschi Architecture.

MICROFARMING

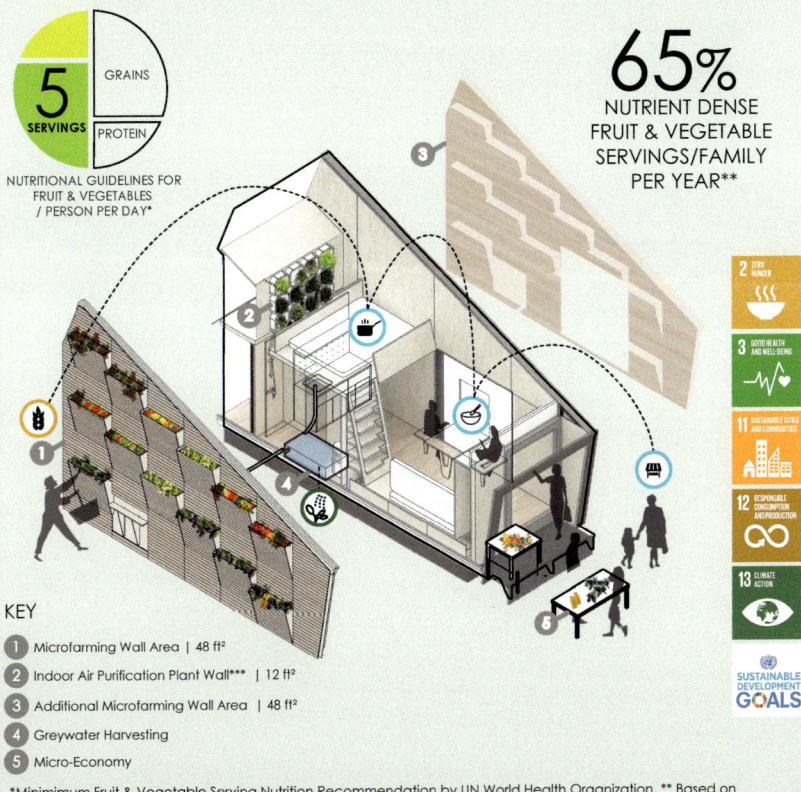

5 SERVINGS

GRAINS

PROTEIN

NUTRITIONAL GUIDELINES FOR
FRUIT & VEGETABLES
/ PERSON PER DAY*

65%
NUTRIENT DENSE
FRUIT & VEGETABLE
SERVINGS/FAMILY
PER YEAR**

2 ZERO HUNGER

3 GOOD HEALTH AND WELL-BEING

11 SUSTAINABLE CITIES AND COMMUNITIES

12 RESPONSIBLE CONSUMPTION AND PRODUCTION

13 CLIMATE ACTION

SUSTAINABLE DEVELOPMENT GOALS

KEY

1. Microfarming Wall Area | 48 ft²
2. Indoor Air Purification Plant Wall*** | 12 ft²
3. Additional Microfarming Wall Area | 48 ft²
4. Greywater Harvesting
5. Micro-Economy

*Minimimum Fruit & Vegetable Serving Nutrition Recommendation by UN World Health Organization. ** Based on optimized plant selection for increased harvest yields across total 100 ft² wall areas. ***Use of Indoor Air Purification

Figure 3.28 ELM's Micro-Farming Wall Providing Nutrient-Dense Fruit and Vegetables for the ELM Inhabitants. Source: Yale CEA.

four, proving the possibility of dwelling-integrated agriculture to address hunger and nutritional deficiency (see Figure 3.28). The reuse of resources demonstrated in the irrigation system promotes the circular economy principle of **recovery and recycling**.

SDG 3 – *Ensure healthy lives and promote well-being for all at all ages* – is approached through ensuring adequate air quality through energy-efficient means. ELM employs an Active Phytoremediation System (AMPS) to measure and act against airborne pollutants to ensure fresh air (see Figure 3.29). Located in the upstairs bedroom, AMPS removes volatile organic compounds, released commonly from

AIR PURIFICATION

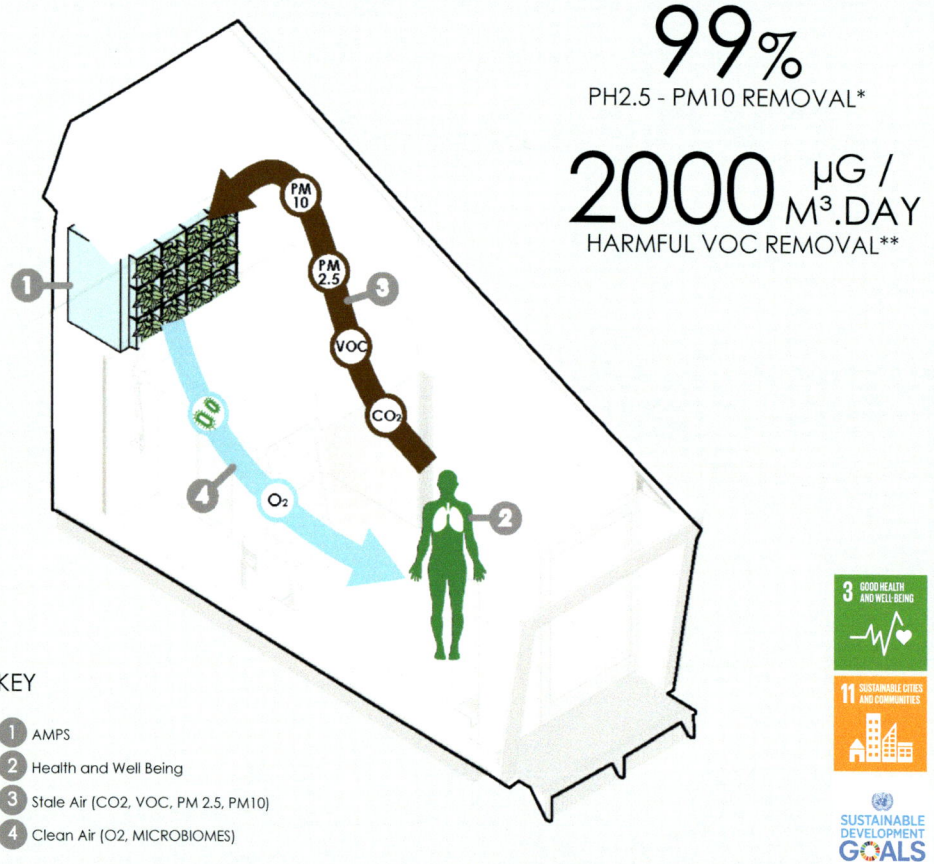

99%
PH2.5 - PM10 REMOVAL*

2000 µG / M³.DAY
HARMFUL VOC REMOVAL**

KEY

① AMPS
② Health and Well Being
③ Stale Air (CO2, VOC, PM 2.5, PM10)
④ Clean Air (O2, MICROBIOMES)

* Liu, X., et al. (2017). "Soy Protein Isolate/Bacterial Cellulose Composite Membranes for High Efficiency Particulate Air Filtration." Composites Science and Technology 138: 124-133. ** Aydogan, A. and L. D. Montoya (2011). "Formaldehyde removal by common indoor plant species and various growing media." Atmospheric Environment 45(16): 2675-2682.

Figure 3.29 The Upstairs Bedroom Features an Air Purifying Plant Wall (FABS) that Provides Fresh Indoor Air. Source: Yale CEA.

technology used in our homes, from indoor air with botanical biofilters by directing airflow through a plant growing medium (Dyson et al., 2020) (see Figure 3.30). This intervention addresses human health and well-being by promoting healthy indoor air, while embodying the circular economy principle of **regeneration** by improving local air quality and health (Pettit et al., 2018).

A solar energy system and efficient morphology strive to *Ensure access to affordable, reliable, sustainable, and modern energy for all* (SDG 7). ELM's electricity needs are 2,600 kWh/yr, compared to a typical New York home which requires 6,860 kWh/yr, which is met solely through the building's solar energy system (Dyson et al., 2020)

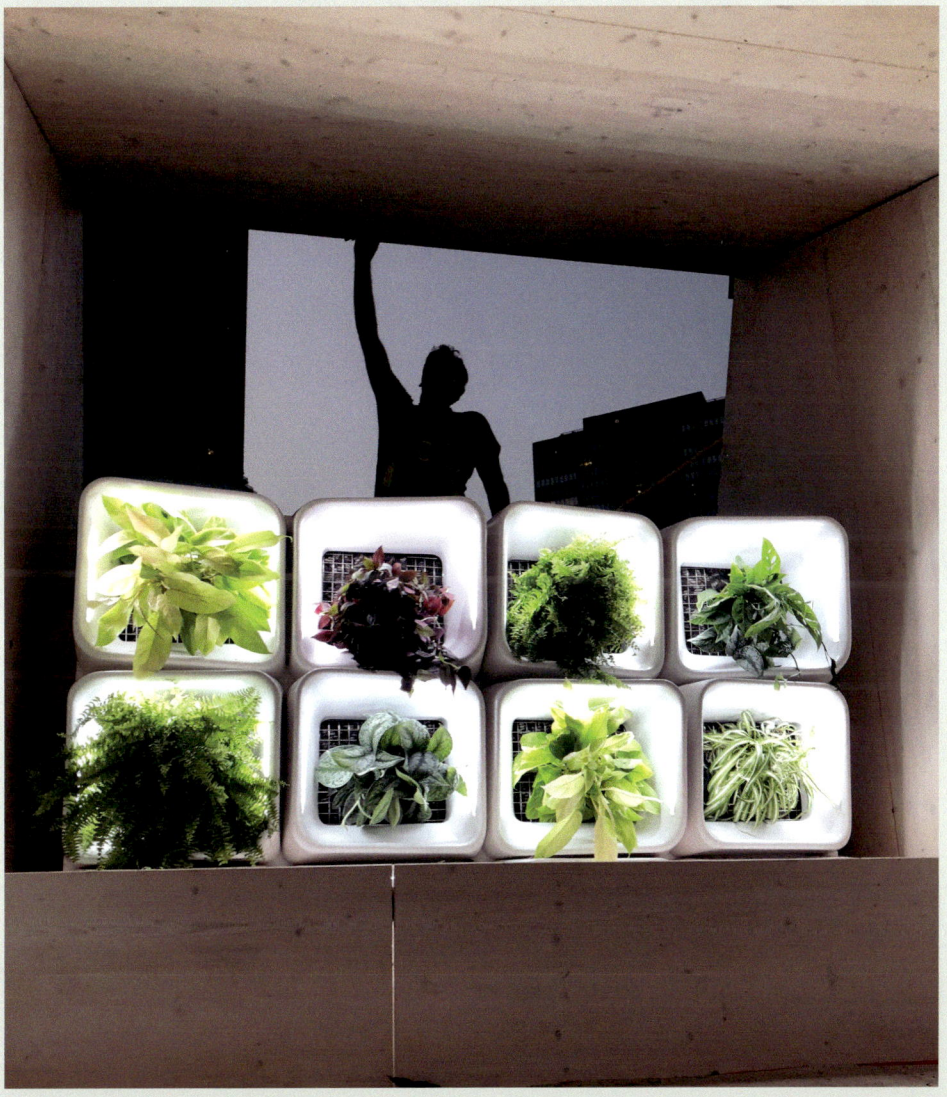

Figure 3.30 The Modular AMPS System Being Assembled on Site. Source: Keena.

(see Figure 3.31). An Integrated Concentrating Solar Façade is incorporated within the roof light and captures direct solar radiation, transforming it into electricity while allowing only glare-free, diffused light into the interior (see Figure 3.32). On-site energy production allows ELM to be off-grid and energy self-sufficient (Raugei et al., 2021). This energy system, as well as other systems vital to ELM such as air filtration, is **virtually** monitored to ensure performance during use and to contribute to future research and circular thinking (see Figure 3.33).

CLEAN ENERGY

2kW

OF CLEAN, FREE, ON-SITE ENERGY GENERATED, RENDERING THE HOUSE ENERGY SELF-SUFFICIENT FOR FOUR PEOPLE*

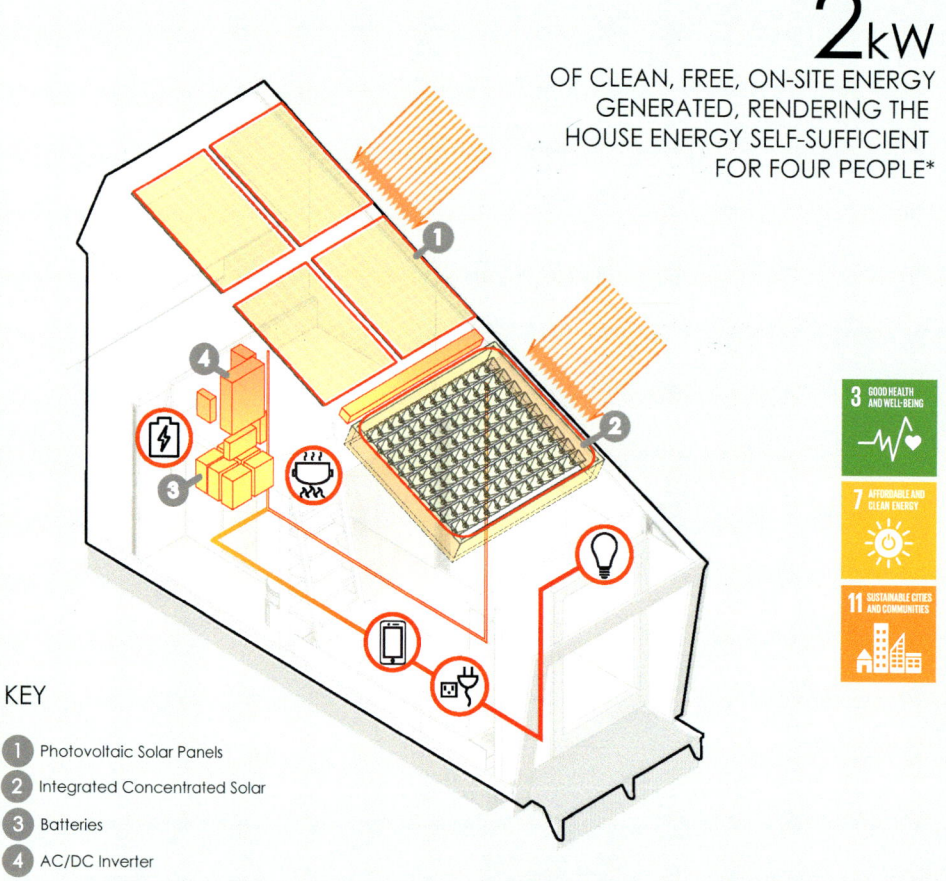

KEY

1 Photovoltaic Solar Panels

2 Integrated Concentrated Solar

3 Batteries

4 AC/DC Inverter

* Clean energy generated from combined PV solar panels and Integrated concentrated solar panel

Figure 3.31 Solar Energy Powers ELM. Clean Energy Is Generated from Combined PV Solar Panels and Integrated Concentrated Solar Facade. Source: Yale CEA.

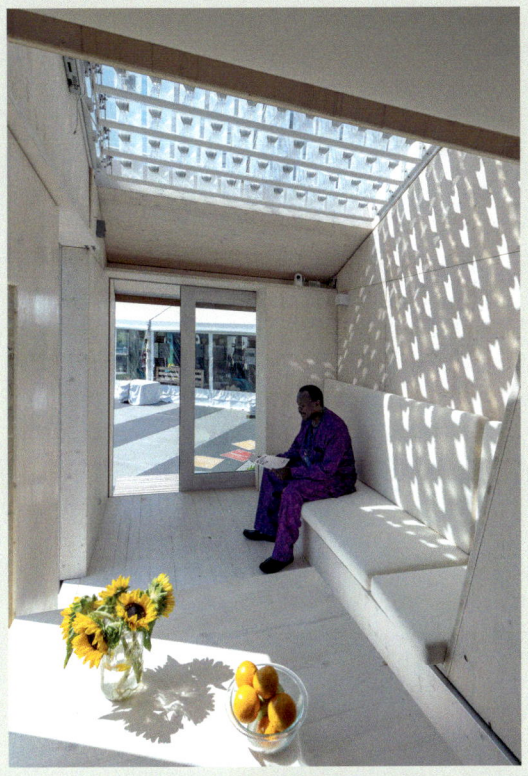

Figure 3.32 Interior View with a Shadow of HeliOptix (an Integrated Concentrating Solar System) Allowing Natural Daylight. © David Sundberg/Esto.

DATA POINTS

Figure 3.33 Data Points: ELM's Environmental Systems Performance Is Monitored and Recorded via Internet of Things and Visualized with SEVA Visual Analytics Environment. Source: Yale CEA.

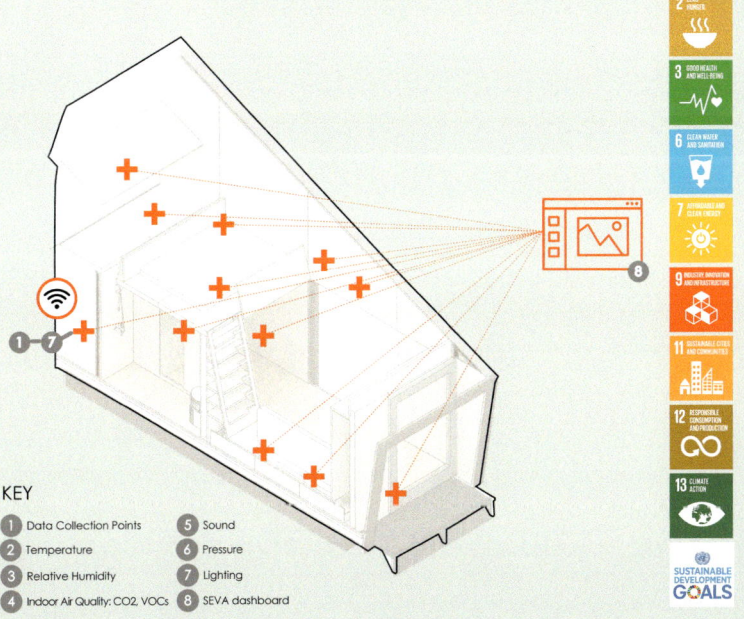

KEY

1. Data Collection Points
2. Temperature
3. Relative Humidity
4. Indoor Air Quality: CO2, VOCs
5. Sound
6. Pressure
7. Lighting
8. SEVA dashboard

*Monitoring occurs via the Mote air quality sensors, the HoBo CO2 logger, and Future Air SAM. Data being collected for Temperature, Relative Humidity, Indoor Air Quality, Sound, Pressure and Lighting is uploaded to the SEVA platform for visual analytics

An additional focus to meet UN SDGs was material life cycle considerations, which targeted SDG 9: *Build resilient infrastructure, promote inclusive and sustainable industrialization and foster innovation.* Cross-laminated timber (CLT) was used to create a modular structure, façade, and interior that is easily assembled and disassembled. This prefabrication technique, made possible through **digital** modeling, encourages the **recovery and recycling** of the CLT as well as integrated mechanical systems due to precisely documented and visible joints. Products and materials within ELM therefore have a **longer life** and can be used to create housing in another location or in another context altogether. The locally sourced CLT was chosen due to its ability to perform as a biomaterial in large-scale buildings, as the design team wished to demonstrate the possibilities at the scale of communities and cities. The biomaterial not only encourages sustainable industrialization, but it also sequesters carbon from the atmosphere, contributing to the **regeneration** of our geo-biosphere (see Figure 3.34).

Finally, toward meeting SDG 6: Clean water and Sanitation. The ELM has a dehumidifier system that produces potable water from capturing the humidity in the air (see Figure 3.35). In addition, as noted above, water collection from rainwater capture on the roof enables a closed-loop water cycle. Twenty liters of water per person was produced per day which is enough for drinking, cleaning, cooking, and bathing as illustrated in Figure 3.36.

The SDGs outlined above are just a few of the targets that the project demonstrated. The ELM is a compact but far-reaching example of the power of circular principles in achieving sustainable urbanization across the globe. The self-contained and self-sufficient dwelling exhibits how approaching housing design with a systems-thinking approach, considering resources and materials as flows and cycles, can create a healthier and more viable future.

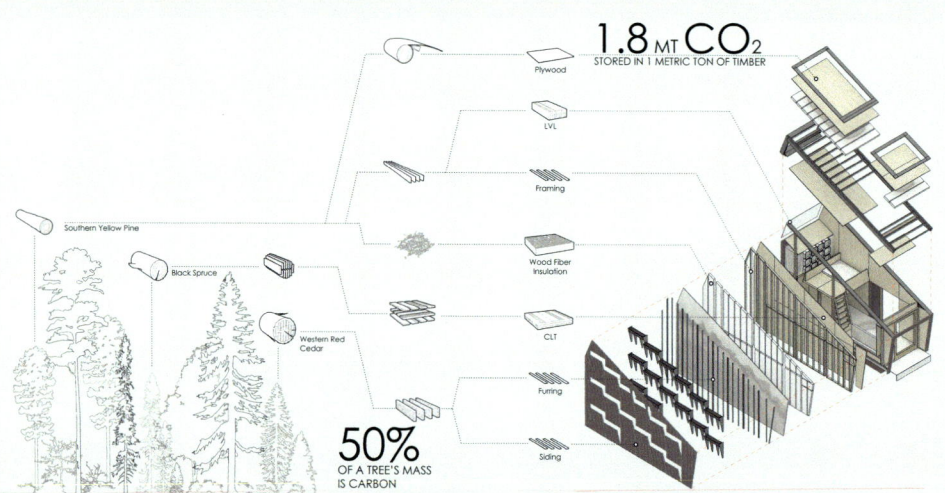

Figure 3.34 ELM Is Constructed of Bio-Based Renewable Materials Which Act as a Carbon Sink During the Building Use Phase. Source: Gray Organschi Architecture.

WATER CAPTURE

Figure 3.35 ELM's Water Capture Assuming Water Generation from Dehumidifier and Water Collection from Rainwater Roof Capture. Source: Yale CEA.

20LITERS
PER PERSON PER DAY;
ENOUGH FOR
DRINKING, CLEANING,
COOKING, & BATHING

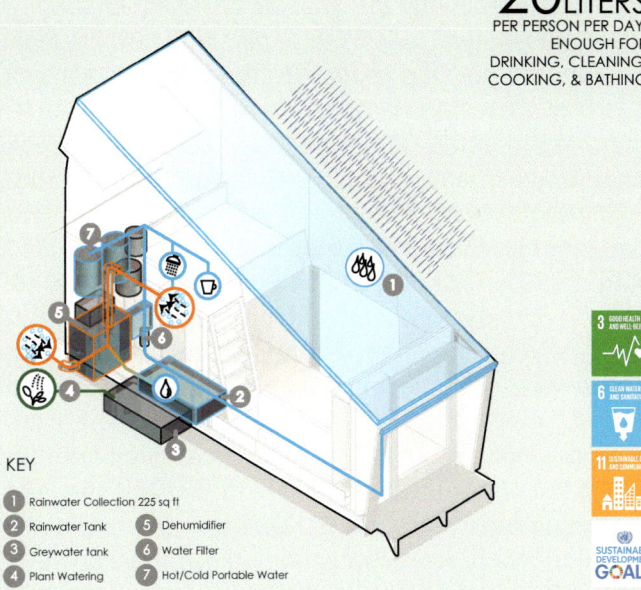

KEY

1. Rainwater Collection 225 sq ft
2. Rainwater Tank
3. Greywater tank
4. Plant Watering
5. Dehumidifier
6. Water Filter
7. Hot/Cold Portable Water

* Assuming water generation from dehumidifier and water collection for rain water roof capture

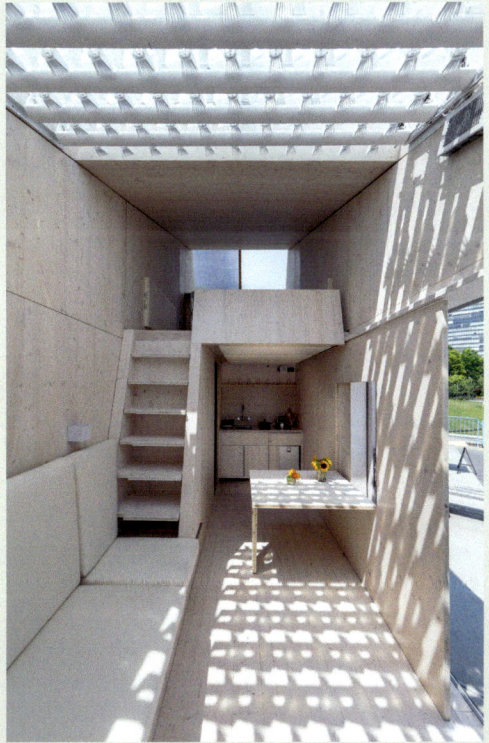

Figure 3.36 Interior View of Kitchen and Bathroom Shower. © David Sundberg/Esto.

3.7 Conclusion

Our new circular economy framework aims to incorporate the concepts discussed in this chapter. While Chapters 1 and 2 focused on why the circular economy should be implemented into the built environment, this chapter begins to understand how circularity can be successfully implemented into the building sector. Multiple dimensions and stakeholders are needed in a shift to a circular framework, including the government, consumers, designers, and the technology sector. Circular economy principles seek to achieve sustainability through an economic lens, and thus, the five business models touch on the six dimensions needed to achieve circularity. Not only are these five business models economically advantageous for multiple stakeholders, but they also align with the ReSOLVE framework by the Ellen MacArthur Foundation, which state six realms that must be met to transition to a circular economy. *Regenerate* connects with the Circular Supply-Chain Model, *Share* with the Sharing Platform business model, *Optimize* with the Product Life Extension business model, *Loop* with the Recovery and Recycling business model, and *Exchange* with the PaaS business model. The sixth criterion, *Virtualize*, is featured in all business models. Not only must circularity be attractive to businesses and consumers but also must touch on the three main pillars of sustainability – environment, economy, and equity. The UN SDGs are an important reference point for stakeholders who want to incorporate circular economy principles into their built environment to follow. Lastly, the existing building certification systems give a good idea of how sustainability is currently being assessed in the built environment. Clearly, these certification systems approach assessing construction projects differently. As a result, we created a comprehensive assessment method that encompasses the circular economy framework principles outlined by the Ellen MacArthur Foundation, concepts discussed in the five business models, the UN SDGs, and positive criteria outlined in existing certification systems. Our circular economy framework is a helpful guide for building design professionals to use to assess whether their building is not only sustainable but specifically incorporates ideas of circularity.

References

Adams, K. (2016, March 8–10). Important factors to consider for applying circular economy in buildings including a focus on reclamation. Presented at the #BuildCircular learning hub, EcoBuild 2016, London.

AIA. (2020). *AIA framework for design excellence*. American Institute of Architects.

Allford Hall Monaghan Morris Architects. (2016). *White collar factory*. Retrieved June 12 from https://www.ahmm.co.uk/projects/office/white-collar-factory/

Antonini, E., Boeri, A., & Giglio, F. (2020). Beyond emergency towards circular design: Building low tech. In *Emergency driven innovation* (pp. 59–86). Springer.

Archello. (2016). *The circular economy building: Arup associates*. Retrieved January 23, 2023 from https://archello.com/project/the-circular-economy-building

Bhatia, N., & Steinmuller, A. (2018). *Spatial models for the domestic commons*: Communes, co-living and cooperatives. *Architectural Design, 88*, 120–127. https://doi.org/10.1002/ad.2329

BRE Group. (n.d.). *BREEAM whole life performance*. Retrieved January 24 from
https://bregroup.com/products/breeam/breeam-solutions/breeam-whole-life-perfomance/

Carra, G., & Magdani, N. (2017). *Circular business models for the built environment*. Ellen
MacArthur Foundation.

CBRE+Streetsense. (2020). *Innovation watch: The rise of co-living*. https://www.cbre.us/-/
media/cbre/countryunitedstates/media/images/multifamily/innovation-watch/co-living/
021420_innovationwatch_january-2020-fw.pdf

Corbey, S., Cullen, J. M., Sansom, M., & Fishwick, R. (2016, March 8–10). Overcoming
the barriers to steel reuse in construction. Presented at the #BuildCircular learning hub,
EcoBuild 2016, London.

Dyson, A., Keena, N., Organschi, A., Gray, L., Novelli, N., Bradford, K., Aly-Etman, M.,
Gindlesparger, M., Wildman, H., & Duwyn, J. (2020). Built environment ecosystems framework towards sustainable urban housing infrastructure. In *IOP Conference series: Earth
and environmental science*.

Fernandez, C. (2016). *The circular building: The most advanced reusable building
yet*. Arup. Retrieved January 23, 2023 from https://www.arup.com/news-and-events/
the-circular-building-the-most-advanced-reusable-building-yet

globechain.com. (n.d.). *How it works*. Retrieved January 24 from https://globechain.com/
how-it-works

GXN, & Assets, R. (2018). *Circle house: Denmark's first circular housing project* (1st ed.,
Vol. 248). GXN.

IFC. (n.d.). *Edge: Certify green and change your world*. Retrieved January 24 from
https://edgebuildings.com/

IKEA. (2014). *IKEA group sustainability report FY14*. https://res.ikeaddict.com/misc/l/IKEA_
EN_Group-Sustainability-Report-FY14/IKEA_EN_Group-Sustainability-Report-FY14.pdf

International Living Future Institute. (2019). *Living building challenge 4.0* (Version 4).
https://living-future.org/wp-content/uploads/2022/08/LBC-4_0_v14_2_compressed.pdf

International Living Future Institute. (n.d.). *Declare. The nutrition label for Products*.
Retrieved January 24 from https://declare.living-future.org/

International Well Building Institute. (2016). *The WELL building standard*. https://standard.
wellcertified.com/sites/default/files/The%20WELL%20Building%20Standard%20v1%20
with%20May%202016%20addenda.pdf

Iyer-Raniga, U., & Huovila, P. (2020). *Global state of play for circular built environment.
A report on the state of play on circularity in the built environment across Africa, Asia,
Europe, Gulf Cooperation Council countries, Latin America and the Caribbean, North
America and Oceania*. Final report. United Nations One Planet Network Sustainable
Buildings and Construction Programme. https://www.oneplanetnetwork.org/knowledge-
centre/resources/global-state-play-circular-built-environment-united-nations-un-one

Keena, N. (2017). *Towards a comprehensive visual analytics environment for the assessment of socio-ecological factors within architectural design*. Rensselaer Polytechnic
Institute.

Keena, N., Friedman, A., Parsaee, M., & Klein, A. (2023). *Data visualization for a circular
economy: Designing a web application for sustainable housing*. Technology | Architecture
+ Design, 7:2, 262–281, DOI: 10.1080/24751448.2023.2246803.

Khoo, J. (2015). Service design. I don't need a drill I need a hole. In *The circular economy
in organisations* (Vol. 11). University College London.

Lacy, P., & Rutqvist, J. (2015). *Waste to wealth: The circular economy advantage*. Palgrave
Macmillan. https://doi.org/10.1057/9781137530707

McKinsey Global Institute. (2017). *Reinventing construction: A route to higher productivity*. https://www.mckinsey.com/business-functions/operations/our-insights/reinventing-construction-through-a-productivity-revolution

Nguyen, B. K., & Altan, H. (2011). Comparative review of five sustainable rating systems. *Procedia Engineering*, *21*, 376–386. https://doi.org/10.1016/j.proeng.2011.11.2029

Pettit, T., Irga, P., & Torpy, F. (2018). Towards practical indoor air phytoremediation: A review. *Chemosphere*, *208*, 960–974.

Pomponi, F., & Moncaster, A. (2017). Circular economy for the built environment: A research framework. *Journal of Cleaner Production*, *143*, 710–718. https://doi.org/10.1016/j.jclepro.2016.12.055

Raugei, M., Keena, N., Novelli, N., Aly Etman, M., & Dyson, A. (2021). Life cycle assessment of an ecological living module equipped with conventional rooftop or integrated concentrating photovoltaics. *Journal of Industrial Ecology*, *25*(5), 1207–1221. https://doi.org/10.1111/jiec.13129

Schnaars, C., & Morgan, H. (2012). In U.S. building industry, is it too easy to be green? *USA Today*. https://www.usatoday.com/story/news/nation/2012/10/24/green-building-leed-certification/1650517/

Swanson, K. (2018). *Sustainable architecture: A critique of LEED and the potential of biomimicry* [Senior Comprehensive Project]. Department of Urban and Environmental Policy, Occidental College.

Thelen, D., Van Acoleyen, M., Huurman, W., Tom, T., can Brunschot, C., Edgerton, B., & Ben, K. (2018). *Scaling the circular built environment: Pathways for business and government*. World Business Council for Sustainable Development & Circle Economy.

Thomas, M. A. (2016). The Living Building Challenge: Roots and Rise of the World's Greenest Standard. In.

UN General Assembly. (2015). *Transforming our world: The 2030 agenda for sustainable development*. United Nations. https://sdgs.un.org/publications/transforming-our-world-2030-agenda-sustainable-development-17981

USGBC. (2009). *Leadership in energy and environmental design (LEED)*. Retrieved January 24 from http://www.usgbc.org/leed

World Business Council for Sustainable Development (WBCSD). (2018). *Scaling the circular built environment: Pathways for business and government*. W. B. C. f. S. Development.

Wheeler, S. (2004). *Planning for sustainability: Creating livable, equitable and ecological communities* (1st ed.). Routledge. https://doi.org/10.4324/9780203300565

Zimmerman, R., O'Brien, H., Hargrave, J., & Morrell, M. (2016). *The circular economy in the built environment*. Arup. https://www.arup.com/perspectives/publications/research/section/circular-economy-in-the-built-environment

PART 2

Applications of Circular Economy Principles to Housing

Chapter 4

Housing Passports

4.1 The Synthesis of Data and Housing

The building sector is one of the greatest exploiters of resources and producers of waste. The sector is responsible for around 40 percent of global material resource use (by mass) and produces approximately one-third of global greenhouse gas emissions (Hertwich et al., 2020). While the circular economy holds important potential in reducing such harms to the environment, this economic approach still faces many obstacles, the most prominent being a general lack of knowledge concerning the exact process of implementation. For instance, the multiple stakeholders involved in the building process may have varying education on residential building materials, architectural approaches, or on their complementary stakeholder's roles in different stages of the building's life cycle. Even with this knowledge, information about the construction and building material of existing sites is often unknown or not shared in an easily accessible format. While some attempts have been made to collect and handle building information, such as the material and Building Renovation Passports (BRPs), a more holistic approach is required.

Our solution is the housing passport (HP): a standardized digital description of material flows, building compositions, and general building characteristics. The HP aggregates material and building data to create one standardized resource. Just as a person may own a passport that holds necessary information about their identity, a similar standard document should exist for housing. Its aim is to bridge the gap between the building sector and their many relevant stakeholders, presenting housing data in an easily digestible format, guiding users in all phases of a building's life cycle. This form of documentation promotes circularity, as extensive knowledge of how a building is constructed can help actors properly deconstruct, or disassemble, a building, facilitating recovery and recycling. Moreover, this initiative presents opportunities to support affordable and sustainable housing by incorporating circular economy principles which can enhance adaptability and flexibility in housing design. Thus, by making knowledge more accessible, the hope is for owners – and other stakeholders – to be encouraged to make decisions that follow circular economy values. Given the major contribution of the building industry to waste production, transforming the protocol – especially regarding the end-of-use phase – would promote sustainability.

This chapter will outline existing passports that currently exist in the housing sector and will introduce guidelines for creating an HP, such as the importance of incorporating a multi-scalar approach when developing HPs and it will highlight how HP can promote circular design.

DOI: 10.4324/9781003333975-6

4.2 Life Cycle Phases and Multi-Scalar Digital Descriptions

There is a wide variety of approaches to formatting a building passport, which makes it difficult to identify a singular standard (Global Alliance for Buildings and Construction and the United Nations Environment Programme, 2021). However, from analyzing stakeholder's ideas, proposals, and needs from current passports, there are three main circularity goals that a building passport should achieve: measure circularity, manage and maintain objects (i.e., buildings), and facilitate future reuse and value retention (Platform CB'23, 2020). In order to accomplish these aims, data needs to be collected at different building phases, meaning that the passport needs to interact with different scales. In other words, to achieve a comprehensive reflection of a building requires an HP's digital representation to capture a building's multi-scalar complexity and life cycle phases (Keena et al., 2023).

One key challenge with building passports is that information pertaining to various levels of scale is required, ranging from raw materials to an actual building. An effective building passport will collect data at different phases in the lifespan of a building – ranging from material extraction, all the way to the end-of-use phase of a building. The building life cycle goes through various phases and scales, starting with materials, then building elements, then the building, and back to materials. Building passports for specific scales are called "passport versions", which provide data on structural management, construction components, raw materials, etc. (Platform CB'23, 2020). Passports need a structure that enables various scales and facilitates how they are documented. Data is inherited and then supplemented with data added at this scale – for instance, raw material data pertains to the manufactured component data which subsequentially will pertain to its use in a construction assembly. A passport's multi-scalar format is key as it ensures that data does not have to be repeatedly entered and is appropriately linked. In other words, there is a trace of the material flow through the life cycle of a building.

Furthermore, in order to ensure that passports are comprehensive, minimum information requirements are set for the construction, operation, and end-of-use of a building. The passport collects data at different phases of a building's lifespan and this data needs to be continuously updated throughout the building processes, as new information about the building's construction, retrofitting updates, or renovations have been accomplished. Therefore, the passport's structure needs to be easily modified. For a building passport to be continuously modified, it needs to monitor updates. One method that is often leveraged to document the key phases of the building life cycle when data entry is needed is life cycle assessment (LCA) which makes objects easily traceable. The LCA tool quantifies the environmental impacts of the raw materials use, by linking environmental performance to a material's functionality (Olivier et al., 2016). This is particularly relevant to sustainability, as it covers the building's entire life cycle.

In developing the HP, the goal was to address both scale and life cycle phases; the HP has a "nesting" structure, meaning that information at more macro-scales is composed of information at more micro-scales (see Figure 4.1). A nested structure, often used in data science, is a structure that contains one or more members that

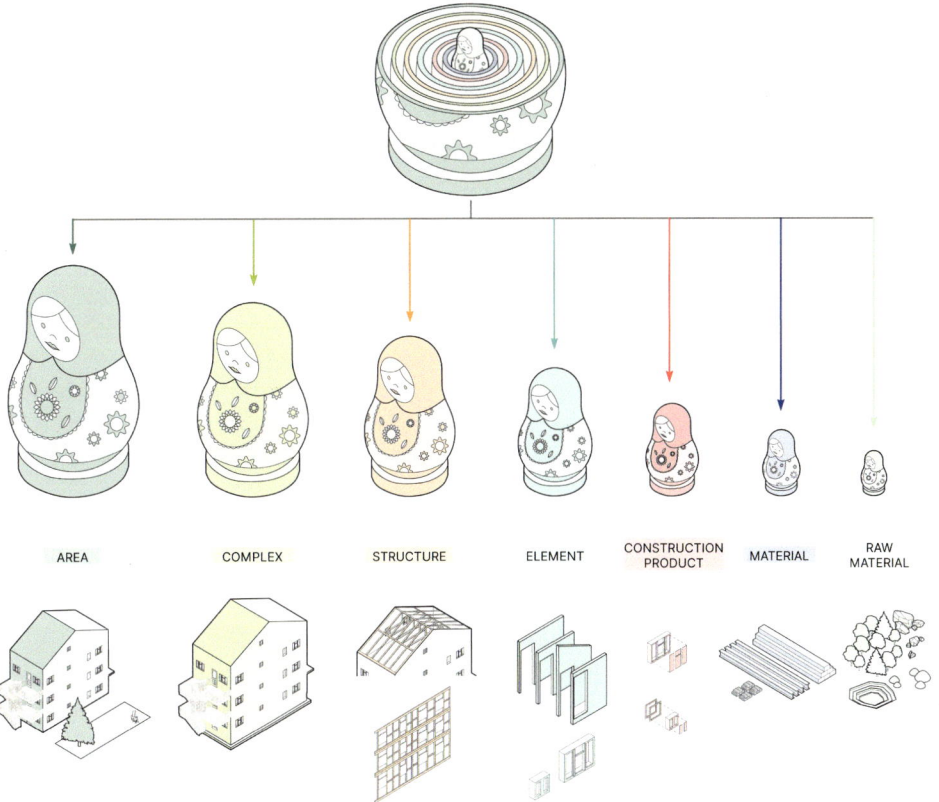

Figure 4.1 Housing Passport's Nesting Structure.

are themselves structures. Nested structures help in organizing complex data and can help with the readability and maintenance of the HP. The HP's nesting structure also considers life cycle phases by including both static elements, such as object snapshots or performance records, and dynamic elements, such as adjustments over time (Keena et al., 2023).

4.3 Existing Passports for the Building Sector

Establishing a circular economy requires a large amount of information, much of which remains unknown or inaccessible. A crucial goal of the circular economy is to promote the reuse and recycling of materials. Currently, downcycling is the norm: our current state of recycling reduces the value and quality of a material (Heinrich & Lang, 2019). Circular economy, however, promotes upcycling: reusing by-products to create a product of higher quality (see Chapter 3). The goal is that construction by-products, which would otherwise be considered waste, be repurposed into new and functional goods. Recycled concrete is an example of upcycling – minerals are aggregated from demolition and used to produce concrete. Despite its various benefits, recycled concrete – along with upcycling in general – has a low uptake, compared to the production of concrete from primary sources (Heinrich & Lang, 2019). This is mainly due to gaps in information, financial risks, liabilities, skepticism about reuse, etc. Passports can fill these gaps of information, thus lessening worries of financial risk or failure. While there are existing approaches to this issue, including the material and BRPs as outlined below, they tend to be too narrow and limited to ultimately support transitioning to a circular economy in housing.

4.3.1 *Material Passport*

As well as being responsible for 40 percent of global material resource use (by mass), the building sector is also one of the largest producers of waste, contributing to 40 percent of global waste production by volume (Heinrich & Lang, 2019). Thus, to promote a circular economy and resource efficiency in the construction industry, information is required pertaining to the material composition of building stock and material flows (including raw materials, building materials, and waste). As discussed in Chapter 3, maintaining the value of materials is crucial in a successful circular economy. Materials remain valuable if they are accessible, functional, and aesthetically pleasing. To achieve this, materials and building products need to be capable of smooth and fast removal from their building after use, with minimal effort, no contamination, and without loss of quality. If the construction of a building is well-documented, and the quality of its materials is recorded, when it comes time to disassemble the building, professionals have a clear guide to follow, salvaging all building material quickly and with little to no damage to the existing building products. This allows that material to be successfully reused in a new construction effort, contributing to the circularity of a product.

Material passports (MPs) represent a current attempt to categorize material information to promote sustainability. The MP consists of a digital report containing relevant circular economy data that is entered into, and then extracted from, a centralized database in the form of reports which are customized to the needs of a diverse user-base (see Figure 4.2) (Heinrich & Lang, 2019). Within an MP, there are hierarchical levels, comprising materials, components, products, and systems (in that order) that make up a building. The MP covers data on a material's physical properties, chemical properties, biological properties, material health, unique product and system identifiers, design and production, transportation and logistics, construction, use and operational phase, and disassembly and reversibility. This passport's dataset composition is facilitated by Environmental Product Declarations (EPDs). By standardizing documentation procedures through MPs and digital technology, time is optimized, and information is accessible to all stakeholders.

MPs have been implemented in various situations. Cradle to Cradle, for instance, is one kind of MP that acts as a form of the environmental certification system, aiming to create a global standard for products that are safe, circular, and responsibly made (Cradle to Cradle, 2022). It assesses these characteristics across five categories of sustainability performance – material health, product circularity, clean air and climate

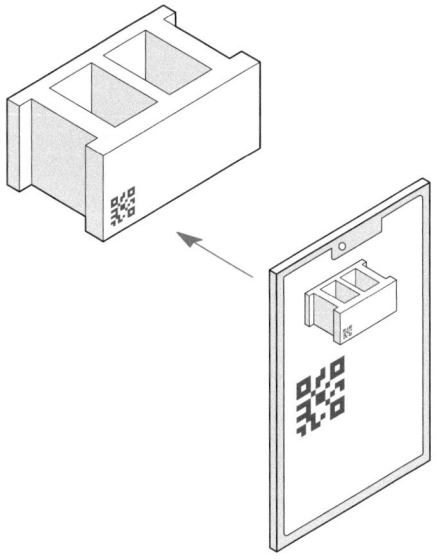
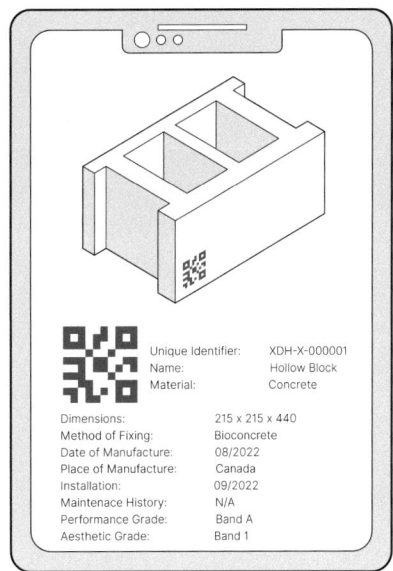

Source: ORMS, "Material Passports"

Figure 4.2 The Material Passport.

production, water and soil stewardship, and social fairness. Other MPs are utilized for health and well-being. The open-source database Quartz, for instance, promotes healthy buildings by focusing on environmental and health parameters of specific building products (Quartz, 2015). This database promotes transparency in building products, with the goal of transforming the market by driving it toward less toxic and lower impact materials for better buildings and healthier communities. Commonly used building products' profiles are provided and include their descriptions, general composition, impurities, health profile, environmental profile, and sources. This aggregation provides stakeholders with a truly open, vendor-agnostic mechanism, which they can utilize to compare, contrast, and evaluate materials based on their impact on the environment and human health (Flux, 2015).

Komproment has developed an entirely reusable, lightweight, ventilated façade solution composed of clay shingles. With Cradle to Cradle certification, the company supplies an MP along with the product, allowing its materials and subcomponents to be documented and eventually reused (GXN & Responsible Assets, 2018). This example illustrates how an MP can record products' important data and ensure subsequent use cycles. This concept could be applied to large-scale buildings if it included energy data.

Overall, information pertaining to materials within a building is key for sustainability. In order to optimize reuse and circular principles, construction processes necessitate documentation of material and product locations, as well as how these are connected to one another. The MP represents a good initiative – it considers multi-scalar conditions and offers a platform of repository for storing, linking, and providing information on materials to relevant actors along the value chain. While the MP does take steps in reducing obstacles associated with a circular economy, it has limitations and on its own it is not sufficiently comprehensive to achieve real change across the building life cycle. Initiatives that employ an MP are successful but only address specific issues of a building at a time. Thus, supplementary information and systems are required to complete the MP. This is why BRPs and Building Passports, as addressed in the next sections, have been developed.

4.3.2 Building Renovation Passport

In an effort to ensure highly efficient and fully decarbonized building stock by 2050 and meet the 1.5°C scenario outlined in the Paris Agreement targets, annual renovation rates need to increase to a total of 2.4 percent (Camarasa et al., 2022). This can be achieved through deep renovation, raising the level of ambition for achieved energy performance, ensuring consistency between short- and long-term measures, as well as aligning individual building's performance targets with long-term targets for the entire building stock (Fabbri, 2017). There are existing methods to facilitate renovations, like the energy performance certificate (EPC), which grades buildings based on energy performance (Sayigh, 2014). However, such approaches have limited market penetration as they fail to cover the most important benefits and drivers of renovation (Fabbri, 2017).

Thus, the BRP has emerged as an evolved EPC. The BRP is a document outlining a long-term step-by-step renovation roadmap for a specific building, resulting from an on-site energy audit and fulfilling specific quality criteria and indicators established in dialogue with the building owners (Buildings Performance Institute Europe, 2016, 2017; Fabbri, 2017). BRPs involve two steps: first, on-site data gathering and, second, data processing that is adaptable to each model. This results in a comprehensive renovation roadmap, with tailored solutions that aim to achieve deep-staged, user-friendly, and personalized renovation, which contains benefits beyond just environmental, such as reduced heating bills, comfort improvement, and carbon dioxide reduction (Fabbri, 2017). To enhance the BRP, a logbook is included, which contains information about energy consumption and production. Furthermore, BRPs are innovative in that they are tailored to each homeowner, adapting renovation strategies to a specific user's financial situation, age, or household composition, for instance. These customized recommendations are presented in an attractive and motivating layout.

At its core, the BRP has five key principles. First, long-term thinking is essential to help owners plan for renovations in a consistent manner, achieve a high level of energy performance over time, and better control total cost (Fabbri, 2017). Second, the timing and sequencing of actions are important for both short- and long-term measures in order to avoid lock-ins, increase building owners' confidence, and enhance the rate of deep renovations. Customer engagement represents another important principle. Occupants' particular needs (e.g., comfort) and contexts (e.g., financial situations) need to be considered. The fourth principle is that BRPs should be attractive and user-friendly. For owners to understand the renovation process, clear visual aids are essential. Lastly, the fifth principle states that automation is a valuable tool that can be used to improve the efficient conduction of audits, and to create automated information sheets upon the completion of a building, which can be filled with specifics of the building renovation roadmap.

There are various cases that demonstrate the successful implementation of the BRP. In Belgium, for instance, the Flemish Energy Agency is developing a "Renovation Pact" that should lead to a thorough improvement of energy performance (Buildings Performance Institute Europe, 2017). They hope to integrate "renovation advice" with a digital logbook. The former will provide a roadmap to help building owners make thoughtful, forward-thinking renovation plans, while the latter collects data on energy performance, housing quality, building features, etc. This scenario promotes effective stakeholder engagement and inter-institutional cooperation. Examples of BRP implementation are most successful when they occur on the government-wide level. Moreover, an important trend among all implemented cases is the ability to add new elements and additional information to the passport over time. Hence, successful BRPs have a modular structure, which can be fed new inputs and be constantly updated. BRPs fulfill what EPCs lack – specifically, their inability to provide personalized recommendation concerning renovation options. The result is higher and deeper renovation rates, utilizing a circular logic and contributing to a more sustainable building practice.

Ultimately, both MPs and BRPs aim to make circular concepts more accessible and attractive to people. However, both are restricted to defined areas of application. For example, the MP has a focus on materials and the BRP has a focus on operational energy performance. Data on material and energy associated with renovation are equally important and need to be understood collectively. While the respective implementation of these approaches is evidently more sustainable, they may not necessarily convince stakeholders that they are beneficial. For these concepts to be more accessible and attractive, a more holistic approach is required, in which information from various fields is included, providing solid data sources for a circular built environment.

4.4 Promoting a Circular Economy through Housing Passports

Both material and building data are crucial in promoting a circular economy within the building sector. Circular materials and construction require design-for-disassembly (i.e., designing a building to be easily taken apart and put back together), as well as material efficiency and reuse. The HP aims to provide an alternative to overcome the limitations of current initiatives; it goes beyond material and energy passports by including circular implementation, policy, and economic and financing considerations, as well as social life cycle information within its structure (see Figure 4.3). Along with these supplementary concepts, the HP gathers significant components from both the material and building passports, to produce a complete digital document.

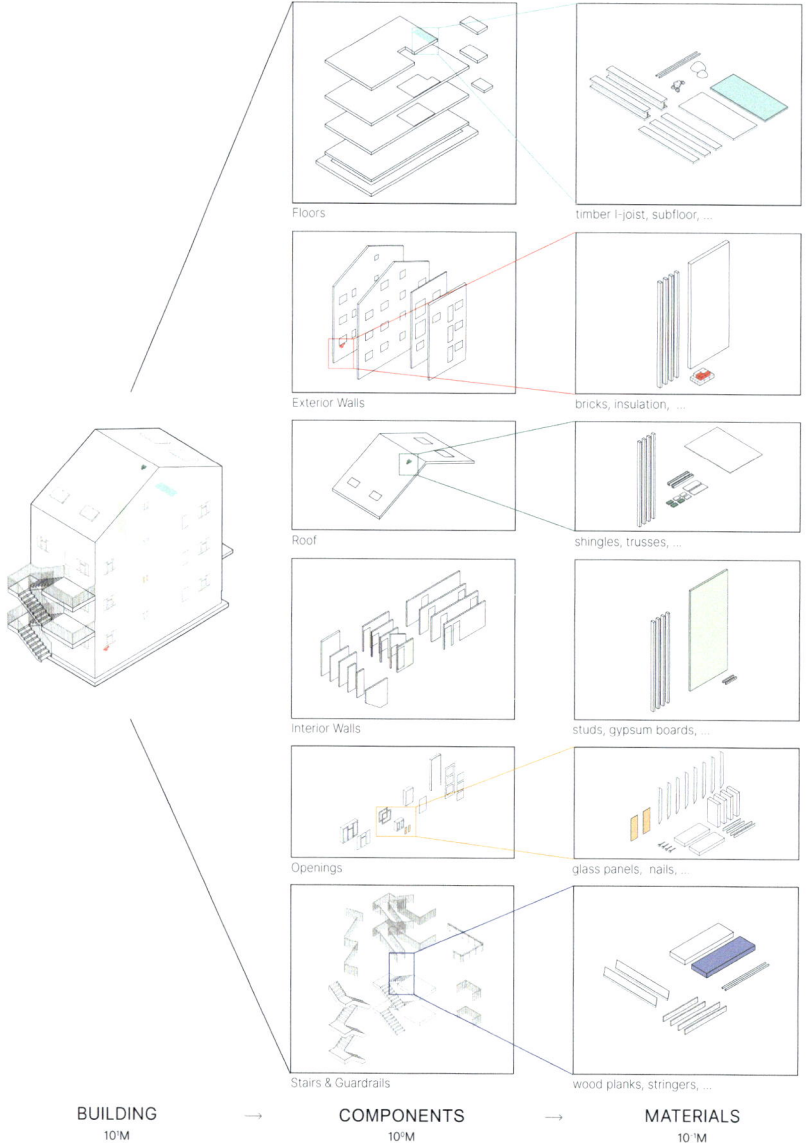

Figure 4.3 A Housing Passport (HP) Is Multi-Scalar, Documenting from the Scale of the Building to the Component and Material Scale.

4.4.1 Material and Building Characteristics within a Housing Passport

The HP utilizes information concerning materials found within the materials passport. However, beyond simply listing material characteristics, the HP demonstrates how it pertains to related circular concepts. These concepts are divided into the following categories: Health, Embodied Carbon, Operational Energy, Supply Chain, Circularity, EPDs, and Design-for-Disassembly (see Figure 4.4) (Keena & Friedman,

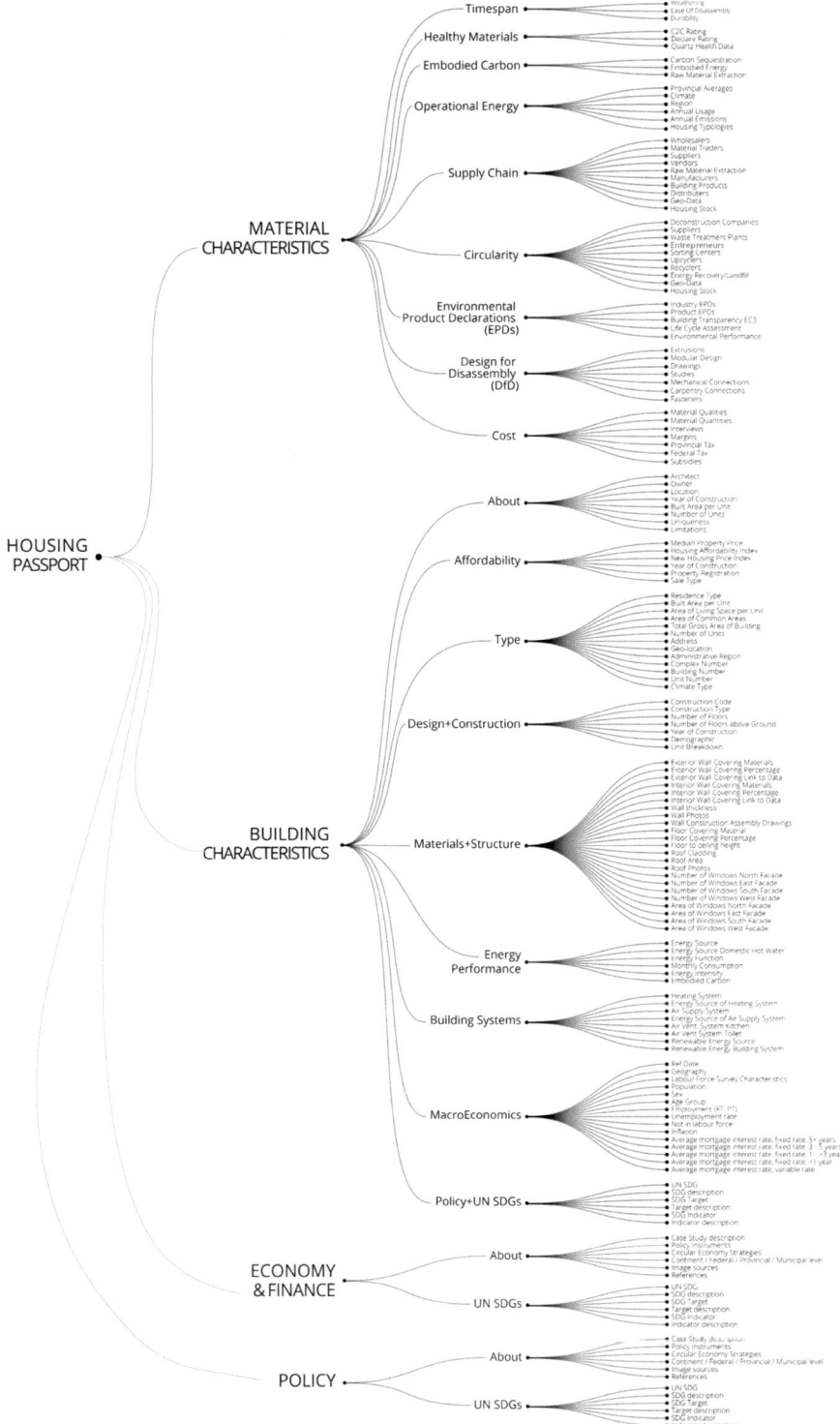

Figure 4.4 The Data Structure of a Housing Passport Toward Greater Standardization of Residential Buildings and Their Characterization.

2021; Keena et al., 2023). To achieve standardization, the HP contains an extensive number of materials, organized by material characteristics (see Figure 4.5). The HP's format permits anyone to consult any material available in the database. This allows individuals to understand a material's characteristics and to compare it to others, all within the framework of a circular economy.

Moreover, concepts found within the BRP are categorized through a standardized circular framework within the HP. Building information is distributed among the following categories: About, Affordability, Type, Size, Location and Climate, Design and Construction, Materials and Structure, Energy Performance, Building Systems, Macroeconomics, and UN Sustainable Development Goals (see Figure 4.6) (Keena & Friedman, 2021; Keena et al., 2023). Building characteristics are broken down into various types of data that potentially pertain to different individuals, are tailored to specific needs, and, therefore, render circular information more accessible and attractive.

4.4.2 Integrating Economy, Finance, and Policy within the Housing Passport

Beyond aggregating material and building characteristics, the HP includes supplementary information that contributes to, as well as benefit from, a circular economy. This diverse yet unified data allows stakeholders along the value chain to grasp the

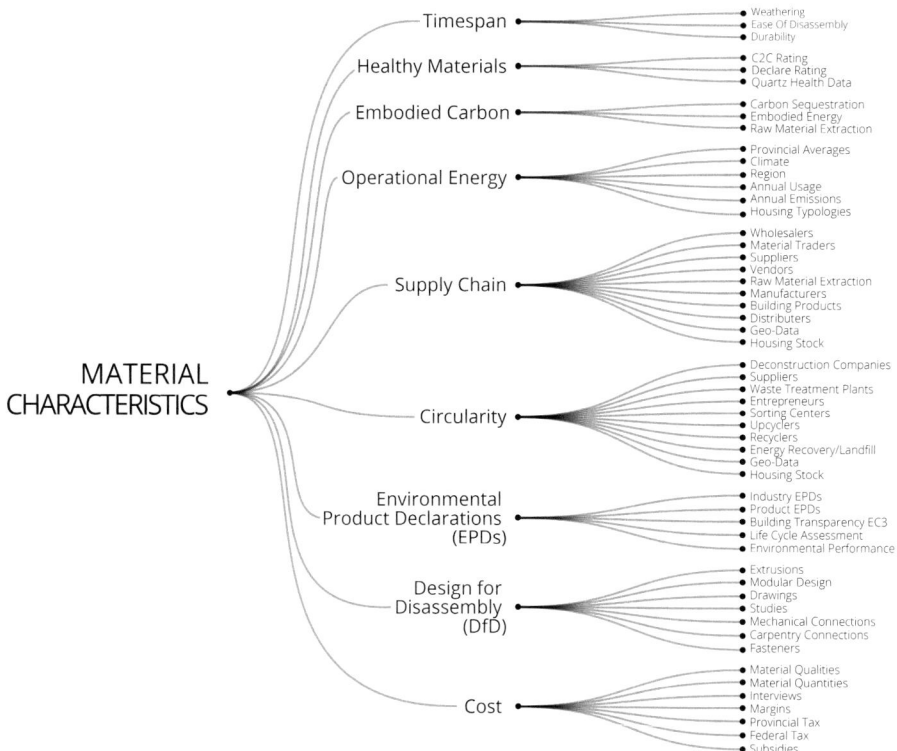

Figure 4.5 Descriptions of Material Characteristics.

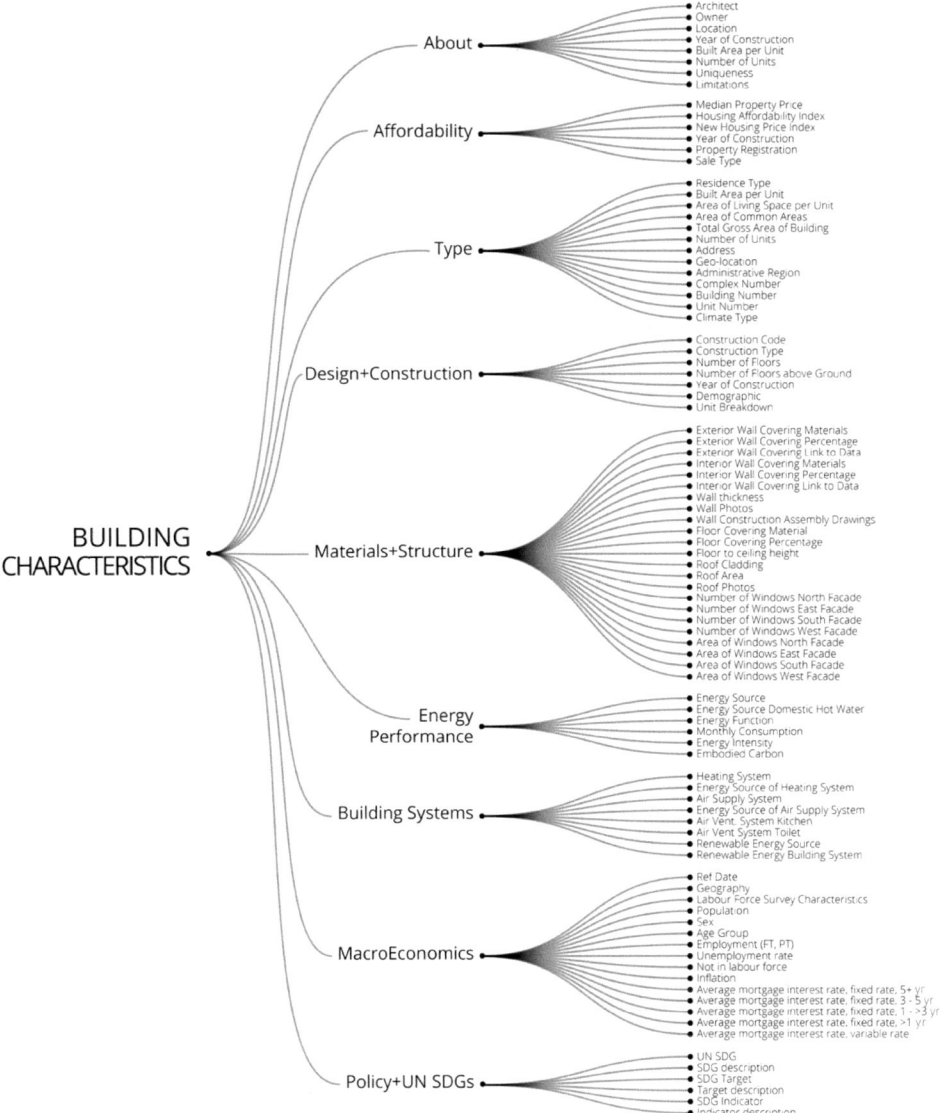

Figure 4.6 Descriptions of Building Characteristics.

significance and advantages of a circular logic. Hence, the HP integrates concepts of economy and finance, as well as policy, as illustrated in Figure 4.7, and demonstrates how a circular economy is mutually beneficial to all related actors.

Economy and Finance

HPs have the potential to render a circular economy financially desirable for building owners. Circular Financing aims to incentivize borrowers to improve the energy efficiency of their buildings or purchase energy-efficient properties through preferential

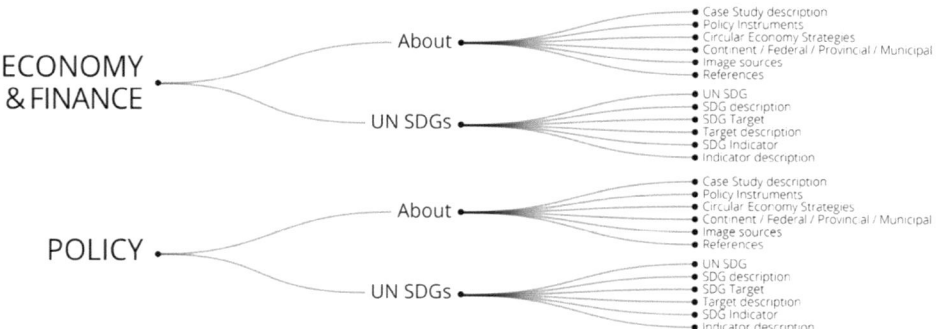

Figure 4.7 Descriptions of Economy, Finance, and Policy Characteristics.

mortgage or larger loan amounts. Energy efficient improvements are beneficial both for the clients and the financial authority involved, making it a mutually beneficial strategy going forward (Keena & Friedman, 2021).

HPs can help with financing. Various financing and economic approaches utilize building and material characteristics. From the bank's perspective, "green" homeowners prove to be lower risk borrowers (Musić, 2021). This is because, by purchasing a home that is deemed at low risk from climate change effects (e.g., poor energy performance, contributes to life cycle carbon emissions, at risk from wildfires, flooding or prolonged drought), this investment is considered safer. In North America, for instance, the US Federal Housing Administration (FHA) recently introduced the Energy Efficient Mortgage scheme, which seeks to incentivize green homebuilding by offering part of the mortgage loan to go to energy efficiency improvements that will lower an occupant's utility bills (Jensen & Sommer, 2016). Users need only to be approved for a loan amount necessary to purchase the house, not for extra energy efficiency improvement costs. This option can be attractive to some homeowners who are willing to put the effort and money into upfront energy saving renovations that will save money down the line. However, such initiatives require certain standards to be followed to lower risks for financial institutions. Before a loan can be approved, the property needs to be inspected by a certified energy specialist to ensure that green improvements will save more money than they will cost. This approach is gaining popularity in various parts of the world, most notably Europe. ABN AMRO – a leading bank in the Netherlands – provides "green loans" and sustainability discounts for applicable users. Green loans pertain to sustainable investments, including solar panels, insulation, and high-efficiency central heating boilers (ABN AMRO, 2019). Moreover, they provide customers with a "Green Guide" that shares advice and practical tips on the financial benefits of "greening up" houses. Their sustainability discount provides rebates on mortgage interest rates when purchasing a new build and for renovations.

Mortgage rates for increased affordability are implemented to incentivize and channel private capital into energy-efficient investments. While financing for energy-efficient dwellings clearly benefits the homeowner, the rationale for banks to provide such financial support is less obvious. There are two main assumptions that justify such financial incentives from the bank's perspective. First, improving a property's energy efficiency has a positive impact on the property value and, therefore, reduces a bank's asset risks. Second, the borrowers have a lower probability of default because of a household's more disposable income (due to lower energy bills), reducing the bank's credit risk. In brief, providing environmental financing options is believed to lower financial risk for banks. ABN AMRO and Barclays are two financial institutions that have initialized such programs (Keena & Friedman, 2021). Despite their growing popularity in Europe, there is hesitance to implement these policies in North America due, in part, to the uncertainty of the risk associated with the programs. To tackle this, initiatives such as Energy Efficiency Data Protocol and Portal (EeDaPP) prep reports on the correlation between energy efficiency and risk, market needs and gaps, along with other issues that would incentivize institutions.

The green financing approach demonstrates how financial institutions can incentivize their services and encourage customers to transition into energy-efficient homes. The relationship between HPs and financial institutions could be mutually beneficial. Information on HPs could provide a construction material inventory as well as data regarding the carbon performance and decarbonization potential of a property. Such information is aligned with addressing imminent new factors for funding and investment as banks and financial institutes work to achieve their climate targets for net zero emissions by 2050 (UNEP Finance Initiative, 2021). One key method to scale up and achieve sustainable development is to link the need for funding of new and renovation developments with the need to address and demonstrate the project's climate reduction strategies. Circular economy is one valuable path toward decarbonization in housing which can be monitored and tracked via HPs. Along with "green" financial, policy is key toward transitioning to a circular economy in housing.

Policy

As discussed in Chapters 1 and 3, infrastructure, construction, and design sectors all interact with the 17 UN SDGs. The building industry plays a key role in sustainability, and as seen in recent years, policies and targets are being set to reduce environmental degradation, particularly coming from the built environment. For instance, achieving the objectives agreed in the Paris Agreement to limit global temperature increase to well below 2°C from pre-industrial levels and striving for 1.5°C will require ambitious actions within the building sector. Circular economy and HPs can be a fruitful tool for policymakers to hit such targets. Bringing together housing sector stakeholders and facilitating knowledge sharing across this vast array of stakeholders (including policymakers) on the state of the built environment is critical (Keena & Friedman, 2023; Keena et al., 2023). A circular economy facilitates policymaking and incentivizes initiatives that cut greenhouse gas emissions, monitor energy performance indicators, and support mapping of building information to UN SDGs (see Figure 4.8). Moreover, policymakers can utilize HPs to gain accessible and reliable data and information on housing. Policymakers and housing sector actors alike require data to capture, administer, and manage buildings. There are currently data gaps and data barriers in the housing sector regarding building data from across the whole life cycle (Global Alliance for Buildings and Construction

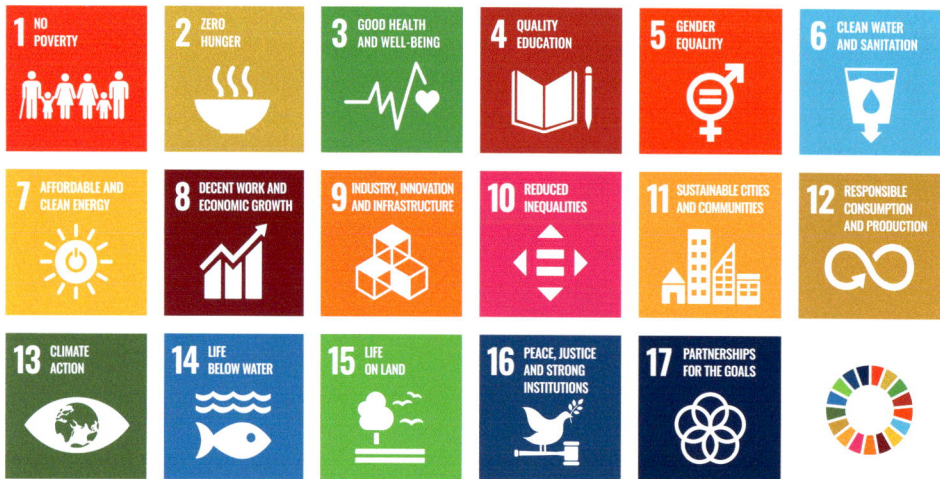

Figure 4.8 United Nations Sustainable Development Goals (UN SDGs).

and the United Nations Environment Programme, 2021). Such data is necessary for evidence-based policymaking that can facilitate sustainable policies that reduce carbon emissions and meet affordable housing demands. By promoting HPs, a more systematic and coherent approach to building-related data and information may emerge which can subsequently support a circular economy in the building industry and assist in addressing various UN SDGs. This is significant as is pointed out in Chapter 3, the housing sector contributes to almost all of the 17 UN SDGs.

4.5 Housing Passport's Semantic Data Structure and Ontology

Given the depth of data required for an HP, a data management strategy is needed that delivers an aggregation of data from multiple sources in one space. For knowledge to be widely available, such a system would need to promote accessible and searchable information. This is where metadata (i.e., information about the data) is valuable as it contextualizes the data. In addition, using semantic web technologies assists in encoding the data with metadata (Pinheiro et al., 2018). This enhances data by providing a rich collection of contextual knowledge (Keena & Friedman, 2021; Pinheiro et al., 2017). Combining acquisitions of both data and metadata to manage, organize, semantically annotate, and link circular economy housing-related data and metadata allows for the creation of a Housing Passport Knowledge Graph (HPKG). This format allows for a semantic web language, aimed to represent complex knowledge about things, groups of things, and, especially, relations between things (Beetz, 2018). Metadata is both human and machine readable and, effectively, reduces data redundancy, enables interference of the data, and facilitates complex data querying. The metadata consists of two main documents – the data dictionary (a document containing terms with their definitions, which is human readable) and a semantic data dictionary (metadata repositories) (Pinheiro et al., 2017).

HPKGs are used to support flexible representation, which can promote improved understanding and data analysis in similar settings. With data for HPs coming from different sources and different stakeholders across the housing life cycle, it's validity and accuracy lays in the fact that they typically originate from primary and secondary sources – including, architects' plans and descriptions or material manufacturers EPDs. This data structure aims to eliminate the risk of losing data accuracy associated with handoffs or data transfer points along a data life cycle.

4.6 Sensing, Tagging, and Certifying

The HP has the potential to revolutionize the building industry; however, in order to be successfully implemented, it requires tools that promote documentation, certification, as well as testing and monitoring. To promote a circular economy, the HP needs to be integrated within each phase of the building life cycle and value chain. By employing standardized policies and innovative technology, the HP can be effectively implemented.

Certification is crucial to promoting a circular economy and, therefore, needs to be implemented in the HP. Information needs to be certified, maintained, and updated with accuracy guaranteed. The use of materials with low-embodied carbon is not only beneficial for the environment, but by having valuable information on the carbon emissions associated with the manufacturing of a construction material, the process of documentation and certifying the contents of material for their future reuse is greatly facilitated. Thus, selecting materials that have an EPD, or are Cradle to Cradle certified facilitates documentation, ensures that all products only enter the final component if their contents are known. To be certified by Cradle to Cradle, for instance, contents need to be documented and accounted for down to parts per million (Jensen & Sommer, 2016). This method divides tasks of certification among many authorities, creating a dense system of certifications – contrary to the current singular general certification of building elements, which promotes a monopoly (Jensen & Sommer, 2016). Hence, if all referenced links are certified, then thorough documentation is guaranteed, allowing the production chain to verify certification of all used contents. This documentation would begin early on in a building's construction phase and would remain certified throughout its life cycle.

Furthermore, for the HP to track materials and energy during a building's use phase, it requires proper testing and monitoring. Current systems are generally manual and passive monitoring. Manual monitoring is the most common and basic technique, done through visual inspection. This technique only applies to obvious or surface-level damages and is time-consuming. Passive monitoring is quicker and more favorable, as data is obtained through low-tech measures. By attaching sensors to elements, a status is constantly measured and when affected, sensors give simple visual clues

(Jensen & Sommer, 2016). Ideally, a building's status would be constantly measured, allowing information about material – such as temperature and moisture – to be accessible in real time. This would require building components be embedded with sensors that can communicate the state to the passport. However, this would require a high level of technological input and overhaul of the construction sector which is notoriously sluggish to change. While certain successful tagging systems have emerged – namely using radio frequency identification, such as with ear tags for cattle – building components require more complex and long-lasting technology that has yet to be developed, as depicted in Figure 4.9. Optimizing monitoring and testing would make thorough documentation achievable and certification facilitated, effectively promoting recycling and reuse, ultimately, circular economy in the building sector.

Finally, for the HP to be effectively implemented, a global and unified approach needs to be taken. Standardization of the HP, and its implementation, is required, preferably at the government level. Luxembourg's Product Circularity Data Sheet (PCDS) is a good example of the potential of implementing a standardized document at the government level. The hope is for each product to have an internationally accepted dataset that describes all relevant circular information in controlled and auditable statements (+ImpaKT Luxembourg, 2020). This system standardizes data through PCDS, making it accessible and allowing others to establish how circular a product is. The PCDS helps avoid reintroducing no longer accepted chemicals – according to Cradle to Cradle – allowing for a closed and clean loop. Hence, Luxembourg's initiative represents a method of achieving standardization. For the HP to succeed, a cohesive approach and regulation in building practices needs to be adhered to.

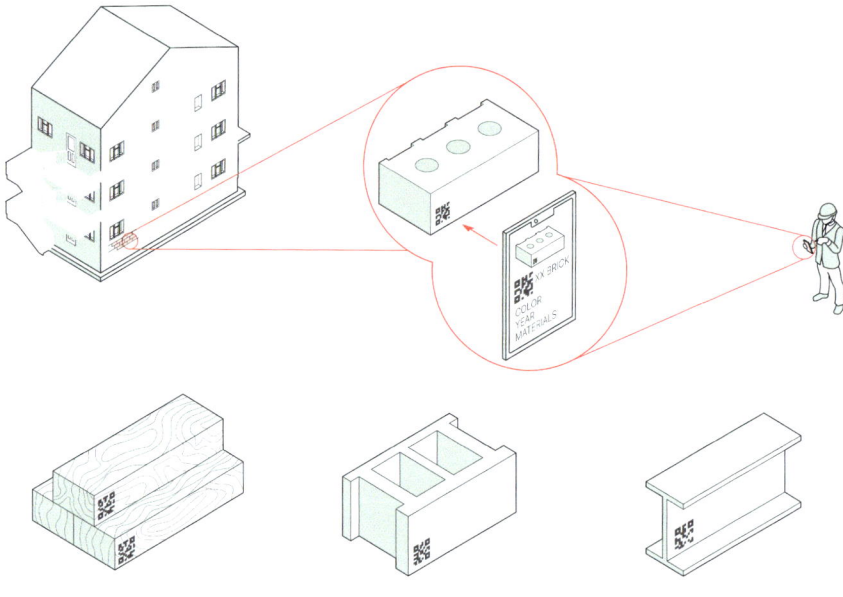

Source: ORMS, "Material Passports"

Figure 4.9 Sensing and Tagging Materials and Components Via QR Codes Can Facilitate Their Regulation and Certification throughout Their Life Cycle.

4A

Project:
BAMB – Buildings as Material
Banks

Location:
Europe

Year:
2015–2019

Team:
European Horizon 2020
Research Project with 15
partners from 7 European
countries.

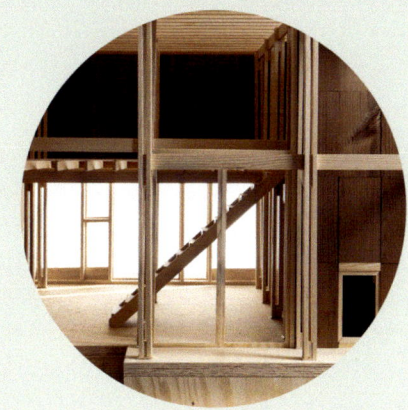

**Mapping to Circular
Economy Framework:**

CIRCULAR ECONOMY PRACTICES

LIFE CYCLE PHASES

Recovery · Life Extension · Sharing Platforms · Service Models · Regenerate · Virtualize

- Work of Geobiosphere
- Sourcing
- Manufacturing
- Design & Construction
- Use
- End-of-Use

LAYERS + LIFESPAN
Structural Layers | Long Life
Skin, MEP Layers | Medium Life
Interior Layers | Short Life

Site 100+yr   Structure 50+yr
Exterior 25+yr   System 15+yr
Partition 10+yr   Stuff 1+yr

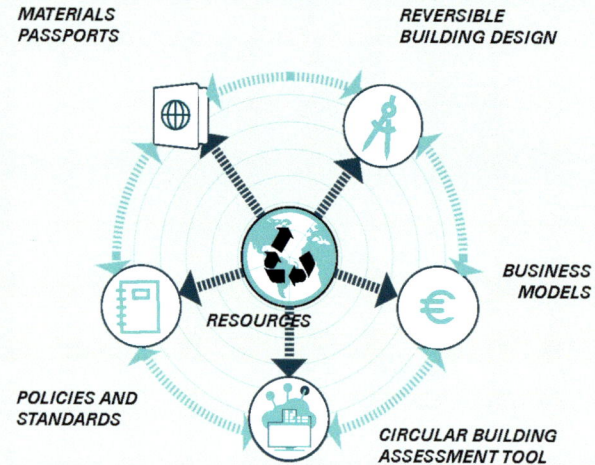

**MATERIALS
PASSPORTS**

**REVERSIBLE
BUILDING DESIGN**

**BUSINESS
MODELS**

RESOURCES

**POLICIES AND
STANDARDS**

**CIRCULAR BUILDING
ASSESSMENT TOOL**

**Figure 4.10 BAMB's
Framework for a Circular
Construction Ecosystem.**

BAMB, or Buildings as Material Banks, is a European research project that sought to increase circular practices in the construction industry and increase material value by promoting and facilitating the recycling of building components (see Figure 4.10). The project was a collaboration between 15 partners from across Europe, funded in their research by the European Commission within Horizon 2020, which aims to create sustainable development throughout the continent. The BAMB project has contributed to the possibility of a circular built environment through an exploration of circular business models, policies, and standards, reversible building design, building assessment, and crucially, MPs.

Electronic MPs developed through BAMB aim to provide "suppliers, builders, architects, users, and next users" a set of all necessary information regarding a material's characteristics to aid in recovery and reuse (see Figure 4.11) (BAMB2020, 2018).

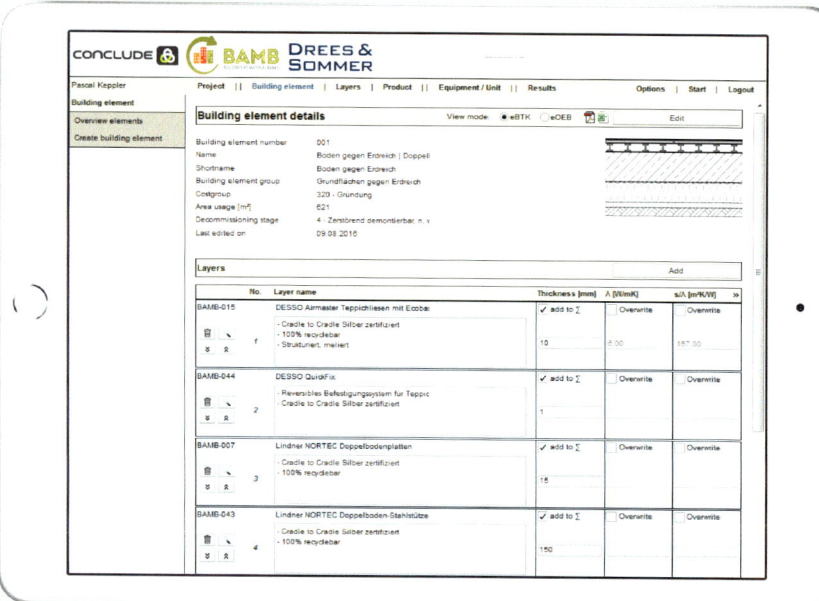

**Figure 4.11 A Page
from the Online
BAMB Tool Showing
Building Element
Details.**

Through standardizing currently scattered data into digital descriptions, the passport equips stakeholders with the knowledge to generate effective circular economy decision-making. BAMB's passport allows for the integration of circular economy principles across all building life cycle phases, with four key stages of intervention being (1) design, (2) construction, (3) use, and (4) end-of-use (Debacker et al., 2017).

MPs promote environmentally favorable material sourcing and design by giving stakeholders involved in the process a better understanding of the potential effects of product, material, and design decisions. This tool was put to the test in one of BAMB's six pilot projects: BRIC – Build Reversible in Conception – a wood-based structure designed to be assembled, disassembled, reconfigured, and reassembled multiple times (see Figures 4.12 and 4.13). All components on the structure were marked with

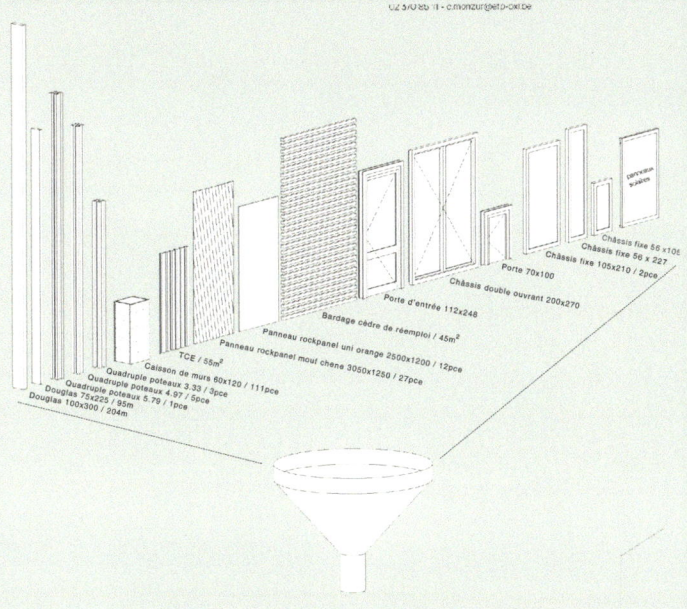

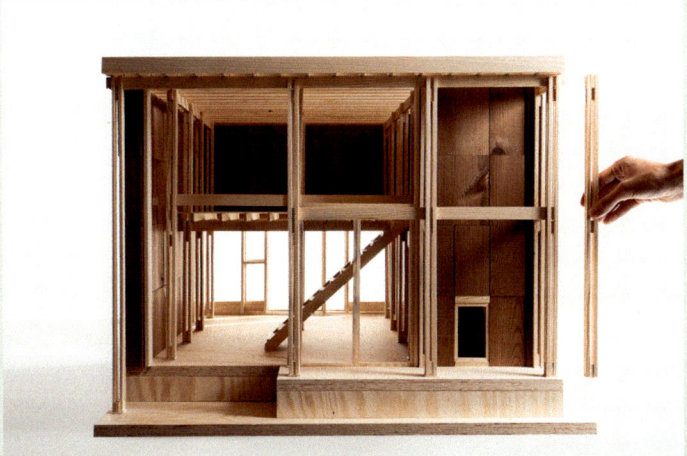

Figure 4.12 Example of Material Inventory for Build Reversible in Conception (BRIC) Design.

117

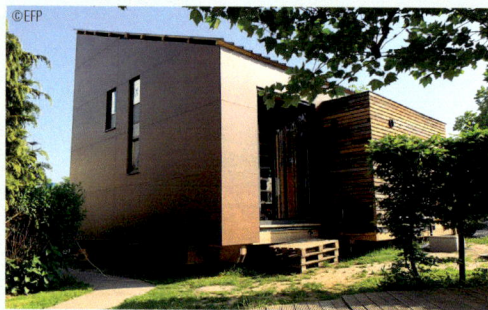

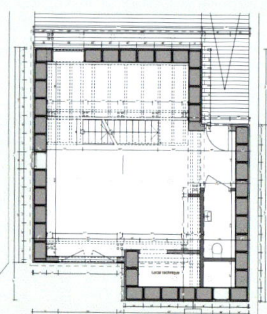

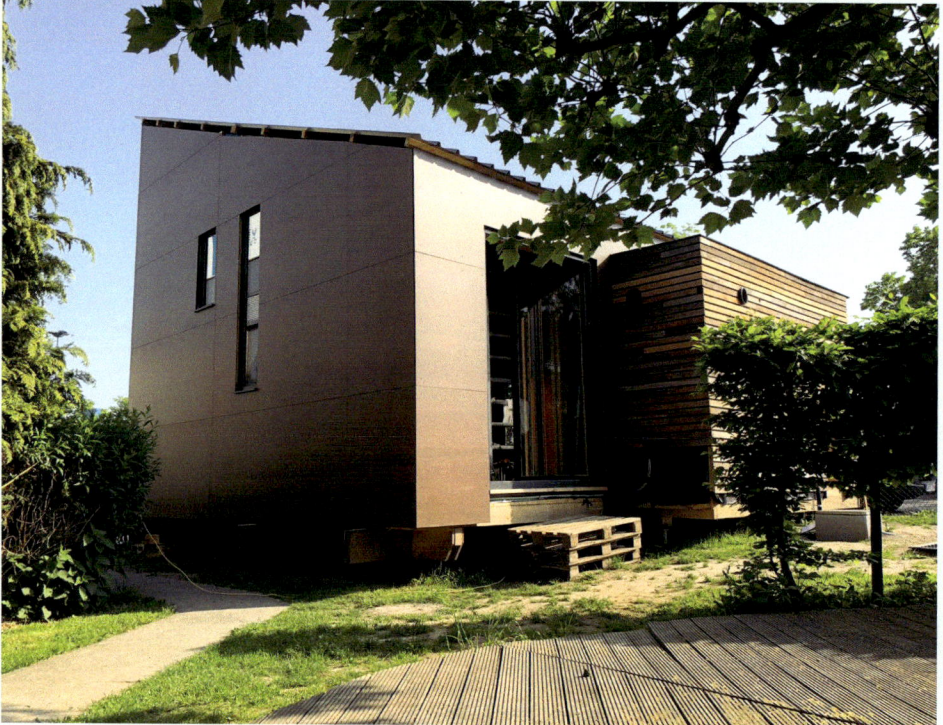

Figure 4.13 View of West and South Facades (left) and BRIC Ground Floor Plan (right).

a barcode to provide material information and were assembled in a digital database to describe the materials of the entire system (see Figure 4.11). By introducing the MP during the project conception, architects and designers are encouraged to consider future uses of materials, ideally selecting products and systems with high reuse and recyclability potential. MPs also empower stakeholders involved in the design phase to ensure long-term quality and deliver dwellings capable of repurpose, resulting in product life extension.

The results of increased **recovery and recycling** and **product life extension** are similarly observed in the **construction** phase of a project. MPs developed by BAMB have an accessible design, featuring a product's illustration, description, color, dimensions, price, name, and contact of seller. The user-friendly design improves material efficiency and organization on construction sites and provides instruction for material connections and construction practices that ensure future reuse (see Figure 4.12).

Conventionally, the actors involved in these earlier life cycle phases are not connected to the **usage** and operation, or **end-of-life** of a dwelling. MPs transfer valuable information about construction, maintenance, and reuse opportunities to residents, who may replace products or take on renovations, as well as to parties involved in repurposing or demolishing efforts. Through considering circular material and design choices from conception of a project, reuse is optimized throughout a building's life. A **virtual** platform and user-friendly barcodes allow communication and connections between stakeholders involved in housing (Figure 4.14). The connection formed between life cycle phases, creating open information transfer, is what makes BAMB's MP such a powerful tool to achieve circularity in the building sector.

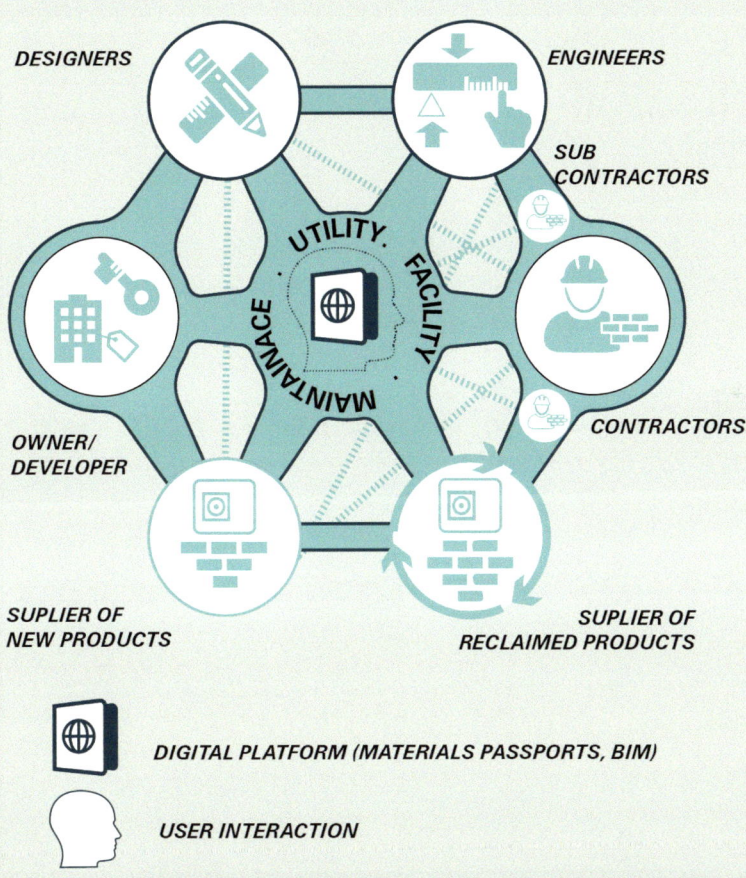

Figure 4.14 A Value Network that Enables Collaboration via the Use of Digital Tools.

4B

Project:
Circle House Demonstrator

Location:
Lisbjerg, Denmark

Year:
2018

Team:
Lejerbo (Client), GXN
Innovation, MT Højgaard,
Danish Building Research
Institute (SBi), The Danish
Association for Responsible
Construction.

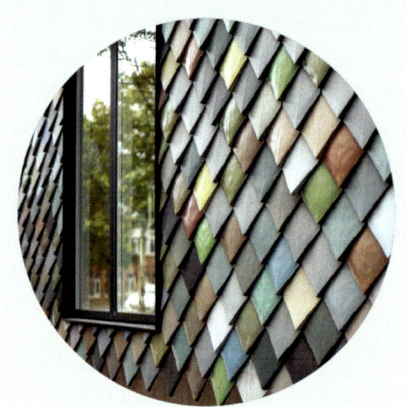

**Mapping to Circular
Economy Framework:**

CIRCULAR ECONOMY PRACTICES

LIFE CYCLE PHASES

	Recovery	Life Extension	Sharing Platforms	Service Models	Regenerate	Virtualize
Work of Geobiosphere						
Sourcing						
Manufacturing						
Design & Construction						
Use						
End-of-Use						

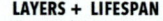
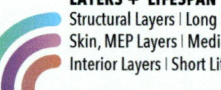

LAYERS + LIFESPAN
Structural Layers | Long Life
Skin, MEP Layers | Medium Life
Interior Layers | Short Life

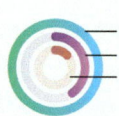

Site 100+yr Structure 50+yr
Exterior 25+yr System 15+yr
Partition 10+yr Stuff 1+yr

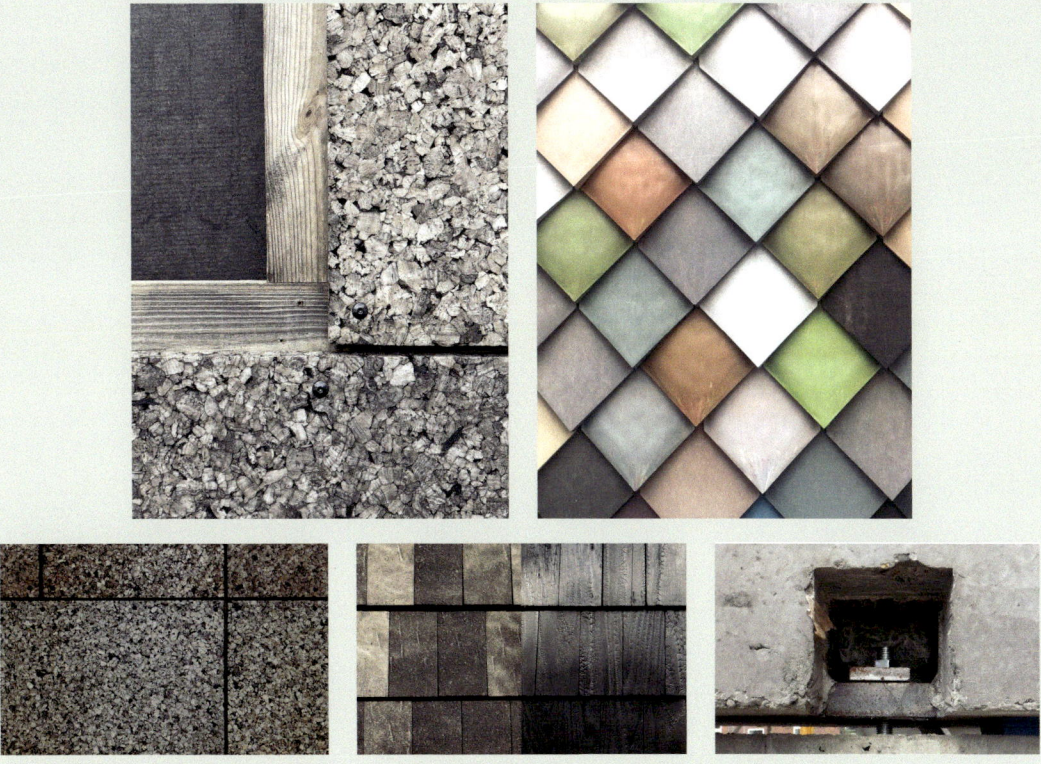

Figure 4.15 (Top left) Reclaimed Cork, (Top right) Recycled Plastic Shingles, (Bottom left) Expanded Cork Boards, (Bottom middle) Reclaimed Wood, and (Bottom right) Design-for-Disassembly Concrete Detail.

GXN Innovation, in collaboration with Lendager Group, Vandkunsten, and 3XN architects, is another group at the forefront of the circularity movement, working to implement MPs. The team utilized a digital model using BIM software to be used as an interactive information bank accessible to all stakeholders. Circle House Demonstrator is a dwelling prototype used as a case study by GXN to explore a 3D MP as a method to implement circular design and practices for affordable and sustainable housing (GXN & Responsible Assets, 2018). Named the "demonstrator", the unit explores the circular economy frameworks of **recovery and recycling**, **product life extension**, and **service models**, each facilitated by the **virtualization** of material information in the form of MPs.

GXN implements **recovery and recycling** through the selection of materials with the possibility of reuse and connections designed for disassembly and reassembly (see Figure 4.15). The documentation of all material and product choices achieves these goals by encouraging architects and construction contractors to consider circular products and construction techniques. Figure 4.16 illustrates the overall general system of the demonstrator design. Circle House features many instances of repurposed materials, including recycled plastic siding, reclaimed wood and cork partitions (see Figures 4.15 and 4.17), and upcycled furniture. Through the implementation of MPs, environmentally sensitive material sourcing becomes the

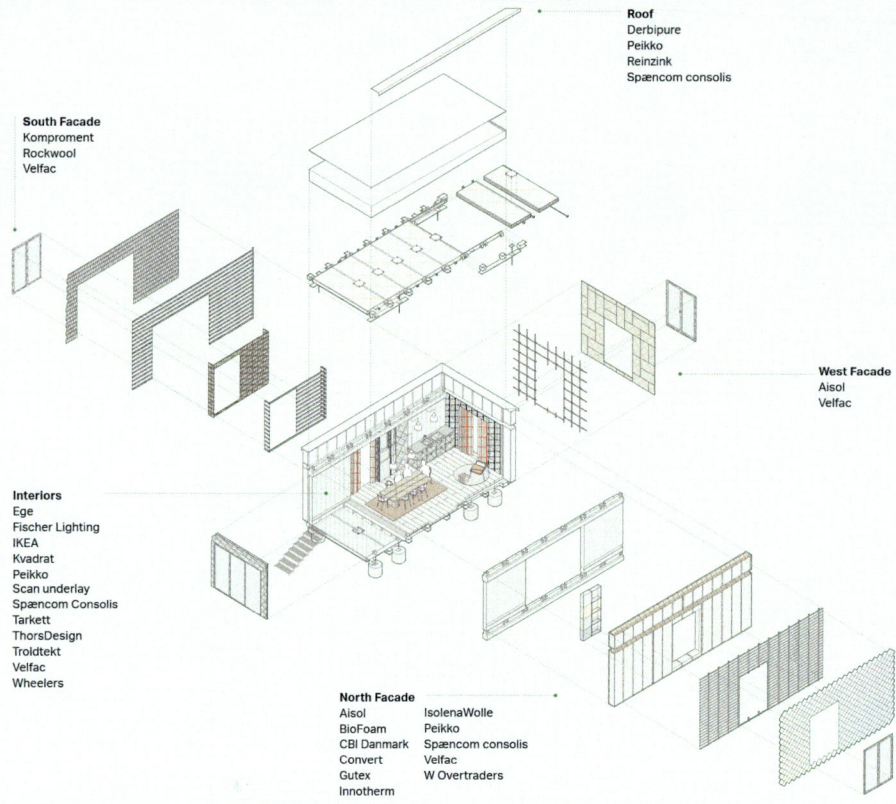

Roof
Derbipure
Peikko
Reinzink
Spæncom consolis

South Facade
Kromproment
Rockwool
Velfac

West Facade
Aisol
Velfac

Interiors
Ege
Fischer Lighting
IKEA
Kvadrat
Peikko
Scan underlay
Spæncom Consolis
Tarkett
ThorsDesign
Troldtekt
Velfac
Wheelers

North Facade
Aisol   IsolenaWolle
BioFoam   Peikko
CBI Danmark   Spæncom consolis
Convert   Velfac
Gutex   W Overtraders
Innotherm

Figure 4.16 Circular House Demonstrator: General System.

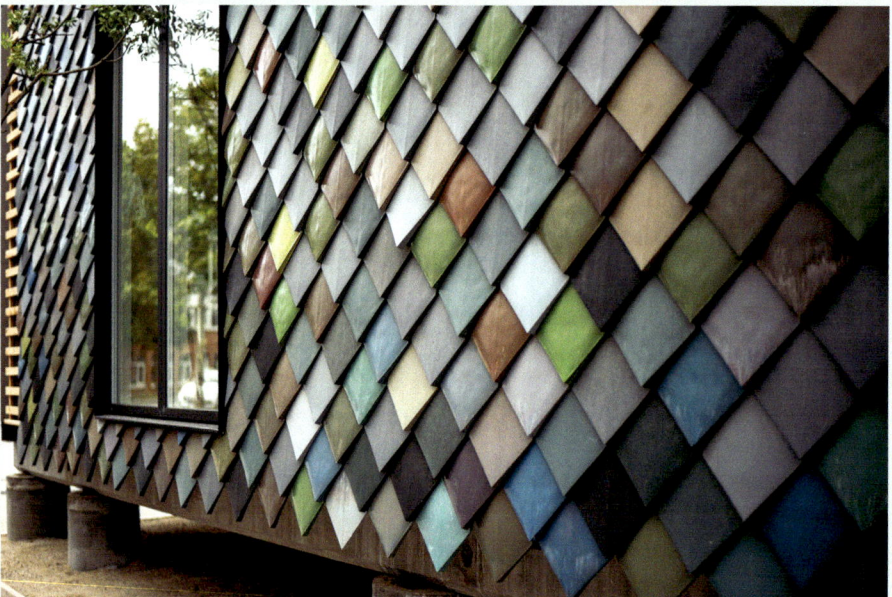

Figure 4.17 Each Façade of the Circle House Showcased a Potential Reuse Facade System; Here Recycled Plastic Shingles.

responsibility of architects, who are connected virtually to all life cycle phases of a building. The housing development is composed of six basic concrete elements designed for easy construction, disassembly, and reuse. Irreversible construction techniques like welding are avoided, and visible joints are designed to limit waste at the end-of-use phase (see Figure 4.18).

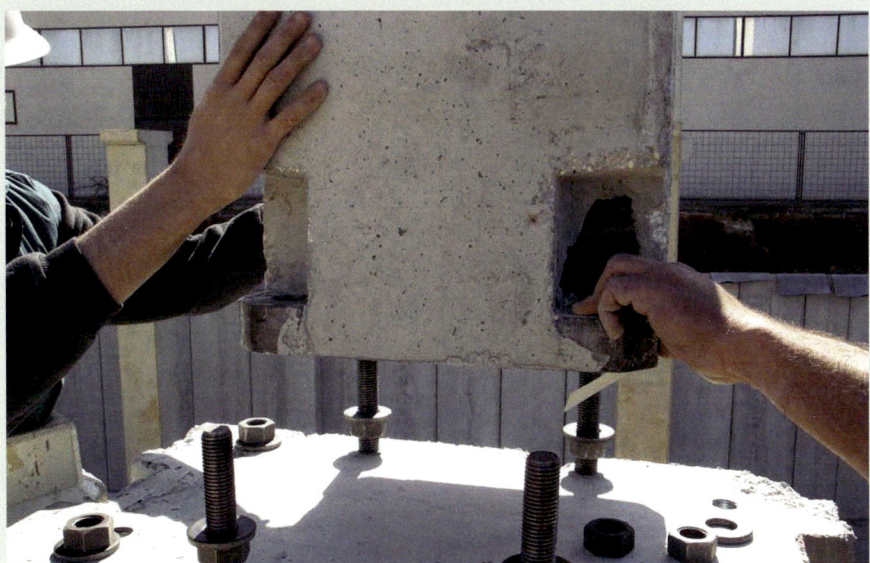

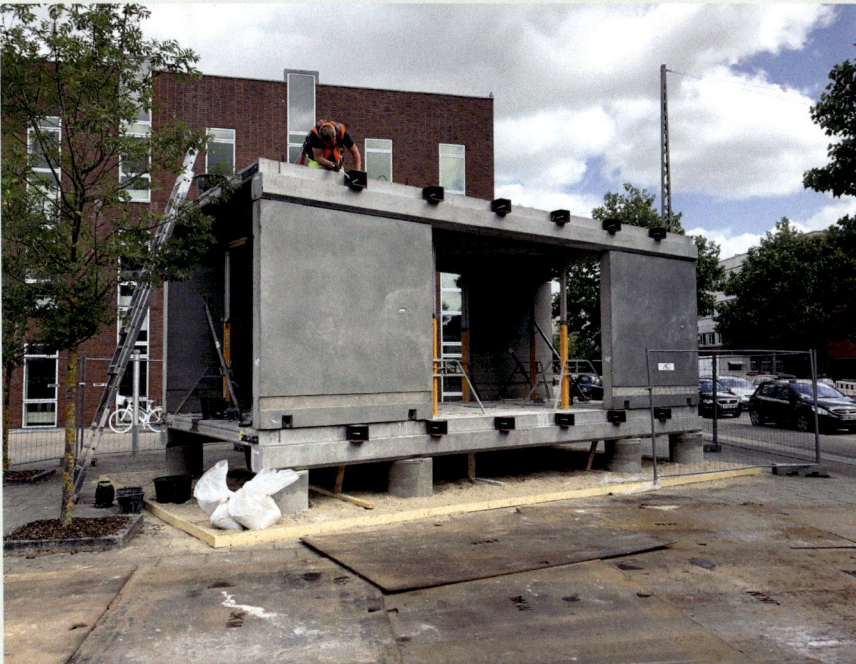

Figure 4.18 The Circle House Under Construction Including a De-constructable Mechanical Connection for Prefabricated Concrete Elements.

The circular economy principle of **product life extension** is achieved through the team's goals to achieve standardization, maintenance, and transition of material information through the Circle House case study. The project is wonderfully simple and succinct as a dwelling form, which lets the materials shine while allowing the building to fit into a larger system of units in the future. The simplicity of form allows for interior adaptations when required by residents and promotes a flexible arrangement of units to provide multifamily housing. These future changes are taken into consideration in the design of the dwelling, promoting renovation and repurposing rather than demolition at the end-of-use phase. MPs contain all necessary information regarding a project's material and systems, including instructions for correct maintenance during the use phase. Proper maintenance is essential to preserving the value of materials. The virtual datasets also ensure the smooth transition between ownership, meaning all information regarding handling of materials is gathered and easily transferred.

The digital tracking of materials facilitates GXN's integration of **service models** within Circle House. By framing a business model as service-centric instead of product-centric places the responsibility of material quality and longevity on the manufacturer. Circle House demonstrates the possibility of service models to provide carpeting and flooring on a *return-to-seller* basis (GXN & Responsible Assets, 2018). Floorboards are typically fit for reuse at the end-of-use phase of a building but are often scrapped and incinerated following demolition. GXN, in contrast, partnered with local manufacturers who agreed to accept returned floorboards and upcycle them as wall panels. Similarly, carpeting within the dwelling is returned to the manufacturer after use to be regenerated as new yarn and reused. A circular approach to manufacturing through service models is economically viable and beneficial for all parties involved and minimizes unnecessary and all-too-common waste. Circle House is an illustration of the possibilities that occur from proper collaboration within the housing sector. This sharing of information is vital to achieve wide reaching change within the construction industry and transition to a sustainable built environment.

4.7 Conclusion

The building industry plays a vital role in sustainability. It has the power to influence the environmental impact of a building positively or negatively. Achieving a circular economy is key but requires a shift in how stakeholders approach building. While there are currently initiatives aimed at optimizing materials and energy after their end-of-use phases, the lack of an aggregated, standardized, and universal approach makes it difficult to achieve change. Thus, the HP represents an innovative concept, capable of achieving a unified circular logic within the building industry. Through documentation, tracking, and certifying, all building components can ultimately be repurposed after use. The HP's "nesting" structure allows for facilitated and organized data. Through proper organization, it has the potential to benefit all related stakeholders along the value chain. This concept reaches far beyond the building industry and can contribute to financial institutions, as well as global policies. However, HP is currently limited by a few factors. First, it requires tools and technology capable of tracking building components throughout their life cycle. Moreover, for this concept to be effective, it requires a standardized HP with unified implementation. The largest barrier, however, remains a general lack of knowledge and understanding of the topic. Therefore, by shedding light on the varied and vast benefits of a circular logic, and making this information easily accessible, the HP has the potential to become a major contributor to a circular built environment. By promoting cost-reduction strategies, as seen in the following chapter, stakeholders will be more inclined to unite on a standardized approach to housing.

References

+ImpaKT Luxembourg. (2020). *Product circularity data sheet (PCDS) v3.2s*. Retrieved January 24 from https://pcds.lu/wp-content/uploads/2020/11/20200214_Light_PCDS_v3.2s_FORM.pdf

ABN AMRO. (2019). *ABN AMRO Groenbank: Green savings, green financing*. Retrieved January 24 from https://www.abnamro.com/en/news/abn-amro-groenbank-green-savings-green-financing

BAMB2020. (2018). *Material passports* [Video]. YouTube. Retrieved January 24, 2023, from https://www.youtube.com/watch?v=9pB6axd7gQk

Beetz, J. (2018). *Structured vocabularies in construction: Classifications, taxonomies and ontologies*. Springer International Publishing.

Buildings Performance Institute Europe. (2016). *Building renovation passport – Customised roadmaps towards deep renovations and better homes*. http://bpie.eu/wp-content/uploads/2017/01/Building-Passport-Report_2nd-edition.pdf

Buildings Performance Institute Europe. (2017). *Building renovation passports: Consumer's journey to a better home*. https://www.bpie.eu/publication/building-renovation-passports-consumers-journey-to-a-better-home/

Camarasa, C., Mata, É, Navarro, J. P. J., Reyna, J., Bezerra, P., Angelkorte, G. B., Feng, W., Filippidou, F., Forthuber, S., Harris, C., Sandberg, N. H., Ignatiadou, S., Kranzl, L., Langevin, J., Liu, X., Müller, A., Soria, R., Villamar, D., Dias, G. P., ... Yaramenka, K. (2022). A global comparison of building decarbonization scenarios by 2050 towards 1.5–2 °C targets. *Nature Communications*, *13*(1), 3077. https://doi.org/10.1038/s41467-022-29890-5

Cradle to Cradle. (2022). *What is cradle to cradle certified?* Retrieved January 24 from https://www.c2ccertified.org/get-certified/product-certification

Debacker, W., Manshoven, S., Peters, M., Ribeiro, A., & De Weerdt, Y. (2017). Circular economy and design for change within the built environment: preparing the transition. In *Proceedings of the International HISER Conference on Advances in Recycling and Management of Construction and Demolition Waste* (p. 114). 2017, June 21–23, Delft University of Technology, Delft, The Netherlands.

Fabbri, M. (2017). *Understanding building renovation passports: Customised solutions to boost deep renovation and increase comfort in a decarbonised Europe.* In *ECEEE 2017 summer study on energy efficiency: Consumption, efficiency and limits*, France. https://www.eceee.org/library/conference_proceedings/eceee_Summer_Studies/2017/6-buildings-policies-directives-and-programmes/understanding-building-renovation-pass-ports-customised-solutions-to-boost-deep-renovation-and-increase-comfort-in-a-decar-bonised-europe/

Flux. (2015). *Flux, HBN, thinkstep and Google collaborate to launch the quartz database at VERGE 2015 – Quartz project.* https://healthybuilding.net/blog/203-flux-hbn-thinkstep-and-google-collaborate-to-launch-the-quartz-database-at-verge-2015

Global Alliance for Buildings and Construction and the United Nations Environment Programme. (2021). *The building passport: A tool for capturing whole life data in construction and real estate – Practical guidelines*. https://globalabc.org/news/new-report-building-passport-practical-guidelines

GXN & Responsible Assets. (2018). *Circle house: Denmark's first circular housing project* (1st ed., Vol. 248). GXN.

Heinrich, M., & Lang, W. (2019). *Materials passport – best practice – innovative solutions for a transition to a circular economy in the built environment*. Technische Universität München.

Hertwich, E., Lifset, R., Pauliuk, S., Heeran, N., & United Nations Environment Programme. (2020). *Resource efficiency and climate change: Material efficiency strategies for a low-carbon future*. United Nations Environment Programme. https://www.unep.org/resources/report/resource-efficiency-and-climate-change-material-efficiency-strategies-low-carbon

Jensen, K. G., & Sommer, J. (2016). *Building a circular future* (3rd ed.). GXN Innovation. http://www.buildingacircularfuture.com/book

Keena, N., & Friedman, A. (2021). *Circular economy and the housing supply change – toward affordability and sustainability*. McGill School of Architecture.

Keena, N., & Friedman, A. (2023). *Data homebase*. https://datahomebase.research.mcgill.ca/

Keena, N., Friedman, A., Parsaee, M., & Klein, A. (2023). *Data visualization for a circular economy: Designing a web application for sustainable housing*. Technology I Architecture + Design, 7:2, 262–281, DOI: 10.1080/24751448.2023.2246803

Musić, R. (2021). Building the business case for green affordable housing. *Enterprise Development and Microfinance*, *32*(3), 179–191. https://doi.org/10.3362/1755-1986.21-00013

Olivier, J., Saadé-Sbeih, M., Shaked, S., Jolliet, A., & Crettaz, P. (2016). *Environmental life cycle assessment*. CRC Press. https://doi.org/10.1201/b19138

Pinheiro, P., McGuinness, D. L., & Santos, H. (2017). *Human-aware sensor network ontology: Semantic support for empirical data collection*. https://doi.org/10.48550/arXiv.1704.01806

Pinheiro, P., Santos, H., Liang, Z., Liu, Y., Rashid, S. M., McGuinness, D. L., & Bax, M. P. (2018). *HADatAc: A framework for scientific data integration using ontologies*. In Proceedings of the ISWC 2018 Posters & Demonstrations, Industry and Blue Sky Ideas Tracks Co-Located with the 17th International Semantic Web Conference (ISWC 2018) (p. 2180). http://ceur-ws.org/Vol-2180/paper-49.pdf

Platform CB'23. (2020). *Passports for the construction sector*. https://platformcb23.nl/images/downloads/Platform_CB23_Guide_Passports_for_the_construction_sector_2.0.pdf

Quartz. (2015). *The quartz common products database*. Retrieved January 24 from https://quartzproject.org/

Sayigh, A. (2014). *Sustainability, energy and architecture: Case studies in realizing green buildings* (1st ed.). Academic Press. http://www.sciencedirect.com/science/book/9780123972699

UNEP Finance Initiative. (2021). *Guidelines for climate target setting for banks*. https://www.unepfi.org/industries/banking/guidelines-for-climate-target-setting-for-banks/

Chapter 5

Cost-Reduction Strategies and Material Re-Use

5.1 Introduction

Substantial global increases in property prices have made home ownership out of reach for many, especially younger generations. Affordable housing has slightly different definitions around the world, but in general, housing should not impede households from meeting other basic costs of living and should be adequate in quality and location (UN Habitat for a Better Urban Future, 2019). In Canada, for example, affordable housing is defined as costing less than 30 percent of a household's income before taxes (see Figure 5.1) (Canada Mortgage and Housing Cooperation, 2018). The affordability crisis affects not only buyers but renters as well, as rent prices have followed a similar trend and are soaring in many cities. Governing bodies have put in motion a variety of proposed solutions with little success, as the market continues to be driven upward by increased demand and the rise of construction and infrastructure costs. The issue of affordability is fundamentally tied to environmental issues, and unfortunately, our current linear economic system prioritizes profit at the expense of citizens' financial and environmental security. This chapter will explore our current affordability crisis through the lens of a circular economy, proposing circular thinking as a holistic solution to this multifaceted issue. This chapter begins by observing housing at the scale of community development, moving in closer to the scale of single lots or developments, and finally at the scale of products and materials.

Designing communities with affordability and accessibility as priorities inevitably leads to designing neighborhoods that last, with less consumed material and lower environmental impacts. In scaling cities to the human scale, thoughtfully designed dense housing becomes an affordable solution without compromising comfort, privacy, and livability. In careful and knowledgeable site selection, costs related to environmental challenges of a site and infrastructure are greatly reduced. Planning communities with appropriate allocation and design of residential lots, open spaces, and streets can lower costs and avoid early demolition with harmful financial and environmental impacts. Infill housing, being the redevelopment of empty lots or existing buildings, utilizes the established infrastructure of existing urban neighborhoods to create affordable housing within a community.

The idea of density is carried through to affordability at the scale of individual projects, as a decrease in the footprint of a dwelling is closely connected to decreases in the cost of construction and maintenance. With creative design, smaller homes can provide comfort and privacy while being more sustainable and affordable. A simplification of form and the attachment of multiple dwellings can considerably lower costs of materials and achieve greater energy efficiency. In employing these strategies as

DOI: 10.4324/9781003333975-7

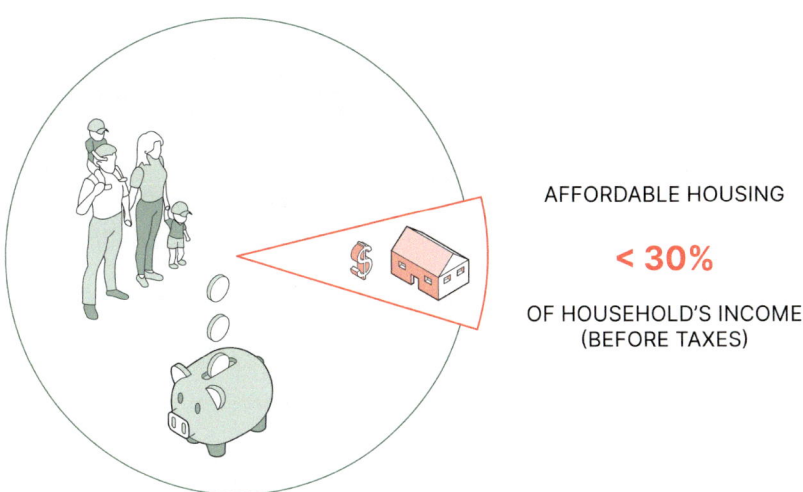

AFFORDABLE HOUSING

< 30%

OF HOUSEHOLD'S INCOME
(BEFORE TAXES)

Figure 5.1 The Canadian Mortgage and Housing Corporation Defines Affordable Housing as Costing Less than 30 Percent of a Household's Income before Taxes.

they will be further explained, as well as utilizing appropriate building composition depending on site conditions, dwellings can be affordable, environmentally considerate, and comfortable all at once.

Using circular economy strategies, costs can be reduced while benefitting the environment. The reuse of materials and urban mining is cost-effective circular economy strategies, seeing construction, renovation, and demolition debris as untapped resources rather than waste. These strategies will be defined and explored in this chapter, with an in-depth look at the obstacles and the potentials of implementing strategies for the reuse, recycling, and upcycling of materials in the construction sector. As seen employed locally, material passports and inventories have the potential to bridge the affordability gap.

5.2 Planning Affordable Communities

Tackling the issue of affordable housing begins with the design of communities to support dense living with adequate infrastructure and amenities. Affordable housing is a broad term that can include housing initiated by the private, public, and non-profit sectors and may come in the form of temporary permanent rental, ownership, and cooperative ownership (Canada Mortgage and Housing Cooperation, 2018). The planning of communities to provide opportunity for affordable housing can and should, therefore, be considered in any new or existing developments, to promote equal opportunity among groups in a diversifying market. The Benny Fam residential development in Montreal, Canada, is a strong example of such an affordable and equitable development (see Case Study: Benny Farm). Indeed, the once homogeneous client base of the housing market is changing from the traditional nuclear family to a mixed demographic of single parents, individual buyers, and seniors, among others (see Chapter 1). The widening gap between household income and home price supports the need for cost-effective planning and development strategies.

5.2.1 Infrastructure and Land Use Designations

Significant cost reduction occurs when densely populated residential areas share common infrastructure. Urban infrastructure includes utility services such as water, waste management, and electricity, as well as transportation, parks and open spaces, community services for emergencies, and public and social health (Raghav et al., 2019). Linear infrastructure like roads, transit, electricity, and water distribution have a great potential for cost reductions when serving a high population density as they require fewer kilometers of costly road or pipeline construction and maintenance to serve a large community (see Figure 5.2). Single loading roads, having roads with development on only one side, result in higher costs per resident, and therefore, double loading should be the objective in an affordable development.

A dense development lowers cost, both financial and environmental, in material and construction that can result in great savings for residents. A dense neighborhood, though, necessitates appropriate public and commercial amenities (e.g., schools, parks, entertainment, and grocery) to be integrated into its initial planning so that the original development can be successful and therefore long lasting. The division of land use to include adequate services and commercial opportunity is an integral process that can avoid costly and wasteful demolition and construction to keep up with the needs of a dense population.

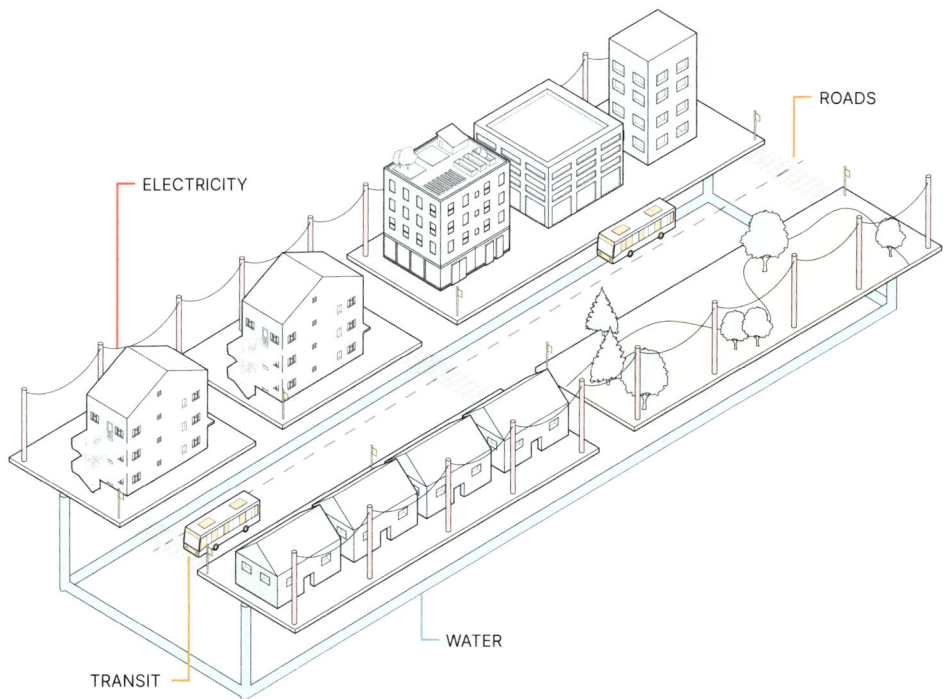

Figure 5.2 Result of Density on Linear Infrastructure Needs.

5.2.2 Residential Lots and Density

As rising land value is one of the main causes of high-priced housing, a key aspect of building affordably is utilizing space efficiently. Lot sizes, and the placement of homes on them, can greatly affect cost. Understanding measures of housing density can aid in estimating a project's affordability and environmental impact (see Figure 5.3). *Gross density* can be measured for an entire neighborhood or for a specific project and

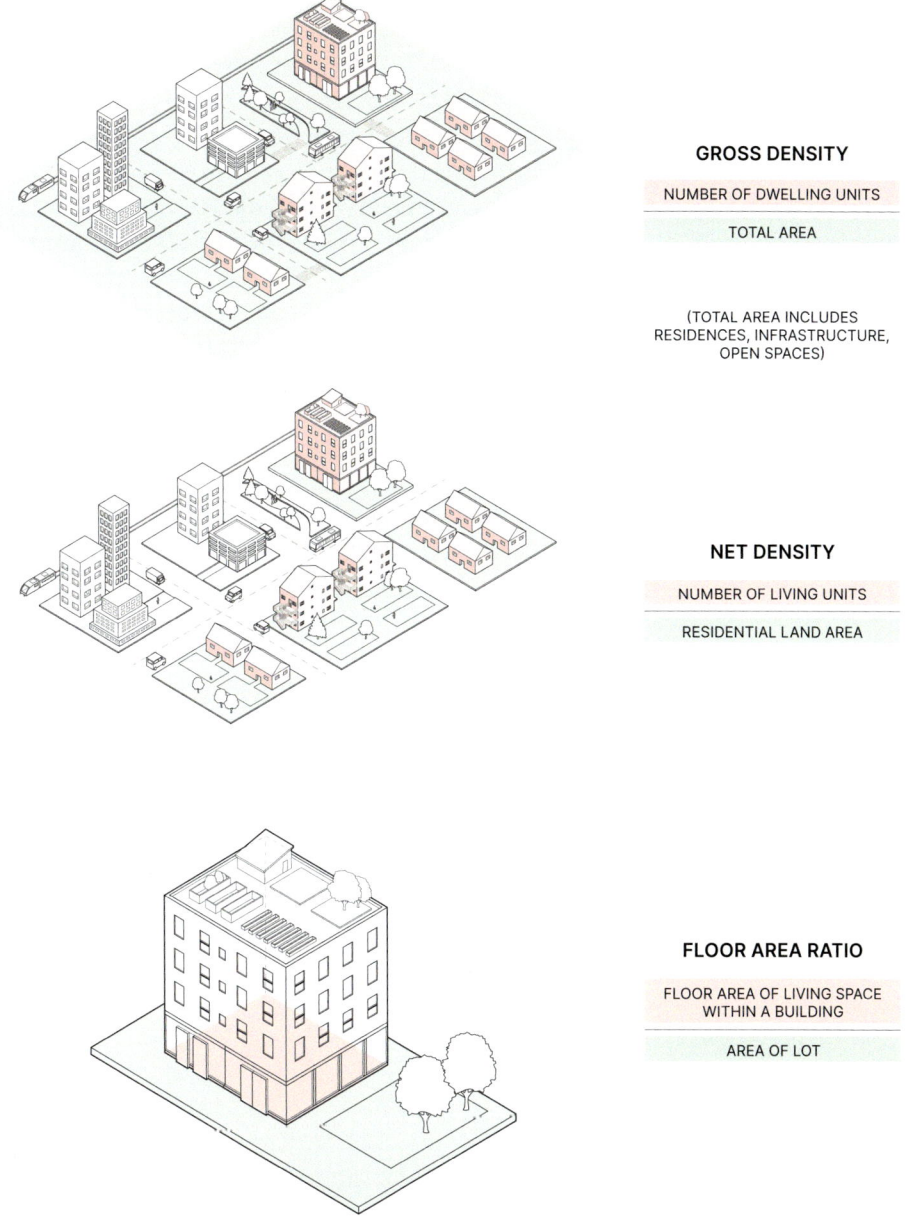

GROSS DENSITY

NUMBER OF DWELLING UNITS

TOTAL AREA

(TOTAL AREA INCLUDES RESIDENCES, INFRASTRUCTURE, OPEN SPACES)

NET DENSITY

NUMBER OF LIVING UNITS

RESIDENTIAL LAND AREA

FLOOR AREA RATIO

FLOOR AREA OF LIVING SPACE WITHIN A BUILDING

AREA OF LOT

Figure 5.3 Comparison of Density Indices.

refers to the number of built living units divided by the total land area, including residences, infrastructure, and open spaces. *Net density* is another index that considers the number of dwelling units divided only by the residential land area (therefore, excluding any public functions). Finally, *floor area ratio (FAR)* measures the enclosed floor area of living space within a building divided by the area of the lot. These three indices are helpful tools in approximating the potential for savings in the design stage of a housing project and should be thoughtfully maximized to cut costs while maintaining quality and livability.

5.2.3 Circulation and Parking

In high-density housing, the efficiency of its circulation system is of great importance in reducing costs and ensuring safe and equal access to services. Intentional street design can also reduce carbon emissions, as their design should promote energy conservation and prevent motorists from driving unnecessarily long distances. This efficiency is achieved through understanding the hierarchy of components in a movement system. Low traffic roads, such as a *place*, a *lane*, or a *way*, should be designed with narrow footprints as they support only limited local access, while *arterial roads* provide regional circulation and must be designed to support high traffic inherent to dense neighborhoods. Thoughtful circulation design avoids the expensive over-design of local streets, can facilitate the integration of public transport as an affordable transportation method, and can support the walkability of a city. Walkability, which is often defined as the ability within a region to walk safely to amenities within 30 minutes or so, allows consumers to save on vehicle expenses. Households in walkable regions devote 50 percent less money to transportation than those in communities dependent on automobiles (Litman, 2017).

Another aspect of circulation design that affects the affordability of communities is parking. Parking currently consumes significant space in cities, with multistory parking structures, open lots, and street-spaces taking up valuable land in urban centers. The current practices regarding parking design prioritize space allocated to empty cars rather than housing or open spaces that could benefit communities. The solution to this issue is not straightforward, and cultural change in automobile dependence needs to occur so that long-term solutions such as vehicle sharing can be adequately implemented. The "sharing" business model is a key circular economy concept as outlined in Chapter 3. Vehicle sharing has been introduced in many cities through taxis and online transport companies (e.g., Uber, Lyft), demonstrating the possibility of mobility without car ownership. Promoting public transportation through the integration of sufficient infrastructure and walkability can reduce the need for personal automobiles. Before this shift occurs though, one must strategically design parking solutions to reduce allocated land area and costs of construction when a parking structure is involved. An independent structure for parking is the most expensive option, and integrating parking space into residential and commercial structures minimizes construction costs and materials.

5.2.4 Open Spaces and Nature-Based Design

As density of development increases, so does the need for open spaces. Open space is a broad term that includes parks and green spaces, serving as recreation and pause in an otherwise developed area (see Figure 5.4). Open spaces are vital for their psychological and physical health benefits, which become particularly important in a dense urban area. A strong correlation has been observed between the quality of green spaces and physical health (Mullenbach et al., 2018). Proper allocation of the property toward communal or private green space also carries environmental benefits, promoting biodiversity and providing ecosystem services such as storm water management, improvement of air quality, promoting biophilia, and the reduction of sound pollution (Cilliers, 2015). In dense residential areas, a hybrid system of both community and private green spaces including shared urban farming should be considered to realize these benefits in a cost-effective manner. Utilizing roofs and facades as spaces for increased living green systems can provide environmental benefits to a city while also promoting the health and well-being of its occupants. It enhances biophilia which is the concept that humans have an innate desire to connect and spend time in nature. The design of green spaces in a city and neighborhood can be enhanced by nature-based design solutions (IUCN, 2023). This design approach focuses on the circular economy principle of "regeneration" by leveraging the power of nature and healthy ecosystems to address societal challenges such as climate change, food and water security, biodiversity loss, and human health, in a way that benefits both people and non-human living systems.

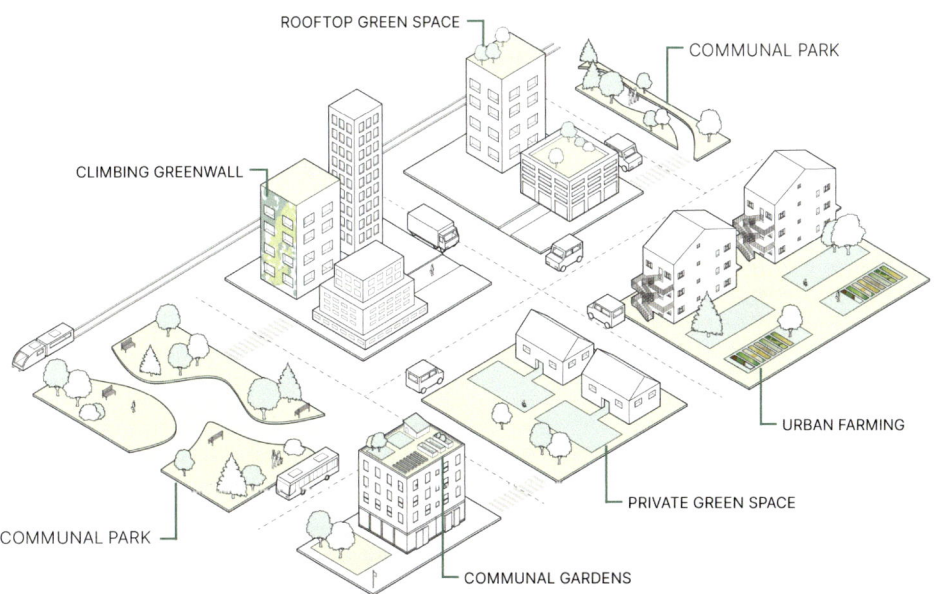

Figure 5.4 Combined Model of Open Space and Nature-Based Solutions in a Design Development.

In a housing development, small outdoor living spaces attached to units are often very attractive as they provide opportunities for private relaxation and outdoor activities such as gardening and exercise. This private model also provides cost benefits, as the care of the space falls under the responsibility of the resident alone. A purely private green system, though, does not have the same social benefits as a system that incorporates communal areas. Communal parks serve as gathering spaces for neighborly connection and children's play and development, becoming places to foster social capital and support active lifestyles in a shared space. The incorporation of urban agriculture in communal spaces can help address food security by offering a community a sustainable supply of local fruit and vegetables. To achieve affordability in a housing development, a blend of private and communal open spaces can limit costs as it maximizes the use of valuable land by sharing it, while conserving privacy through small private spaces. Additionally, park design need not be expensive or ecologically intrusive. A minimal design approach, conserving the landscape, including some trees and land variation, can encourage creativity in children's play and maintain the natural beauty of a site.

5.3 Designing Affordable Dwelling

Within communities, individual housing projects must be designed with affordability in mind to limit the cost of living. Sufficiency is an important concept that relates to both the sustainability and affordability of a dwelling. Sufficiency, in this regard, is the appropriate amount of something based on one's requirements, meaning enough to satisfy one's needs without having a surplus. In the current age of consumption and excess, consumption often far outweighs need. This is seen across industries, with exorbitant waste associated with fashion and food industries, for example. The building sector is no exception. To achieve affordability in the housing market and reduce the building sector's environmental impact, a revaluation of current values must occur, closing the gap between the market's needs and the built reality.

5.3.1 *Minimizing Footprint*

Housing trends have seen a constant growth in its carbon footprint in high-income countries. This growth is contributed to lifestyle expectations, industrial design trends, and the commercialization of homes but has little basis in the realized needs of modern households (Cohen, 2021). Between 1950 and 2015 in the United States, for instance, newly constructed houses have nearly tripled from 91 square meters (979 square feet) to 255 square meters (2745 square feet). In conflict with growing house sizes, household size has been declining during the same period, indicating a disconnect between the needs of modern homebuyers and the current market. Re-evaluating the real requirements for comfortable living is key to achieving sustainability and affordability in housing, as the current mindset of "bigger is better" has unnecessary and harmful impacts on the economy and on the environment. Minimizing the footprint of a dwelling increases its energy efficiency, producing significant savings on heating and cooling as well as limiting associated greenhouse gas emissions. A smaller footprint also requires less envelope, resulting in material, construction, and carbon savings.

Research suggests that a sufficient home size for a single person is between 14 and 20 square meters (150 and 215 square feet) and between 42 and 80 square meters (452 and 861 square feet) for a four-person household to meet healthy living standards (Cohen, 2021). When compared to the US's average of 255 square meters per new home, this target suggests a 70-percent reduction in floor area to achieve sufficient space for a comfortable lifestyle. This means that there is tremendous opportunity in reducing cost and environmental impact of housing through downsizing (see Figure 5.5). A smaller footprint does not necessarily compromise the comfort, privacy, and flexibility that many homebuyers seek, it just needs a careful design approach to maximize the livable space.

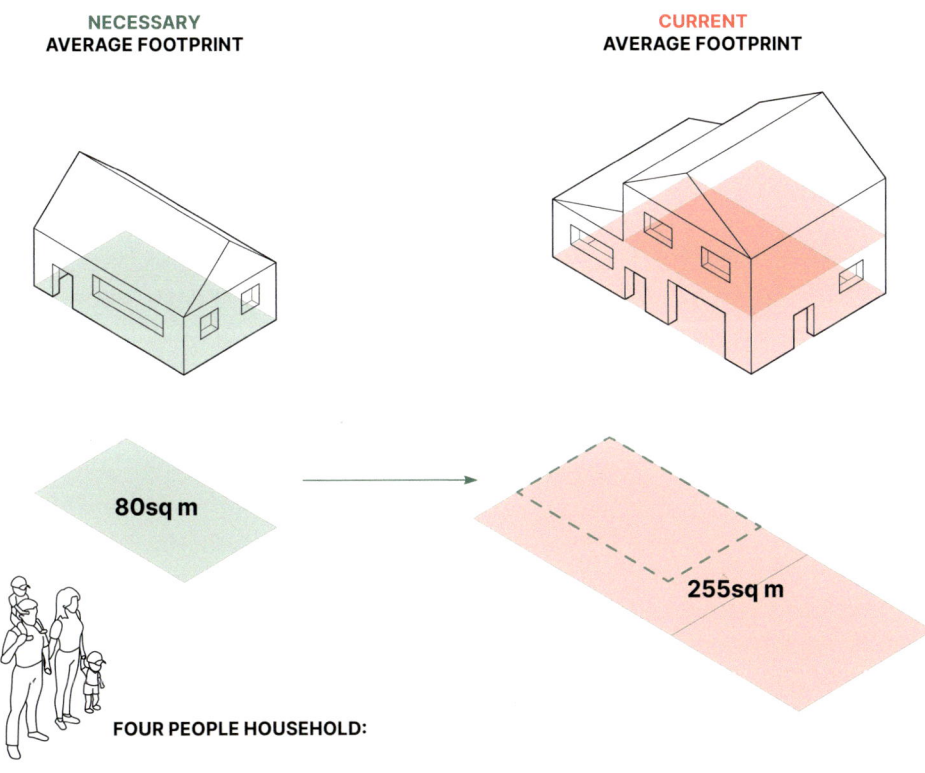

NECESSARY
AVERAGE FOOTPRINT

CURRENT
AVERAGE FOOTPRINT

80sq m

255sq m

FOUR PEOPLE HOUSEHOLD:

Figure 5.5 Current Area vs Necessary.

5.3.2 Simplifying Form

Complex building configurations, while perhaps visually interesting, contribute to additional costs in material and energy through increased surface area where heat transfer can occur. With a simple overall shape and few projections, less exterior wall and roof surface are necessary for the envelope, minimizing heat absorption during the day and heat loss at night. *Form Factor* is an index developed to measure the efficiency of a building type and is calculated by dividing the total heat loss area (external faces of the building: walls, roofs, floors, and openings) by the habitable floor area of a dwelling (Cutland Consulting Ltd, 2016). A lower Form Factor indicates higher energy efficiency, as there is less heat loss (or unwanted heat gain) for a given floor space. A simplified building form also imposes the use of fewer windows to provide daylight to the same area. Windows and openings are typically the weakest points in the envelope in terms of efficiency, so this reduction results in lower energy costs as well as unnecessary material and construction.

Inefficient configurations can be avoided while maintaining visual appeal. For example, a protruding entrance volume can be replaced by an awning to achieve the same effect, and a façade can be decorated with variation in cladding material to add dimension instead of adding costly protrusions. A simple building form also typically results in more regularly shaped interior spaces that lend themselves to different uses based on an occupant's needs. A flexible interior results in cost reductions because it requires less remodeling while a household ages. This flexibility also brings long-term savings as it can extend the useful cycle of a building and avoid costly and environmentally harmful demolition.

5.3.4 Attachment

As mentioned, energy losses in a home occur in the external faces and openings of a building. The attachment of multiple dwelling units is an effective solution to further lower a dwelling's form factor since shared walls or floor/ceilings are not exposed to the outdoor temperature. A townhouse employs attachment horizontally, with dwellings sharing common walls, while an apartment-style dwelling shares walls and floors, further minimizing exposed surfaces per household. This reduction in heat loss area can dramatically lower energy costs (see Figure 5.6). Attached dwellings also require less materials and construction to complete their envelope and reduce infrastructure needs as the proximity of households requires less length of linear infrastructure (roads, water pipes, and electricity lines).

The attachment of dwellings will ultimately lead to a higher residential density. As mentioned as a solution to affordability at the community scale, density can result in savings at many levels. An environmental advantage to attached living is that the increased density allows more land to be allocated to open spaces and public areas that are vital in developing a comfortable living environment when the floor area of a residence is minimized. Clustering units as such also results in the disturbance of less land and thus the preservation of ecosystem services.

APARTMENT STYLE **SINGLE FAMILY HOUSE**

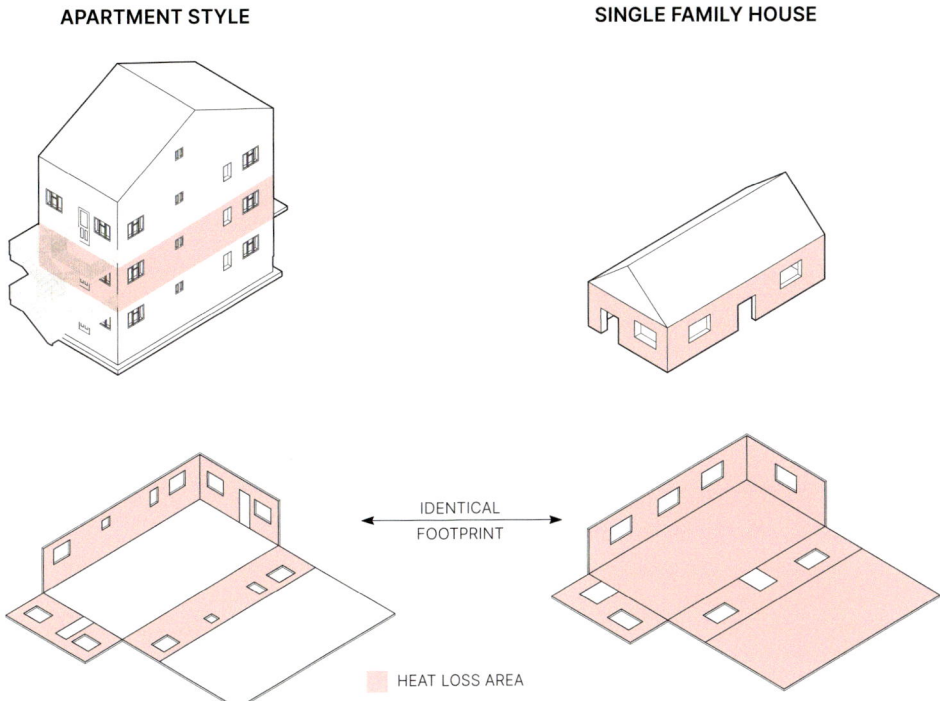

IDENTICAL
FOOTPRINT

HEAT LOSS AREA

Figure 5.6 Floor Area vs Heat Loss Area.

5.3.5 Compact Interior Design

A small dwelling has tremendous potential for energy, environmental footprint, and cost savings. The success of small footprint and attached living, though, relies on the efficient and flexible design of its interior spaces. An important consideration in optimizing space within dwellings is minimizing the area designated for circulation. Defined hallways eat up valuable space. Programming the interior to decrease the length of circulation paths increases the functional and livable space in a home. Grouping similar functions within a layout is another cost-reduction strategy in housing design. Plumbing and electrical costs can be greatly reduced when placing adjacent wet functions: bathrooms, kitchens, laundry. Additionally, an open-plan approach is energy efficient, as there are less barriers to prevent airflow throughout the space, additionally cutting costs in material and construction.

When planning for a small footprint, design approaches can be used to give the illusion of a larger space to improve comfort. Employing an open-plan layout will facilitate the reduction of circulation while opening traditionally closed-off spaces to make a small volume feel open and airy. Designing the interior with light colors and creative lighting solutions can make rooms look and feel larger. Additionally, flexible furniture can allow spaces to transform based on the needs of the resident at a given time. A retractable table, for example, can allow for a dining space that can be employed only when needed, allowing an open space for most of the day that can be used for another function.

5.4 Circular Economy Strategies and Terminology at the End-of-Use Phase

Circular economy strategies, while certainly being environmentally friendly alternatives to our current industry norms, can produce cost reductions in housing construction to begin to close the affordability gap. Circular economy is a model of production that recognizes the value of built projects as resources rather than eventual demolition sites and landfills. Eco-design is an established approach to sustainability in the built sector that strives to reduce waste and other harmful effects of production, but the newer circular economy approach strives toward a closed material loop and therefore redefines some well-known sustainability terms such as recycling, reuse, remanufacturing, and product use cycle and lifetime (see Figure 5.7) (den Hollander et al., 2017). Understanding these terms in relation to circular economy points to significant cost-reduction potential.

5.4.1 Recycling

As our environmental and sustainability crises worsen, the reduction in demand for new materials must be considered. Circular economy seeks to reduce this demand and therefore avoid the extraction of non-renewable raw materials through extending the lifetime of a resource through recycling. This concept is familiar to most of the public, and its definition in terms of circular economy is not unlike the popular

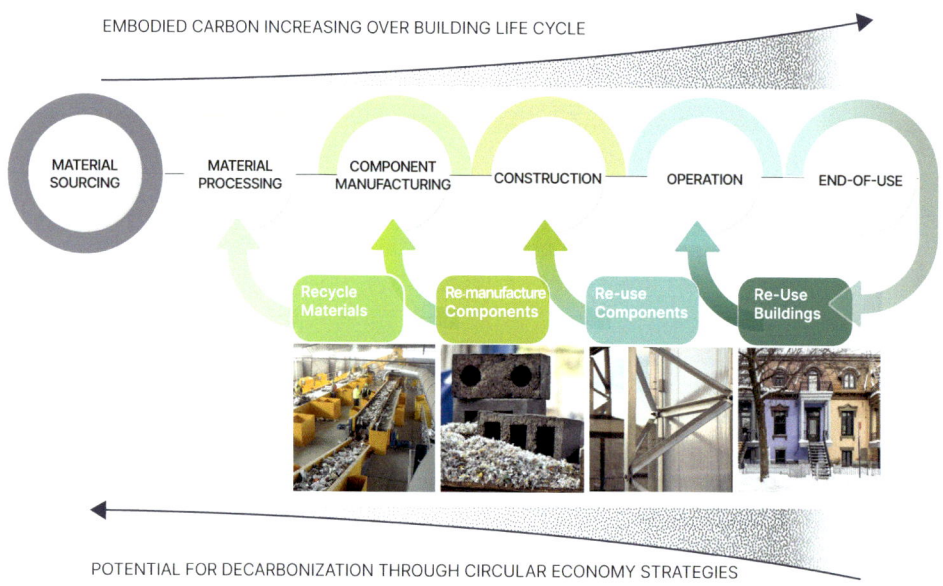

Figure 5.7 Hierarchy of Circular Economy Strategies Toward Decarbonization in the Housing Sector from Reuse of an Entire Building (Life Extension) to Recycling Materials.

conception: "the dismantling and disintegration of a product and its constituent components and the subsequent reprocessing of the product's materials" (den Hollander et al., 2017). Through the carefully supervised disassembly of building components at the end of their current use, waste and cost can be significantly reduced (GXN & Assets, 2018).

Steel in the construction industry is a great example of the potential of recycling for a smaller environmental footprint and lower costs. Currently, an estimated 98 percent of structural steel avoids landfills and is reused in new projects (CSSBI, n.d.). The concept of recycling materials for cost savings is not new. Brick, stone, and timber have also been reused historically in cases of shortage, but recycling is not used to its full potential. For example, drywall is theoretically 100 percent recyclable, but demolition practices usually do not value the integrity of this material and it ends up in landfills unnecessarily. Circular building design strives to incorporate the possibility of recycling in the design stage through the selection of recyclable materials, visible joints, and the development of accurate material logs (material passports) (see Chapter 4) (GXN & Assets, 2018). Recycling, though, is the least preferred method of extending a component's lifetime as it does not maintain original integrity.

5.4.2 Re-Manufacturing

Before recycling is considered, the possibility of remanufacturing should be explored as it involves lower associated waste and cost. Remanufacturing is the act of combining components of obsolete systems or building components, with as few new parts as possible, to manufacture a product to as-new standards (GXN & Assets, 2018). The implementation of remanufacturing should fall under the responsibility of the original equipment manufacturer or a contracted third party in a factory environment to achieve a final product of equal quality and warranty to the completely new product. Remanufacturing therefore minimizes the extraction of natural resources as it maximizes the use of functional parts of a component that has served its useful cycle, to create a product that is as good as new. In addition to this reduction in environmental footprint, cost of manufacturing decreases with less need for raw materials.

5.4.3 Reuse or Re-Contextualization

The optimal next step for a building component or material that has passed its useful cycle in its original form, before considering recycling or remanufacturing, is its reuse. When a building component is reused, no change occurs to the product, only its context. When a product is no longer useful in its originally intended use, it may very well be put to good use in exactly the same state but in a different location or setting that better suits it. Re-contextualizing is another name for the popular term reuse that emphasizes the shift in context of a repurposed object rather than the object itself. The scale of re-contextualizing can vary from the material to system scale, as hardwood flooring, as well as entire door or window systems, has the potential to be reused. Reuse, as opposed to remanufacturing or recycling, has little to no associated costs.

5.4.4 *"End-of-Use" Rather than "End-of-Life"*

Previous eco-design approaches have used the term *end-of-life* to describe what was thought of as an inevitable final stage of a product or material as waste. Circular economy, however, functions on the notion that producing waste is avoidable. Circular economy design instead uses the term *end-of-use* to describe the stage in which a product or material becomes obsolete in its current use (see Chapter 3). It is not yet reality, but a circular economy strives to achieve an infinite lifetime of materials through many different cycles (see Figure 5.8). A product's obsolescence can be brought on by physical factors like damage, aesthetic factors such as wear and tear, and factors relating to its wider context. Social conventions and trends are changing constantly and may accelerate the obsolescence of certain product uses, but obsolescence is not permanent or universal. Therefore, re-contextualizing material is so powerful and effective; its perceived value may be vastly different for different uses over time. In considering the value of materials as cyclical, cost savings may increase even as value does.

5.5 Implementing Material Reuse in the Building Sector

To see the benefits of circular economy in the "end-of-use" phase, strategies must be established to implement it in the construction industry. Circular reuse strategies such as recycling, remanufacturing, and re-contextualization are not being utilized to their potential, despite their demonstrated cost and environmental benefits.

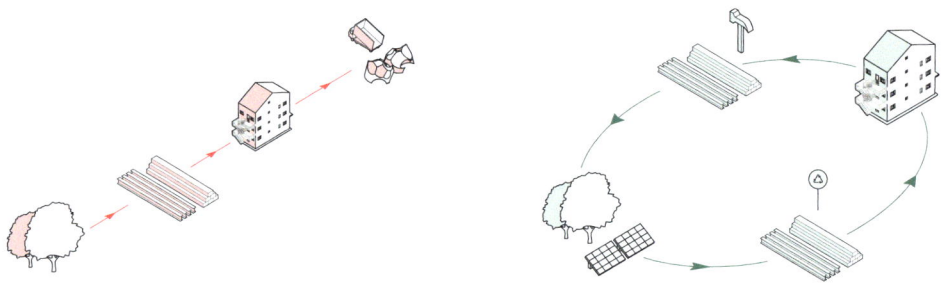

LINEAR ECONOMY   **CIRCULAR ECONOMY**

Figure 5.8 A Linear (Ending in Obsolescence and Waste) Versus a Circular Cycle (Looping).

Education within the building industry and the public, efficient and standardized documentation, and public certification processes can facilitate the transition to circularity and reuse.

5.5.1 Material Inventories and the Deconstruction Phase

When a building is to undergo major changes, whether it be aesthetic renovations, a full gutting of the interior, or a full destruction and redevelopment, current construction methods generate extreme waste at high costs. Buildings which are perceived to have reached the end of useful life are, in our current practices, an expensive barrier to new construction. Through the lens of circular economy though, existing buildings are valuable resources that can contribute to the success of a new construction through material reuse, as demonstrated in Resource Rows, a housing project from Denmark designed by Lendager Group and outlined in the below case study. A key aspect to realizing sufficient reuse in the building sector is the maintenance of material inventories. Material inventories can be created for new projects in their conception, or for existing buildings when renovations or demolitions have been planned. A material inventory serves to identify materials that could possibly have value in the interest of cutting construction costs and reducing the project's footprint.

A material inventory of a building is completed through the careful inspection of an existing structure to identify any materials or building components that have the potential to be recovered and reused in some way. Prior to a construction period, while the building is unoccupied, such inspection can be carried out non-invasively and at a low cost. This method can improve the affordability of a construction process by cataloging a building's assets to be repurposed, sold, or even donated instead of paying for their demolition and transport to landfill (see Figure 5.9). Materials such as structural steel or masonry, cladding like hardwood and tiles, or complete systems like doors and windows can be noted in a material inventory

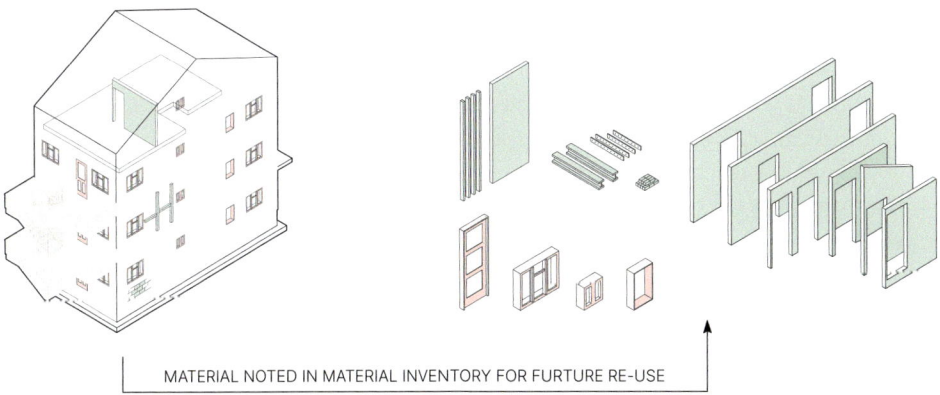

MATERIAL NOTED IN MATERIAL INVENTORY FOR FURTURE RE-USE

Figure 5.9 Elements of a Previous Structure Are Reused in a New Building.

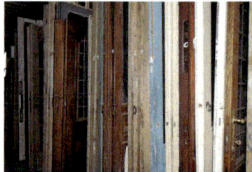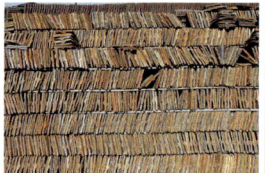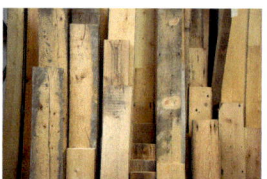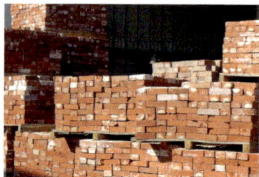

Figure 5.10 Examples of Material Inventories from Rotor's Opalis Project Where Materials Are Sorted for Easy Reuse.

if they are deemed reusable. There are several factors in a material/component's potential to be reused. Ease of disassembly and durability are to be considered, as not all products are designed to maintain integrity after dismantlement. Valuable materials can then be specified and quantified in an online platform so they may be reallocated for future functions.

Rotor is a design cooperative in Brussels working toward the efficient reuse of construction materials through the development, both conceptual and practical, of material inventories. Driven by sustainability, Rotor's work also holds great economic advantages (Idenburg, 2022). The cooperative practices design and is heavily involved in research in this emerging field. Numerous publications, such as their 2015 handbook "How to Extract Re-usable Materials from Public Buildings" (Rotor, 2015b), act as valuable tools for designers and developers globally, exploring the potential of common materials to cut demolition and construction costs, and the application of material inventories to achieve this (see Figure 5.10). It is these initiatives that are needed to advance reuse in the construction industry; as the process becomes the norm, it only becomes more efficient, more straightforward, and more cost-effective.

5.5.2 *Heritage Designation*

Obsolescence of a material, component, product, or even building is dependent on many factors and can be subjective, as discussed in Section 5.4.5. With the same thinking, a material's value changes over time depending on its physical properties (durability, strength), aesthetic qualities (finish, color), but also contextual factors such as its relevance in design trends, popular opinion, and heritage value. All this to say, value of a material is closely tied to its perceived importance. While the significance of physical properties is certain, it is contextual qualities that can change with little to no material or cost input. Heritage value, as mentioned, is commonly associated with historic monuments or places. Heritage conservation projects, in which culturally significant buildings are renovated to meet modern needs, are great examples of the value that history and time can add to a project. Heritage conservation not only preserves important historic, aesthetic, or cultural reminders, but it is also a holistically sustainable approach that limits demolition, waste, and associated costs. The benefits of considering heritage have long been established at the scale of buildings, but it can also play a role at the material level by increasing reuse.

Companies have begun to recognize the value of the past in selling products, increasing profits while maximizing reuse. One example of this initiative is Genbyg, a Danish company specializing in the resale of building materials (GXN & Assets, 2018). Since 1998, Genbyg has sourced and purchased used doors and windows among other materials with unique qualities to give them a second life. In the company's model, materials or components that cannot be reused in their found state are recycled, or upcycled, to become modern furniture. Floorboards, for example, can be converted into modern tables or shelving. Genbyg's storefront in Copenhagen, as well as their online store, allows consumers to browse and purchase items with low environmental impact and unique histories. Rotor Deconstruction, or Rotor DC, is a Brussels-based cooperative that runs Reuse Made Easy, which facilitates reuse of materials among local professionals, as discussed in the following case study. Over time, Western culture has learned to value aesthetic perfection as a sign of quality and sanitation, but the rising popularity of upcycling indicates an important shift in this thinking (see Chapter 3). Abandoning unfounded aesthetic requirements will allow the growth of reuse in the building sector to give way to more cost-effective and sustainable practices.

5.5.3 Certification

Vital in promoting reuse in the building sector is certification. So that more private companies turn to these circular economy practices, standardized guidelines and documentation need to be established. This process has begun under some government organizations and allows professionals in the construction industry to verify the circularity in their chosen products and methods. Luxembourg, for example, has developed a Product Circularity Data Sheet (PCDS) with the goal of documenting the qualities and potential for reuse of all products and materials (+ImpaKT Luxembourg, 2020). The PCDS can then serve as an invaluable tool in the industry to maximize a project's circularity. Databases such as this would then allow for the assessment and ranking of projects' sustainability in circular economy terms, hence promoting and incentivizing these methods. With the further development of certification tools across governments, standards for reuse can eventually be enforced to achieve environmental goals. The cost savings and environmental benefits of reuse are clear, but certification can give a clear path to achieving these things to more participants in the industry and be a tool to educate the public.

5A

Project:
Benny Farm

Location:
Montreal, Canada

Year:
2006

Team:
L'OEUF and Saia Barbarese
Topouzanov architects

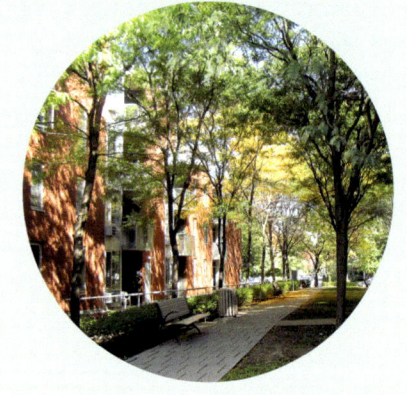

Mapping to Circular Economy Framework:

CIRCULAR ECONOMY PRACTICES

LIFE CYCLE PHASES

	Recovery	Life Extension	Sharing Platforms	Service Models	Regenerate	Virtualize
Work of Geobiosphere						
Sourcing						
Manufacturing						
Design & Construction						
Use						
End-of-Use						

LAYERS + LIFESPAN
Structural Layers | Long Life
Skin, MEP Layers | Medium Life
Interior Layers | Short Life

Site 100+yr   Structure 50+yr
Exterior 25+yr   System 15+yr
Partition 10+yr   Stuff 1+yr

As climbing property prices are affecting most major cities worldwide, it becomes ever more difficult for an increasingly diverse household population to buy property or find affordable living situations. Montreal, Canada, is no exception to this crisis, as renting and ownership prices are estimated to continue to increase substantially in the coming years (CMHC et al., 2022). To provide accessible housing during this difficult time, Montreal's unique and diverse built environment includes a variety of affordable and social housing solutions designed for low-income families, most commonly single-parent households, elderly citizens, and people living with disabilities. One prime example that illustrates the capacity cost-reduction strategies of circular design discussed in this chapter is Benny Farm, an affordable residential development in Montreal's Notre-Dame-de-Grace neighborhood (see Figure 5.11).

The community has been an urban landmark since its conception as a public residential development for veterans and their families following World War II, and it continues to serve a crucial role in the city's social fabric after firms L'OEUF and Saia Barbarese Topouzanov Architectes' redevelopment beginning in 1996 and completed in 2006. The project is a hybrid community, with social housing, private ownership, and non-profit organizations linked by a common green area. A total of 570 units are dispersed within simplified brick-cladded structures on 7.3 hectares (18 acres) of land. The project houses diverse groups, including senior citizens, people with disabilities, young families, and single-parent families. The award-winning project shows

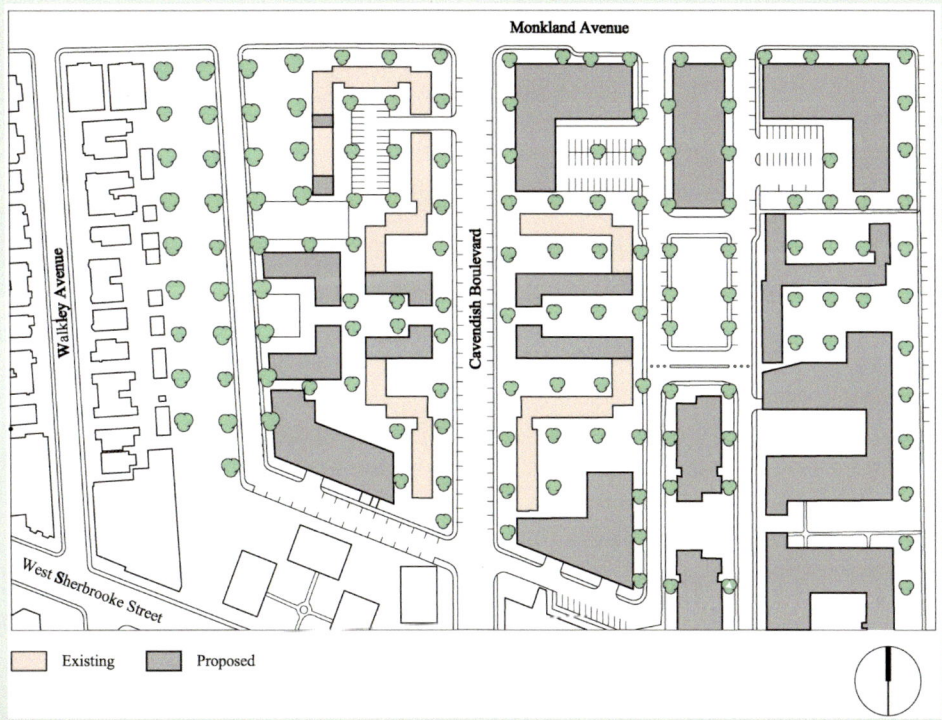

Figure 5.11 Plan for Benny Farm.

the interrelation of economic, environmental, and social issues. Benny Farm is an established example of the power of affordability techniques discussed in this chapter and employs **recovery and recycling**, **product life extension**, **sharing platforms**, and **regeneration** across the building's life cycle phases to achieve affordable quality at a reduced environmental footprint.

First, Benny Farm displays the circular economy principles of ***recovery and recycling.*** In the 1940s, farmlands on what were then outskirts of Montreal were transformed into a close community composed of 64 three-story walk-ups (Pearl & Wentz, 2014). Totaling 384 apartments, the original Benny Farm buildings were wood-frame and brick veneer construction with no elevators or air conditioning. This community thrived as a well-organized and integrated development for many years, but in later years, an aging population saw many buildings vacated and left to deteriorate. In 1994, L'OEUF proposed a rehabilitation plan involving renovations and additions to continue the life of the established social housing and provide accessible and comfortable living. With the help of community participation, these revised master plans were eventually chosen over plans for privatized demolition and redevelopment that would erase the important social history of Benny Farm and value profit over the accommodation of low-income households.

Local firms L'OEUF and Saia Barbarese Topouzanov Architects led the large-scale project, renovating the remaining apartments to contemporary safety and accessibility standards, constructing new units, updating existing infrastructure, and creating vibrant common green spaces. To maintain heritage, affordability, and offset the project's environmental impact, the architects maintained as much of the original site as possible and sourced materials from demolished portions of the community. For example, as illustrated in Figure 5.12, much brick from the existing buildings were reclaimed, kept on site, sorted, and repurposed for use on the newly renovated facades. Samples of the brick were laboratory tested for water resistance and compressive strength, and the results showed they were of higher performance than many of the new bricks on the market at the time (Pearl & Wentz, 2014). Some of the new buildings used salvaged brick, while some of the renovated buildings used new brick – the result is a blurring between old and new buildings on site. Careful evaluation and organization ensured that materials and systems deemed reusable were utilized in the newly constructed units. The new buildings, simplified in form to achieve energy and material efficiency, were also cladded using original bricks, and a new geothermal system was adapted to use the original radiators (see Figure 5.12).

Second, Benny Farm utilizes ***product life extension*** and ***virtualization***. Responsible material sourcing, inherent to the original proposal and carried through to the final construction stage, extended the useful life of bricks, glass blocks, salvaged floorboards, radiators, other materials, and completed structures of the original development. Through re-contextualizing these materials as part of a highly important and successful social housing system and taking advantage of their associated heritage, the team added value to the project at a lower cost than new construction. Additionally, newly constructed high-efficiency building envelopes were designed and

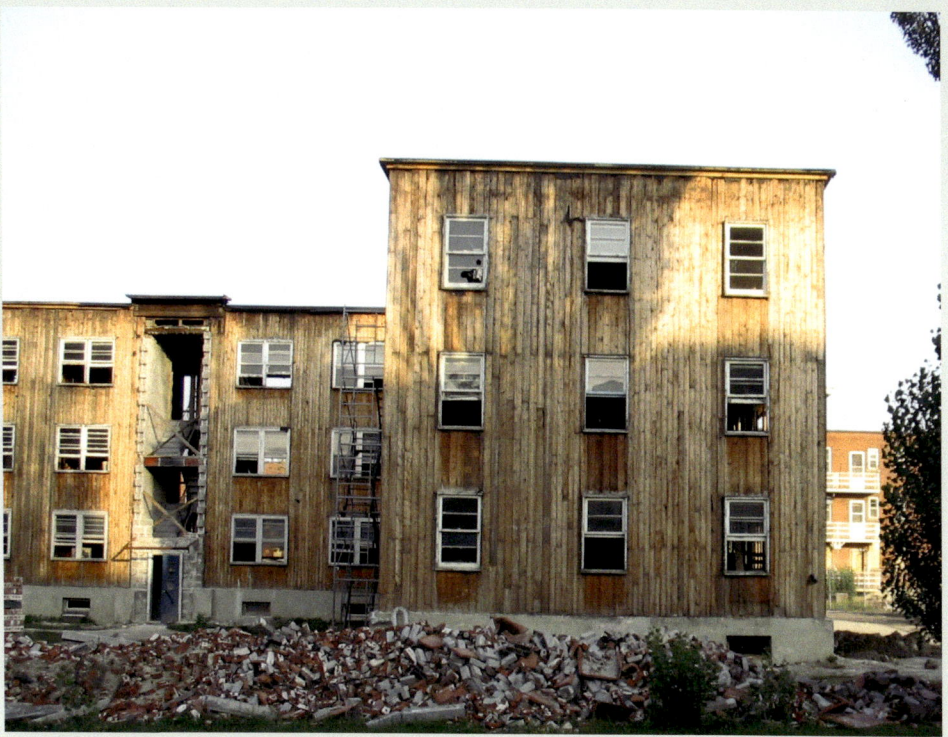

Figure 5.12 Benny Farm Façade Under Renovation with the Salvaged Brick to the Forefront.

tested using EE4 software, an energy simulation software developed by National Resources Canada (NRCan, 2015). The façade design aimed to reduce energy needs for heating and cooling via airtightness and effective R-insulation values that considered thermal bridging. In addition, the strategic placement of vapor barriers took longevity and durability into account to avoid unnecessarily early repairs or demolition and thereby extending the building lifetime (Pearl & Wentz, 2014). The use of virtual energy simulations allowed the team to test the most efficient solutions. EE4 automates energy use assessments and helps verify that a design is at least 25 percent more energy efficient than if constructed to meet Model National Energy Code for Buildings (MNECB) 1997 requirements (NRCan, 2015).

Lastly, Benny Farm features *regeneration* and the *sharing platform*. Currently, Benny Farm offers rent and ownership opportunities for low-to-moderate-income households in addition to hosting cooperative and social housing for disadvantaged communities (Pearl & Wentz, 2014). Through the operation of different social programs that house single mothers going back to work, seniors, and people with limited mobility on the same site, material and construction needs in infrastructure are greatly reduced. People with common needs in terms of building programs and services have shared access and find other housing solutions once financially possible, promoting efficient use of the buildings and infrastructure. The incorporation

147

of green energy production, water management, and community gardening on site (see Figure 5.13) ensured long-term cost savings while achieving sustainability and generating resources. Water collection and treatment systems, as well as an integrated geothermal system, take pressure off municipal infrastructure and create self-reliance within the community. Similarly, community gardens and ample green spaces preserve and regenerate natural resources of the geo-biosphere and promote community development.

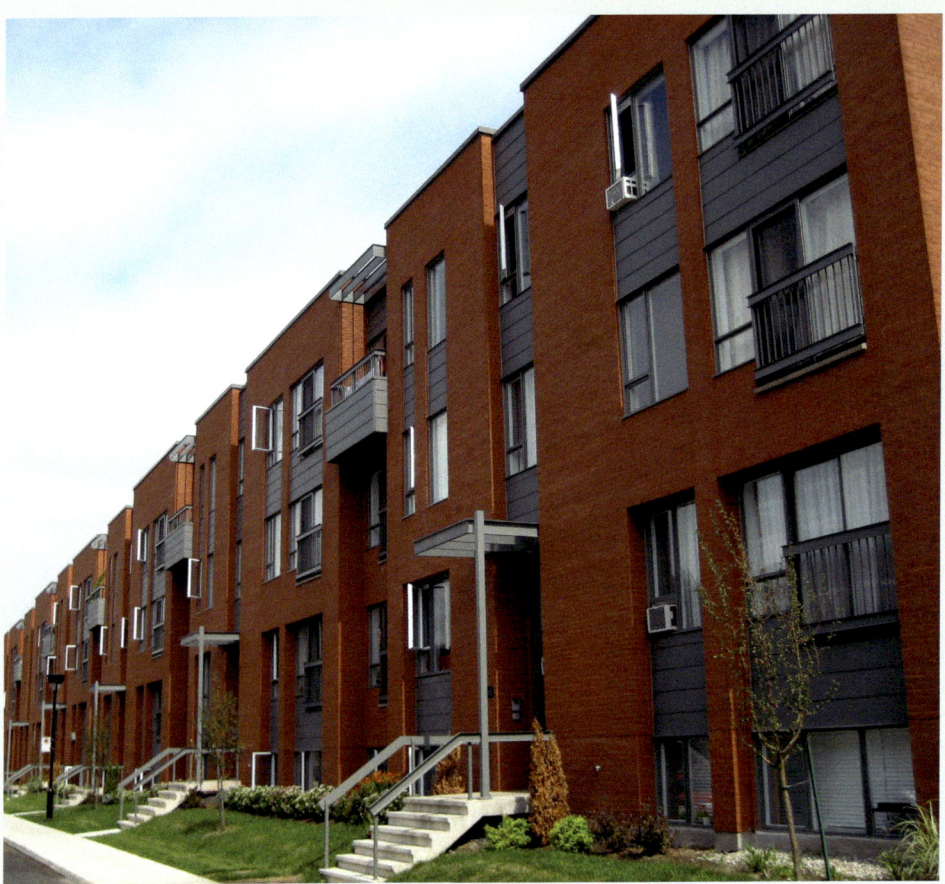

Figure 5.13 New homes in Benny Farm.

5B

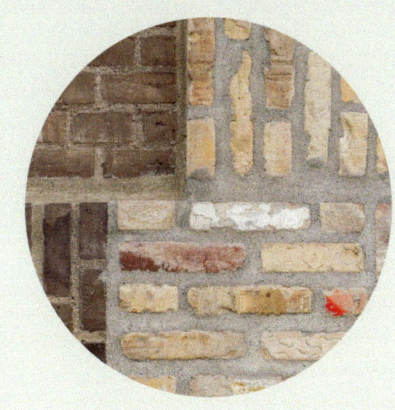

Project:
Resource Rows

Location:
Copenhagen, Denmark

Year:
2019

Team:
Lendager Group

**Mapping to Circular
Economy Framework:**

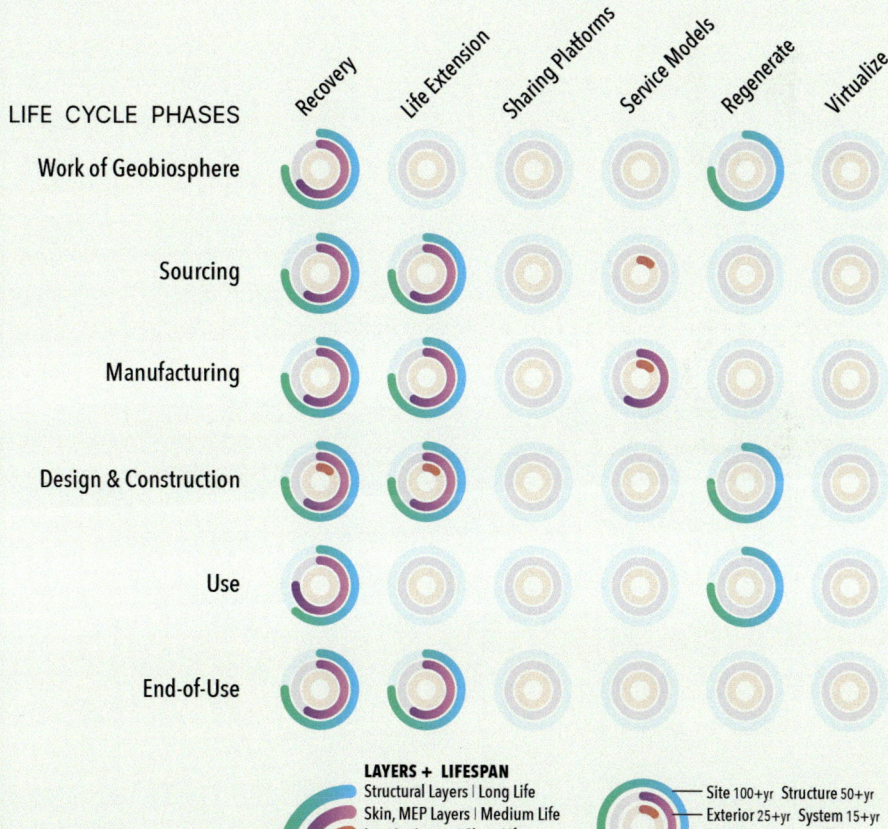

CIRCULAR ECONOMY PRACTICES

LIFE CYCLE PHASES

Recovery · Life Extension · Sharing Platforms · Service Models · Regenerate · Virtualize

Work of Geobiosphere

Sourcing

Manufacturing

Design & Construction

Use

End-of-Use

LAYERS + LIFESPAN
Structural Layers | Long Life
Skin, MEP Layers | Medium Life
Interior Layers | Short Life

Site 100+yr   Structure 50+yr
Exterior 25+yr   System 15+yr
Partition 10+yr   Stuff 1+yr

Resource Rows is a housing project in Denmark that implemented material reuse to achieve affordability, aesthetic quality, and environmental benefits (see Figure 5.14). Designed by Danish firm Lendager Group, it won the 2022 Mies van der Rohe Award (EU Mies Award, 2022). The project is part of a larger ongoing development in the area Ørestad Syd, on the outskirts of Copenhagen, and was completed in 2019 by local Danish firm Lendager Group. The upcycling of materials was a central philosophy in the project, and the thoughtful expression of mismatched brick facing created from "waste" at local demolition sites makes this apparent (see Figure 5.15). The site features a shared rectangular courtyard, around which two five-story apartment blocks are placed at the end of two rows of three-story townhouses. The 92 units, 29 being row houses and 63 being apartments, also share common open area with rows of small green-house huts on the row house rooftops. A bridge connects the two rows of roofscape to optimize the utilization of outdoor space and its benefits within a dense development.

Anders Lendager, founder of the Lendager Group, understands that a key aspect of sustainable architecture is economics. For environmentally friendly construction techniques to be adopted, they must be economically feasible, bringing cost benefits to the project (Wilson, 2019). The Lendager Group designs with the knowledge that affordability and sustainability are two fundamentally connected ideas, and Resource Rows employs material reuse through upcycling of potential waste, high density with thoughtful allocation of open space, as well as a regimented and simplified form to achieve sustainability at a low cost.

The high density of Resource Rows brings cost and environmental footprint savings through the use of shared infrastructure and green space, decreasing the need for cladding materials and the energy-efficient qualities of attachment (see Figure 5.16) (Heward, 2019). The units are compact but have been designed with ample natural light and open plans to give the impression of a large space. Public greenery also

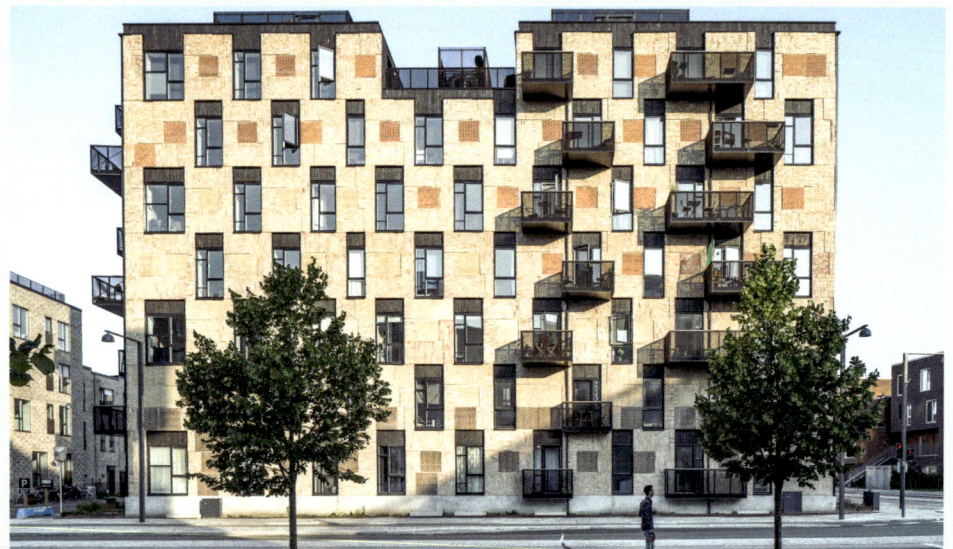

Figure 5.14 East Façade of the Resource Rows in Denmark. The Façade of Salvaged Brick Panels Reads Like a Tapestry or Quilt-Work.

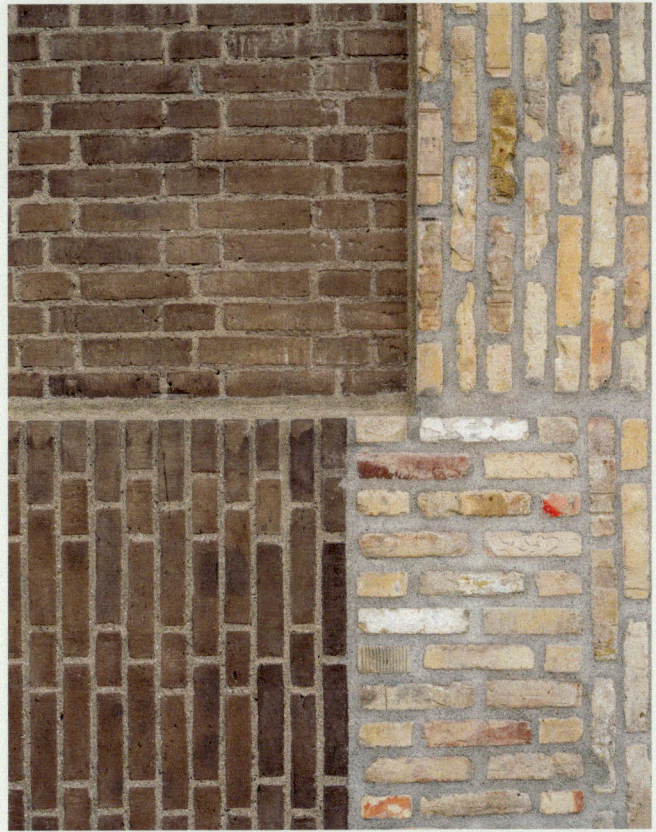

Figure 5.15 A Close-Up of Reused Brick in the Construction of Resource Rows.

invites tenants into common areas where community connections are strengthened, and physical and psychological health is benefited (see Figure 5.17). Areas for indoor and outdoor gardening also encourage community and health while enlivening the dense development. The integrated underground parking garage eliminates the need for inefficient street parking, maximizing the use of valuable land that is a large contributor to housing prices.

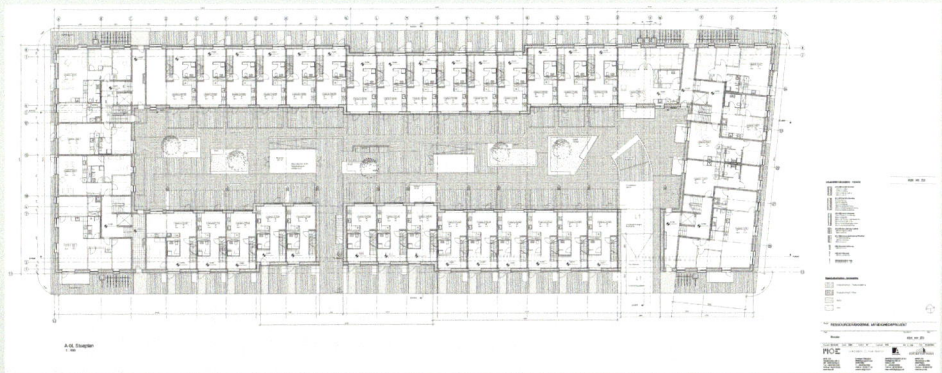

Figure 5.16 Ground Floor Plan of the Resource Rows.

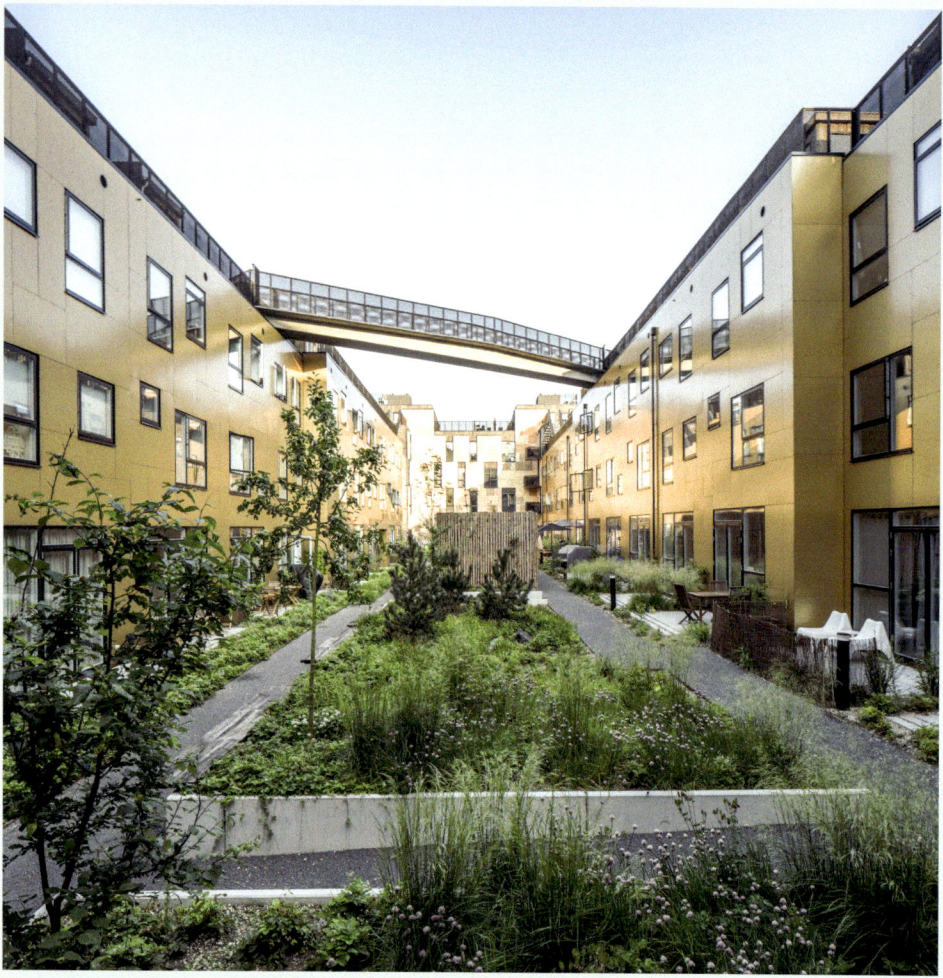

Figure 5.17 Public Greenery at Resource Rows. The Steel Bridge Connecting the Parallel Terrace Rooftops Is a Recycled Roof Truss.

The housing project's unique and striking brick façade is composed of panels of original brick and mortar. These panels of salvaged material were cut from the walls of buildings targeted for demolition at three different local demolition sites, including Denmark's own Carlsberg Brewery (Lendager, 2022). Modern mortar is strong enough to remain intact throughout this cutting process at the demolition site, allowing a greater decrease in cost and carbon footprint than more common brick reuse techniques. The reuse of bricks typically involves individually detaching each brick from the mortar, cleaning and repurposing it for reuse (see Figure 5.18). The innovative panelized technique used in Resource Rows saves time, money, and material while adding local historical heritage to the project. The distinctive façade also adds visual interest to an otherwise-simple elevation (see Figure 5.19). Lendager also diverted waste from other local projects, using timber crates used for the Copenhagen Metro expansion as exterior window frames and decking, and a roof truss designed for another project

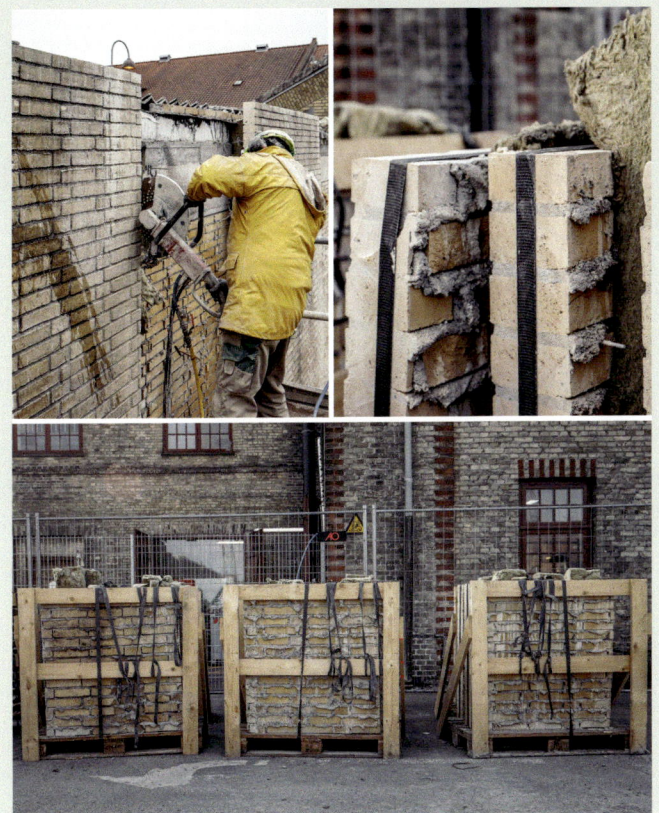

Figure 5.18 Salvaging and Fabricating Wall Panels from Cut-Out Segments of Old Brick Walls Complete with Mortar.

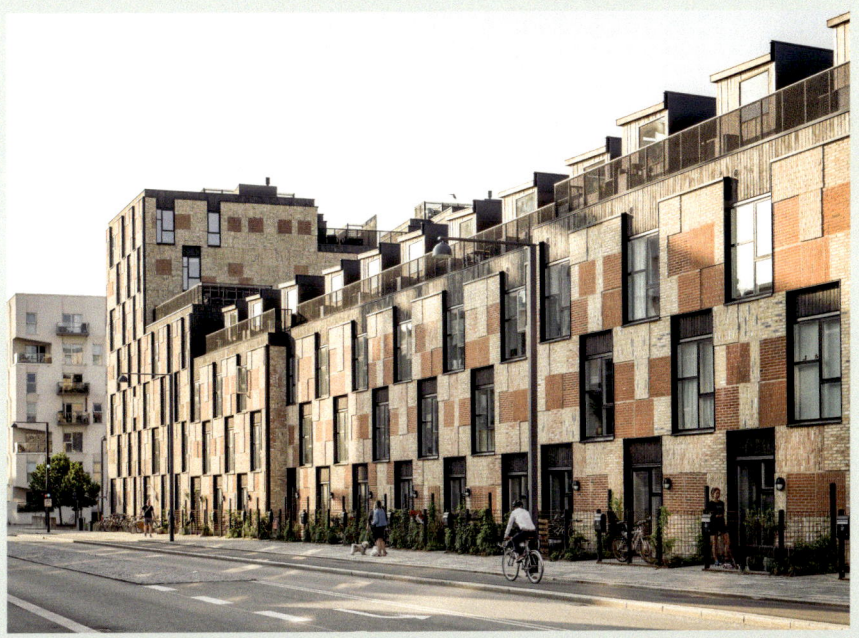

Figure 5.19 A View of the Three-Story Terraced Houses Which Have Direct Access to the Roof Top Green House. All Exterior Wood in Upcycled from Waste Wood and Impregnate for Fire Proofing via Charring – an Old Japanese Technique.

as the steel bridge stretching across the courtyard. Through tapping into the valuable and underutilized resources of previous construction, Resource Rows diverted 463 metric tons of material from landfills. This amounts to 29 percent savings in carbon dioxide equivalent per square meter of construction and has proved to be cost-neutral in terms of maintenance (Lendager, 2022). In terms of brick construction alone, the project saved 500 g of carbon dioxide equivalent per brick, which equates to a 70 percent carbon reduction compared to typical (new) brick construction (EU Mies Award, 2022). The project was built at a lower cost than a non-upcycled equivalent, and the architectural firm believes that cost benefits of reuse strategies in the building sector will only improve as they become more standard within the industry.

5C

Project:
Reuse Made Easy

Location:
Brussels, Belgium

Year:
2019

Team:
Rotor DC

**Mapping to Circular
Economy Framework:**

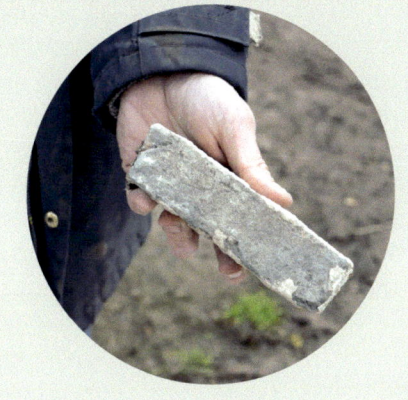

CIRCULAR ECONOMY PRACTICES

LIFE CYCLE PHASES

	Recovery	Life Extension	Sharing Platforms	Service Models	Regenerate	Virtualize
Work of Geobiosphere						
Sourcing						
Manufacturing						
Design & Construction						
Use						
End-of-Use						

LAYERS + LIFESPAN
Structural Layers | Long Life
Skin, MEP Layers | Medium Life
Interior Layers | Short Life

Site 100+yr   Structure 50+yr
Exterior 25+yr   System 15+yr
Partition 10+yr   Stuff 1+yr

155

Rotor Deconstruction, or Rotor DC, is a cooperative based in Brussels that specializes in the reuse of construction materials (Rotor, n.d., 2015a, 2015b). This organization is an offshoot of the non-profit architectural firm Rotor that promotes reuse in design and has been involved in dismantling, processing, and trading recovered building components since 2016. Rotor DC's project Reuse Made Easy was conceived from ten years of knowledge and research on material flows and material reuse within the construction industry, which made apparent the lack of reuse organization facilitators within the sector. Figures 5.20–5.23 depict the reuse material

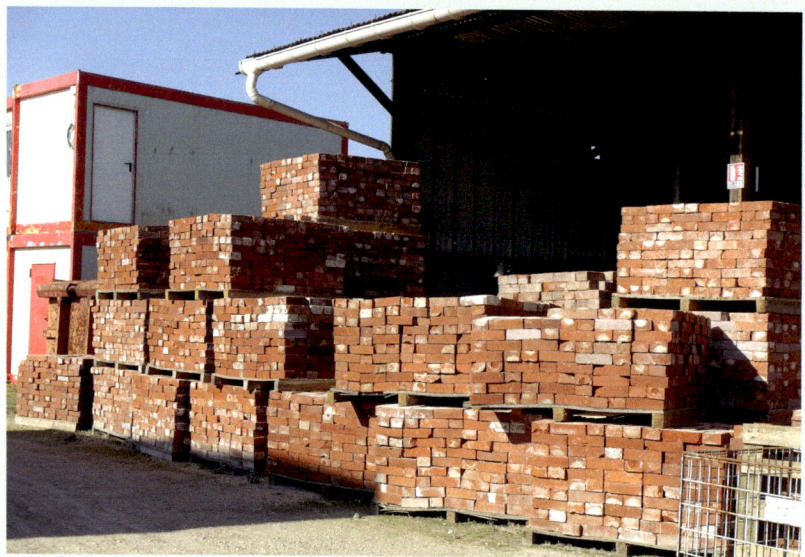

Figure 5.20 Salvaged Reused Brick.

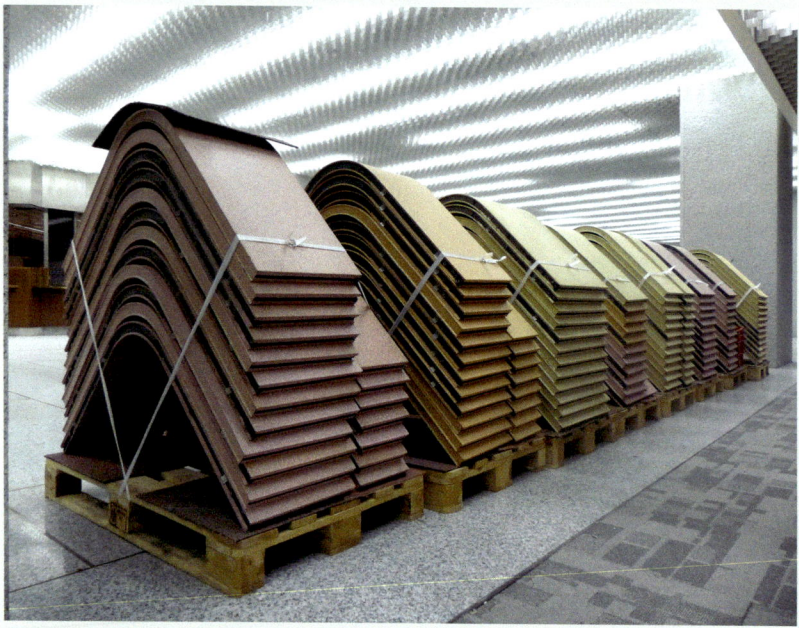

Figure 5.21 Reclaimed Insulation.

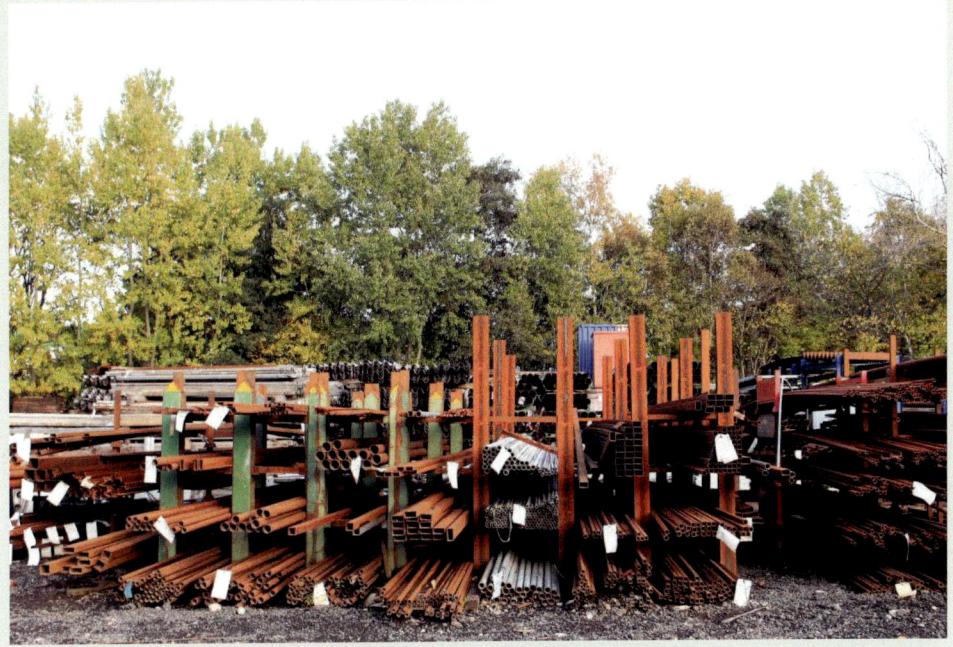

Figure 5.22 Collected Reclaimed Steel Frames and Other Building Materials.

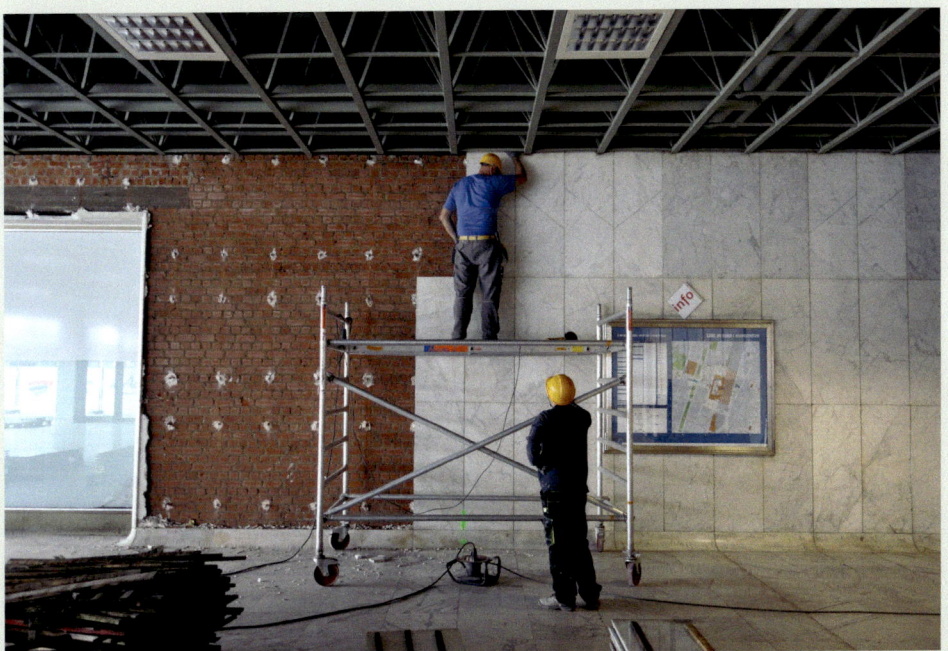

Figure 5.23 Careful Deconstruction Practices Allows for Materials to Be Recovered on Site at the End of a Buildings Use, and Hence, Avoiding Demolition.

and collection that Reuse Made Easy acquires. The team actively generates and manages a stock of salvaged building components, as well as providing guidance to building owners, contractors, and architects on how to best integrate these materials and elements into new building projects as consultants.

Reuse Made Easy educates local professionals in the evaluation, cataloging, and extraction of reusable material while operating extraction efforts, consultation services, and a storefront in their own reuse efforts. Upcycling of materials is not new, but Rotor DC recognized that most existing dealers handle "rustic" materials within the rural market despite construction materials from large building compounds making up most of the material waste in landfills (Baker-Brown, 2019). The company is at the forefront of **recovery and recycling** efforts within the construction industry, working to divert waste from local landfills and eventually become a key figure in a regional building market to facilitate reuse of materials.

Rotor DC's efforts not only reduce demolition waste, but they also provide high-quality building materials that would be previously overlooked in conventional demolition practices. The organization's **virtual** and in-person storefront offers the majority of their reclaimed materials cheaper than market value, even though they are typically the same, if not better, quality as new. Other materials sold by Rotor are equally expensive or more expensive than new but carry aesthetic or cultural heritage and feature beautifully aged surfaces that add value. This successful business model shows that reuse can contribute to affordability within the construction industry, while also illustrating the value that time can add to materials (Wang et al., 2017). Figure 5.24 depicts how these reused materials can be implemented successfully in a business.

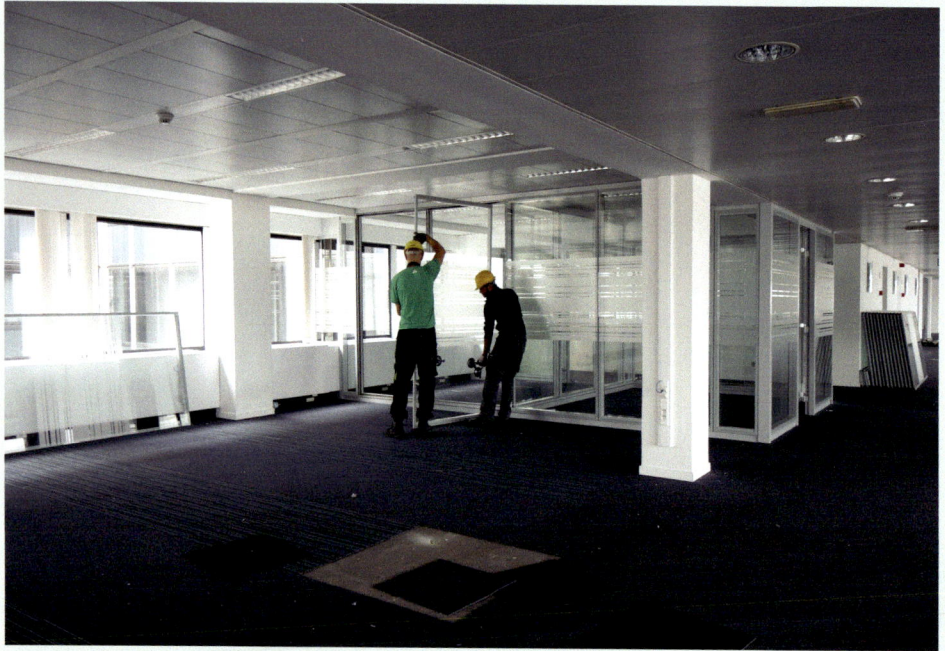

Figure 5.24 Reclaimed Materials Being Used to Create an Office Space.

In recognizing demolition sites as potential extraction and recovery sites, Rotor DC contributes to achieving the circular economy framework of **product life extension**. Large-scale reuse efforts contribute to the adoption of this attitude that appreciates the value of materials throughout their entire life cycle, which benefits the sector both economically and environmentally.

The reuse of construction materials is not a new concept, but contemporary building materials and techniques have evolved in a way that neglected this powerful tool. Rotor DC is pioneering the development of new skills to increase recycling in contemporary buildings, creating new deconstruction techniques and systems to empower other professionals in the industry. Through the repair and cleaning of lighting equipment, furniture, hardware, and plumbing components, mortar removal from ceramic tiles, the reprocessing of wood, and the planning of salvage operations, the project contributes to the **regeneration** of a diminishing resource and material supply. The increased use of reclaimed materials avoids reliance on non-renewable materials extracted from our geo-biosphere that has proved to be unsustainable and harmful to our environment. Reuse Made Easy illustrates the possibility of material sourcing for housing that does not harm our natural landscape while adding value, beauty, and clear conscience.

5.6. Conclusion

Excessive material and energy waste and high costs occur in current linear practices within the building sector. The linearity of our existing model ensures the generation of waste while depleting renewable resources, cementing challenges for future generations and their environment. Moving toward circular economy principles in the conception, design, and evaluation of housing can vastly reduce waste and expenses, putting affordable and sustainable houses on the market. In a time of economic and environmental uncertainty, affordability and sustainability are crucial issues in the well-being of future generations. In the appropriate provision of land and infrastructure at the community scale, affordability can be increased regionally to create savings for homeowners and renters while diminishing the industry's environmental footprint and maintaining quality. Closing the gap between our built environment and our needs in terms of space, aesthetic quality, and quantity of materials/products can bring about affordability in the design of homes and buildings. Another solution that the circular economy offers to the affordability crisis is the implementation of reuse and its many forms to decrease the demand put on raw materials and energy. Finally, material inventories, along with heritage value and certification, are three methods of achieving reuse in the building sector to realize its many benefits. As affordability and sustainability go hand-in-hand, the circular economy model strives for both; the possibility of a future where all may have access to housing that does not come at the expense of their environment.

References

+ImpaKT Luxembourg. (2020). *Product Circularity Data Sheet (PCDS) v3.2s*. Retrieved January 24 from https://pcds.lu/wp-content/uploads/2020/11/20200214_Light_PCDS_v3.2s_FORM.pdf

Baker-Brown, D. (2019). Rotor & RotorDC. In *The re-use atlas* (pp. 82–85). RIBA Publishing.

Canada Mortgage and Housing Cooperation. (2018). *About affordable housing in Canada*. Retrieved January 24 from https://www.cmhc-schl.gc.ca/en/professionals/industry-innovation-and-leadership/industry-expertise/affordable-housing/about-affordable-housing/affordable-housing-in-canada

Cilliers, E. J. (2015). The importance of planning for green spaces. *Agriculture Forestry and Fisheries*, 6. https://doi.org/10.11648/j.aff.s.2015040401.11

CMHC, Bond, E., & Cortellino, F. (2022). *Housing supply report*. https://assets.cmhc-schl.gc.ca/sites/cmhc/professional/housing-markets-data-and-research/market-reports/housing-supply-report/housing-supply-report-2022-05-en.pdf?rev=e66a4117-594f-4b3e-8477-c33fbe1e7766

Cohen, M. J. (2021). New conceptions of sufficient home size in high-income countries: Are we approaching a sustainable consumption transition? *Housing, Theory and Society*, 38, 32, https://doi.org/10.1080/14036096.2020.1722218

CSSBI. (n.d.). *Sustainable steel*. Retrieved January 25 from https://cssbi.ca/mid-rise-construction/sustainable-steel

Cutland Consulting Ltd. (2016). *The challenge of shape and form: Understanding the benefits of efficient design*. NHBC Foundation. https://www.nhbcfoundation.org/wp-content/uploads/2016/10/NF-72-NHBC-Foundation_Shape-and-Form.pdf.

den Hollander, M., Conny, C., Bakker, A., & Jan Hultink, E. (2017). Product design in a circular economy. *Journal of Industrial Ecology*, *21*, 9.

EU Mies Award. (2022). *The Resource Rows*. European Union Prize for Contemporary Architecture Mies van der Rohe Award. Retrieved June 20 from https://www.miesarch.com/work/4305

GXN, & Assets, R. (2018). *Circle house: Denmark's first circular housing project* (1 ed., Vol. 248). GXN.

Heward, J. (2019). *Resource Rows, ørestad syd by Lendager*. Retrieved January 23, 2023 from http://danishdesignreview.com/kbhnotes/2019/1/25/resource-rowe

Idenburg, F. (2022). By redrawing the way we design, build, and "unbuild," circularity could reduce forced labor in the building industry. *The Architect's Newspaper*. https://www.archpaper.com/2022/05/by-redrawing-the-way-we-design-build-and-unbuild-circularity-could-reduce-forced-labor-in-the-building-industry/

IUCN. (2023). *Nature-based solutions*. International Union for Conservation of Nature. Retrieved June 19 from https://www.iucn.org/our-work/nature-based-solutions

Lendager. (2022). *Resource rows*. Retrieved January 23, 2023 from https://lendager.com/project/resource-rows/

Litman, T. A. (2017). *Economic value of walkability*. Victoria Transport Policy Institute.

Mullenbach, L. E., Mowen, A. J., & Baker, B. L. (2018). Assessing the relationship between a composite score of urban park quality and health. *Preventing Chronic Disease: Public Health Research, Practice, and Policy*, *15*(*E136*), 8.

NRCan. (2015). *EE4*. Natural Resources Canada. Retrieved June 20 from https://natural-resources.canada.ca/energy/ee4/7453

Pearl, D., & Wentz, D. (2014). *Community-inspired housing in Canada: Benny Farm and Rosemont*. Holcim Foundation for Sustainable Construction. https://src.holcimfoundation.org/dnl/4b638d42-a390-492e-bfb3-23d481dab507/CommunityHousingCanada-lowres.pdf

Raghav, S., Kasraian, D., & Miller, E. J. (2019). Literature review of the costs of infrastructure provision for different development forms. *iCity: Urban Informatics for Sustainable Metropolitan Growth*, 22, Article Project 2.4.

Rotor. (n.d.). *Rotor deconstruction – Reuse of Building Materials Made Easy*. Rotor deconstruction scrl. Retrieved January 23, 2023, from https://rotordc.com/

Rotor. (2015a). Vade-mecum pour le réemploi hors-site: Comment extraire les matériaux réutilisables de bâtiments publics? https://www.vademecum-reuse.org/Vademecum_extraire_les_materiaux_reutilisables-Rotor.pdf.

Rotor. (2015b). *Handbook for reuse off site. How can reusable materials be extracted from public buildings?* https://opalis.eu/sites/default/files/2022-02/Vademecum_offsite_reuse-Rotor.pdf

UN Habitat for a Better Urban Future. (2019). The Global Housing Affordability Challenge: A more Comprehensive Understanding of the Housing Sector. *Urban Data Digest, Version 2*(May 2019 Edition), 8.

Wang, K., Vanassche, S., Ribeiro, A., Peters, M., & Oseyran, J. (2017). *Business models for building material circularity: Learnings from frontrunner cases. The Netherlands*: Delft University of Technology: Delft.

Wilson, R. (2019). *Old into new: Recycled bricks form facade of Copenhagen housing project*. Retrieved January 23, 2023 from https://www.architectsjournal.co.uk/buildings/old-into-new-recycled-bricks-form-facade-of-copenhagen-housing-project

Chapter 6

Design for Flexibility and Choice with Space as a Resource

6.1 Space as a Resource

Space is a resource to be conserved. Yet, current design and building practices do not treat it as such. Inefficiencies, especially in housing, render space inadequate and, ultimately, result in waste. There exists a disparity between people's evolving spatial needs and the rigid spatial conditions of housing. Current social factors – including demography, mobility, and new technologies – make dwellings inadequate, leading to inefficient renovations and constant moving. Beyond people's comfort, this disparity contributes to a large amount of waste. Therefore, in an effort to promote a circular economy, the design and construction of housing need to be rendered flexible.

Over time, residents' needs evolve and require their space to evolve simultaneously (see Figure 6.1). In recent times, there has been a rise in the number of diverse household structures beyond the nuclear family, including seniors, singles, same-sex couples, and single parents. For example, surveys show that the elderly prefer to age independently at home (see Chapter 1) (Friedman, 2002). In the United Kingdom, retrofitting homes for people who become disabled costs around 350 million pounds per year (Schneider & Till, 2007). As people's mental and motor abilities decline with age, homes need to be adaptable to the aging process. These changes may include small or large ones – for instance, adding a guest room, skylights, converting a room into an office, and updating bathrooms. Another trend is the rise in mobility. North Americans, in particular, have a higher mobility compared to people in other continents – households move every ten years, on average (Friedman, 2002). New jobs, social upgrading, and a desire to live closer to other family members, for example, motivate residents to move. However, in certain cases, the house itself causes moving. With certain changes, such as a growing family, a change in status, or a desire for a new interior arrangement, there is a tendency to relocate rather than to adapt. This presents a conflict: homes are designed and built at a particular point in time, characterized by specific tendencies and technologies, and as time progresses, the factors and decisions that shaped the original design become increasingly dated.

Common residential design and construction characteristics – including room proportions, lighting and socket locations, and window sizes – restrict adaptability. Rooms have clear and defined functions, making it difficult to allow post-occupancy adaptability in the production of mass housing. Therefore, modern households are left with conventionally designed interior layouts, which are rigid and outdated. There is a growing demand for adaptable units that accommodate varying spatial needs and facilitate the introduction of new building systems without compromising functionality

DOI: 10.4324/9781003333975-8

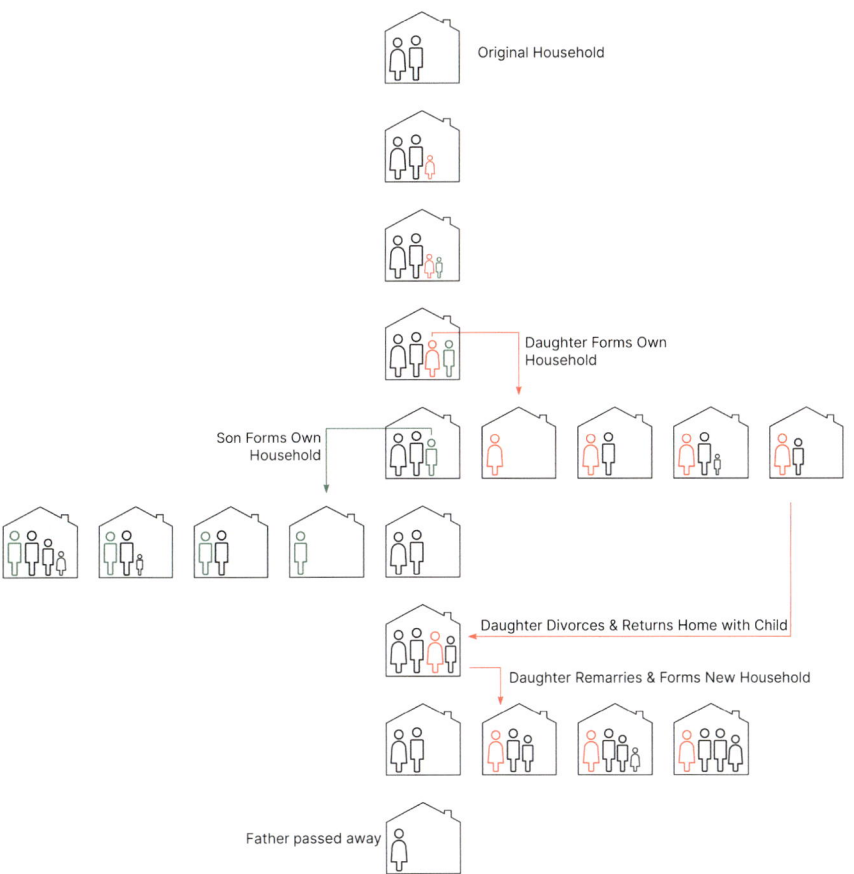

Original Household

Daughter Forms Own Household

Son Forms Own Household

Daughter Divorces & Returns Home with Child

Daughter Remarries & Forms New Household

Father passed away

Figure 6.1 Family Tree.

or comfort. Architects need to assume not only the profile of the occupants but also their evolving needs.

While it is difficult to make accurate predictions in a society that is continuously changing, it *is* possible to predict that homes will continue to reflect inhabitants' tastes, habits, needs, and lifestyles and will be influenced by new technologies. Thus, flexible housing is presented as a solution; it responds to the volatility of dwelling by being flexible or adaptable, or both. These two terms are distinct – adaptability involves issues of use while flexibility covers issues of form and technique. Adaptable design – namely rooms accommodating various uses – can solve social issues (Groak, 2002). Flexibility, on the other hand, requires different physical arrangements, such as joining units by extending them or through movable partitions. In other words, flexibility makes physical changes, whereas adaptability does not (Schneider & Till, 2007). Moreover, from an economic standpoint, flexibility limits obsolescence in the housing stock (Schneider & Till, 2007). Homes last longer and will be more inexpensive in the long run, as they reduce the need and frequency of refurbishment. The ability to adjust to different circumstances allows it to avoid considerable long-term capital costs. Overall, employing these design solutions gives buyers more freedom, allowing those with modest means to have a better fit between dwelling, household composition, lifestyle, and resources. Achieving a close fit between occupants' evolving space needs and their homes can and *should* be simpler than it is at present.

6.2 History of Contemporary Design for Flexibility

The concept of adaptability in housing is not new. Residents have been adapting their shelters to suit their varying needs for as long as human habitation has existed. Back when societies were overwhelmingly nomadic, the ability to adapt was relatively easy because dwellings were light and simple in order to facilitate their transportation (Friedman, 2002). The three archetypes of housing – the primitive hut, the cave, and the tent – all consist of a single space, where various activities take place (Schmidth & Austin, 2016). Then, as people settled, adaptability slowed. Dwelling conditions changed; permanent walls marked the boundaries of homes, and interior and exterior walls could not easily be altered. The Industrial Revolution marked one of the first major turning points in housing. Technology emerged and played a large role in building construction, and rapid urbanization drew more people from the countryside to the city (Friedman, 2002). Urbanization transformed lifestyle, and mobility emerged as people moved and settled where work was available (Schmidth & Austin, 2016). The meaning of adaptability shifted in this context – homeowners could now find more suitable space in another residence.

The end of World War II marked another major shift as society underwent an accelerated pace of change due to demographic transformations, rapid technological evolution, and new lifestyle tendencies. Initially, after World War II, builders knew the demographic makeup of their clients – working fathers, stay-at-home mothers, and children. Housing reflected this: the standard was homogeneity with mid-rise, mass-produced housing dominating the urban scene (Friedman, 2012). However, the rise of automobiles, and subsequently suburbs, as well as the rise of the women's liberation movement, jeopardized the "traditional" household. Shifts in the cultural context, and a rise in divorces and unconventional family structures, expanded the definition of a family. Houses, thus, needed to accommodate a wide range of households over their lifespan and required spatial arrangements that permitted moving from one status to another. Beyond social changes, post-war conditions created a high demand for housing that vastly outweighed supply. There was a growing need to house a large portion of the population efficiently and cost-effectively. The increasing demand for housing placed pressure on builders to improve speed and efficiency, which led to important technological breakthroughs. This introduced the concepts of full-scale mass production and prefabrication. Alongside the acknowledgment of diverse needs, architects recognized that conventional and monotone mass housing was inadequate, and design sought to provide individuals with the opportunity to influence design according to particular personal requirements.

Since then, contemporary designs for flexibility have continued to grow. In 1994, Stuart Brand's *How Buildings Learn* suggests that one ought to "examine buildings as a whole" and analyze what happens in buildings over time (see Figure 6.2) (Brand, 1995). He argued that it was critical to conceptualize a building beyond material

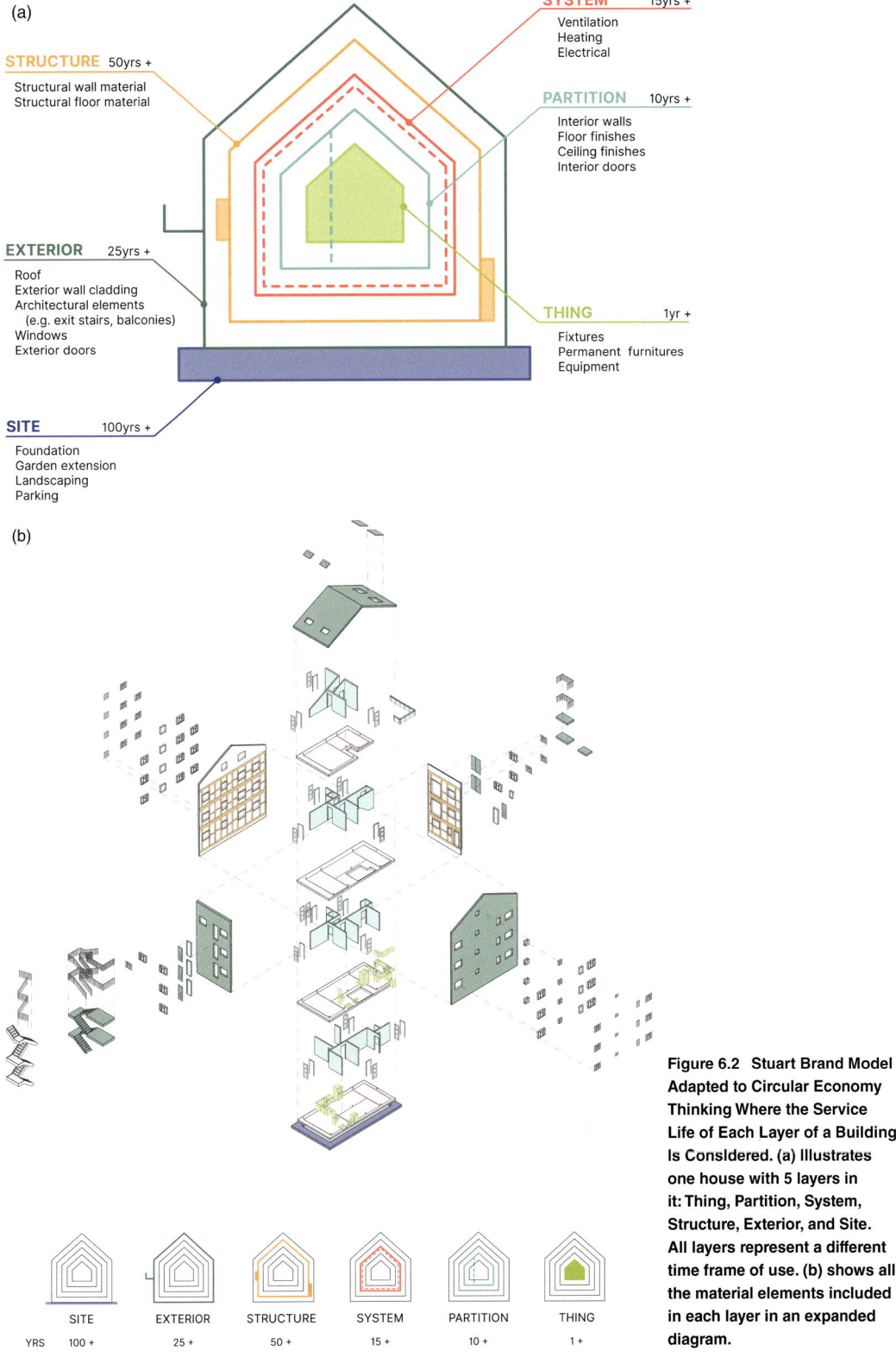

(a)

SYSTEM 15yrs +
Ventilation
Heating
Electrical

STRUCTURE 50yrs +
Structural wall material
Structural floor material

PARTITION 10yrs +
Interior walls
Floor finishes
Ceiling finishes
Interior doors

EXTERIOR 25yrs +
Roof
Exterior wall cladding
Architectural elements
   (e.g. exit stairs, balconies)
Windows
Exterior doors

THING 1yr +
Fixtures
Permanent furnitures
Equipment

SITE 100yrs +
Foundation
Garden extension
Landscaping
Parking

(b)

SITE	EXTERIOR	STRUCTURE	SYSTEM	PARTITION	THING
YRS 100 +	25 +	50 +	15 +	10 +	1 +

Figure 6.2 Stuart Brand Model Adapted to Circular Economy Thinking Where the Service Life of Each Layer of a Building Is Considered. (a) Illustrates one house with 5 layers in it: Thing, Partition, System, Structure, Exterior, and Site. All layers represent a different time frame of use. (b) shows all the material elements included in each layer in an expanded diagram.

terms, but rather as units of time. Brand's model has since been expanded to cover a broader interpretation of the layered concept, adding two layers that are crucial when considering the building in time. His concept has evolved into building decomposition, which envisions a building as a set of "shearing" layers that change at different rates – the more the layers are connected, the greater the difficulty and cost of adaptation (Schmidth & Austin, 2016). As illustrated in Figure 6.2, the Stuart Brand diagram has been adapted to circular economy thinking where each layer represents the service life of the materials and components used within that layer. For example, from a circular design perspective site and structure, which can last for well over 50 years, should be designed with life extension in mind. Whereas its common for exterior materials to be reused or recycled every 25 years. Additionally, interior partitions, as well as "stuff" such as furniture and fixtures and fittings, will typically have a more dynamic life cycle with many reuses and repurposing turnover everyone to ten years. Such consideration of materials and component service life can sync nicely with adaptability principles in design that meet shifting societal trends.

Over the course of history, major shifts in societal trends have demanded shifts in housing strategies. While these changes are unpredictable and varied, one thing remains: there will continue to be change, and the only way to address it is by creating adaptable homes that can be modified to accommodate all. Thus, the concept of flexibility has emerged and has been associated with progress.

6.3 Adaptability

While many understand adaptability to be desirable, its meaning is not entirely understood. Adaptability can be interpreted as "providing occupants with forms and means that facilitate a fit between their space needs and the constraints of their homes either before or after occupancy" (Friedman, 2002). The stereotypical design characteristics that are often associated with adaptability include generous floor-to-floor heights, movable walls, and open-plan spaces (Schmidth & Austin, 2016). While these do represent important design characteristics, specific user needs, and a broader range of tailored solutions are not expressed. A house's subcomponents, such as utilities, partitions, and rooms, can be made flexible in order to enable occupants to achieve adaptable homes and lifestyles.

Adaptable buildings are desirable because they rely on the premise that they will be easier to alter in the future, which subsequently reduces costs (see Figure 6.3). Buildings that are not adaptable will eventually fall out of use or be demolished. Adaptability provides a solution to extending the life cycle of a building and, therefore, contributes to sustainable solutions. For instance, flexible buildings can be adapted, resulting in less material waste, and effectively reducing carbon emissions. Despite the various benefits of an adaptable design, there are certain obstacles. Initial cost is a primary issue, given that adaptable solutions are more expansive than non-adaptable alternatives; however, this is not always the case. The majority of adaptability's benefits are long-term, which is difficult for people to appreciate.

It is critical for clients, as well as all stakeholders along the value chain, to understand terminology and issues relating to building, in particular as it relates to adaptability. Through clarifying the topic, the objective is to simplify the implementation of more appropriate design solutions, by recognizing opportunities for adaptability and avoiding costly and inefficient solutions. Adaptable buildings have immense opportunities but require a shift in the way in which architecture is approached. One cannot simply choose from a list of off-the-shelf flexible design characteristics – adaptability requires challenging the ways in which stakeholders approach building (Cheshire, 2021; Schmidth & Austin, 2016). Figure 6.3 illustrates how the service life of a building layers, as shown in Figure 6.2, directly connects to changes in occupancy and adaptable principles. Information on the service life of building layers can greatly inform the occupants and designers on what circular strategies could be best employed.

During construction, adaptability involves employment of strategies or building components that allow builders or occupants to make changes to the design as the building progresses. This is crucial for tract developments, which refers to when a client's identity and preferences are unknown at the time of design. Adaptability enables builders to offer choices to buyers by allowing them to select between alternative layouts. Moreover, changes during the construction period are permitted and common. Once occupants move into a home, the life cycle process that generates ongoing needs for adaptability begins. Life cycles change based on trends and changes in social agendas (Schmidth & Austin, 2016). The need for adaptability is driven by various areas, with one important aspect being functional needs in accordance with the family life cycle. These include simple changes such as painting, expanding the kitchen, demolishing a wall, as well as more elaborate alterations such as joining two levels or building an addition.

An example of adaptable strategies is seen in the Next Home, constructed at McGill University in 1996 and later adopted by private sector builders (Rohe & Watson, 2007). The Next Home is based on the belief that housing can be designed to evolve beyond configuration and appearance, by adapting to use. The project allows prospective buyers to purchase one, two, or all three of the floors in a three-story structure. Moreover, buyers can choose from a catalog of interior components to further tailor the design to their budget. Ultimately, the Next Home is designed to be subdivided and rearranged in both pre- and post-occupancy in an effort to achieve both flexibility and affordability – a strategy that will be further explored in the remainder of the chapter.

Forms of adaptability depend on various factors, including the type of home, method of construction, and procedure used to make changes. Four main areas of intervention have been identified as essential in achieving adaptability in housing (Friedman, 2021). First, manipulation of volumes: considerations that a designer, builder, or occupant will give to the use of the entire volume (such as floors in multistory buildings). Second, spatial arrangement: considerations of use of spaces themselves within the volume (e.g., floor or single room). Third, growth and division: design strategies or means that allow expansion or reduction of a space's volume, either during construction or occupancy. Fourth, manipulation of subcomponents: elements employed in the construction and use of a building, which may be as large structural

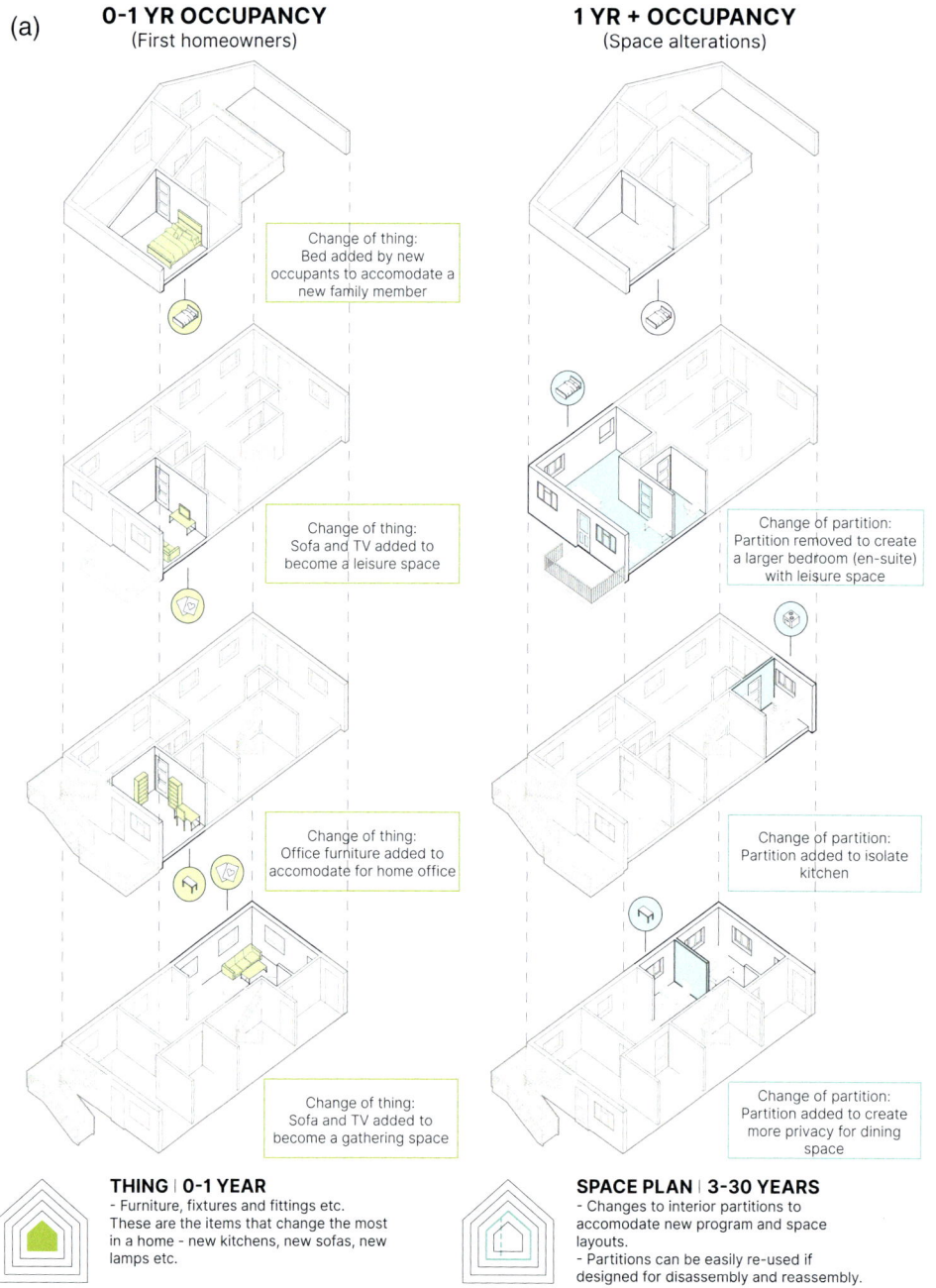

(a)

0-1 YR OCCUPANCY
(First homeowners)

1 YR + OCCUPANCY
(Space alterations)

Change of thing:
Bed added by new occupants to accomodate a new family member

Change of thing:
Sofa and TV added to become a leisure space

Change of partition:
Partition removed to create a larger bedroom (en-suite) with leisure space

Change of thing:
Office furniture added to accomodate for home office

Change of partition:
Partition added to isolate kitchen

Change of thing:
Sofa and TV added to become a gathering space

Change of partition:
Partition added to create more privacy for dining space

THING | 0-1 YEAR
- Furniture, fixtures and fittings etc. These are the items that change the most in a home - new kitchens, new sofas, new lamps etc.

SPACE PLAN | 3-30 YEARS
- Changes to interior partitions to accomodate new program and space layouts.
- Partitions can be easily re-used if designed for disassembly and reassembly.

Figure 6.3 Adaptability and the Service Life of Building Layers Work Hand-in-Hand When Implementing Circular Design. (a) Adaptability and the Service Life of Building Layers Work Hand-in-Hand When Implementing Circular Design. (b) one floor plan is shown across four different periods of time: 0 to 1 year of occupancy, 1 or more years of occupancy, 5+ years of occupancy, and 100+ years of occupancy. The space can be adapted and reconfigured according to the needs of an evolving household or new homeowners.

(b)

5 YRS + OCCUPANCY
(New family members)

100 YRS + OCCUPANCY
(Fifth homeowners)

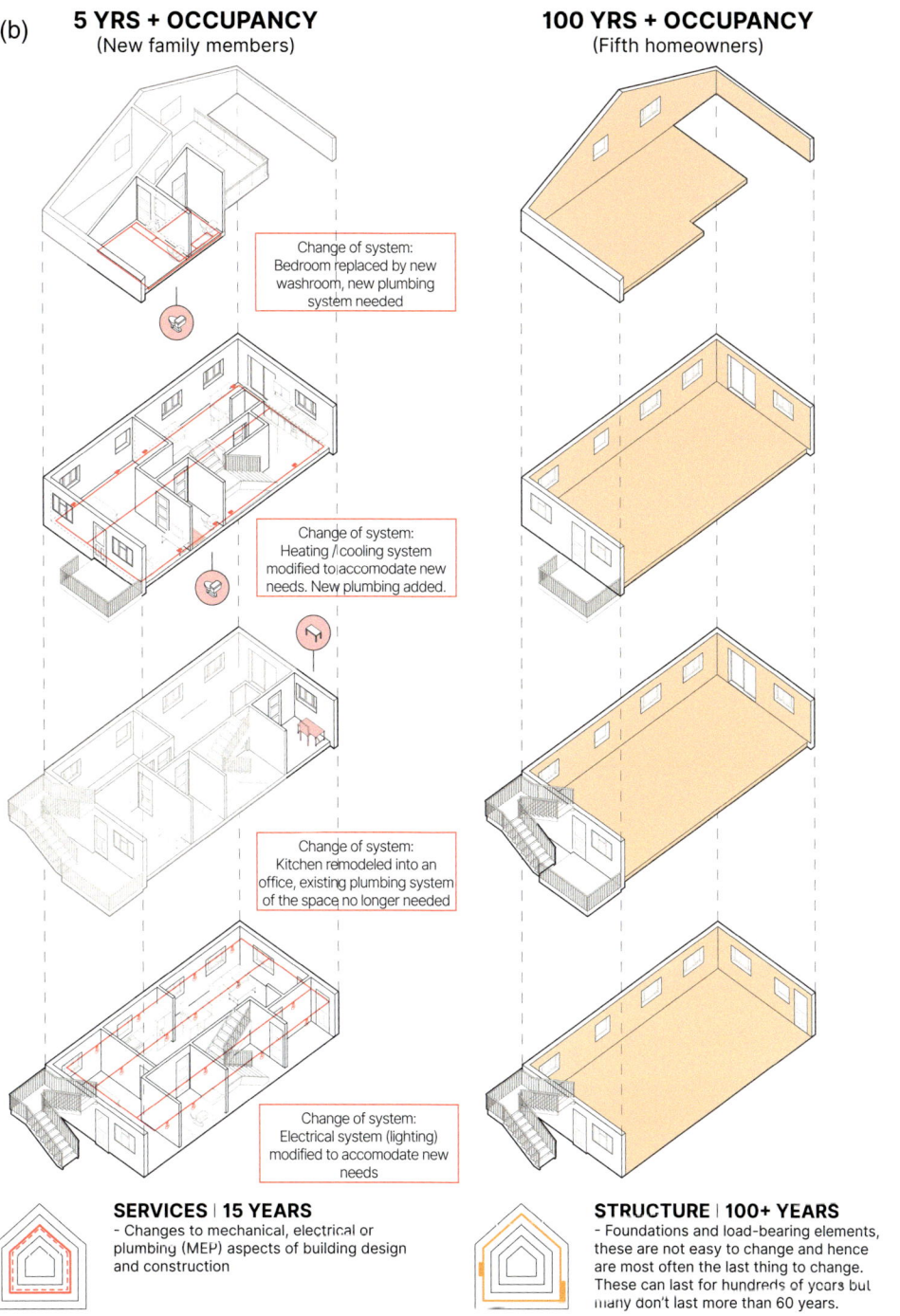

Change of system:
Bedroom replaced by new washroom, new plumbing system needed

Change of system:
Heating / cooling system modified to accomodate new needs. New plumbing added.

Change of system:
Kitchen remodeled into an office, existing plumbing system of the space no longer needed

Change of system:
Electrical system (lighting) modified to accomodate new needs

SERVICES | 15 YEARS
- Changes to mechanical, electrical or plumbing (MEP) aspects of building design and construction

STRUCTURE | 100+ YEARS
- Foundations and load-bearing elements, these are not easy to change and hence are most often the last thing to change. These can last for hundreds of years but many don't last more than 60 years.

Figure 6.3 (*Continued*)

169

components or as small as a waterpipe. Adapting a building is not restricted to its interior – a building's envelope also participates in flexibility. Changes in the external environment of a dwelling unit involve work at the macro level. This generally begins at the scale of a building. Internal changes arise at the micro-scale and involve individual housing or unit levels (Schneider & Till, 2007). The two are interrelated; however, for the sake of clarity, they will be treated separately in this chapter. Within each entity, four main groups of topics will be explored: manipulation of volumes, spatial arrangement, growth and division, and manipulation of subcomponents.

6.4 Macro Design Decisions

A home's macro aspects – including volume, envelope, and systems – can be effectively designed and altered to promote flexibility. The type of unit, a house's dimensions, utilities' location, and modularity, all currently play a role in inhibiting flexibility. However, by properly planning and implementing flexible approaches, a home's macro design decisions can greatly contribute to its adaptability.

6.4.1 Dwelling's Typology

The unit typology influences the amount of choice and adaptability in a home. It affects both the appearance and the function. Major unit types are outlined below, with their characteristics and their ability to allow adaptability (see Figure 6.4).

The bungalow consists of a home in which all habitable rooms are on one level (Friedman, 2002). Its low-pitched wide roof extends out over the verandah. Originally from England in the late 19th century, a bungalow is a northern-summer translation of British colonial homes in India (Brand, 1995). Designed for the growing middle class, it was the standard expansion housing of the 1910s and 1920s. Bungalows are commonly built as single-family detached homes, which simplifies expansion. The bungalow became known for its diversity. The main level offers possibilities for open interior planning. Its spread-out nature represents an advantage for adaptability, as the unit perimeter allows for a greater choice in locating each function, given the

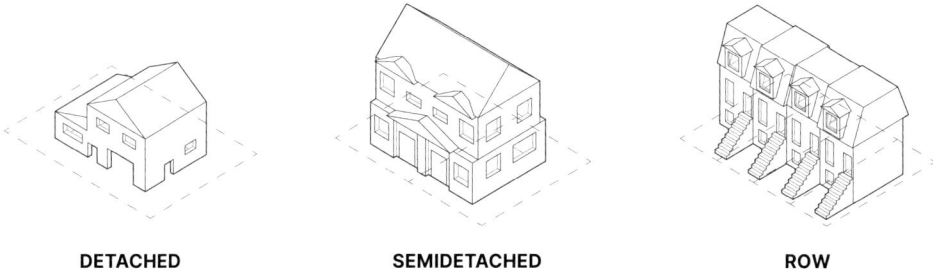

DETACHED   SEMIDETACHED   ROW

Figure 6.4 Macro Design Decisions Considering Different Residence Typologies.

better exposure to natural light, but, consequently, raises the cost of land and infrastructure due to the large roof area.

The bungalow is known as the direct parent of the ranch house. The rancher represents one of the most adaptable types of dwellings (Friedman, 2002). It spreads the bungalow horizontally, on larger lots of automobile suburbs of the 1940s and 1950s (Brand, 1995). This housing type is built entirely on a single level above grade. Having all functions located on the same floor permits many options for open-space planning and post-occupancy adaptability. The rancher's often flat roof allows for relatively easy addition of a second floor.

The split-level represents a hybrid between the bungalow and rancher, enjoying the advantages of both. Since the unit is designed on different levels, it is possible to arrange the spaces within it according to different zones and functions. Additionally, this offers the possibility of eventually dividing the structure into smaller units – each level could become an independent dwelling with its own entry. Ultimately, depending on the housing type, different degrees of flexibility are afforded.

The one-and-a-half story's adaptability potential lies in the attic. It represents an opportunity for add-in expansion. This, however, requires preparing the top level for expansion in the initial construction stage. Moreover, this unit's interior demonstrates remarkable versatility; given that the top level does not have bearing partitions, its interior can be arranged in a variety of configurations and can easily be modified later. The two-story is preferred when more than two bedrooms are needed on the upper floor. One of this prototype's advantages is its versatility in the use of floors; the two-story house can easily be transformed into a three-story when the basement is introduced as a living area. Each level can be designed to become an independent dwelling unit either at pre- or post-occupancy stages.

The row house – also known as the terraced house – has proved to be an infinitely adaptable form of building. It is not particularly technological nor innovative; however, its size and shape fit well into context (Schmidth & Austin, 2016). Individuality is confined behind the decorum of its façade. This housing type allows for growth and adaption; additions to the back of terraced row houses show how social and economic growth can be manifested.

The high-rise building is typically known to be ill-suited for modular construction and, subsequently, flexibility. Contractors often work separately from designers until construction begins and, by then, they are not willing to make changes to accommodate adaptability (Farnsworth, 2015). However, the projected global urban population growth urgently demands high-rise housing, suitable for dense urban development. Thus, high-rise buildings have been made more adaptable with the help of modular construction. For instance, in 2016, a volumetric modular system was adapted to a 32-story apartment in Brooklyn, New York designed by SHoP architects (SHoP Architects, 2016; Wallance, 2021). Similar to a modular approach, the concept of a volumetric modular system is that three-dimensional volumes or chunks of buildings are fabricated off-site in a factory and then brought to site where the pieces are assembled. In the case of the Brooklyn tower, the developer set up a factory within miles of the site. Although, once on-site there were issues with traffic congestion getting to the site, the volumes were very large and difficult to maneuver given constraints of the tight site, and issues arose with tolerances between the prefabricated volumes and the on-site built steel structure. Despite these difficulties, it is still an example of how an ambitious architectural high-rise modular tower was made possible (Wallance, 2021). Given the modular design construction efficiency was increased, it reduced noise and traffic impacts associated with on-site construction in urban areas. In addition, it avoided waste via fabrication off-site in a controlled environment which increases material efficiency (SHoP Architects, 2016).

There are numerous housing typologies, each with their own attributes and limitations. A housing style has a unique configuration, with its own sets of possibilities for future modification. It is useful to have housing types, as they can be most appropriate for the needs of a specific location or family. However, despite its initial characteristics, a housing unit should always possess the ability to evolve into a different style or into a generally more adaptable space. No matter the specific characteristics of a style, with proper planning strategies, virtually all styles can lead to greater flexibility.

6.4.2 Dimensions

The dimensions and proportions of a home or of a single floor of a home heavily influence choice and adaptability in housing. Building proportions affect both appearance and function and should, therefore, be designed with care. Today's conventions define buildings based on functions, including labeling rooms with prescribed dimensions, which accommodate a specific arrangement of furniture (Schmidth & Austin, 2016). In order to accommodate change, the relationship between program and space needs to be loosened. Design choices can be made to influence configuration and yield the greatest number of variations of the structure, or spaces within it.

The placement of openings in a building's exterior, for instance, significantly impacts the proportions of interior space and, subsequently, potential changes in layout and use. The placement of the main entrance is critical; the decision to have a front or side main entrance is one that must be considered early in the design process. In the case of a single-family detached home, the functional and spatial configuration of its front elevation is critical. When an entry door is located at the center of the front façade, the interior space is naturally divided into two areas with circulation in between – this configuration severely limits adaptability. Thus, in the event of a house being divided, placing a door near one of its wide walls is ideal, as it provides greater exposure to natural light and circulation to the upstairs levels (Friedman, 2012). Alternatively, having a side entrance provides greater opportunity for division of the space from the rest of the unit, as it prevents access and circulation. Furthermore, the placement of windows is also important to consider. To accommodate specific needs, window placement should accommodate individuality, but this often comes at the price of understanding a single module as a unified whole. According to the Next Home concept, a combination of random order and composition is ideal to obtain a proper balance between flexibility and a unit's identity (Friedman, 2002).

With the right dimensions and proportions, a space can be adapted to different styles. Currently, certain factors lead to housing being identical and unsuitable. For instance, houses are often designed for tract developments, in which many consider repeating the same dwelling type and design to be most efficient. Moreover, due to zoning regulations, very little choice and diversity of configurations are offered, which leads to a demographic and economic similarity of buyers. With proper planning and consideration, however, one building could be built in a variety of housing types. When a multistory dwelling is constructed, the area of each floor must be sufficient to accommodate self-contained and independent living. Thus, space needs to be designed to adapt to all basic functions. The maximum size of floor area will depend on the client's means and the minimum size will depend on its desired livability. Thus, by incorporating flexibility into the planning stages – in a large development especially – units can be arranged to form a variety of configurations, allowing greater choice and producing a community's desired urban character.

6.4.3 Utilities and Their Location

Utilities and their location play a significant role in a dwelling's achievement of adaptability. Manipulating utilities is difficult and costly, due to utility conduits (Friedman, 2002). The adaptable home, therefore, needs to permit such processes, which requires various initiatives.

To tackle this issue, a systems-based approach is crucial. Owners need to be able to locate subcomponents to easily replace or upgrade them when desired. For this to be achievable without interrupting the occupants' daily lives (as it generally does, today), a system is required. These initiatives need to be taken early in the design process to instill better practices in constructing for change. For instance, having raised floors or suspended ceilings allows for quick rerouting of ventilation pipes or the insertion of new computer cables (Friedman, 2012). By developing a method of systematically laying utilities, they can be concentrated into a single known location, effectively simplifying future renovation projects. Moreover, when utilities branch out to different rooms, their chase (i.e., location of passageway) should be identified. Thus, through concentrating on the location of utilities and simplifying access to them, builders' choices are widened at the pre-occupancy stage, effectively expanding the variability of possible layout configurations.

Wet functions (e.g., kitchen, bathroom) represent a utility that requires particular attention, given its impact on flexibility. Essentially, the location of wet functions influences the exchange of areas among zones. Moving wet functions is difficult and costly. Therefore, when the kitchen or bathroom are integral components of the zones, it becomes difficult to alter a zone's use and character. A solution is to place these functions in neutral areas, such as between zones. As a result, if occupants decide to expand their home while adapting old uses in the future, the bathroom and kitchen will not pose any issues. Another solution is incorporating a prefabricated utility pod for the shower and kitchen, which can be easily relocated as needed. Both prefabricated bathroom pods and utility cupboards are beginning to be regularly utilized in housing (Bayliss & Bergin, 2020).

For a systematic approach to utilities to be widely implemented, a defined and universal guide should be available. For instance, a user manual effectively simplifies the process for all those involved. Several North American housing authorities and publishers have authored manuals, which provide guidance on the general maintenance and upkeep of homes. The Next Home initiative, for instance, suggests confining mechanical systems to a vertical shaft and horizontal chaser (Schneider & Till, 2007). This arrangement permits access to building systems through the floor, which facilitates all changes without disrupting neighboring units.

6.5 Micro Design Decisions for Flexibility

A house's micro details – including interior space and functions – play a major role in flexibility. While macro design decisions manage significant and general architectural features, secondary issues are just as crucial in solidifying an adaptable house. Decisions regarding how to plan a space, the size of rooms, and the placement of stairs can significantly influence a dwelling's future possibilities.

6.5.1 Open Plan and Room Sizes

Flexibility of a space requires large, open areas. Generous dimensions and ambiguity facilitate adapting a space to other uses. This does, however, come with associated costs and regulations (Schmidth & Austin, 2016). With the rise of non-traditional households, open-space design has become more common. Wide open space ensures sufficient room for change and should, therefore, be employed as a strategy in designing homes. Moreover, one could argue that a single person might need a minimal number of walls, as there is less of a concern for acoustic separation or privacy. Loose-fit spaces and spatial variety create flexible spaces; non-hierarchal standard room sizes provide a variety of activities and avoid bureaucratic issues allowing improved interchangeability. With that being said, extremely large or small sizes should be avoided. Room sizes of 3.7 by 3.7 m (12 by 12 ft) up to 4.6 by 4.6 m (15 by 15 ft) should be sufficient to accommodate any future adaptions (Friedman, 2021).

In order to achieve these large spaces, structural considerations need to be planned for. Large spaces require structures with little to no internal bearing support. This can be achieved in narrow houses, in which floor joists span between two exterior longitudinal walls, or by using products that allow for greater spanning distances, such as I-joists or open-web wood joists (Friedman, 2021). The result is large, open floor spaces, optimal for adaptability. Moreover, returning to the Stuart Brand model, by keeping as many elements as possible outside of the structural layer, a building's infrastructure can better receive change. For instance, a framed solution effectively separates the function of structural elements, internal partitions, and the exterior's façade. A load-bearing solution, on the other hand, combines at least two layers (Schmidth & Austin, 2016).

Once achieved, the space itself needs to be arranged to maximize adaptability. There needs to be a strategy in establishing zones, as they determine how space will be adaptable at pre- or post-occupancy stages. The decision in determining which spaces ought to be left open is dependent on the dwelling type. For instance, as seen in the case of the rancher – in which all functions are located on the same level – combining its public functions is relatively simple and optimal for allowing future changes. In the case of the two-story home, open-space design is also achievable, especially in the lower level where public uses can be located and combined. If that level is eventually turned into an independent unit, then partitioning the space will not require extensive demolition nor change. Thus, an open floor plan maximizes the potential range of uses within a restricted space. This, effectively, allows occupants to define space according to their own specific needs, contrary to the common approach of designers dictating the definition of space.

6.5.2 Location of Stairs

The placement of a stairs is important and challenging, as they possess the ability to control, and potentially limit, a space's function. While stairs can open space to a range of flexible uses, they similarly have the power to restrict it. It is, therefore, important to plan the location of stairs in order to achieve an adaptable dwelling.

Stairs allow for the division of a volume into a range of configurations, either before or after occupancy. Once placed, their location influences a house's entire layout, as well as movement across all levels throughout its life cycle. Future adaptability and functionality are sometimes at odds. For instance, if a prime objective is to shorten the length of a corridor, stairs should be placed closer to the entrance in order to free up the rest of the space for manipulation. Other factors, however, need to be considered. For instance, placing the stairs against the front façade will limit the view and natural exposure from this elevation (Friedman, 2002). Thus, compromises and careful planning need to be implemented. Using stairs as wedges between rooms effectively limits restrictions to changes within these spaces. In a multistory house, stairs should be placed along the longitudinal wall rather than in the middle of the room. Some strategies include placing stairs close to the entrance, in between two zones. Alternatively, creating a stair shaft – both within and outside of the structure – frees up the interior space, which simplifies dividing a multilevel structure into independent units. Moreover, a space can be made more adaptable to accommodate possible future installation of stairs. For instance, CUB Housing at BRE Innovation Park's modules include a removable ceiling panel, allowing stairs to be installed if additional modules are added to the top of the original one (Lawson et al., 2014).

Not only should the location of stairs be carefully considered, but the design of a home also needs to accommodate potential future stairs. It is difficult to introduce stairs to an upstairs level after a unit has been constructed. It becomes costly to build stairs perpendicularly to joists when the joists' direction is from wall to wall. It is, therefore, desirable to frame the floor in advance, in such a manner that facilitates future introduction of stairs.

6.6 Modularity at the Micro-Scale

At the small scale, modularity is common in design. Some considerations of modular design are as follows: standardization of usage components, modularization of structure, kit packaging, interchangeability, and part identification (Gullo & Dixon, 2021). Recently, the opportunity to apply these strategies to architecture has emerged as it allows architecture to be more flexible. Modularity is defined as the "separation of the physical parts of the building into defined functional entities" (Schmidth & Austin, 2016). Modular characteristics include reversibility, movable components, component accessibility, and functional separation. Thus, modularity entails the capacity for the construction to be separated into its constituting parts. Components, such as furniture, equipment, and fixtures, can support modularity by being easily movable and accessible.

6.6.1 Demountable and Movable Partitions

As stated previously, open-plan houses are popular and flexible options. However, the lack of enclosed rooms may become problematic. As a family grows, additional partitioning may become necessary. These changes can be expensive and disruptive. Thus, prefabricated, demountable walls represent an appropriate solution (see Figure 6.5). There exist three basic types of demountable wall systems. First, mobile, or operable, systems, which have a sliding mechanism that enables a wall panel to move along a ceiling track. Second, demountable systems, which are similar to the traditional dry-wall system. And third, portable partition system, which is made of prefabricated panels, brought to a desired location, and held in place by channels in the floor and ceiling (Friedman, 2021). Other movable strategies for creating interior partitions include sliding screens and furniture partitions.

There are various precedents of movable partitions being installed and successfully fulfilling the needs of occupants, all the while promoting adaptable spaces. In Carasso, Switzerland, for instance, Luigi Snozzi installed high-quality movable partitions into a residential context in order to provide a greater degree of adaptability in his 1973 project, Casa Patriziale di Carasso Ti. Post-occupancy studies show that residents did not attempt to alter or cover up the partitions, indicating that the implementation was well received (Friedman, 2002).

6.6.2 Modular Strategies

Various strategies can be implemented in design to promote modularity and, ultimately, flexibility. The multiple flexible elements and decisions can be integrated

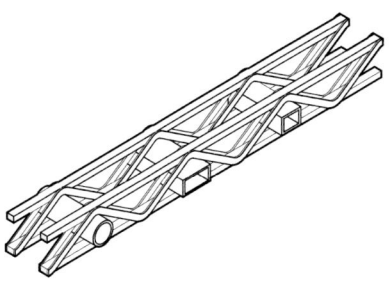

SPACE JOIST

- Allow wide spans which eliminate the need for additional support walls
- The open web allows for easy "fishing" of utility conduits

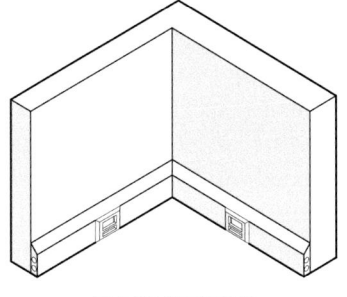

FLOOR MOLDING

- Allow flexibility in the installation of recepticals and avoids the need to pass wires through the walll

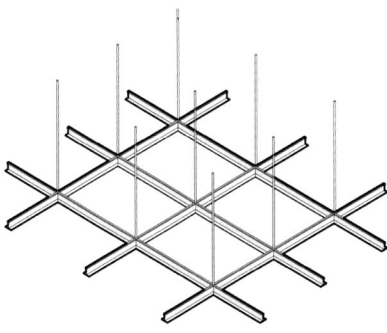

SUSPENDED CEILING

- Allow for quick covering of exposed joists and easy access to conduits for their future alteration

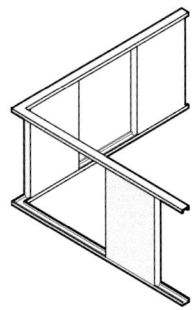

DEMOUNTABLE PARTITION

- Allow easy placement of partitions anywhere on a floor and their dismantle & reuse

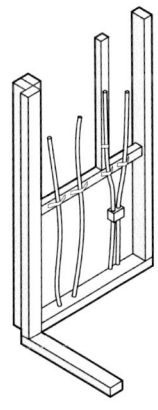

FLEXIBLE COLD WATER TUBING

- Allow easier installation and replacement of plumbing fixtures

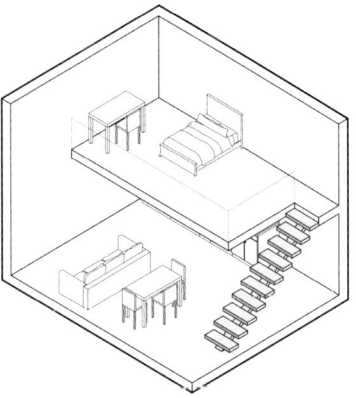

LOCATION OF STAIRS

- Ability to control space function - potential to increase and/or restrict flexibility

Figure 6.5 Demountable and Movable Partitions Allow for Modularity at the Micro-Scale.

177

to provide modular strategies for building. Given that potential residents are not known, this systematic approach simplifies the extent of internal configurations and ensures compatibility with the structure. In order to efficiently accommodate future occupants, modular coordination is implemented.

Since the 1960s, modular strategies have been developed in an attempt to support flexibility and adaptability. In 1965, Dutch architect John Habraken introduced a design methodology to engage users into the design process, by enhancing their choice and adaptability in mass housing. Habraken's "support and infill" system refers to permanent elements and elements that can be detached from the support (Kumar Dhar et al., 2013). Thus, infills – which are any combination of partition, drain, waste, ventilation, water supply, heating, etc. – can be assembled by occupants within a general support structure. These classified systems combine to create permutations of dwelling configurations, recognizing the individuality of the occupants' needs (Friedman, 2021). This approach is distinct from traditional mass housing, with façades varying according to the internal design, for instance, and became popular in many North American and European cities, as well as Japan and China. An example of such implementation is the Molenvliet-Wilgendonk project, presented in a competition design in 1969 (Schneider & Till, 2005). Its support structure consists of a cast-in-place concrete framework, with openings in the slabs for vertical mechanical chases and stairs. To maximize adaptability, the location of support elements was determined through a series of capacity studies. The resulting design supports variation and changeability in unit designs. The use of support structure, both technically and socially, allows for dwellings that can be built, altered, and taken down independently of others.

To support the "support and infill" strategy, the Matrix Tile and Baseboard Profile were developed to allow adaptability to occupants' needs in pre- and post-occupancy stages. The Matrix Tile is a modular floor plan (see Figure 6.6). It possesses grooves, which provide room for the distribution of primary building services (including drains, water, heating electricity, as well as pipes and wiring). The Baseboard Profile runs the wires for appliances. Habraken's use of prefabricated package of off-the-shelf subsystems and parts that are integrated into the Matrix Tile and the Baseboard Profile. This system effectively allows for adaptability, as it provides fast on-site installation and future changeability in concrete buildings (Friedman, 2002).

The Modular Ceiling and Partition System is another strategy that promotes modular partitions in a holistic manner (Blanc, 2014). With the help of a ceiling grid, panels can be integrated with flexibility. The ceiling's framework consists of extruded aluminum alloy channels, which are suspended by rods to the ceiling's main span members. The ceiling grid offers a dimensional relationship with the partitioning, therefore promoting complete adaptability within the modular layout. Moreover, this system integrates modular storage by including various brackets that screw into the framing and provide anchorage for shelves.

Finally, a complete modular approach to housing requires a system that enables all related actors access to design. A common structure of systems and interfaces is required to efficiently produce a stream of products (Halman et al., 2008). Repetition, maximization, interchangeability, and increasing reusability – standardized components and production allow modular strategies to be effectively implemented.

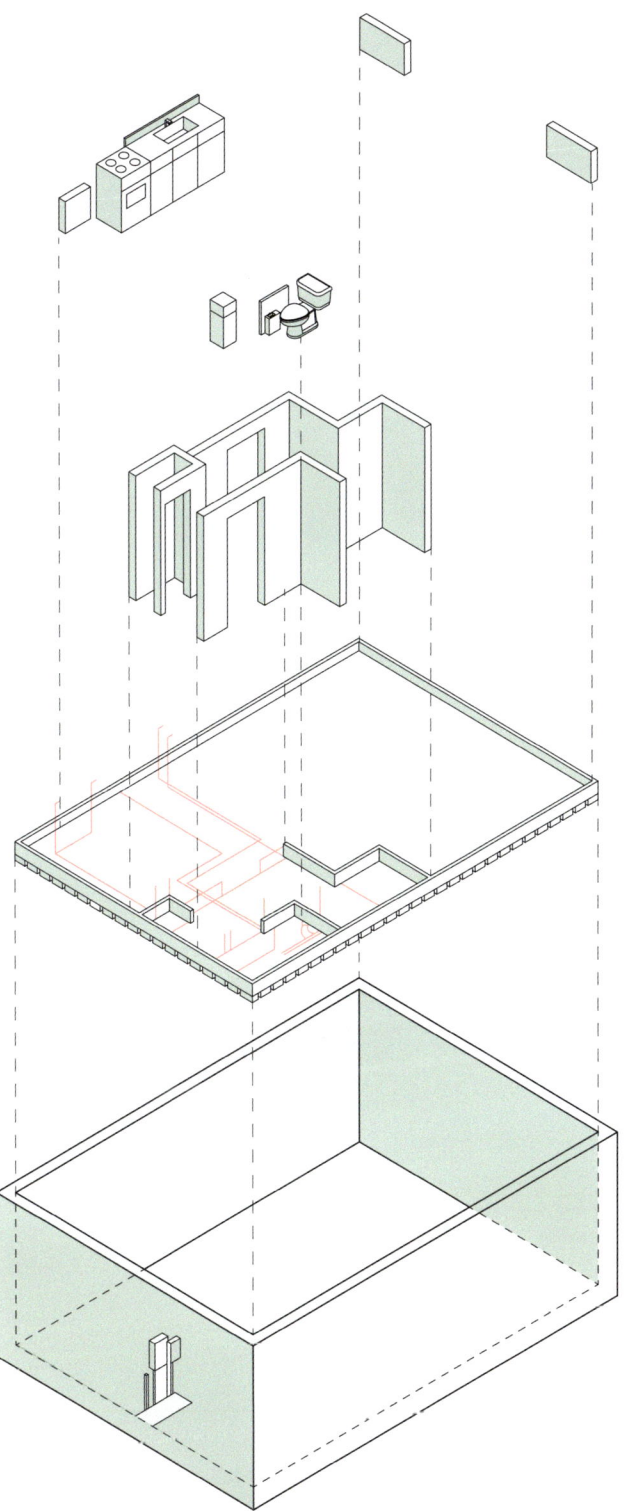

Figure 6.6 Modular Strategies – Example of Matrix Tile and Baseboard Profile.

6A

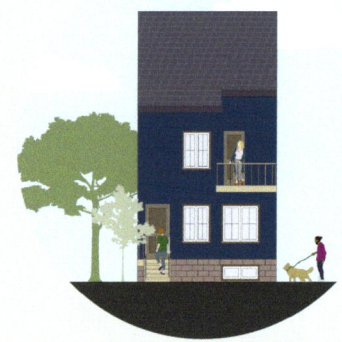

Project:
Circular Multi-Family and
Single-Family Housing
(CMF and CSF)

Location:
Montreal, Canada

Year:
2021

Team:
McGill's Circular
Homebuilding Team

**Mapping to Circular
Economy Framework:**

CIRCULAR ECONOMY PRACTICES

LIFE CYCLE PHASES	Recovery	Life Extension	Sharing Platforms	Service Models	Regenerate	Virtualize
Work of Geobiosphere						
Sourcing						
Manufacturing						
Design & Construction						
Use						
End-of-Use						

LAYERS + LIFESPAN

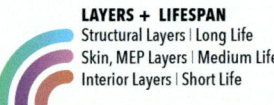

Structural Layers | Long Life
Skin, MEP Layers | Medium Life
Interior Layers | Short Life

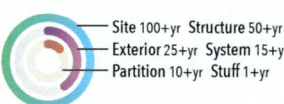

Site 100+yr   Structure 50+yr
Exterior 25+yr   System 15+yr
Partition 10+yr   Stuff 1+yr

Conventional construction and design practices have demonstrated wide-ranging negative social, economic, and environmental effects. Globally, the construction sector consumes the greatest number of natural resources (IRP, 2020). To achieve a sustainable future in which waste and pollutants are limited and community, health, and affordability are promoted, our building practices require radical change. Circular Homebuilding Team at McGill University, based in Montreal, Canada, sought to address this crucial reassessment of building norms with their 2021 design project Circular Multi-Family and Single-Family Housing (CMF and CSF) (Keena & Friedman, 2022). CMF and CSF are designs that exist as basic flexible footprints, adaptable to the needs and budget of any potential occupant. The flexible design also considers material choices and energy efficiency to provide environmental impact estimates during the early planning stages of construction. Figures 6.7 and 6.8 show the different layout options for a CMF dwelling that are easily accessible via a web application designed by the team named Data Homebase (see the Data Homebase case study in Chapter 10). The innovative design project employs the circular economy principles of recovery and recycling, product life extension, sharing platforms and virtualizing to achieve sustainable dwelling that uses flexibility of space as a resource.

The design demonstrates the circular economy principle of product life extension by considering the differences in needs of different populations and family types that may inhabit the space. The form may be rearranged and subdivided prior to occupancy in the design and construction phases, as well as post-occupancy at the end-of-use phase when needs and number of occupants change. One example of how a flexible footprint is achieved is the placement of stairs along the longitudinal side wall next to the front entrance. This simple choice increases the sense of open space and allows the space to be easily adapted for different functions. The design

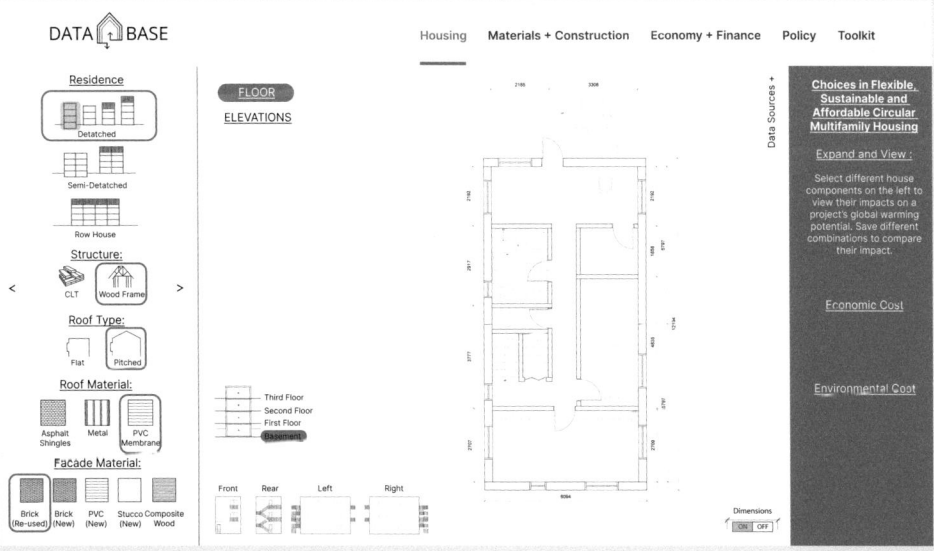

Figure 6.7 Floor Plan for Circular Multifamily Housing.

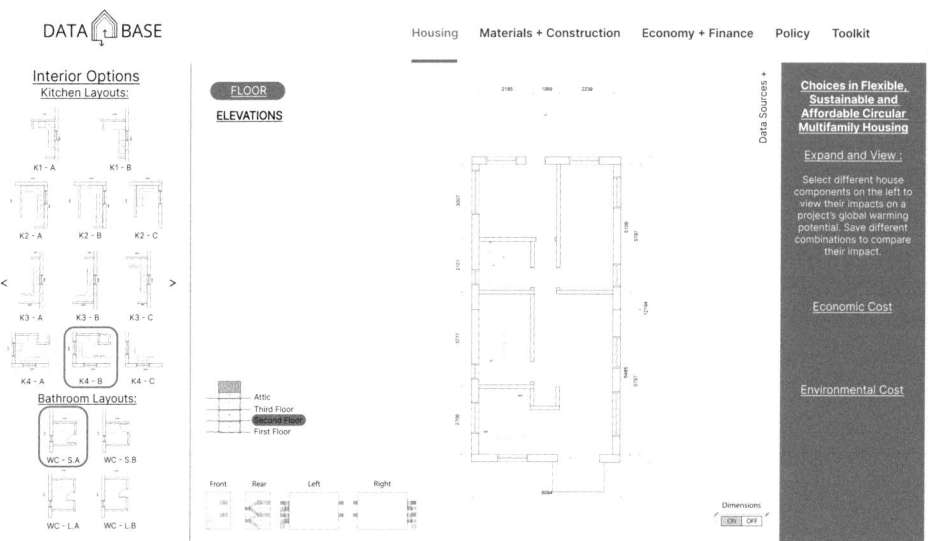

Figure 6.8 Alternative Kitchen Layout Floor Plan for a CMF Dwelling.

also incorporates a pre-occupancy choice menu targeted toward developers or future occupants to accommodate diverse demographics, lifestyles, and budgets. Through providing a basic footprint with a variety of interior component options, occupants are empowered to consume only what they need and can afford, and people with reduced mobility can choose components to help them live independently. For example, bathrooms in the CMF design can range from small powder rooms to complete bathrooms with walk-in showers for seniors. The adaptability inherent to the project extends the useful life of the dwelling and therefore of the materials and components consumed.

The flexible design, using stacked utilities and space-efficient layouts, illustrates the circular economy sharing platforms approach by allowing for co-living (Lacy & Rutqvist, 2015). Circular Homebuilding Team aimed to design inclusive environments that meet the diverse needs of people living in Canada today. To do this they considered the needs of various demographics, including young professionals, low-income individuals, nuclear families, LGBTQ2+ couples, indigenous communities, domestic violence survivors, multi-generational households, as well as people with physical and mental disabilities, who all may have differing dwelling requirements. Configurations of CMF and CSF can exist as communal row houses, semi-detached houses, as well as private houses, with the aim of providing safe and healthy interiors for a diverse demographic of all occupants as illustrated in Figure 6.9. Co-living is facilitated by providing more common space for many occupants who may welcome this community approach. For example, studies show that this can be particularly valuable for domestic violence survivors as well as those with mental disabilities as it allows for independence with private space but also gives the opportunity for more shared kitchens and living areas (Keena & Friedman, 2022).

Through the CMF prototype design, the team tested their methodology toward supporting revolutionary circular economy decision-making. They developed a digital

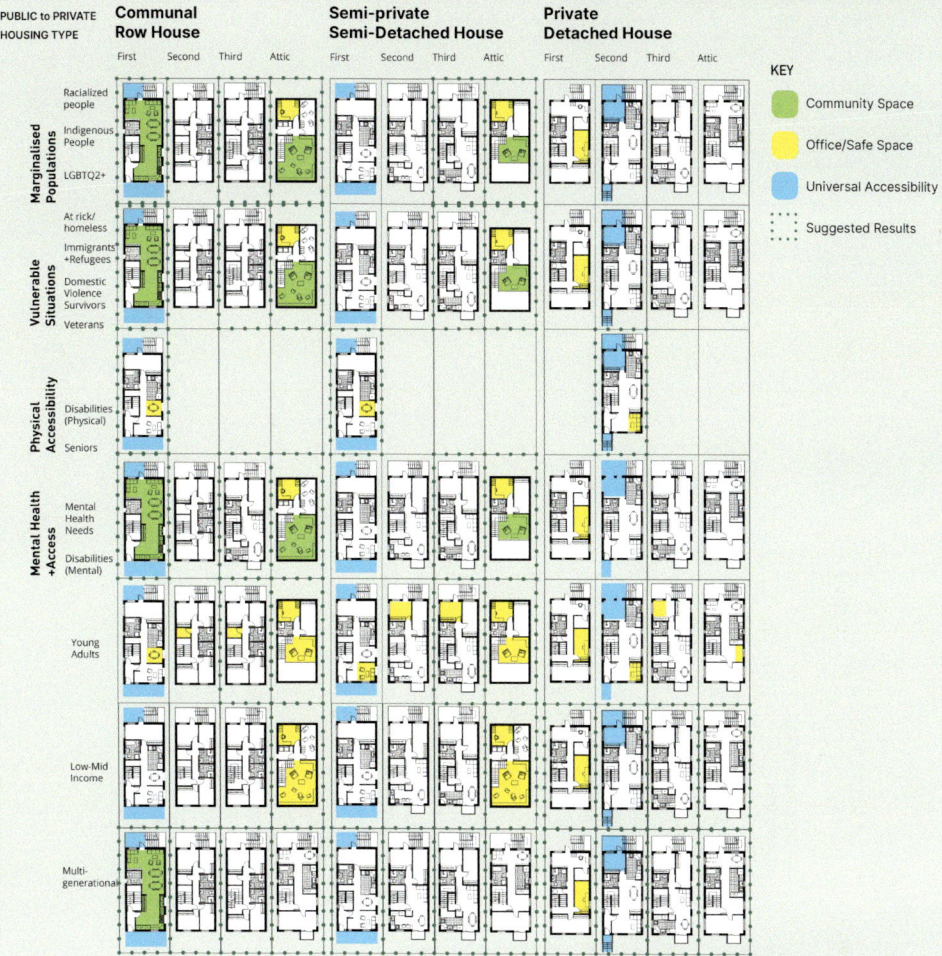

Figure 6.9 Diversity, Inclusion, and Reconciliation Considerations: Permutations and Combinations of a CMF Demonstration Project Illustrating How Circular Economy Design Principles of Flexibility, Sustainability and Affordability Reflects the Diverse Needs of Multiple Groups Living in Canada.

twin of the CMF prototype and had an accompanying web application. Through the web application, a user can simultaneously understand the environmental and economic costs associated with different housing designs that use circular economy best practices (see Figures 6.7 and 6.8). The first step involved generating a series of building information modeling (BIM) models for the demonstration of CMF housing project using the Autodesk Revit software. This virtualization allowed the environmental assessment and comparison of various layouts and configurations using Tally (Bates et al., 2013; Tally, 2023), a life cycle assessment (LCA) plugin for Autodesk Revit. Nine options of the CMF demonstration project were developed to test and validate the prototype and methods. As illustrated in Figure 6.10, 27 permutations and combinations of these nine design options were explored by changing three key parameters: (1) geometry, (2) material, and (3) components. For example, geometry options included housing with or without a basement, or with a pitched versus a

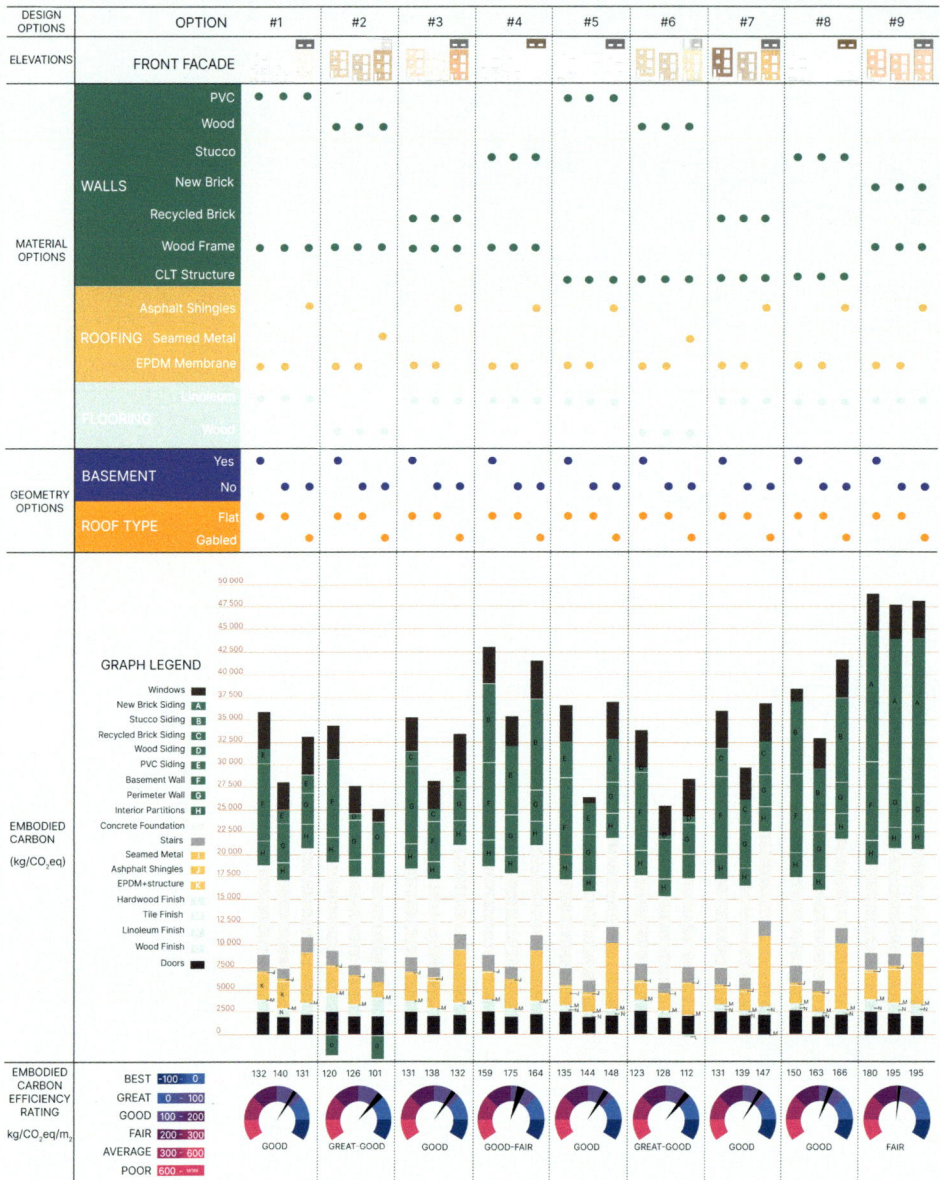

Figure 6.10 Embodied Carbon Analysis of a Circular Multifamily Housing Demonstration Project with Various Material and Geometry Changes for 9 Different Design Options with 27 Combinations.

flat roof; examples of material options included different façade material types such as brick, stucco, and composite wood; also the material of the structural system, such as a timber frame or cross-laminated timber (CLT); and the inclusion of a balcony or a particular window assembly reflected component options. The LCA analysis boundary included a cradle-to-gate logic, with material use across the life cycle from material extraction, manufacture, building construction considered, based on prior methodological approaches to understanding embodied energy and carbon in buildings (Keena & Dyson, 2017; Keena et al., 2022). The different embodied carbon impacts of the different CMF design options can be easily accessible via the web application as illustrated in Figure 6.11.

The BIM model was used to leverage a bill of materials which was used to conduct a life cycle cost assessment (LCCA) comparing the cost difference between using new versus secondary materials in the CMF and CSF construction, as shown in Figure 6.12. An overview of the environmental and economic costs associated with different versions of CMF based on a user's choice of geometry, material, and components is illustrated in Figure 6.13.

The BIM model was labeled as illustrated in Figure 6.14 to facilitate prefabricated construction, occurring in a controlled setting off-site toward economic and material savings. This method was chosen because it allows for simple assembly and disassembly, encouraging the recovery and reuse of materials in the end-of-use phase. Design-for-disassembly maximizes material reuse in a new building cycle through employing reversible connections and visible joints (Durmisevic, 2019). These housing prototypes demonstrate a circular economy framework and pave the way for a socially and economically conscious zero-waste future. The demonstration projects accompanying digital twins with web apps showcase how adaptability and flexibility in design can be empowered through digital technology offering choice and agency to the home occupants.

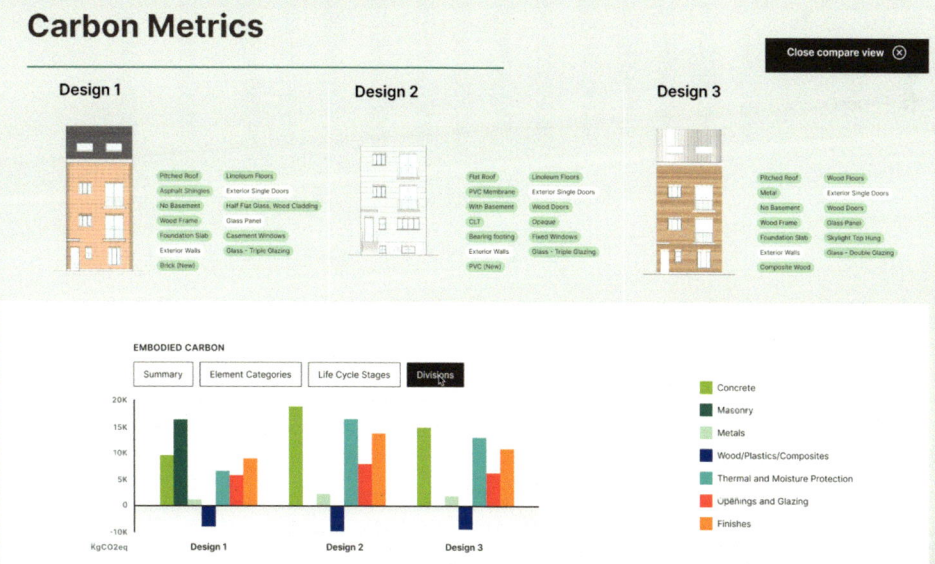

Figure 6.11 The Data Homebase Web Application Allows Users to Compare the Environmental Impact of Different CMF Design Options Based on Their Choices.

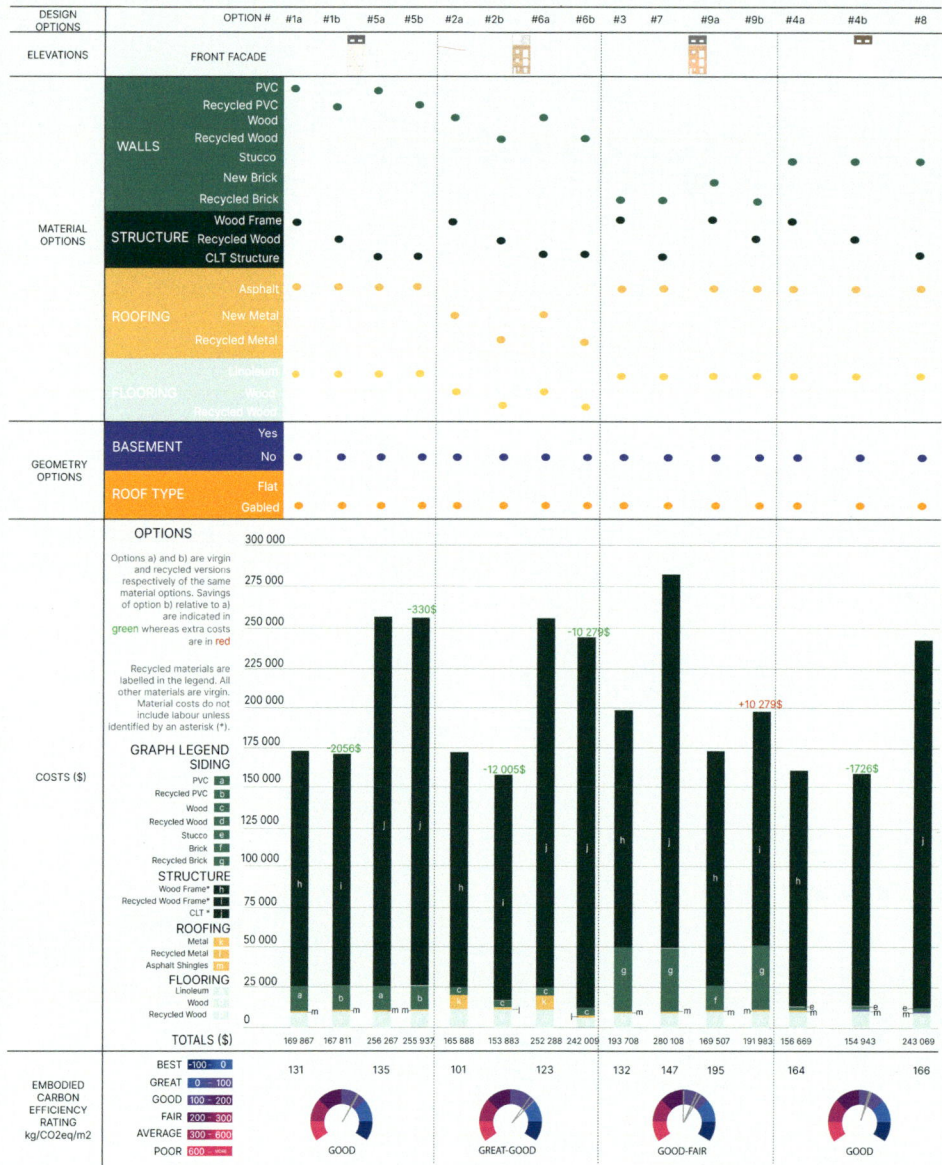

Figure 6.12 Cost Analysis of Multiple Design Options for a Circular Multifamily Housing Demonstration Project Comparing New and Reclaimed Materials and Their Associated Costs. All Cost Values in CAD.

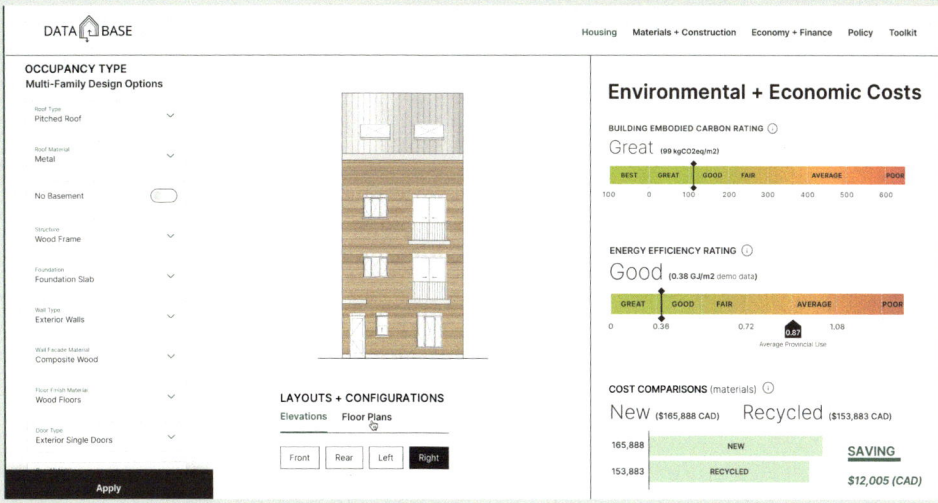

Figure 6.13 The Data Homebase Web Application Allows Users to Compare the Embodied Carbon, Energy Performance, and Cost Impacts of Different CMF Design Options Simultaneously Based on Their Choices.

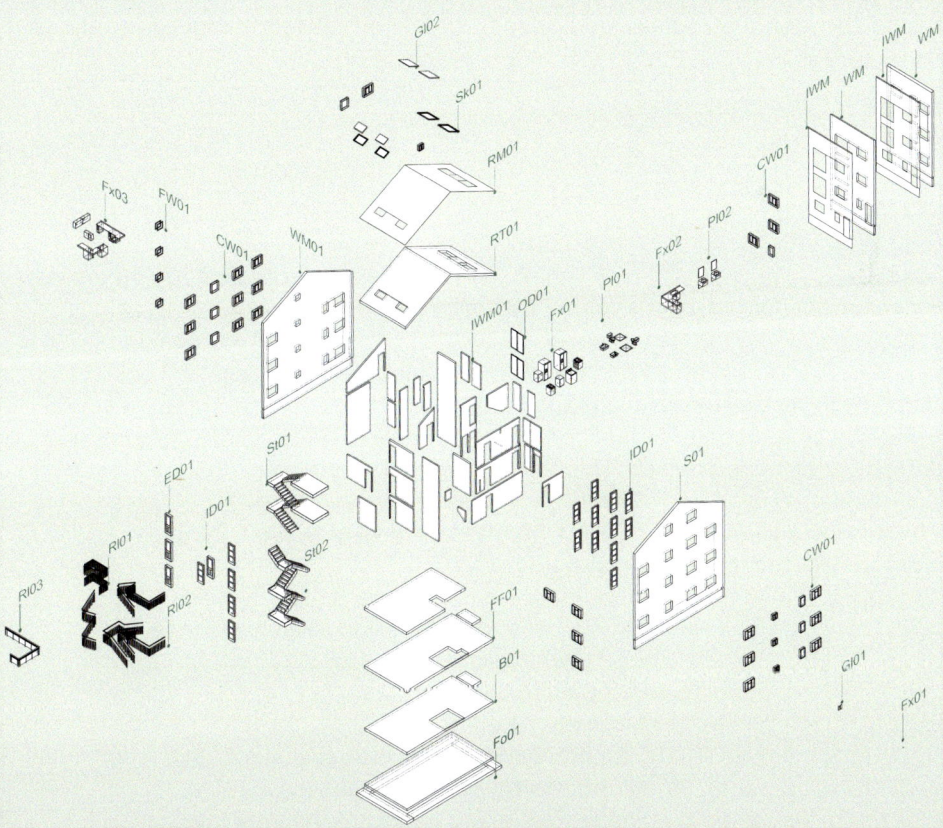

Figure 6.14 An Exploded Axonometric of Panelized Prefabricated Method.

6.7 Conclusion

Lifestyles are constantly changing, in accordance with dynamic life cycle processes. To offer people homes most suitable for their needs – and effectively reduce waste associated with complex renovations and moving – flexible design strategies need to be implemented. Flexible housing requires proper planning and needs to be addressed both in macro and micro features. As seen in this chapter, there are various details and decisions that can and need to be considered in designing adaptable homes. Designing flexibly can be aided with the use of innovative products and strategies. Together, these initiatives allow building components and systems to be adaptable during the operational phase, as well as provide a calculated approach to dismantling building parts for easy recovery at the end of the building life.

In order to promote a circular economy, space ought to be understood as a resource; a valuable product, which, without careful planning and use, can quickly contribute to waste. To limit wasteful consumption, systems and strategies need to be implemented. However, occupants' specific and changing needs must be considered. Universal and systematic approaches cannot fulfill evolving households' needs and, ultimately, lead to more waste. Thus, a balance between individuality and flexibility is ideal as it allows a building's life cycle to advance alongside occupants or, alternatively, is adaptable to the needs of new occupants. These flexible strategies create alternatives to the deconstruction of houses, which effectively reduces waste and promotes circular logic.

References

Bates, R., Carlisle, S., Faircloth, B., & Welch, R. (2013). *Quantifying the embodied environmental impact of building materials during design*. PLEA.

Bayliss, S., & Bergin, R. (2020). *The modular housing handbook*. RIBA Publishing. https://www.taylorfrancis.com/books/9781003106296 http://search.ebscohost.com/login. aspx?direct=true&scope=site&db=nlebk&db=nlabk&AN=2564174 https://www.vlebooks. com/vleweb/product/openreader?id=none&isbn=9781000217148

Blanc, A. (2014). *Internal components*. Routledge. http://public.ebookcentral.proquest.com/ choice/publicfullrecord.aspx?p=1829408

Brand, S. (1995). *How buildings learn: What happens after They're built*. Penguin. https://books.google.com.pe/books?id=zkgRgdVN2GIC

Cheshire, D. (2021). *The handbook to building a circular economy*. Routledge.

Durmisevic, E. (2019). Circular economy in construction design strategies for reversible buildings. *BAMB, Netherlands.[Online] Available at: bamb2020. eu/wp-content/ uploads/2019/05/Reversible-Building-Design-Strateges.pdf [Accessed 18 October 2021]*.

Farnsworth, D. (2015). Ask a CTBUH expert: David Farnsworth: Modular construction in tall buildings. *CTBUH Journal*(4), 58–58. http://www.jstor.org/stable/44154476

Friedman, A. (2002). *The adaptable home: Designing homes for change*. McGraw-Hill.

Friedman, A. (2012). *Fundamentals of sustainable dwellings*. Springer.

Friedman, A. (2021). *Pre-fab living*. Thames & Hudson.

Groak, S. (2002). *The idea of building: Thought and action in the design and production of buildings*. Taylor & Francis.

Gullo, L. J., & Dixon, J. (2021). *Design for maintainability*. John Wiley & Sons, Inc. https://search.ebscohost.com/login.aspx?direct=true&scope=site&db=nlebk&db=nlabk&AN=2899200 https://doi.org/10.1002/9781119578536

Halman, J. I. M., Voordijk, J. T., & Reymen, I. M. M. J. (2008). Modular approaches in Dutch house building: An exploratory survey. *Housing Studies*, 23(5), 781–799. https://doi.org/10.1080/02673030802293208

IRP (2020). *Resource efficiency and climate change: Material efficiency strategies for a low-carbon future*. International Resource Panel.

Keena, N., & Dyson, A. (2017). Qualifying the quantitative in the construction of built ecologies. In D. Benjamin (Ed.), *Embodied energy and design: Making architecture between metrics and narratives*. Columbia University GSAPP Lars Müller.

Keena, N., & Friedman, A. (2022). Circular economy in the built environment: Towards housing affordability and sustainability. In W. Leal Filho, A. M. Azul, F. Doni, & A. L. Salvia (Eds.), *Handbook of sustainability science in the future: Policies, technologies and education by 2050*. Springer International Publishing Cham.

Keena, N., Raugei, M., Lokko, M.-l, Aly Etman, M., Achnani, V., Reck, B. K., & Dyson, A. (2022). A life-cycle approach to investigate the potential of novel biobased construction materials toward a circular built environment. *Energies*, 15(19), 7239. https://doi.org/10.3390/en15197239

Kumar Dhar, T., Sk. Maruf Hossain, M., & Rubayet Rahaman, K. (2013). How does flexible design promote resource efficiency for housing? A study of Khulna, Bangladesh. *Smart and Sustainable Built Environment*, 2(2), 140–157. https://doi.org/10.1108/SASBE-10-2012-0051

Lacy, P., & Rutqvist, J. (2015). *Waste to wealth: The circular economy advantage*. Palgrave Macmillan. https://doi.org/10.1057/9781137530707

Lawson, R. M., Ogden, R., & Goodier, C. I. (2014). *Design in modular construction*. CRC Press, Taylor & Francis. https://doi.org/10.1201/b16607

Rohe, W. M., & Watson, H. L. (2007). *Chasing the American Dream: New Perspectives on Affordable Homeownership*.

Schmidth, R., & Austin, S. (2016). *Adaptable architecture: Theory and practice*. Routledge.

Schneider, T., & Till, J. (2005). Flexible housing: Opportunities and limits. *Architectural Research Quarterly*, 9(2), 157–166. https://doi.org/10.1017/S1359135505000199

Schneider, T., & Till, J. (2007). *Flexible housing*. Architectural Press. http://catdir.loc.gov/catdir/toc/fy0803/2007282780.html http://catdir.loc.gov/catdir/enhancements/fy0808/2007282780-d.html

SHoP Architects. (2016). *Proving the ability of modular construction to meet the pressing demands of our time, B2 was a landmark technological achievement*. Retrieved June 21 from https://www.shoparc.com/projects/b2/

Tally. (2023). *Tally for Revit*. Building Transparency, KT Innovations, Autodesk, Thinkstep. Retrieved June 21 from https://choosetally.com/

Wallance, D. (2021). *The future of modular architecture*. Routledge.

PART 3

Designing Low-Carbon Circular Housing

Chapter 7

Low-Carbon Footprints and Material Efficiency

7.1 Materials, Building, and Climate Change

Human activities are increasingly influencing the climate by adding enormous amounts of greenhouse gases to those naturally occurring in the atmosphere. This increases the greenhouse effect and global warming leading to climate change. Key sources of anthropogenic greenhouse gas emissions are construction and manufacturing-related activities. As depicted in Figure 7.1, the building construction industry is responsible for a significant amount of energy consumption and emissions in comparison to other industries. In 2020, buildings and construction accounted for 36 percent of global final energy consumption, and 37 percent of global final energy and energy-related carbon dioxide emissions (United Nations Environment Programme [UNEP], 2021). While consumption saw drops in 2020, this is largely due to the Covid-19 pandemic. The overarching trend suggests that emissions will continue to increase if business-as-usual approaches persist in the building sector.

However, the percentages illustrated in Figure 7.1 are only considering energy-related greenhouse gas emissions. Although a substantial share of greenhouse gas emissions is energy-related, typically from the burning of fossil fuels, there are other causes. For example, the consumption and use of resources for the production of building materials and components also plays a role in contributing to anthropogenic climate change. The building construction industry is reliant on the manufacturing of construction materials, including steel, cement, and glass. The material manufacturing sector causes direct emissions in its production life cycle, as well as indirect

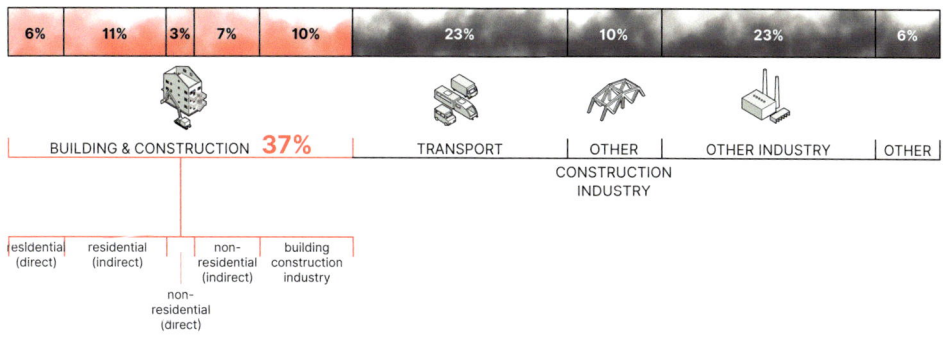

Source: Adapted from IEA 2021a, "Tracking Clean Energy Progress"

Figure 7.1 Building and Construction Sector's Contribution to Global Final Energy and Energy-Related Carbon Dioxide Emissions, 2020. Data Sourced from UNEP (2021).

DOI: 10.4324/9781003333975-10

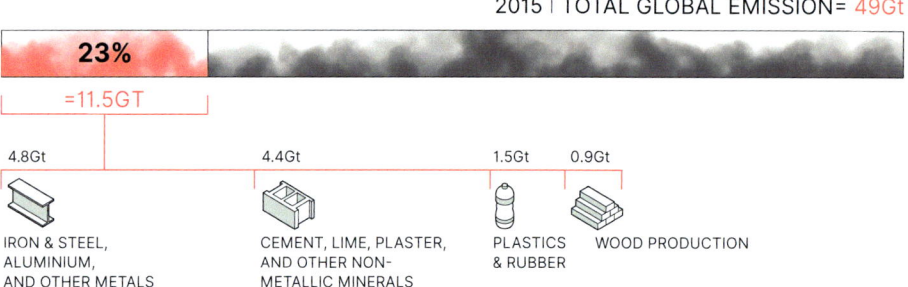

1995 | TOTAL GLOBAL EMISSION = 35Gt

15%

=5Gt

2015 | TOTAL GLOBAL EMISSION= 49Gt

23%

=11.5GT

4.8Gt   4.4Gt   1.5Gt   0.9Gt

IRON & STEEL,   CEMENT, LIME, PLASTER,   PLASTICS   WOOD PRODUCTION
ALUMINIUM,   AND OTHER NON-   & RUBBER
AND OTHER METALS   METALLIC MINERALS

Source: Adapted from IRP 2020

Figure 7.2 Emissions Caused by Material Production, 1995 versus 2015.

emissions, from power generation for electricity and commercial heat (see Chapter 9). According to an IRP 2020 report, in 2015, the production of materials in the global economy contributed 11 metric gigatons of carbon dioxide – equivalent to 23 percent of total greenhouse gas emissions as outlined in Figure 7.2 (IRP, 2020). Over half of the carbon footprint of materials were caused by direct emissions from the material man-ufacturing processes. Energy-related emissions across the supply chain contributed to 35 percent, mining was 2 percent, and other economic processes were 9 percent as illustrated in Figure 7.3 (Hertwich et al., 2019). As shown in Figure 7.2., the material

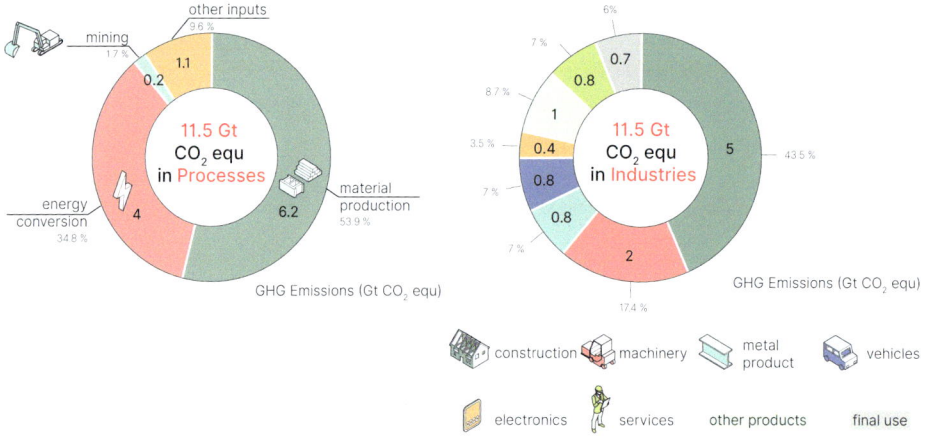

Source: Adapted from IRP 2020 from Hertwich, E.G., Ali, S., Ciacci, L., Fishman, T., Heeren, N., Masanet, E., Asghari, F.N., Olivetti, E., Pauliuk, S., Tu, Q., Wolfman, P., 2019. Material efficiency strategies to reducing greehouse gas emissions associated with buildings, vehicles, and electronics- a review. Environ. Res. Lett. 14,043004. https://doi.org/10.101088/1748-9326/an0fe3.

Figure 7.3 Global Carbon Footprint of Materials, 2015.

production most dominant in terms of contributing to total global emissions included, in descending order, metals (iron, steel, aluminum, and other metals), non-metallic minerals and products (cement, lime plaster, and other non-metallic minerals), plastics and rubber, and finally wood. In terms of the use of the materials, 40 percent of emissions related to material production were for materials used in construction as illustrated in Figure 7.3 (Hertwich et al., 2019). Housing was the most important product of construction.

This trend is not unique to 2015; the IRP Global Outlook Report to 2060 projects a doubling of global material use from 2015 to 2060 due to an increasing global population and a demand for housing (OECD, 2019). This demand for increased resources could have drastic consequences on our climate if a linear building and construction process continues.

7.1.1 Embodied Carbon, Carbon Footprint, Carbon Dioxide Emissions – Which Is It?

A number of terms, "embodied carbon", "carbon footprint", and "carbon dioxide emissions", are used to describe essentially the same thing. The "embodied carbon", "carbon footprint", and "carbon dioxide emissions" of a material are a measure of the accumulative life cycle greenhouse gas emissions associated with the use of energy and material resources in its production. It indicates the materials' global warming potential. It is measured in carbon dioxide equivalent. Carbon dioxide equivalent is the number of metric tons of carbon dioxide emissions with the same global warming potential as one metric ton of another greenhouse gas. Embodied carbon of building materials and components varies substantially based on the type of material and amount of it used in construction. Generally, emissions from materials and their production are more elevated in fossil-based materials as highlighted in Figure 7.4; however, the presentation of data is sometimes misleading. For instance, on a per unit weight basis, carbon emissions from concrete are significantly lower than that of aluminum. However, unlike aluminum, which is lightweight, a significant quantity of cement is required for concrete construction ranking it the third largest source of anthropogenic carbon dioxide production (Lehne & Preston, 2018; OECD, 2019). Needless to say, current material use practices are harmful to the environment. In addition, at the end-of-life, certain materials are often difficult to reuse and are hence disposed of, contributing substantially to greenhouse gas emissions. The longer a building and its component parts last, the less embodied carbon is expended over the life of the building; therefore, extending the life cycle of a building is a vital circular economy approach. Repair and maintenance can reduce building obsolescence and increase the lifespans of buildings. Figure 7.4 illustrates the embodied carbon values of a variety of construction materials.

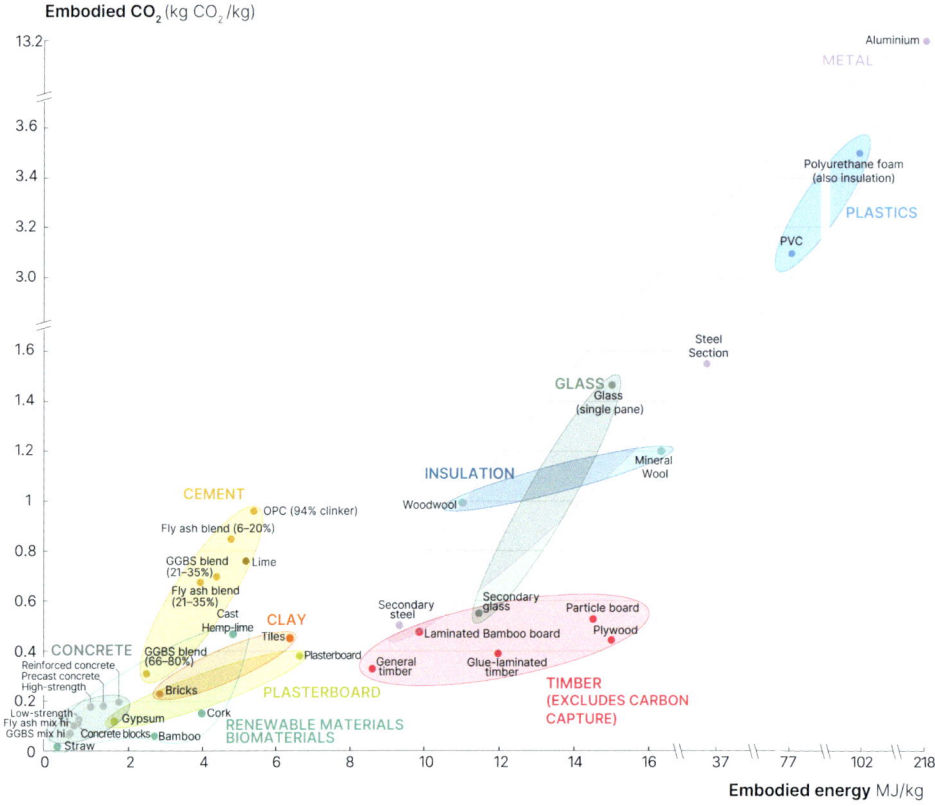

Figure 7.4 The Embodied Carbon and Embodied Energy Per 1 m² of Various Construction Materials. Embodied Energy and Embodied Carbon of a Selection of Common Building Materials. Note that This Data Is on a Per Unit Weight Basis Therefore the Embodied Energy and Embodied Carbon Values Will Vary Substantially Based on the Amount of Material Used. Data Sourced from the Inventory of Carbon and Energy (ICE) Databases (Hammond & Jones, 2008, 2011, 2019).

7.2 Current Global Context and the Growing Demand for Construction Materials

With the world's continuously growing population comes a growing demand for construction materials. Rapid urbanization is emerging and requires buildings. In accordance with the United Nations' Sustainable Development Goals 11th target – *Sustainable Cities and Communities* – an increase in demand for construction materials is required to provide decent and affordable housing. By the year 2050, 68 percent of the world's population is projected to live in urban areas. Overall, 90 percent of this increase is expected to occur in cities of Asia and Africa (United Nations, 2019). To satisfy demands and build an increasingly complex society, more materials are being produced and accumulated. The World Bank estimates that 300 million additional houses will be needed by 2030, primarily in emerging economies (World Bank, 2016). Figure 7.5 illustrates the projections for global resource use by 2060 to meet the needs of a growing global population.

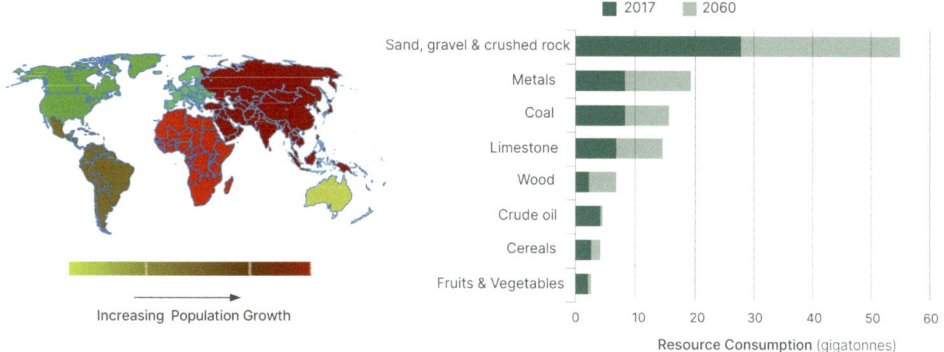

Figure 7.5 Relationship Between Increased Global Population Growth and Global Resource Use, with Projections to 2060. Construction Materials Dominate Resource Consumption. Data Sourced from United Nations (2019) and OECD (2019).

High demand and increased construction are quickly exacerbating environmental impacts. If the current linear material production practices continue, non-renewable resources will be depleted and climate change affects will be increased (OECD, 2019). Yet, the current response to these demands remains a linear approach which is economically and environmentally unsustainable, driving an exponential growth in material production. Economically, our society is approaching certain limits, with respect to not only resource availability but also wider economic systems. From an economic standpoint, there is a strong correlation between resource consumption and economic development (see Figure 7.6). Analysis conducted by Accenture found that, historically, for every 1 percent increase in gross domestic product, there is a

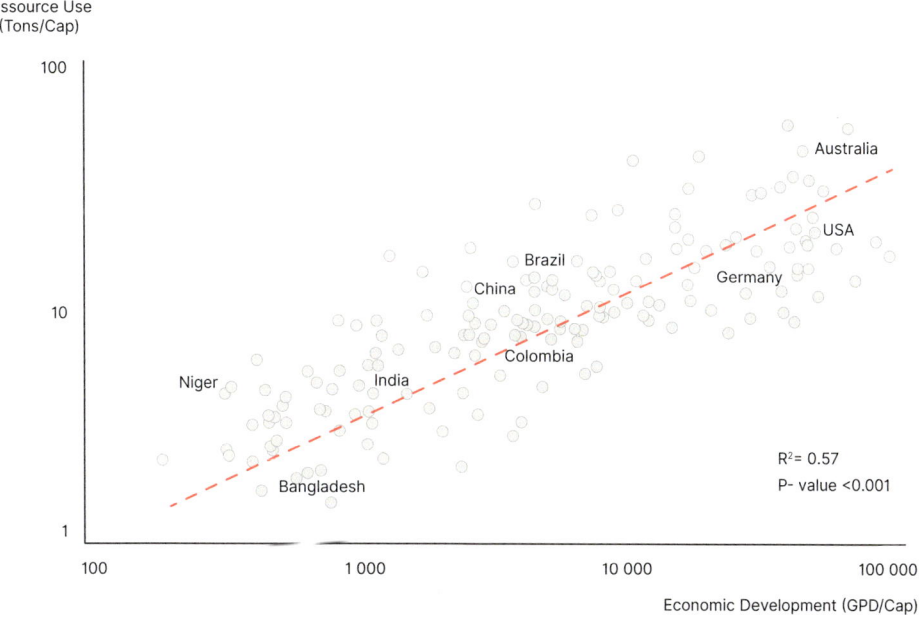

Source: Adapted Accenture Strategy Circular Advantage

Figure 7.6 Relationship Between Economic Development and Resource Use, in 166 Countries.

197

consequential rise of 0.4 percent of resource usage (Accenture, 2014). This results in increasing resource scarcity and mounting waste. As is explained in Section 7.3, historically trends in the use of materials are highly dependent and linked to world events. Events affect the supply and demand for materials and can impact the economy. The distribution to supply chains during the Covid-19 pandemic is a good example of this. Both economically and environmentally, present linear use and choice of materials are unsustainable. A circular economy approach promotes the decoupling of economic activity from the consumption of finite resources. Yet, globally new housing is needed so how can this decoupling be achieved? This is where circular material efficiency approaches hold promise.

Globally there are two key trends; in emerging economies there is typically a need for new construction given that much of the building stock has yet to be built. In contrast, in advanced economies much of the building stock already exists. The focus there, ideally, is on extending the life of these buildings rather than a linear practice of demolition and new construction. The next sections will highlight how reducing the overall demand for primary materials through material efficiency represents a pathway to achieving decarbonization. However, one of the key barriers to shifting to a more circular approach is a social factor. Materials such as steel, concrete, and glass are associated with progressive societies and contemporary living. More low-carbon approaches, such as thatch, mud buildings, even wood, or the reuse of reclaimed materials, are often associated with techniques that are passé and unmodern, not new ("shiny") or desirable. This has its roots in how certain architectural design has shaped our cities.

7.3 Challenges with Resource Use in Building: A Historical Perspective

While there is a consensus that the use of non-renewable materials is harmful to the environment, they remain prevalent within the building industry. Traditionally, bioclimatic designs and the reliance on locally sourced materials were predominant; however, technological innovation and historical events have caused a shift toward a reliance on non-renewable resource use which is quite often associated with a global supply chain. Despite the various benefits of biomaterials, fossil-based materials remain the status quo due to socioeconomic factors. In 2014, only 4 percent of the nearly 3,000 Mt of new materials entering the US economy were renewable – in comparison to the 46 percent in 1900 (Matos, 2017). Both social and economic events throughout history have greatly impacted the use of materials and inhibited change.

From a socio-cultural perspective, certain fossil-based materials – namely steel, concrete, and glass – have been linked to certain societal and aesthetic choices. Some have been associated with progressive and contemporary lifestyles, which ought to be requestioned. Beginning with the Industrial Revolution, diverse technological innovations emerged and affected architecture. During the modernist movement in the mid-1900s, material mass production, as well as structural innovations in steel, reinforced concrete, and glass caused a shift. National and vernacular architecture, which often utilized local and bio-based resources, was lost, along with its associated identity. In its place came the International Style, which celebrated steel, concrete, and glass innovations producing many pioneering, architectural feats of high-rise steel and glass towers, such as Mies van der Rohe's Seagram building in New York. These buildings were typically internally dominated and took the liberty to ignore the environmental context in which they were situated thanks to advancements in heating, ventilation, and air conditioning mechanical systems. Such buildings and their evolved forms have become ubiquitous worldwide. Despite the brilliance of these original buildings in shaping an architectural movement, the proliferation of this building and construction approach has contributed to significant environmental impacts and challenges both from an operational energy standpoint as well as a material use perspective. In addition, as depicted in Figure 7.7, the transition to fossil-based materials has resulted in a worldwide conformity of contemporary architecture and, as Koolhaas exhibited in the 2014 Venice Biennale, with it, the inherent loss of national identities and vernacular (Mackenzie, 2014).

Furthermore, the use of fossil-based materials is inherently tied to the economy. Despite the various concerns associated with raw material construction, trends show resistance to shifting to more sustainable practices – people have become increasingly dependent on non-renewable materials in order to sustain a standard of living. Popular fossil-based materials are associated with established and often global supply chains, which have demonstrated affordable and reliable economies of scale for the construction process (Keena et al., 2022). Trends in the United States from the 20th century to today depict that the use of non-renewable material extraction is synonymous with economic growth (Matos, 2022). For instance, as seen in Figure 7.8, a dip in material consumption is directly related to the 2008 economic recession and with Covid-19 pandemic in 2020.

As stated above, a key principle in a circular economy is decoupling economic growth from non-renewable material consumption. Thus, non-renewable resource use needs to be dissociated with our economy. Culturally, progress needs to be associated with future use architecture which promotes urban mining as opposed to raw material mining. The Resource Rows case study by Lendager Group in Chapter 5 which won the 2022 Mies van der Rohe award is a good example of this. Shifting into a circular economy requires adjusting our relationship with building materials. One promising approach in transitioning away from a linear approach to a circular one is the use of material efficiency strategies as described in the next section.

7.4 Material Efficiencies

The current overuse of carbon-intensive materials, including steel, cement, and glass, results in wasteful and unsustainable buildings. Material efficiency represents one solution toward achieving circularity – i.e., using less materials to provide the

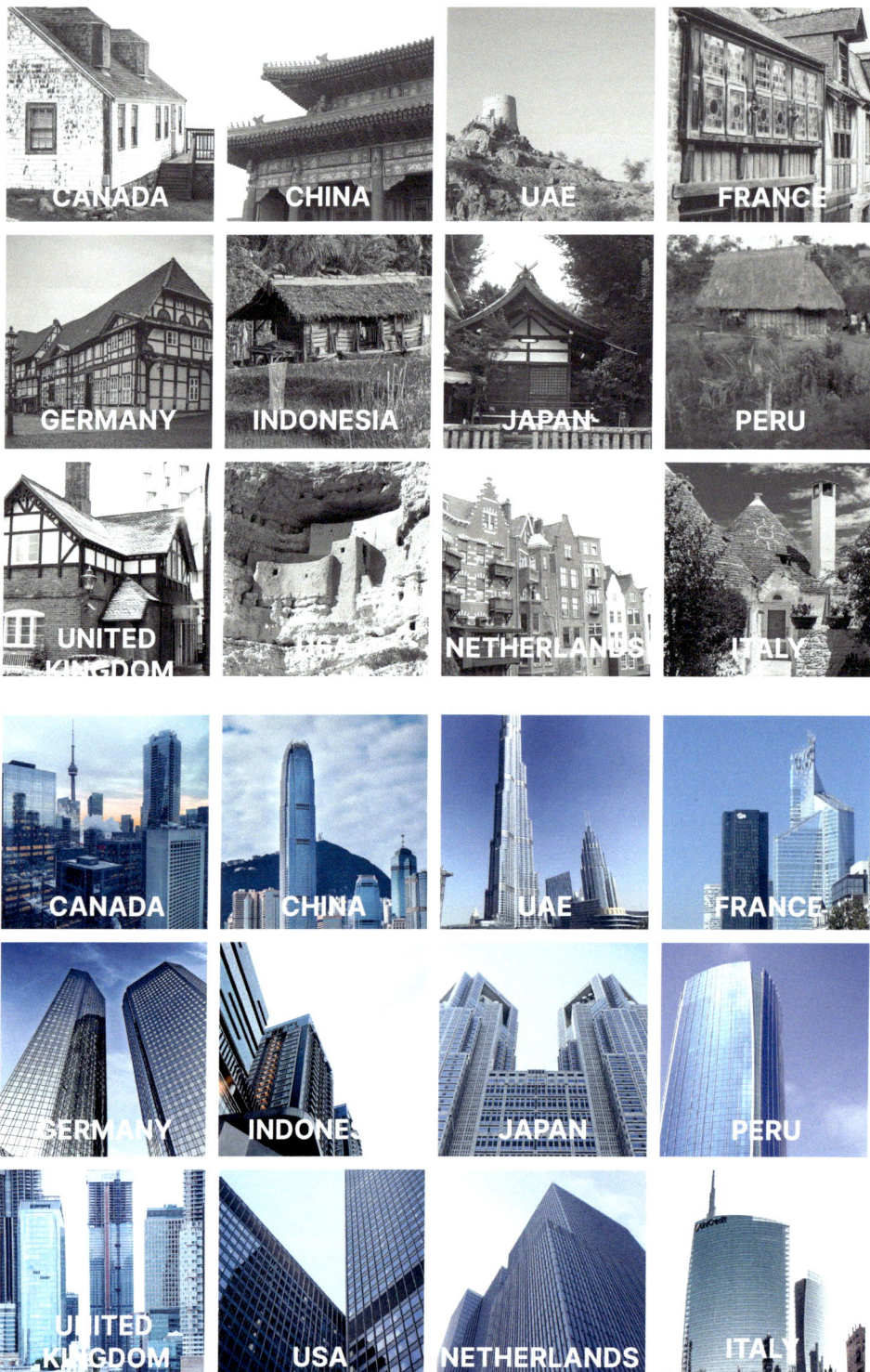

Figure 7.7 Loss of National Identity in Architecture and Conformity of Contemporary Architecture Worldwide.

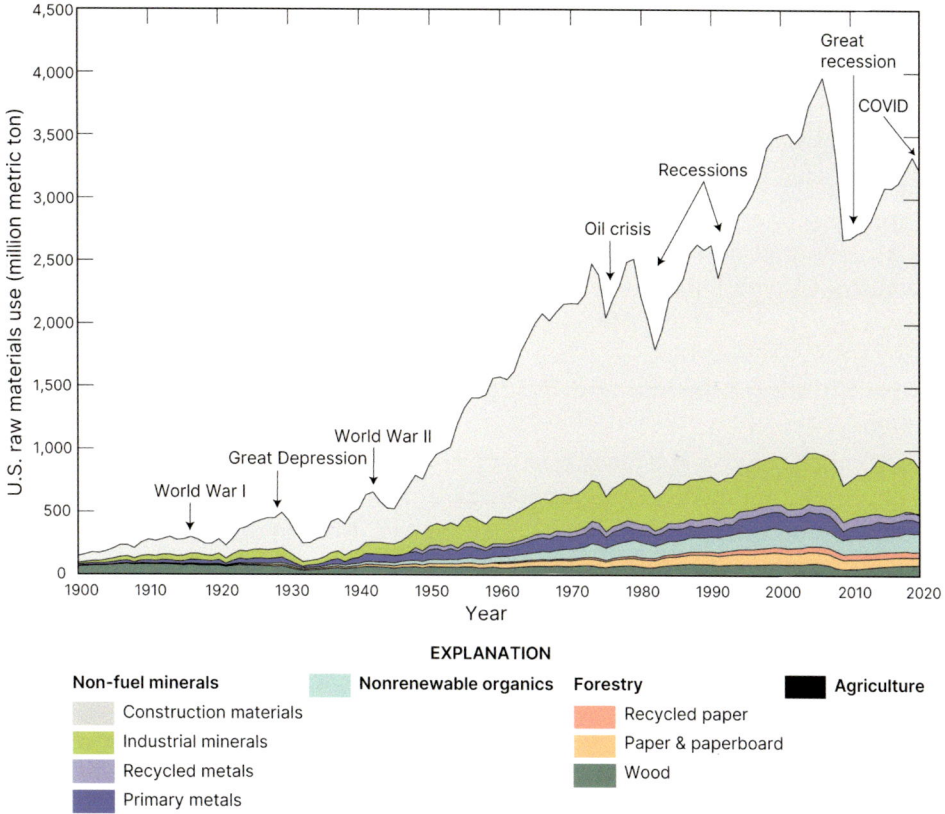

Figure 7.8 Use of Raw Materials, by Category in the United States from 1900 through 2020. The Number of Agricultural Products Is Plotted at the Base of the Graph but Is Not Visible at the Scale of This Figure. Materials Embedded in Imported Goods Are Not Included.

same level of well-being (Hertwich et al., 2020). Material efficiency strategies should ultimately reduce the demand for virgin materials in the construction of new buildings. By making secondary materials available to other markets, the need to produce virgin materials is reduced.

Material efficiency strategies can be implemented at various stages of a building's life cycle – within design, operational strategies during use, and recycling methods at the end-of-use phase. The design represents a particularly important point of intervention as it affects a building's entire potential. Material choice, construction techniques, opportunities for increased building lifetimes, and end-of-use strategies are all determined within the initial phases.

7.4.1 Material Efficiency Strategies for Housing and Policy Options

Design is indirectly, but substantially, shaped by policy, through primary building codes. Therefore, careful attention is required both to a building standards and

201

codes, as well as their adoption and diffusion by public authorities. Given the potential mitigation of material efficiency on climate change, policy targets need to shift in order to include greenhouse gas emission reduction goals. Buildings that are lighter and design closer to technical specifications use less material and can lower emissions. In order to implement these changes, policies play a role in stimulating the adoption of material efficiency strategies through building codes. Codes are ideally performance based (i.e., using design to reduce greenhouse gas emissions and testing its potential effectiveness) rather than prescriptive based (i.e., a one-size-fits-all approach with little to no testing of the design).

Extending the Building Lifetime and Using Less Material(s) by Design

The first question should be if a new building needs to be built at all. The highest percentage of carbon emissions reduced can be achieved at the early planning and design phase as illustrated in Figure 7.9. During this time is when decisions are made concerning if a new build is needed or whether an existing structure can be

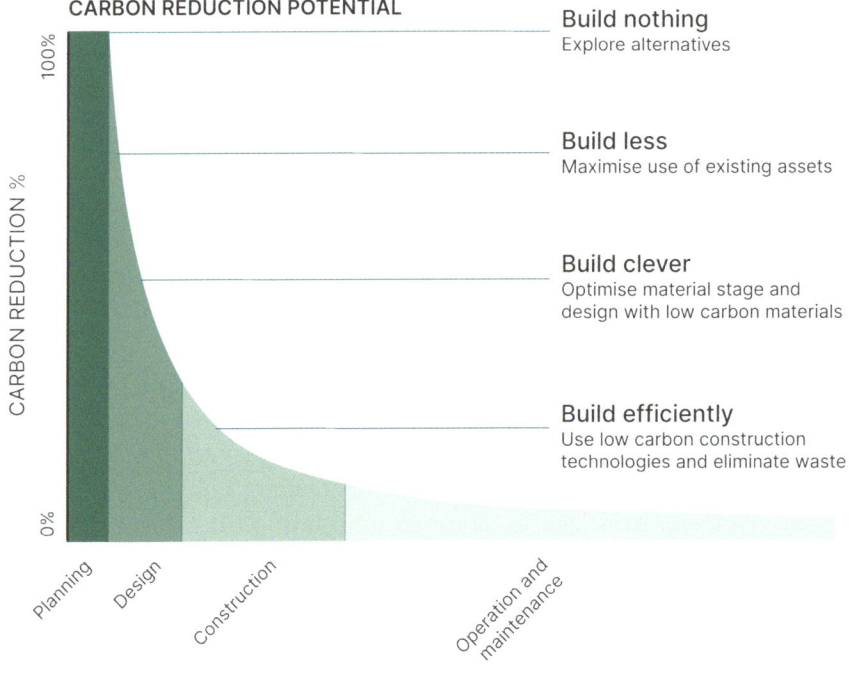

Figure 7.9 Design Is Key in Avoiding Carbon Emissions and Waste. There Are Opportunities to Reduce Carbon in Each Stage of Project Development. The Greatest Potential to Avoid Embodied Carbon Is During the Planning and Design Phases.

adapted for reuse. Overall, 50–75 percent of carbon emissions can be prevented by choosing renovation over demolition and new build (Strain, 2017).

When new construction is necessary, for a new build or renovation, designing lighter and smaller products that deliver the same service allows for reductions in the amount of material and energy used. This can be aided through prefabrication methods and technology. Another option is monolithic construction, which means achieving the same energy requirements for occupant comfort but by using very few material types. This approach can reduce life cycle emissions by reducing the need to manufacture and transport numerous individual materials, e.g., cladding material, insulation material, sheathing materials, waterproofing materials, air barrier materials, and structural materials to site for a hybrid construction. For example, studies show that the monolithic nature of cross-laminated timber (CLT) panels can be multifunctional where the single membrane serves as thermal mass and as both the water-resistive barrier and continuous air barrier (Andersen et al., 2022; Brandner et al., 2016). Hence, design is key in shifting our mindsets toward more tectonic solutions which aim to use less material(s) by design. Policy could promote prefabrication and modular construction, as these tools facilitate light weighting and add more control to the construction process which can also reduce waste (see the 'Fabrication Yield Improvements' section). From a structural standpoint incorporating the use of building information modeling (BIM) during the design phase, areas of medium and low structural loads can be located and help lightweight construction as well as consideration of the correct material which may be multifunctional.

Material Substitution

Another material efficiency strategy is substituting materials which produce more carbon emissions in their sourcing and manufacturing with those that have a lower carbon footprint across their life cycle. For example, replacing cement and steel with bio-based materials could reduce life cycle emissions. There are many options with bio-based materials as explained in Section 7.5.

Despite many bio-based materials' lower relative life cycle emissions compared to concrete and brick, many building codes have limitations on their use in construction especially in relation to high-rise construction with mass timber engineered wood. Moreover, given cement's high contribution to greenhouse gas emissions, innovative policies are needed to enable standards that allow cement with clinker substitutes such as alternative binders. For instance, the European Cement Standardization presents BS EN 197-1: a conformity criterion for common cements. The standard identifies and defines specifications of 27 distinct common cements, and requirements that constituents need to meet (bsi.knowledge, 2019). Building codes can help to address the embodied carbon impact of materials. Performance, rather than prescription-based standards, would facilitate the use of alternative materials. In California, for instance, a low-carbon concrete building code was proposed, which would set limits to the embodied carbon in concrete (King, 2018).

Fabrication Yield Improvements

By reducing material scrap during fabrication and manufacturing processes, the demand for material input from original raw materials is decreased. Additionally, prefabrication in place of on-site construction can avoid or even eliminate construction waste through more controlled planning of production and material use (Chen et al., 2022). This is typically facilitated by BIM which allows potential waste to be identified in the planning stage, given the higher level of collaboration of building planners. This collaboration can expand to enhance circularity. For example, data from the BIM model regarding potential waste can be sent to reuse and recycling centers in advance so they can anticipate the supply of materials they will expect to receive. This can facilitate a new supply and demand model which is inevitable in a circular economy.

Densification of Housing

More intensive use of housing can reduce carbon emissions by designing housing that treats space as a resource to conserve as discussed in Chapter 6. Densification of housing can be promoted by various policies. For instance, the promotion of single-family zoning typically creates land use restrictions on minimum site and structure lifts, limiting construction of multifamily homes and increasing house sizes. Schuetz outlines Minneapolis 2040's strategies to improve housing affordability, and the challenges faced in implementing it (Schuetz, 2022). Its zoning reform includes building more housing, building less expensive housing (particularly in more desirable neighborhoods), and, most notably, ending single-family zoning. Being the first major city in the United States to end single-family zoning in 2018 was particularly noticeable as it had covered almost 75 percent of their residential land. The shift in zoning means that every neighborhood that has currently only single-family houses will now allow duplexes and triplexes to be built with higher density housing along transit lines. By allowing triplexes in all neighborhoods, the city's intention is to offer the opportunity for all to locate to neighborhoods with good schools or jobs, as well as to increase affordability, reduce displacement of lower income residents, and increase both the economic and racial diversity of neighborhoods (Minneapolis, 2023). The Minneapolis 2040's plan to pursue density increases, however, has faced various hurdles. Among them is public resistance, particularly from residents who benefit from low-density, single-family zoning and may not want to see changes in the densification of their neighborhoods. The Minneapolis 2040 Plan is an example of how policy and zoning changes can allow for the more intensive use of housing. The goal of housing densification from a circular economy perspective is to conserve resources and limit environmental impacts while providing the same level of residential service, comfort, and well-being for its occupants.

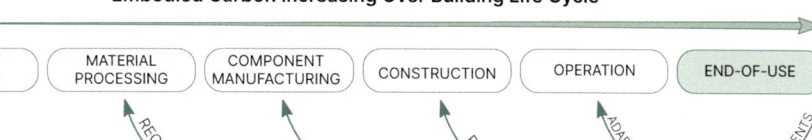

Embodied Carbon Increasing Over Building Life Cycle

| MATERIAL SOURCING | MATERIAL PROCESSING | COMPONENT MANUFACTURING | CONSTRUCTION | OPERATION | END-OF-USE |

RECYCLING OF MATERIALS
REUSE MATERIALS
REUSE COMPONENTS
ADAPTIVE REUSE OF BUILDING ELEMENTS

Potential for Carbon Savings & Embodied Carbon Preservation

Figure 7.10 Embodied Carbon Preservation Along a Building Life Cycle.

Enhanced End-of-Use Processes – Recovery, Reuse, Recycle

The key premise of circularity in buildings is to keep the building and its materials in use for as long as possible. Hence, there is a cascading effect in terms of preserving the embodied carbon at the end-of-use of a building as illustrated in Figure 7.10. The best option is to reuse the building. Next best option is to reuse components or materials. The last resort is recycling. Within recycling there is another hierarchy of options starting from recycling a material back to its original form, to a worst-case scenario of downcycling where a product of lesser value is produced.

Not all materials are made equally, hence, different materials have variant degrees of reusability and recyclability. Figure 7.11 shows the current technological viability of reuse and recycling for different construction materials. Aluminum and steel have excellent ability to be reused and recycled. Material finishes like paint and insulation materials such as polyurethane have very little options when it comes to reuse and recycling. Given this variance in materials end-of-use options, upstream design choices have huge repercussions for potential end-of-use strategies.

Technological Viability for Reuse and Recycling

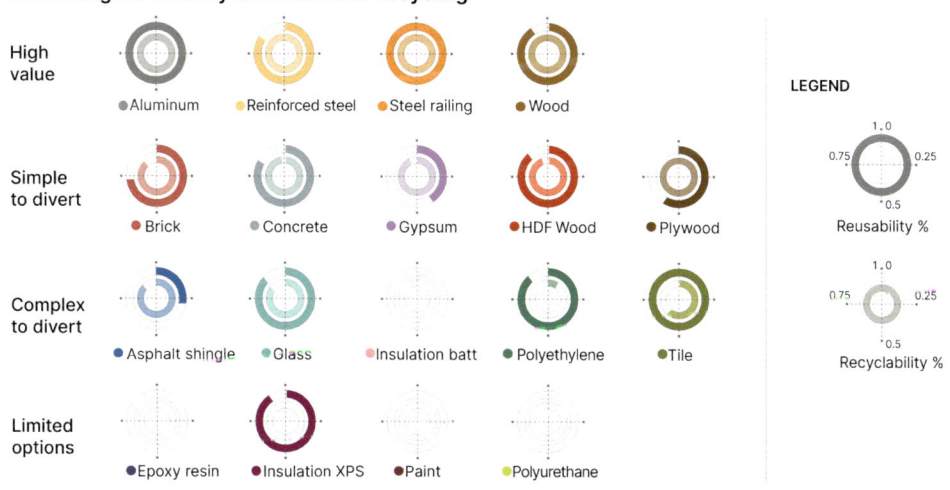

Figure 7.11 The Technological Viability for Reuse and Recycling of a Selection of Construction Materials.

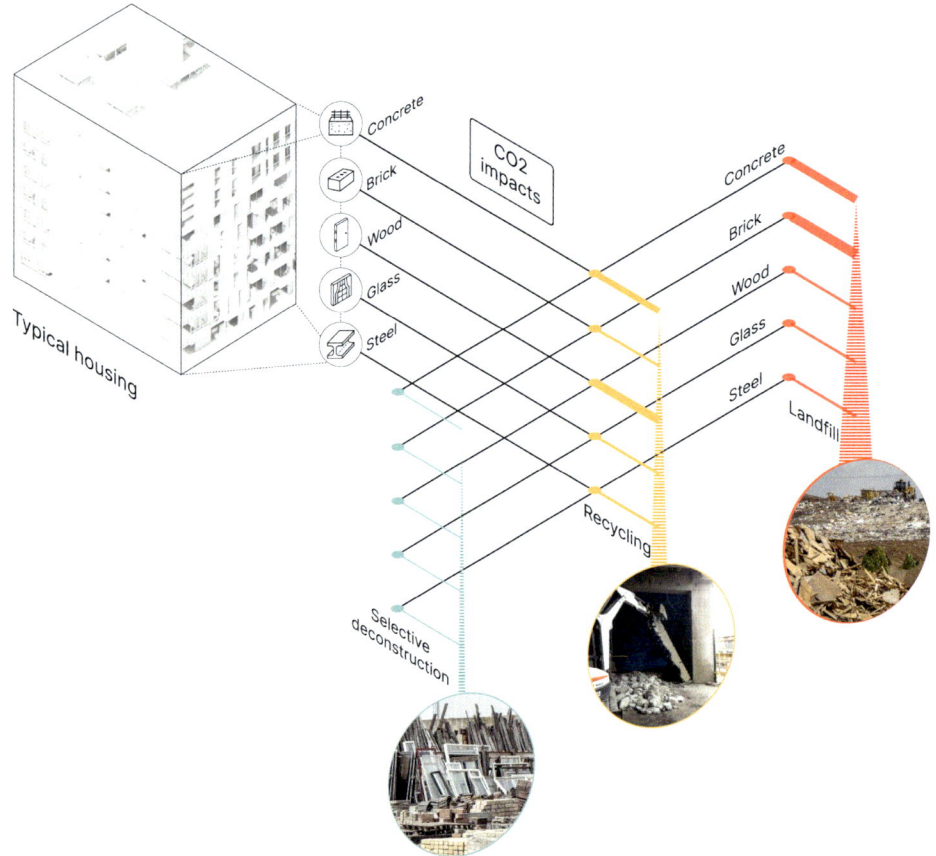

Figure 7.12 Enhancing End-of-Use Circular Economy Strategies of Selective Deconstruction and Recycling to Facility a Transition Away from Demolition and Landfill.

Enhanced end-of-use recovery and recycling of materials requires sorting and processing construction, renovation, and demolition materials (see Figure 7.12). As opposed to demolition, selective deconstruction involves the careful dismantling of a building at its end-of-use. This step is key in promoting on-site sorting where the value of components and materials is maintained, and reuse and recycling is increased. Once sorting has occurred, the widescale availability of reuse and recycling centers is extremely important if circularity is to become the norm in construction. For secondary materials to compete strongly in the construction materials marketplace, technical, operational, social, cultural, regulatory, and economic limitations need to be overcome (Knoth et al., 2022). Policymaking is key in helping to overcome these limitations. Government incentives can encourage both the reuse marketplace as well as the widespread adoption of secondary materials and selective deconstruction practices.

In Japan, for instance, the Construction Material Recycling Law was enacted in order to address issues of waste by ensuring efficient use of resources (Ministry of the Environment, 2000). Aimed at recycling and reusing prospective construction materials, the law requires contractors to sort out and recycle wastes generated in demolition. Appropriate demolition is enforced by a registration system for demolition. Furthermore, mandating landfill bans would further shift the treatment of buildings at the end of its use to a circular economy. Landfill bans are supported by various policies, such as recycling laws. In 2012, Vermont Legislature passed Act 148, a universal recycling and composting law that facilitates reducing waste in landfill (Chittenden Solid Waste District, 2012). The law includes bans on the disposal of certain materials, collection requirements for trash-accepting facilities, etc. Hence, by introducing policies, the end-of-use recovery of materials is enhanced through a series of systems and tools, which reach actors along the entire value chain.

7.4.2 Implementation of Material Efficiency Strategies

Despite the various methods of incorporating material efficiency into construction, there are obstacles that hinder implementation. One challenge is demonstrating to stakeholders that materials have been responsibly sourced. While there are existing evaluations for determining if a material is used responsibly, they do not necessarily account for the behavior of relevant actors.

Policymaking is key to implementing material efficiency and shifting toward bio-materials. Policies enable transformation by regulating the government approval process for materials before they enter the marketplace. Government incentives can encourage both the manufacturing and the widespread adoption of new bio-based and sustainable building products. For instance, by requiring that new materials meet recognized material standards and certification regarding their composition and properties and must also comply with building codes. For example, the BES 6001 responsible sourcing standards for construction products were developed by the BRE Group to provide a holistic approach to managing products from sourcing to delivery (Goodhew, 2016). The standard describes criteria on the organization management, and behavior required for sourcing to be responsible. Using materials manufactured by environmentally responsible companies with external accreditation ensures sustainable materials but also comes at a higher cost. Overall, policy intervention is required in order for material efficiency benefits to be achieved. Along with policy, technology can aid in the implementation of material efficiency strategies. The use of digital tools (such as BIM) and prefabrication facilitate the adoption of these strategies – the role of virtual tools will be further explored in Chapter 10.

Material efficiency strategies require various efforts for effective implementation. However, once applied, significant mitigation of emissions is observed (as depicted in Figure 7.13). The IRP (2020) report demonstrates that material efficiency strategies could significantly reduce greenhouse gas emissions associated with the material cycle of residential buildings by 2060. It projects that between 2016 and 2060, with these strategies, there could be a 350-million-metric-ton reduction in greenhouse gas emissions in China, 270-million-metric-ton reduction in India, and

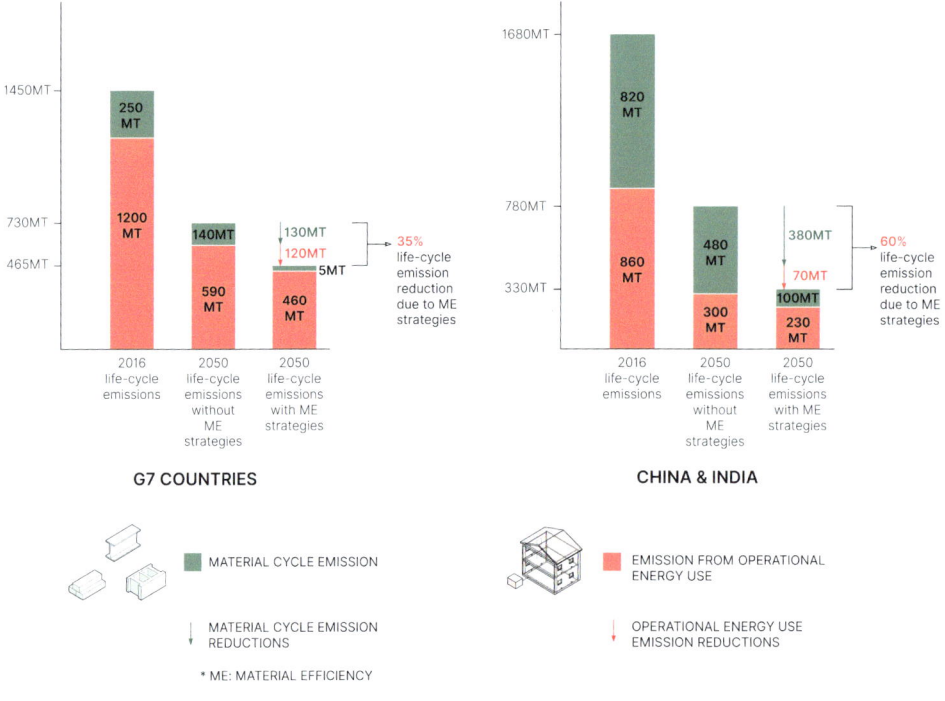

G7 COUNTRIES

MATERIAL CYCLE EMISSION

MATERIAL CYCLE EMISSION
REDUCTIONS

* ME: MATERIAL EFFICIENCY

CHINA & INDIA

EMISSION FROM OPERATIONAL
ENERGY USE

OPERATIONAL ENERGY USE
EMISSION REDUCTIONS

Source: Adapted from IRP 2020 "Resource Efficiency and Climate Change"

Figure 7.13 Life Cycle Emissions from Homes with and without Material Efficiency Strategies in G7 Countries, and China and India, in 2050.

170-million-metric-ton reduction in G7 countries (Hertwich et al., 2020). Ultimately, proper implementation of these strategies results in more sustainable materials and, consequently, lower environmental impacts.

7.5 Transitioning from a Fossil-Based to a Bio-Based Economy

As described above, "material substitution" is a material efficiency strategy. The following sections explore a recent shift in the building and construction industry toward bio-based materials, in an effort to decarbonize buildings. From sourcing and production stages to use, consumption, and disposal, biomaterials have the potential to reduce emissions. The sourcing of such materials does not rely on extractive mineral-based processes, resulting in lower embodied carbon. Biomaterials refer to materials that interact with living systems (Khitab et al., 2016). Their sourcing – including harvesting and forestry – is derived from bio-based renewable resources, which are often biodegradable at the end of their life cycle (see Chapter 9). A fossil-based economy is linear as it fails to close the loop on waste generation, given that it relies heavily on the energy-intensive extraction, manufacturing, and transport of non-renewable, mineral-based resources. Adopting a more sustainable economy may involve shifting away from a fossil-based economy toward a bio-based one. This transition represents a potential solution to answering the demands of rapid urbanization while simultaneously reducing the carbon footprint of cities and infrastructure. This shift, along with material efficiency in general, is critical in meeting the 1.5°C goal of the Paris Agreement and the 2030 Agenda for Sustainable Development. Within a circular economy, the goal is to maintain a continuous flow of materials. As seen in Figure 7.14, there are two main cycles in this process, which should remain separate. The technical cycle involves products and materials being kept in the circular process through reusing, repairing, remanufacturing, and recycling. The biological cycle refers to the biodegradable materials' nutrients being returned to the earth to regenerate nature. If the cycles do not remain distinct, then it becomes difficult to recover all elements at the end of a building's use (Ellen MacArthur Foundation, 2019).

Ultimately, materials are crucial in design – they should not be limited to preservation and aesthetics and instead need to consider performance, circularity, and regeneration. Without significant improvements in resource efficiency, it will be virtually impossible to keep global warming below the targeted 1.5–2°C (Czigler et al., 2020). The result of combining resource efficiency and circular logic is a policy and design framework that can transform our use of materials. Figure 7.15 highlights that in the United States, while slow, there has been a recent increase in the use of renewable materials; more than half of the renewable materials were used during the past 40 years (Matos, 2022). Yet the use of non-renewable raw materials (especially for construction) is still dominant. Although transitioning to a bio-based economy offers significant benefits, such a transition requires special consideration and implementation. Critically, sustainable criteria are required to prevent unsustainable practices and environmental impacts, such as deforestation, loss of biodiversity, and changing land use patterns.

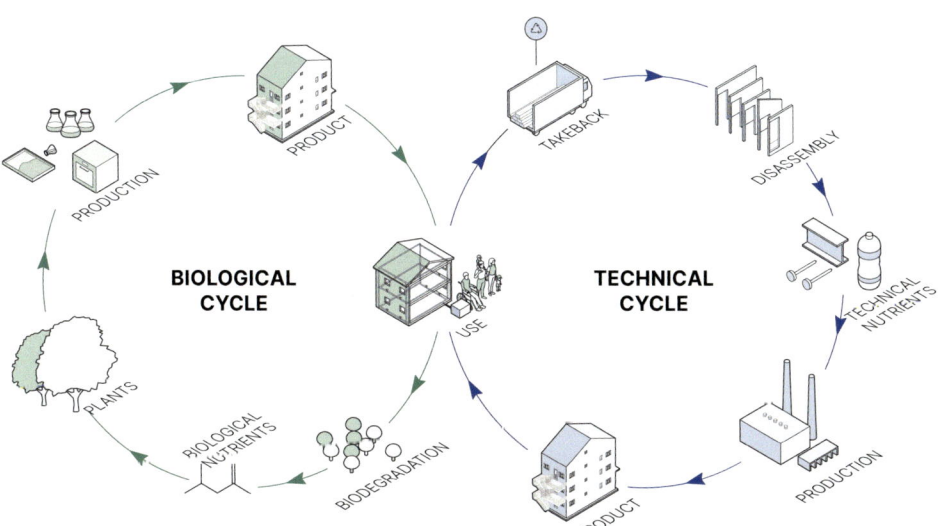

Figure 7.14 Circular Economy Systems – Ellen MacArthur Foundation.

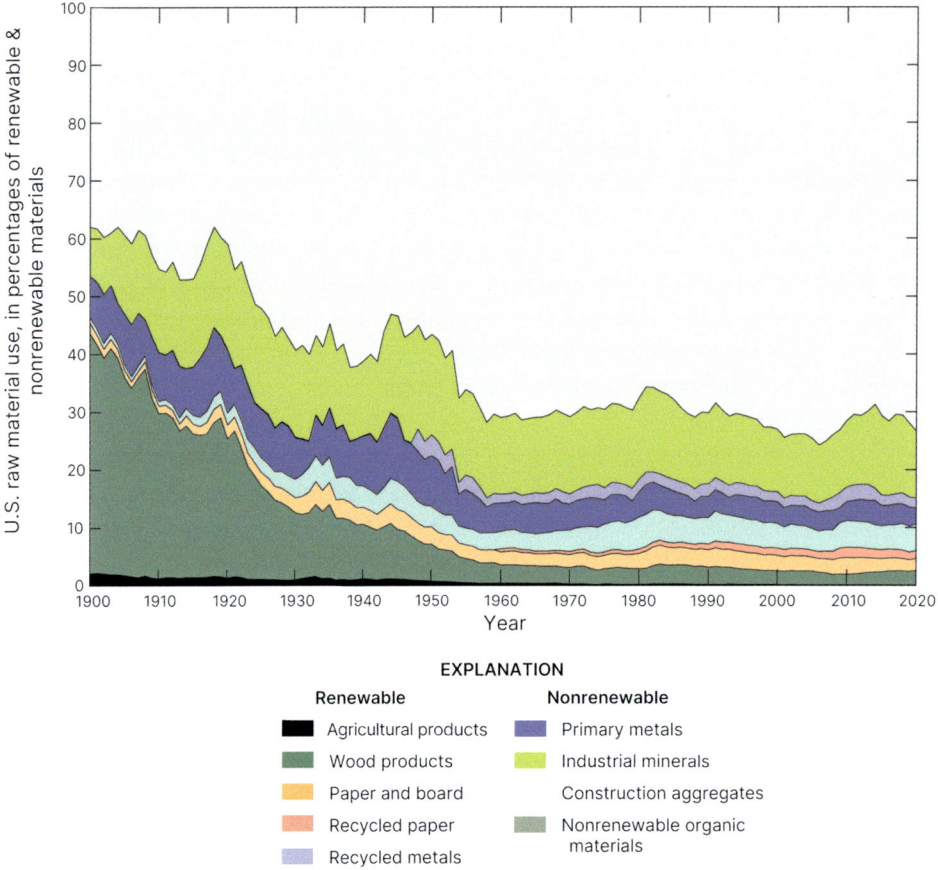

Figure 7.15 Circular Economy Systems – The Percentage Shares of Renewable and Non-Renewable Raw Materials Used Annually in the United States from 1900 through 2020.

7.6 Biomaterials and Circular Economy

While society once shifted away from biomaterials, they have recently begun to regain prominence. Biomaterials offer significant opportunities for reducing emissions associated with the life cycle of building materials, from the sourcing and production stages to the use, consumption, and disposal phases. Biomaterials can be made from various living materials and can be employed in different forms. Each offers unique qualities and can solve a variety of issues.

Certain biomaterials are directly employed. For instance, timber has historically been used as a construction material and was instrumental in framing, roofing, and flooring structures for centuries. Achieved through gluing wooden panels and boards together, CLT has emerged as a popular construction material. Recent innovations allow the use of timber frames in tall buildings, which allows timber to replace more carbon-intensive construction materials. Biomaterials are generally more environmentally friendly, as they produce less carbon emissions. In the case of timber, timber frames have the highest level of carbon storage, which is beneficial as it delays the emission of carbon dioxide. In fact, emissions from the material cycle of construction materials can be reduced by 1–8 percent in the G7 through greater use of timber (Hertwich et al., 2019). With that said, the timber supply is limited, and its climatic benefits are only applicable to sustainably sourced wood products. In addition, bio-based alternatives such as bamboo, CLT, and upcycled agricultural waste (coconut) have been shown to have much lower life cycle impacts per functional unit, compared to traditional timber-frame construction (Keena et al., 2022).

Biomaterials can also be employed indirectly, through chemical modification to optimize material performance. Thus, biomaterials include recycled, or partially recycled, materials in which natural materials are indirectly applied. Bioplastics are a form of such and consist of plastics that are either made from renewable resources, are biodegradable, are made through biological processes, or a combination (Rosenboom et al., 2022). Moreover, bio-based polymers are combined with concrete to mitigate cracking, as will be expanded on later in this chapter.

Furthermore, agricultural waste, or agro waste, represents another indirect use of biomaterial. Alongside the building industry, agriculture is another sector that practices intensive use of non-metal materials – it is responsible for the consumption of 8 percent of phosphate rock and 1.5 percent of potash in overall mineral consumption throughout the 20th century (Pacheco-Torgal et al., 2014). This contributes to emissions and produces a large amount of waste. Thus, making use of agricultural waste not only benefits the building industry but also helps mitigate the impacts of the agricultural sector. Agricultural waste includes waste associated with rice, straw corn, and coconut husk, as well as non-food materials derived from land products, animal products, and fishery products. Traditionally, agricultural waste was used in the generation of heat, biogas, or compost across rural areas. Today, new research employs agricultural waste in the development of materials for the building industry (Matos, 2017). For example, mycelium forms part of the root structure of mushrooms and has emerged as an innovative building material, particularly for panel insulation (see Figure 7.16). Mycelium offers many advantages, including acting as a natural fire retardant, given that it contains chitin, and, of course, that it is a biodegradable product that comes from agricultural waste (Albert, 2021).

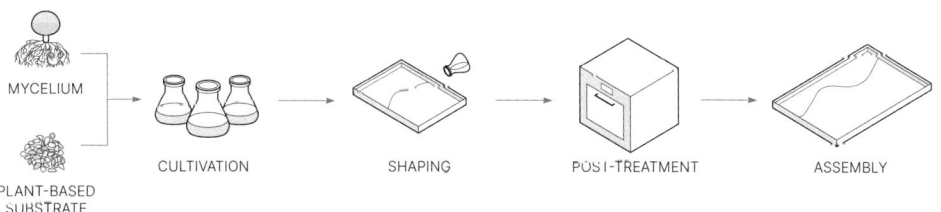

Source: Adapted from fungal Biology and Biotechnology, "A review on architecture with fungal biomaterials: the desired and the feasible"

Figure 7.16 Mycelium Production Process.

Using waste bio-based materials that are derived from plants, including wood and agricultural by-products, means rather than releasing greenhouse gas emissions during biodegradation or when they are burned at their end-of-life, these materials are kept in use to sequester atmospheric carbon over the course of their secondary lifetime (Keena et al., 2022).

Overall, in order to achieve a circular economy within the building industry, the choice and use of materials is critical. Achieving a circular economy involves three principles: designing out waste and pollution, keeping materials and products in use, and regenerating natural systems. Given their recycled nature and extended life cycle, biomaterials represent a viable method in achieving a circular logic within both the sourcing and construction of buildings. Once used, these materials are returned to the earth, rendering the building process circular. However, once biodegrading, they can release greenhouse gas emissions such as carbon or even methane, so the longer they are kept in use for an extended life cycle, the better.

7.6.1 Biomaterials: One Path Toward the Circular Production of Building Materials

The extraction phase of construction materials represents one of the most harmful stages in regard to the environment. Fossil-based materials are typically associated with a linear process that relies on energy-intensive extraction and fails to close the loop on waste generation. Biomaterials, on the other hand, do not rely on extractive mineral-based processes but instead are derived from bio-based renewable resources. They eliminate the need for mining construction minerals, thus reducing extractive processes and offering a typically biodegradable alternative at the end-of-use, which may effectively assist in regenerating natural systems. Moreover, the use of bio-based materials allows engagement in the material production and construction sectors at a local scale. This is due to the fact that effective use of biomaterials involves using those biomaterials which are locally available. Such materials are typically "climate specific", meaning when used in a building they offer appropriate performance characteristics in response to the climate in which the building is located. In addition, local sourcing and production result in providing additional employment and income streams to local economies – biomaterials effectively promote a circular logic both in the environment and economy. Biomaterials offer an alternative approach to construction as they naturally fulfill many of circular economy's criteria.

7.6.2 Using Biomaterials to Promote a Circular Approach to the Manufacturing, Fabrication, and Construction of Buildings

A circular economy requires radically rethinking construction practices by minimizing and controlling the amount of material used and associated waste. During the construction phase, biomaterials are compatible with innovative and cutting-edge construction practices. Combined prefabrication and bio-based building components facilitate construction, such as biomaterial panels, which are manufactured within a controlled environment and transported to site for quick assembly. Technological innovations are also compatible with bio-based materials; three-dimensional printing is consistent with bio-based plastics and ceramics, as well as hybrids. This combination is optimal as it allows for control over the quantity of material used, thereby limiting material waste. Hence, the use of biomaterial during the construction stage offers clean, healthy, and efficient construction sites.

7.7 Challenges in Making Biomaterials More Readily Available

While the benefits of biomaterials are evident, certain factors pose a challenge to their immediate and continuous integration. From a socio-cultural perspective as highlighted in Section 7.3, people need to view biomaterials – and low-tech and "vernacular" building techniques – as desirable and innovative. For biomaterials to compete strongly in the construction materials marketplace, social, cultural, economic, and regulatory limitations need to be overcome (Keena et al., 2022). With housing in many emerging economies yet to be built to meet a rapidly growing population, these countries have the potential to pave the way in the use of circular design techniques.

In order to promote environmental health while preventing unanticipated environmental impacts, two primary issues must be considered: first, avoiding the infringement of land marked for food production and, second, preventing the exploitation of land. The sourcing of raw materials can be harmful as, if not done properly or if done to excess, it has the potential to degrade land and soil nutrients. However, positioning biomaterials as a main source for the construction sector implies an increase in the volume of materials and resources sourced from the cultivation of land. In order for safe sourcing and use of biomaterials, policies and regulations for sustainable practices are critical.

7.8 Hybrid Materials

Hybrid biomaterials are a combination of naturally derived and synthetic materials. The biocompatibility of these materials encourages strong interactions in the host tissue and enhanced cellular interactions. Thus, not only are the sought-after characteristics of synthetic materials conserved, but they can be enhanced with natural processes since many biological features allow for regenerative properties within materials. Emphasis is placed on hybrid biomaterials for concrete, as it offers an innovative solution for a popular and ubiquitous building material.

Indeed, concrete remains a popular construction material given its performance characteristic and the wide availability of limestone, making it likely to remain the global material of choice. The use and production of concrete, in its current state, is unsustainable, requiring an energy-intensive production process at a large volume, to keep up with worldwide demand. In 2015, it was estimated that the annual global cement production was approximately 4100 Mt. With business-as-usual practices, annual global cement production is projected to grow to 4,800 Mt by 2030 (Worrell & Carreon, 2017). The cement industry alone is responsible for approximately one quarter of all industry carbon dioxide emissions and generates the most carbon dioxide emissions per dollar revenue (Czigler et al., 2020). Cement is the binder between aggregates in the formation of concrete. While cement represents only a small fraction of the whole mixture, it is almost entirely responsible for the resulting emissions (Czigler et al., 2020). Given its negative impact, there has been a growing demand for change from society and the government. Investors have shown concern regarding funding of cement, with some requiring environmental impact assessments. This has led to an increasing pressure on the cement industry to decarbonize. Hence, in order to mitigate emissions while retaining the advantages of concrete, certain changes in the concrete industry need to be made.

Bio-concrete has emerged as a hybrid solution. Not only does it possess the qualities of concrete in a more environmentally friendly approach, but it may even surpass it. Despite concrete's high strength, it develops cracks, which decreases the overall durability of a structure. Current practices use synthetic polymers as treatment, which are effective but raise environmental concerns. Hence, a bio-concrete approach known as "autogenic healing" utilizes bacteria to seal cracks. Given the chemical composition of healing products, this bacterium offers improved compatibility with the host matrix. As depicted in Figure 7.17, through the use of pozzolanic

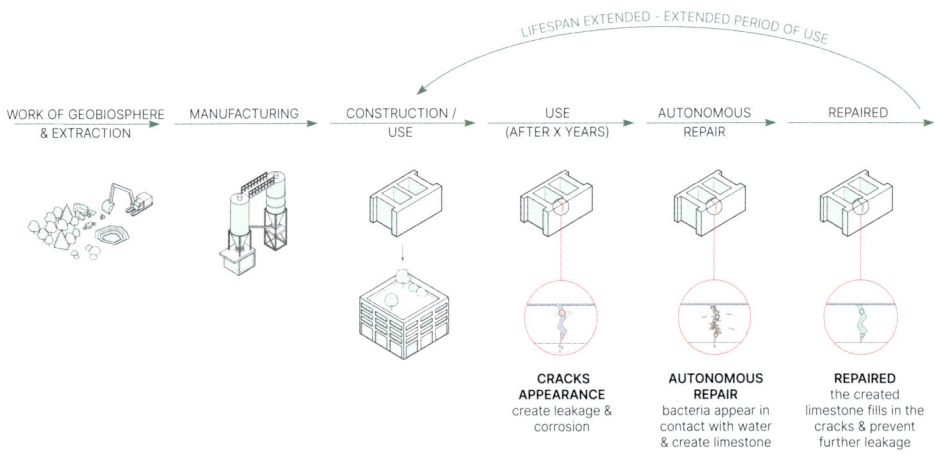

Source: Adapted from Labiotech "Biomaterials Are Making the Building Industry More Sustanaible"

Figure 7.17 How Bio-Concrete Works.

material, the concrete's newfound strength is compared to that of undamaged cement (Gardner et al., 2017). Another alternative is using bio-reinforcement and biochar. This method utilizes agro waste as a partial or full replacement of sand or as a reinforcing material to increase concrete's compressive strength. Moreover, recent research aims to amplify the performance of cement mortar through the use of biochar as a carbon-sequestering additive. The results suggest that bio-char can successfully be employed as a carbon-sequestering admixture in concrete, which also provides a method for recycling waste (Brownell & Global, 2020). Finally, "green charcoal" has emerged, suggesting the possibility of using similar bio-reinforcements and charcoal together to explore a co-existing material with higher environmental performance. Green charcoal effectively looks at a selection of fibers that are pre-engineered by nature in such an arrangement that enhances the structural integrity and permeability of concrete. This results in the development of new construction materials made of soil, charcoal, and air. Hence, the goal of green charcoal is to address the issue of pollution by creating healthy building materials, which are biodegradable, lightweight, and allow for the growth of living plant and insect ecosystems on its surface. Overall, the use of hybrid techniques represents a valid approach to reducing building's emissions; however, with this approach comes new issues. While hybrid materials can lengthen the life cycle of a building, when it comes to end-of-use, the solution could turn into an obstacle. The hybrid approach directly opposes a circular economy's requirement for technological and biological cycles to remain separate. The hybrid nature of these materials would render them difficult to disassociate at their end-of-use and, therefore, difficult to reuse and recycle. Thus, it is critical to remain mindful of this, and to approach the design of a building (including material selection) with the whole life cycle in mind.

7A

Project:
The House of Wood, Straw, and Cork

Locations:
Magnago, Italy

Year:
2016

Team:
Luca Compri Architects

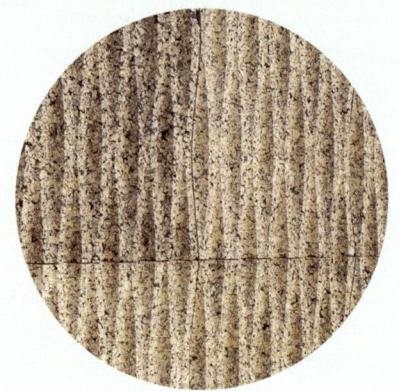

Mapping to Circular Economy Framework:

CIRCULAR ECONOMY PRACTICES

LIFE CYCLE PHASES

	Recovery	Life Extension	Sharing Platforms	Service Models	Regenerate	Virtualize
Work of Geobiosphere	●				●	
Sourcing	●	●				
Manufacturing						
Design & Construction		●		●		
Use		●		●		
End-of-Use	●					

LAYERS + LIFESPAN
Structural Layers | Long Life
Skin, MEP Layers | Medium Life
Interior Layers | Short Life

Site 100+yr   Structure 50+yr
Exterior 25+yr   System 15+yr
Partition 10+yr   Stuff 1+yr

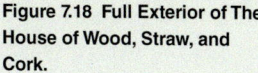

Figure 7.18 Full Exterior of The House of Wood, Straw, and Cork.

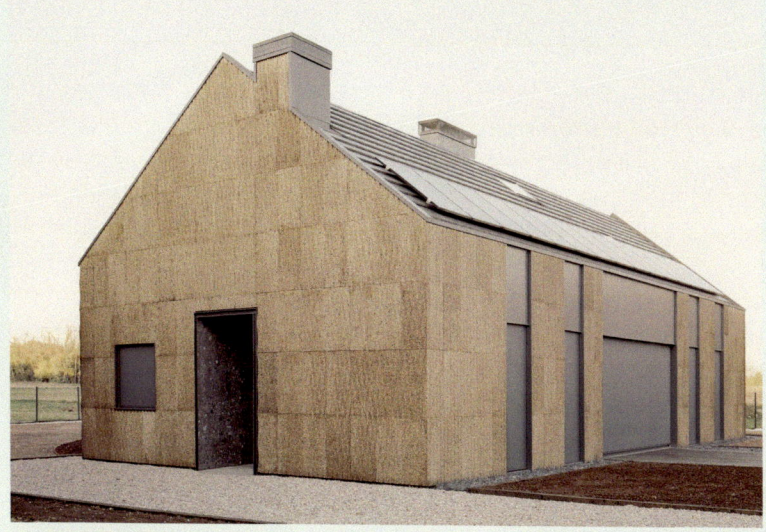

On the edge of a small village near Milan, Italy sits the simple and elegant House of Wood, Straw, and Cork (see Figures 7.18 and 7.19). The two-bedroom home was designed by Italian firm, Luca Compri Architects (LCA) with the goal of showcasing the aesthetic potential of inexpensive, bio-based materials and simplicity of form and expression. The home's design vision valued beauty as well as environmental

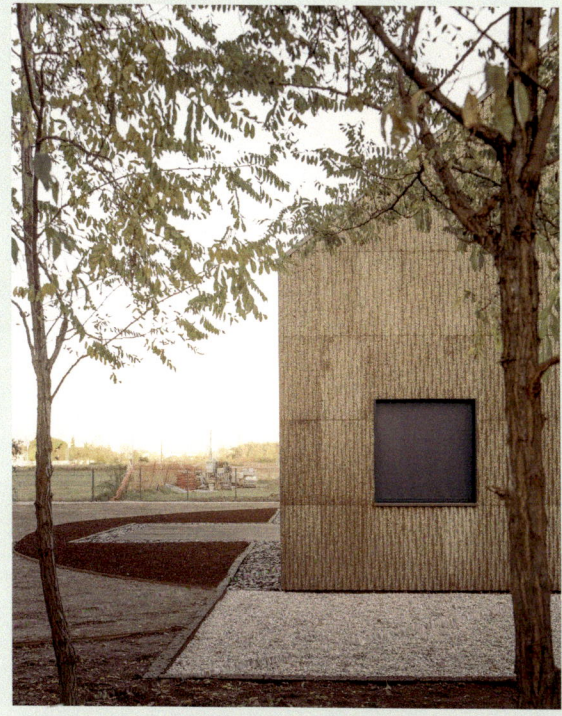

Figure 7.19 The House of Wood, Straw, and Cork.

217

sensitivity, illustrating that efficiency, sustainability, and durability can lend themselves wonderfully to beautiful housing projects. With this project, LCA showcases the circular economy principles of recovery and recycling, product life extension, service models, and regeneration through recyclable, bio-based materials, and passive design strategies.

Material choice was central to the design, with the architects taking on the responsibility of sourcing **recycled** materials to divert waste from local landfills (see Figures 7.20 and 7.21). Straw, sourced from waste at local rice farms, was selected as the main insulation material in the build (Crook, 2020). The material has a strong history as an insulator in housing and provides a low-carbon alternative to conventional insulating materials that are highly processed and difficult to recycle. Cork, another great insulator, clads the house's exterior. Cork is a renewable, resistant, and insulating material that is harvested from the bark of the cork oak tree and has many practical applications in construction (Hirshberg, 2022). This material features the project's only decorative element, a wavy and textured finish carved into the cladding that only strengthens its natural appeal (see Figure 7.22). Wood, the last key material chosen

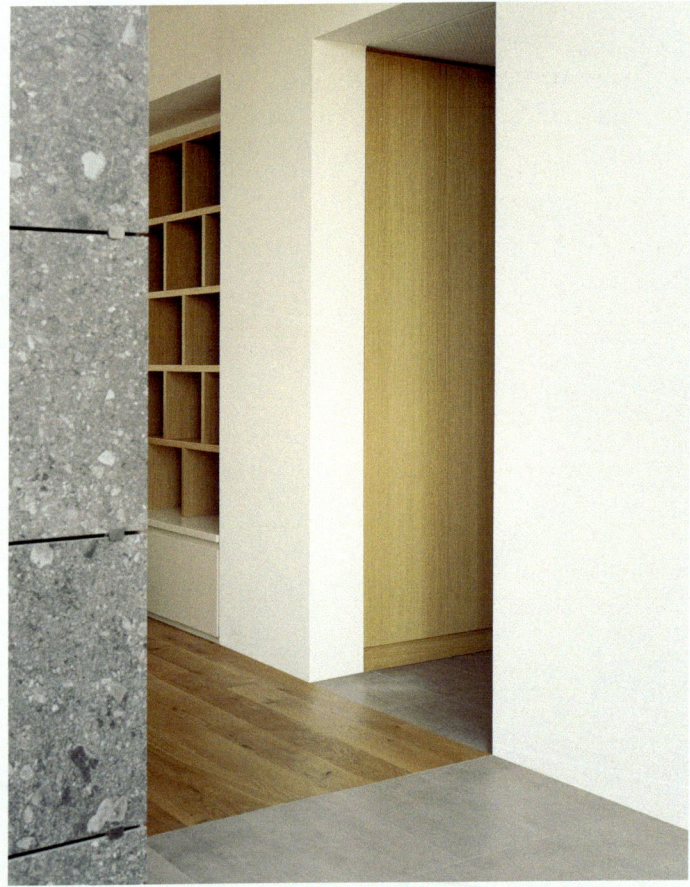

Figure 7.20 The Interior Finishes Also Reflect the Earthy, Natural Material Palette of the Exterior.

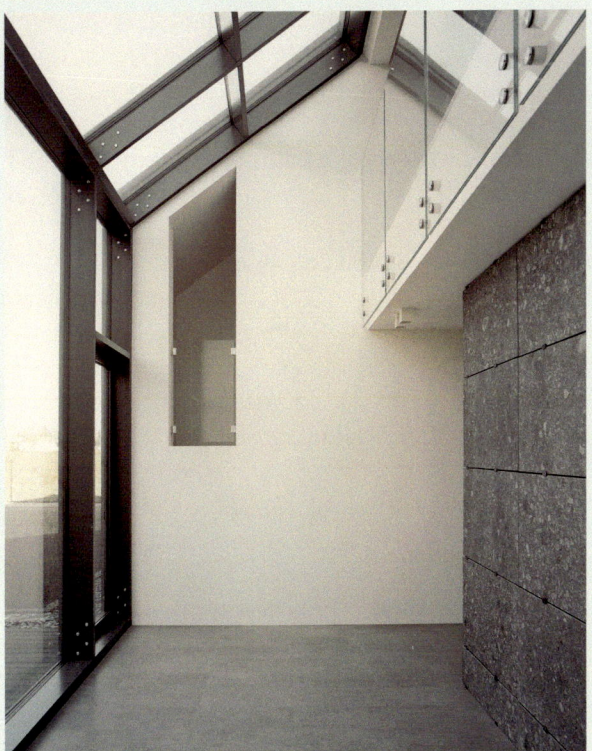

Figure 7.21 View of the Living Room Which Forms the Heart of the House.

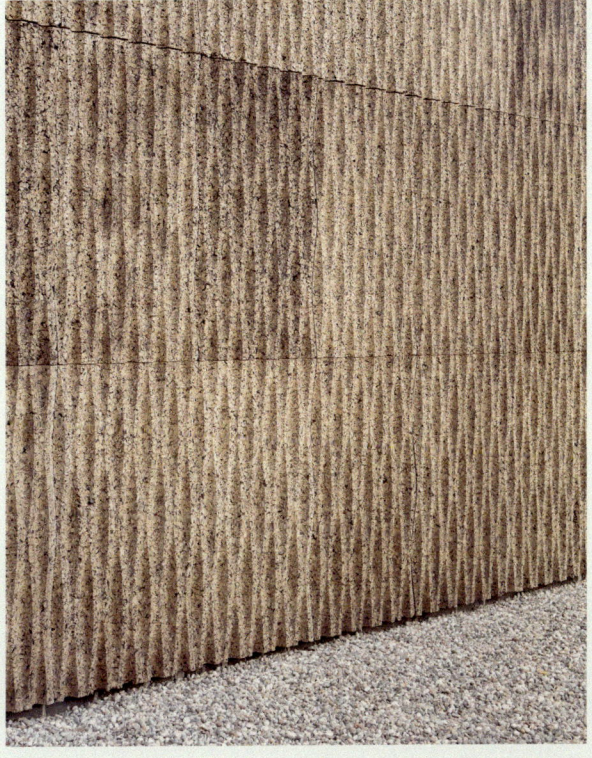

Figure 7.22 Detailed View of the Cork Cladding Finish.

for renewability and recyclability makes up the house's basic structure and is seen in the interior finishing. The use of bio-based materials carries multiple advantages, they can be easily recycled to reduce waste when the house is decommissioned in the end-of-use phase, and wood captures and stores atmospheric carbon dioxide for its use phase and beyond. This process, called carbon sequestration, reduces carbon present in the atmosphere that contributes to the greenhouse gas effect and global warming.

The conscious simplicity represented by material choices is also applied to the building's form to achieve an energy efficient volume, devoid of unnecessary protrusions (see Figures 7.23–7.25). The simple, rectangular plan comfortably supports all living functions on two floors with minimized exterior walls conducive to unwanted temperature loss. This form was inspired by the surrounding farmhouses, acknowledging, and preserving this local heritage while embodying passive design strategies that limit energy needs (Pintos, 2020). Another passive strategy employed is the full glazing on the north facing façade that maximizes diffuse, or indirect, daylighting, coupled with small openings on the south wall to limit direct solar gains that would heat the space. These design choices reduce reliance on energy and carbon-intensive lighting and cooling systems, whose lifespans cannot compare to the longevity of the building's form and fundamental structure. LCA's house is therefore resilient and self-reliant and has an **extended life cycle**. In addition to these fundamental design approaches, an active solar system integrated into the building's roof eliminates reliance on the energy grid, along with carbon dioxide

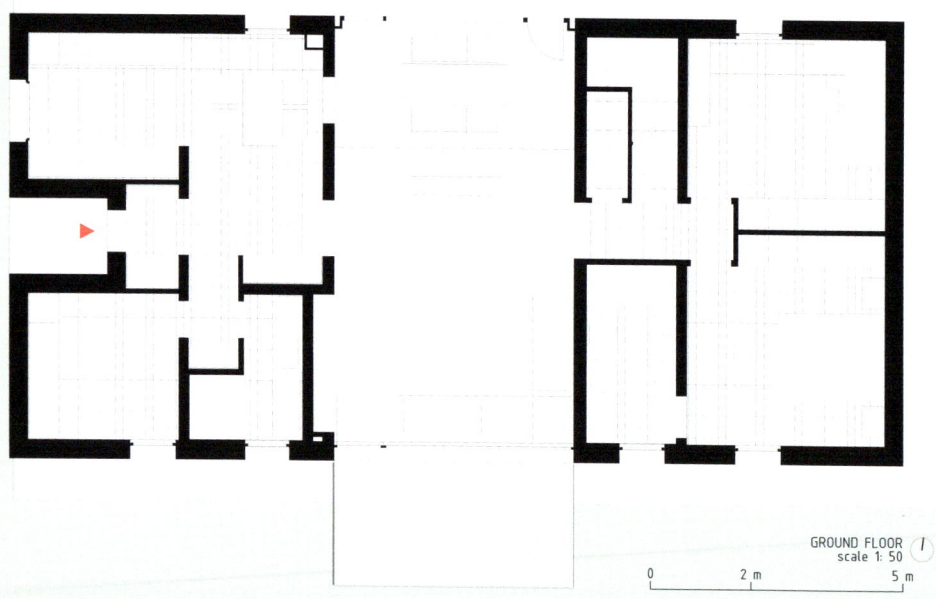

GROUND FLOOR
scale 1: 50

0   2 m   5 m

Figure 7.23 Ground Floor Plan.

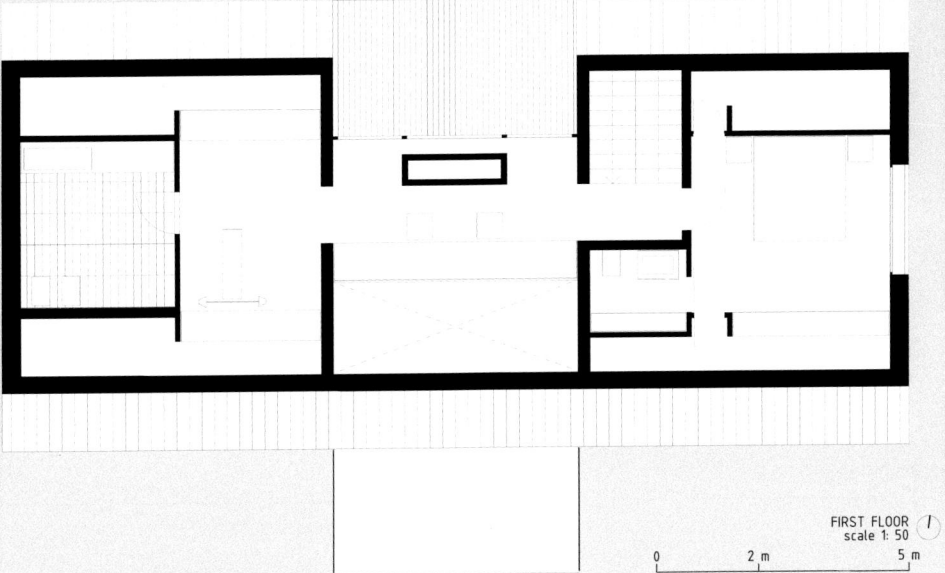

FIRST FLOOR
scale 1: 50

0   2 m   5 m

Figure 7.24 First Floor Plan.

emissions. Any surplus of energy produced by the home can be distributed to the rest of the energy grid. This is an example of a circular economy **service model**, and at a larger scale, this approach can create energy resiliency and limit waste within entire communities. The House of Wood, Straw, and Cork suggest that simplicity and elegance can be achieved through sustainable practices that encourage a circular economy.

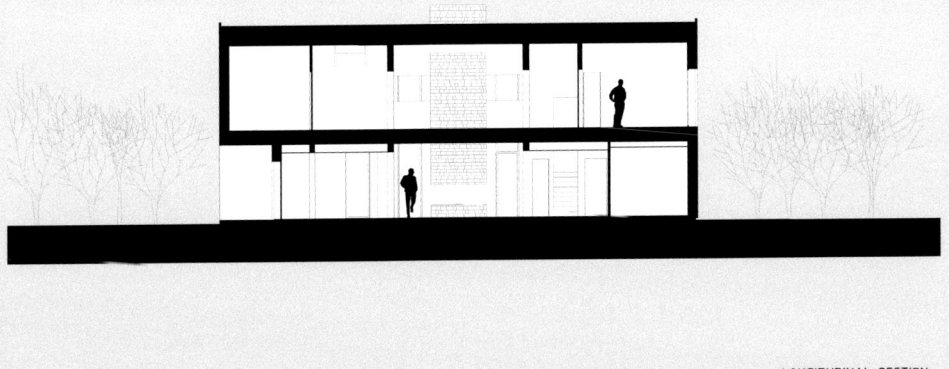

LONGITUDINAL SECTION
scale 1: 100

0   4 m   10 m

Figure 7.25 Longitudinal Section of the House of Wood, Straw, and Cork.

7B

Project:
Loblolly House

Locations:
Maryland, United States

Year:
2006

Team:
KieranTimberlake Architects

**Mapping to Circular
Economy Framework:**

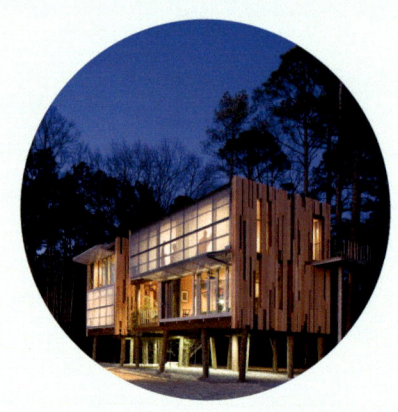

CIRCULAR ECONOMY PRACTICES

LIFE CYCLE PHASES — Recovery, Life Extension, Sharing Platforms, Service Models, Regenerate, Virtualize

- Work of Geobiosphere
- Sourcing
- Manufacturing
- Design & Construction
- Use
- End-of-Use

LAYERS + LIFESPAN
Structural Layers | Long Life
Skin, MEP Layers | Medium Life
Interior Layers | Short Life

Site 100+yr   Structure 50+yr
Exterior 25+yr   System 15+yr
Partition 10+yr   Stuff 1+yr

Today's construction industry, as explored in this chapter, is a major contributor to greenhouse gas emissions. Housing design must adapt low-carbon solutions to work toward eliminating greenhouse gas emissions and decelerating climate change. KieranTimberlake Associates sought to provide sustainable and environmentally ethical housing with their 2006 project, Loblolly House (KieranTimberlake, 2013; see Figure 7.26). The two-story home has a compact area of 2,200 sq. ft. (204 m²) and was designed to minimize the impact on the site and local environment. The dwelling sits inconspicuously within a forest of loblolly pine trees, raised on a series of timber piles erected irregularly and slightly skewed to mimic the natural

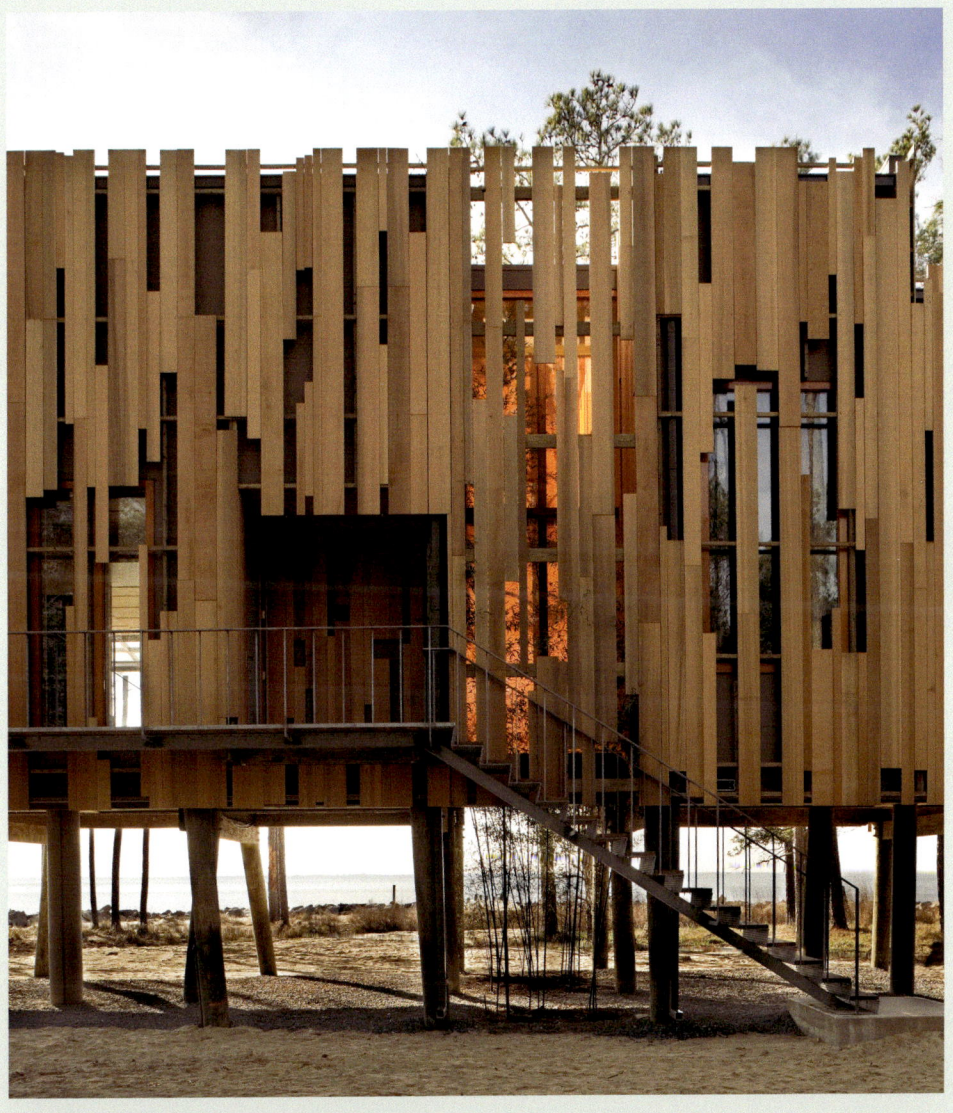

Figure 7.26 Front Façade for the Loblolly House.

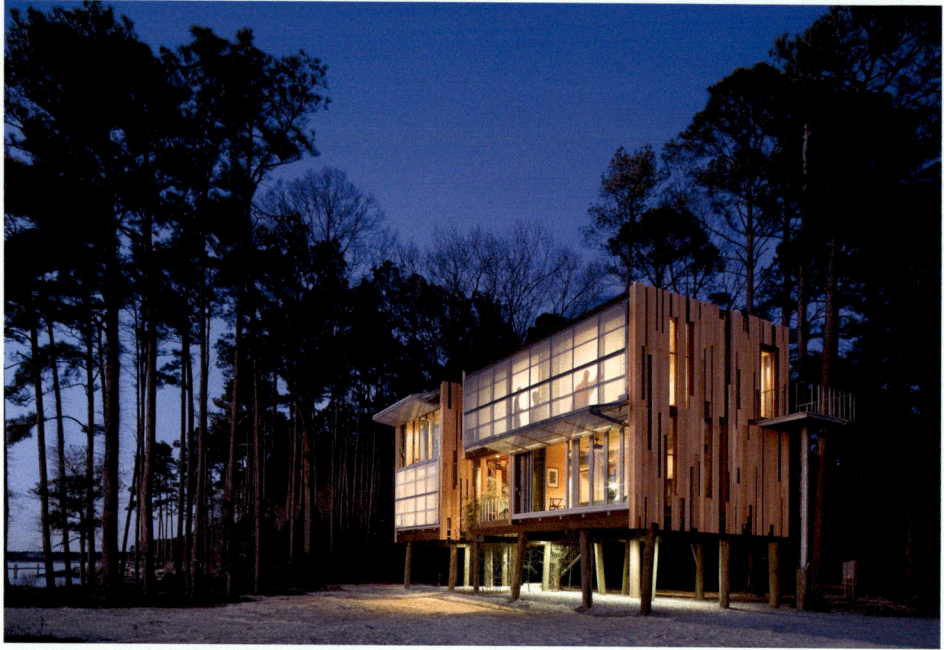

Figure 7.27 Night View of the Loblolly House.

surroundings (see Figure 7.27). Elevating the house was a response to environmental conditions, as the site on Taylors Island in Maryland, United States, can experience flooding which can cause structural damage and shorten a building's lifespan.

A pile foundation is driven into the ground at key points to prevent water infiltration while providing sheltered parking, minimal impact on the site's soil, and a playful and modern interpretation of a treehouse. Through a minimally invasive approach to housing, KieranTimberlake prioritized the health of the natural environment of the site, whose ecosystem components, including the namesake loblolly trees, regulate carbon dioxide within the atmosphere (see Figure 7.28) (*Loblolly House: Prefabricated Architecture Integrated with Nature*). In addition to this low-impact design, the house minimizes carbon output through the strong use of biomaterials, and a prefabrication construction technique that provides energy and material efficiency through virtualization.

The house's façade, interior, and foundation are composed of timber, bamboo, and plywood. These biomaterials were chosen for their aesthetic quality, allowing the house to blend seamlessly to its surroundings and create a comfortable and warm living space. Biomaterials are low-carbon alternatives to common building materials such as brick and cement (see Figures 7.29 and 7.30). These fast-growing, **renewable materials** are sourced using harvesting and forestry practices that ensure maintenance of these ecosystems to support continued growth, contrasting mineral extraction that is energy intensive and resource depleting. Additionally, the materials chosen are durable and long lasting, yet are biodegradable and can be

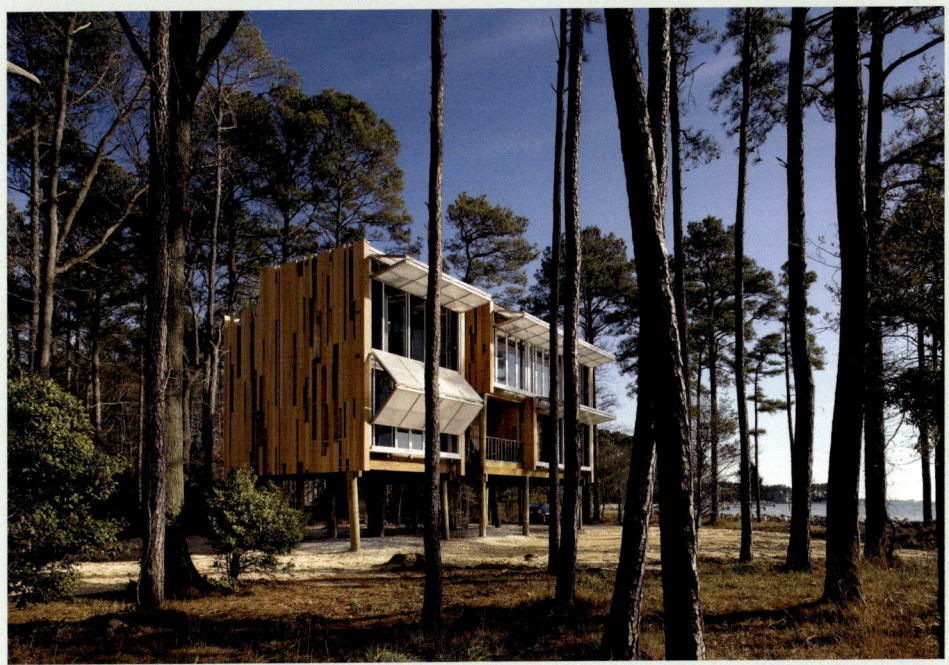

Figure 7.28 The Loblolly House Situated Within Loblolly Trees.

broken down with natural processes at the end-of-use phase (Khitab et al., 2016). The design team further committed themselves to cut carbon emissions, sourcing only materials available within a 500-mile (805-km) radius to cut down on transportation and associated emissions.

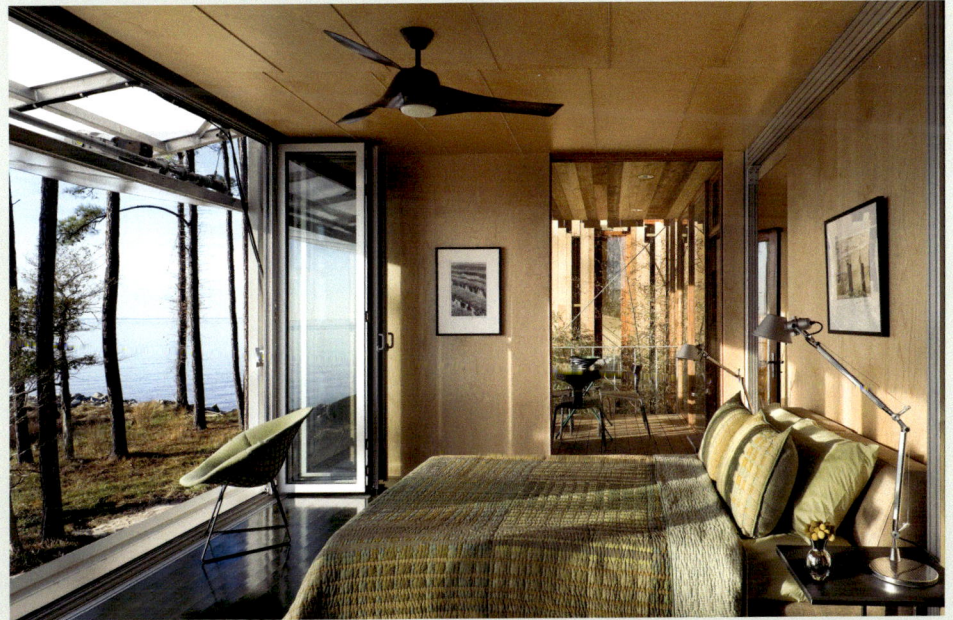

Figure 7.29 Interior View of the Loblolly House.

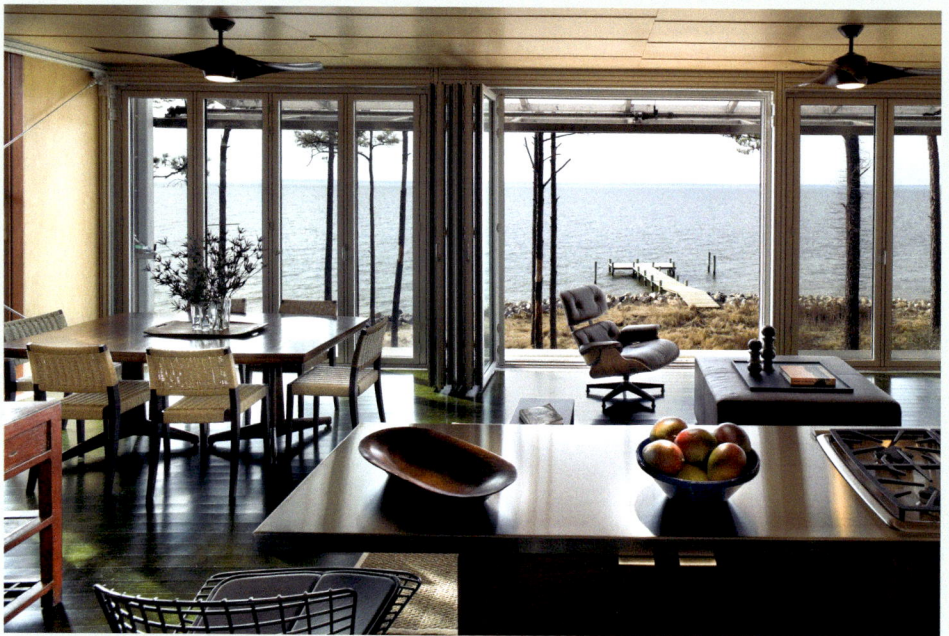

Figure 7.30 Kitchen Interior of the Loblolly House.

Loblolly House featured a ground-breaking use of technology to achieve energy and material-efficient design. A **virtual** model of the site and building was used to design the façade, structure, and interior as an assembly of components that could be prefabricated in a construction facility off-site and simply connected on-site (*Loblolly House: Prefabricated Architecture Integrated with Nature*). Prefabrication allowed the design team to ensure material efficiency, minimizing waste caused by on-site construction practices. The building components were designed so that they could also be easily disassembled and reattached, allowing for complete relocation of the dwelling with minimal impact on the site. This house was also used as a test case in the development, by the architecture firm, of a life cycle analysis (LCA) plugin called Tally® for the Autodesk BIM software Revit (Shapiro, 2016). Using Tally®, the embodied carbon of the project in terms of its component parts can be understood by comparing different construction materials and finishes.

7.9 Conclusion

Construction materials have a significant impact on the environment. Fossil-based materials are currently the leading building material, creating high embodied energy and associated carbon emissions. As the global population rises and demand for housing grows, a shift in material choice must be made to achieve a more sustainable industry. The use of biomaterial offers an innovative solution to the issue of sustainability. Through a series of strategies, tools, and policies, biomaterials can be implemented to create a more efficient – and subsequently more sustainable – building industry. Once efficient building materials are selected, sustainable construction techniques can be employed to promote circular building.

References

Accenture. (2014). *Circular advantage innovative business models and technologies to create value in a world without limits to growth*. https://www.accenture.com/t20150523t053139__w__/us-en/_acnmedia/accenture/conversion-assets/dotcom/documents/global/pdf/strategy_6/accenture-circular-advantage-innovative-business-models-technologies-value-growth.pdf

Albert, H. (2021). *Biomaterials are making the building industry more sustainable*. Labiotech.eu. Retrieved January 24 from https://www.labiotech.eu/in-depth/biomaterials-building-industry-sustainable/

Andersen, J. H., Rasmussen, N. L., & Ryberg, M. W. (2022). Comparative life cycle assessment of cross laminated timber building and concrete building with special focus on biogenic carbon. *Energy and Buildings*, *254*, 111604, https://doi.org/ARTN11160410.1016/j.enbuild.2021.111604

Brandner, R., Flatscher, G., Ringhofer, A., Schickhofer, G., & Thiel, A. (2016). Cross laminated timber (CLT): Overview and development. *European Journal of Wood and Wood Products*, *74*(3), 331–351. https://doi.org/10.1007/s00107-015-0999-5

Brownell, B. E., & Global, I. G. I. (2020). *Examining the environmental impacts of materials and buildings*. IGI Global. https://www.igi-global.com/gateway/book/236583

bsi.knowledge. (2019). *BS EN 197-1:2011: Cement – Composition, specifications, and conformity criteria for common cements*. BSI.

Chen, Z., Feng, Q., Yue, R., Chen, Z., Moselhi, O., Soliman, A., Hammad, A., & An, C. (2022). Construction, renovation, and demolition waste in landfill: A review of waste characteristics, environmental impacts, and mitigation measures. *Environmental Science and Pollution Research International*, *29*(31), 46509–46526. https://doi.org/10.1007/s11356-022-20479-5

Chittenden Solid Waste District. (2012). *Act 148: Universal recycling law*. Retrieved January 24 from https://cswd.net/about-cswd/universal-recycling-law-act-148/

Crook, L. (2020). *The House of Wood, Straw and Cork is an eco-friendly residence in the Italian countryside*. Retrieved January 23, 2023 from https://www.dezeen.com/2020/12/28/house-wood-straw-cork-lca-architetti/

Czigler, T., Reiter, S., Schulze, P., & Somers, K. (2020). *Laying the foundation for zero-carbon cement.* McKinsey & Company. https://www.mckinsey.com/~/media/McKinsey/Industries/Chemicals/Our%20Insights/Laying%20the%20foundation%20for%20zero%20carbon%20cement/Laying-the-foundation-for-zero-carbon-cement-v3.pdf

Ellen MacArthur Foundation. (2019). *The butterfly diagram: Visualising the circular economy.* Retrieved January 24 from https://ellenmacarthurfoundation.org/circular-economy-diagram

Gardner, D., Herbert, D., Jayaprakash, M., Jefferson, A., & Paul, A. (2017). Capillary flow characteristics of an autogenic and autonomic healing agent for self-healing concrete. *Journal of Materials in Civil Engineering*, 29(11), 04017228. https://doi.org/10.1061/(asce)mt.1943-5533.0002092

Goodhew, S. (2016). *Sustainable construction process: A resource text.* John Wiley & Sons. http://swbplus.bsz-bw.de/bsz485065533cov.htm

Hammond, G., & Jones, C. (2008). Inventory of Carbon and Energy (ICE) (Version 1.6a). Sustainable Energy Research Team (SERT), Department of Mechanical Engineering, University of Bath, UK.

Hammond, G., & Jones, C. (2011). Inventory of Carbon and Energy (ICE) (Version 2.0). Sustainable Energy Research Team (SERT), Department of Mechanical Engineering, University of Bath, UK.

Hammond, G., & Jones, C. (2019). Inventory of Carbon and Energy (ICE) (Version 3.0). Sustainable Energy Research Team (SERT), Department of Mechanical Engineering, University of Bath, UK.

Hertwich, E. G., Ali, S., Ciacci, L., Fishman, T., Heeren, N., Masanet, E., Asghari, F. N., Olivetti, E., Pauliuk, S., Tu, Q., & Wolfram, P. (2019). Material efficiency strategies to reducing greenhouse gas emissions associated with buildings, vehicles, and electronics—A review. *Environmental Research Letters*, 14(4), 043004. https://doi.org/10.1088/1748-9326/ab0fe3

Hertwich, E., Lifset, R., Pauliuk, S., & Heeran, N., & United Nations Environment Programme. International Resource, P. (2020). *Resource efficiency and climate change: Material efficiency strategies for a low-carbon future.* United Nations Environment Programme. https://www.unep.org/resources/report/resource-efficiency-and-climate-change-material-efficiency-strategies-low-carbon

Hirshberg, J. (2022). *All About cork – A natural born technology.* Retrieved January 23, 2023 from https://www.greenbuildingsupply.com/Learning-Center/Flooring-Cork-LC/Cork-101

IRP. (2020). *Resource efficiency and climate change: Material efficiency strategies for a low-carbon future.* In E. Hertwich, R. Lifset, S. Pauliuk, & N. Heeren (Eds.), A report of the International Resource Panel. United Nations Environment Programme, Nairobi, Kenya. https://doi.org/10.5281/zenodo.5245528

Keena, N., Duwyn, J., & Dyson, A. (2022). *Biomaterials supporting the transition to a circular built environment in the global South.* Yale Center for Ecosystems + Architecture and UN Environment Programme. https://globalabc.org/index.php/resources/publications/biomaterials-supporting-transition-circular-built-environment-global-south

Keena, N., Raugei, M., Lokko, M.-I, Aly Etman, M., Achnani, V., Reck, B. K., & Dyson, A. (2022). A life-cycle approach to investigate the potential of novel biobased construction materials toward a circular built environment. *Energies*, 15(19), 7239. https://doi.org/10.3390/en15197239

Khitab, A., Anwar, W., Mehmood, I., Khan, M. U. A., Minhaj, S., Kazmi, S., & Munir, M. (2016). Sustainable construction with advanced biomaterials: An overview. *Science International*, *28*, 2351–2356.

KieranTimberlake. (2013). *Loblolly House: Prefabricated architecture integrated with nature*. KieranTimberlake. Retrieved January 23, 2023 from https://kierantimberlake.com/page/loblolly-house

King, S. (2018). *Bruce King PE: A low-carbon concrete building code – Towards a carbon-sequestering built environment*. Retrieved January 24 from https://www.bruce-king.com/building-codes

Knoth, K., Fufa, S. M., & Seilskjær, E. (2022). Barriers, success factors, and perspectives for the reuse of construction products in Norway. *Journal of Cleaner Production*, *337*, 130494. https://doi.org/10.1016/j.jclepro.2022.130494

Lehne, J., & Preston, F. (2018). *Making concrete change: Innovation in low-carbon cement and concrete*. Chatham House. https://www.chathamhouse.org/sites/default/files/publications/research/2018-06-13-making-concrete-change-cement-lehne-preston.pdf

Mackenzie, A. (2014, March 25 2014). Rem Koolhaas: National identity in architecture. *Architecture AU*. https://architectureau.com/articles/national-identity-in-architecture-an-interview-with-rem-koolhaas/

Matos, G. R. (2017). *Use of raw materials in the United States from 1900 through 2014* [Report](2017–3062). (Fact Sheet, Issue. U. S. G. Survey). https://doi.org/10.3133/fs20173062

Matos, G. R. (2022). *Materials flow in the United States—A global context, 1900–2020: U.S. Geological Survey Data Report*. https://doi.org/10.3133/dr1164

Ministry of the Environment. (2000). Construction Material Recycling Law. Japan. https://www.env.go.jp/en/laws/recycle/09.pdf

Minneapolis. (2023). *Minneapolis 2040 Access to Housing: Increase the supply of housing and its diversity of location and types*. Minneapolis City of Lakes. Retrieved June 27 from https://minneapolis2040.com/policies/access-to-housing/

OECD. (2019). *Global material resources outlook to 2060: Economic drivers and environmental consequences*. OECD Publishing. https://doi.org/10.1787/9789264307452-en

Pacheco-Torgal, F., Cabeza, L. F., Labrincha, J., & de Magalhães, A. (2014). 1 – Introduction to the environmental impact of construction and building materials. In *Eco-efficient construction and building materials* (pp. 1–10). Woodhead Publishing. https://doi.org/10.1533/9780857097729.1

Pintos, P. (2020). *The House of Wood, Straw and Cork/LCA Architetti/luca compri architetti*. Retrieved January 23, 2023 from https://www.archdaily.com/952204/the-house-of-wood-straw-and-cork-lca-architetti

Rosenboom, J.-G., Langer, R., & Traverso, G. (2022). Bioplastics for a circular economy. *Nature Reviews. Materials*, *7*(2), 117–137. https://doi.org/10.1038/s41578-021-00407-8

Schuetz, J. (2022). *Minneapolis 2040: The most wonderful plan of the year*. Retrieved January 24 from https://www.brookings.edu/blog/the-avenue/2018/12/12/minneapolis-2040-the-most-wonderful-plan-of-the-year/

Shapiro, G. (2016). *Award: Tally, an app for assessing environmental impact*. Retrieved January 23, 2023 from https://www.architectmagazine.com/awards/r-d-awards/award-tally-an-app-for-assessing-environmental-impact_o

Strain, L. (2017). *Time value of carbon*. https://carbonleadershipforum.org/wp-content/uploads/2017/06/CLF-Time-Value-of-Carbon.pdf

United Nations. (2019). *World urbanization prospects: The 2018 revision* (ST/ESA/SER.A/ 420). https://population.un.org/wup/publications/Files/WUP2018-Report.pdf

United Nations Environment Programme. (2021). *2021 global status report for buildings and construction*: *Towards a Zero-emission, efficient and resilient buildings and construction sector*. Nairobi.

World Bank. (2016). *Housing for all by 2030*. Retrieved June 28 from https://www.worldbank.org/en/news/infographic/2016/05/13/housing-for-all-by-2030

Worrell, E., & Carreon, J. R. (2017). Energy demand for materials in an international context. *Philosophical Transactions: Mathematical, Physical and Engineering Sciences, 375*(2095), 1–13. http://www.jstor.org/stable/44678454

Chapter 8

Construction Practices for Circular Economy and Digitalization

8.1 The Challenge with Existing Construction Methods

As demonstrated in Chapter 6, conventional building practices can no longer support the evolving and dynamic nature of households. As occupants grow, their homes cannot accommodate their changing needs. This inability to adapt to people's changing lifestyles causes inefficiency. Not only are current housing systems unfit for people's needs, but their construction practices are also inefficient in numerous ways. The rigidity of the building industry's linear logic results in the generation of enormous amounts of waste. Waste, within this context, refers to unwanted or undesired materials (Burlinghouse & Ebook Central – Business Ebook Subscription, 2009). Within a single year, an estimated 184.3 million metric tons of building-related construction and demolition debris are generated in the United States. In comparison, the United States creates a total of 268 million metric tons of municipal solid waste per year (US EPA, 2019). Globally, on an annual scale buildings account for 40 percent of primary energy use, use 25 percent of all potable water, and consume 40 percent of the earth's natural resources (IRP, 2017). Hence, any improvement in transportation, water use, energy use, and construction equipment would significantly help reduce a building's life cycle impact. The solution to reducing waste and improving environmental performance is to make use of salvaged, recycled, and local materials, as well as developing a plan for managing construction waste. None of these methods are viable within the current conventional practices.

Moreover, not only are the current practices unsustainable, but they are also expensive. The linear nature of the building industry is inherently costly – materials are constantly obtained and then dismissed (Hebel et al., 2014). When a natural resource is transformed into a product with a limited lifespan, society should ideally make a profit off of its constant reformulation. Thus, there is a growing need for sustainable building practices that are both resource efficient and affordable. While it is generally understood that adaptable housing is necessary, the means by which this is achieved is unclear.

The solution to creating housing fulfils societal needs, as well as reduces waste and cost, is adaptable housing. Adaptability relies on rethinking current building systems, which includes construction methods. In a completely circular building logic, homes would function as material banks. Components could be easily arranged to create a customized and particular home, or completely taken apart to be used for a new project. This could become a reality by rethinking construction, and designing

DOI: 10.4324/9781003333975-11

for disassembly, in which dwellings can be easily broken down into their components, which allows them to be reconfigured or reused at any point in time. Through pre-fabrication and digitalization, homes can become entirely adaptable. These methods can be incorporated into any design and yield benefits in terms of environmental, financial, and social issues.

8.2 Prefabrication: The Fundamentals

Prefabrication is a crucial component of design-for-disassembly and represents a technology that is likely to transform the building industry. Prefabrication generally refers to components being manufactured off-site through automation and trans-ported to the construction site to be assembled (Wang et al., 2018). This method is popular due to its financial, environmental, structural, and time-saving advantages. In terms of construction, prefabrication is favorable as it often occurs in a controlled factory setting, which negates issues related to vandalism, material storage, and weather delays. Additionally, factories require fewer workers and, therefore, offer an economical advantage. Moreover, prefabrication is highly efficient; certain high-tech factories can produce a house in a week, compared to the average five months associated with on-site construction (Friedman, 2021). Thus, prefabrication accel-erates a project's schedule. Finally, waste represents a fundamental advantage of this approach for various reasons. Certain prefabrication methods, such as panel systems, generate far less waste than on-site construction; the assembly of walls in a closed, controlled environment ensures that materials are used efficiently and that scrap pieces of material are easily recovered and reused. Not only does pre-fabrication lower material waste, but this, consequently, results in a lowered cost of clearing and removing debris. While prefabrication refers to the general concept of assembling prefabricated components, within this approach are various techniques, each with particular benefits.

Modular prefabrication represents an advantageous method, particularly for the speed at which dwellings can be erected. It consists of factory-built, nearly complete dwelling sections (Friedman, 2021). This approach enables an entire level of a house to be manufactured, shipped to the site, and positioned on foundations using a crane. Panelized prefabrication represents the most commonly used prefabrication method, as it is similar to traditional on-site building practices. Within this approach, wall panels of varying sizes and stages are produced in a factory. This can be achieved manually or through fully automated methods, and a variety of panel types can be produced, including open-sheathed, structural sandwich, and unsheathed structural panels. Manufactured panels are then stacked in trucks and shipped to the site, where they are assembled to become exterior walls (see Figure 8.1). Interior partition pre-fabrication is also available, giving the option to easily add or remove partitions.

Kit of Parts is another prefabrication system, in which well-marked housing com-ponents, such as studs, floor or roof trusses, doors, windows, stairs, and exterior finishes, are manufactured and delivered to the site where they are assembled and

PANELIZED METHOD

MODULAR METHOD

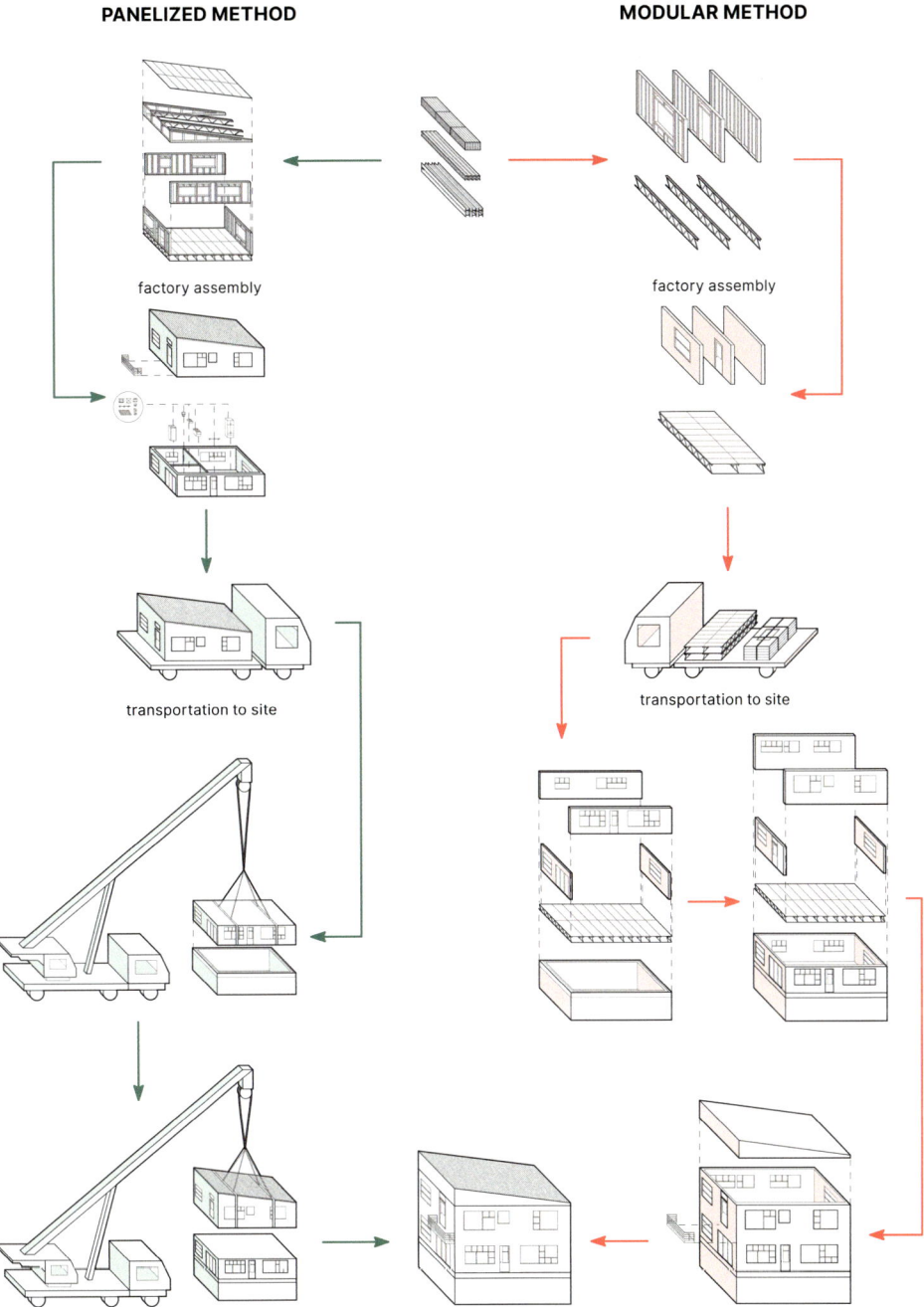

Figure 8.1 Modular and Panelized Prefabrication.

installed to construct a building (see Figure 8.2) (Brütting et al., 2021). The process begins with an architectural consult to understand the program, use, and local requirements. Next, a crate of appropriate kit of parts is prescribed for the particular project. Then, the site is prepared for shipment and assembly. Following the shipment, a team is responsible for assembling and delivering the product. The bias

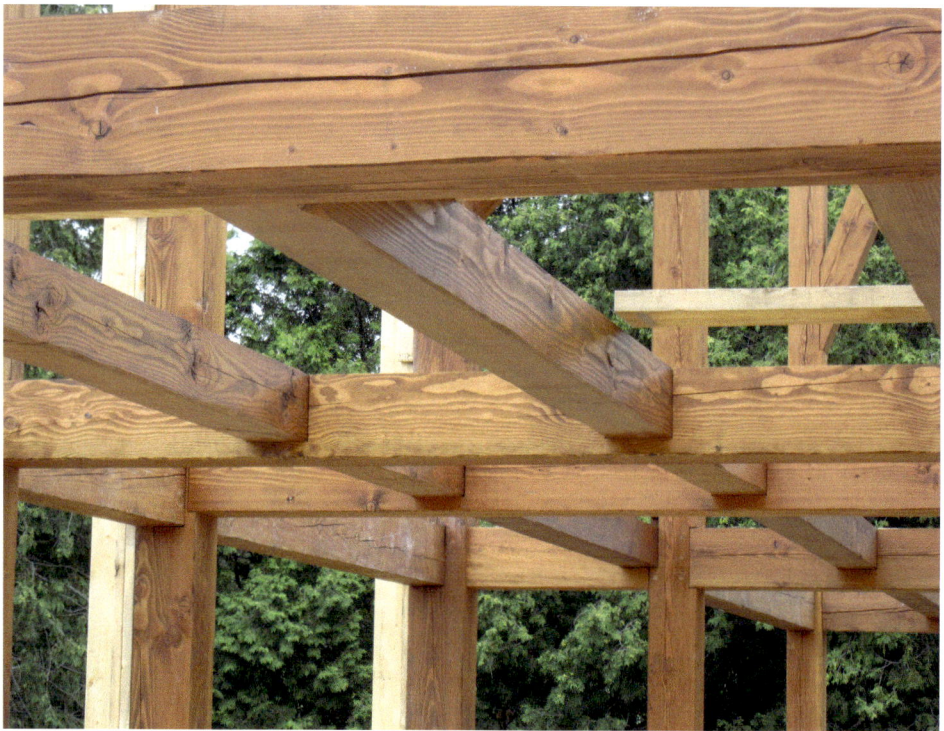

Figure 8.2 Kit of Parts.

that prefabrication inherently entails a lack of customization is defied in Kit of Parts. While elements are prefabricated, they are designed for a specific project and tailored accordingly. Moreover, the variety of assembly options allows for various structural arrangements that can fulfil several purposes, which permits kits to be reused for different projects. This method of prefabrication can be seen in architect Jean Prouve's Maison Tropicale, 1949–1952, a flat-pack house that exemplifies eco-design and mobile design through a Kit of Parts approach. This project is further discussed in Case Study 8A at the end of this chapter.

Among prefabrication systems, panels are among the most used method. Their significant advantage is the quality achieved through its manufacturing process and ease of dismantling (Friedman, 2021). Prefabricated panels are further explored in Case Study 8B of Zufferey House, 2003, by the Swiss-based firm, Nunatak Sàrl Architectes.

8.3 Other Prefabrication Methods

Prefabrication is flexible in that it can create a building type, as well as be applied to various dwelling typologies. The design and structure of prefabricated units and components allow them to be transported or relocated worldwide. While there are often assumptions that modular and transportable units are cheap and uncomfortable, recent technological innovation has created high-tech, aesthetically pleasing structures that are sleek, efficient, and lightweight.

8.3.1 Plug and Play

Plug and Play dwellings consist of products installed by the user and immediately used, without professional help. Products can subsequently be unplugged and removed or repositioned with equal ease (Friedman, 2021). Thus, Plug and Play homes refer to prefabricated modular units, which can be rapidly installed and made ready for immediate homeowner use (see Figure 8.3). By reducing homes to a comprehensive

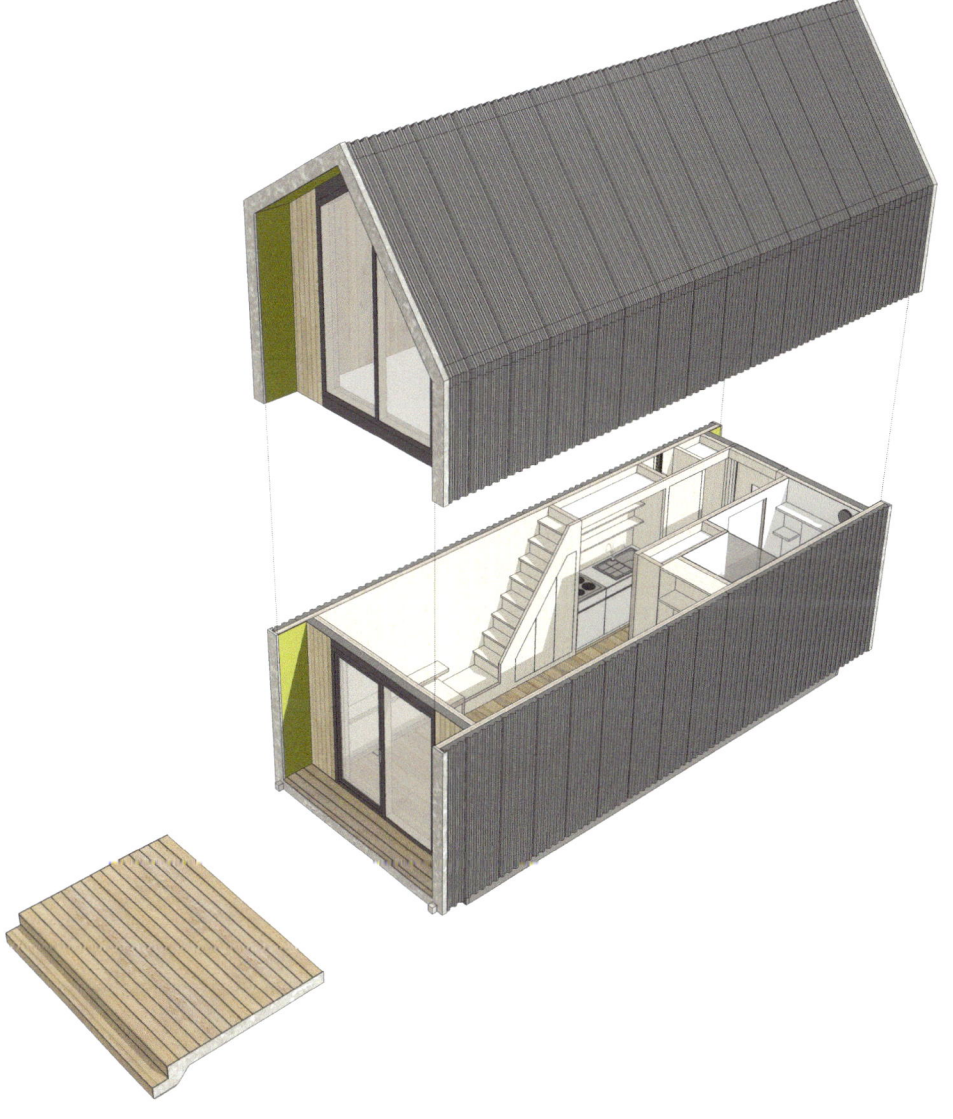

Figure 8.3 Plug and Play.

system of elements meeting at flexible interfaces, pre-assembled chunks can effectively be hoisted in place with a crane and bolted together with little more than a ratchet. The aim of this approach is to achieve heavy units that are capable of sustaining maximum wind drag when erected while remaining light enough as not to exceed the supporting allowance on rooftops. Moreover, these homes are designed to protect external building components. For example, windows are protected by including sliding protective panels in the design. Plug and Play homes embody rapid construction, as joint details are engineered to allow beams, columns, and infill elements to meet at bolted connections (as opposed to welds or adhesives). Due to Plug and Play homes' small size and relatively inexpensive construction, there is the opportunity to use more expensive materials, sophisticated technologies, and customizable features to make them more comfortable and well-suited to modern homeowners' needs. Plug and Play is distinct from typical prefabricated houses because its homes do not require assembly upon delivery – they simply necessitate connecting utilities once on-site. These homes contain convertible rooms, making them receptive to moving panels, folding furniture, and multi-purpose spaces. Plug and Play homes are unique for their ability to balance adaptability and comfort.

8.3.2 Apartment Buildings

Prefabrication is easily employable and highly effective in apartment buildings. Recent developments in the modular industry suggest that mid-rise multi-unit housing represents the primary area of growth for the next decade, in terms of innovation and market (Quale & Smith, 2017). Given the sheer size of buildings, their repetitive nature, and the need for integration into its context, apartments would benefit from prefabrication. While applicable to all sizes, mid-rise apartments, in particular, employ prefabrication methods to achieve both economically and environmentally advantageous homes. While the definition varies, mid-rise apartments are generally understood to be apartments between 4 and 12 stories. Both panelized building and modular prefabricated construction are utilized within this apartment typology. Beyond the general benefits of prefabrication – including precision of factory construction, reduced material waste, and quicker assembly – there are particular advantages within mid-rise apartments. One advantage is that a mid-rise apartment's height range allows it to more easily integrate into existing communities within small- and mid-sized cities. In addition, these apartments have the possibility of offering mixed-density living, suitable for a wide range of living situations and demographics. Design-build firm Onion Flats demonstrates how prefabrication can be adapted to low- and mid-rise housing typologies. In 2012, Onion Flats built Belfield Homes in Philadelphia in the United States. These three row-house units were assembled from wood-frame boxes. Their modular approach quickly expanded into their 147-unit apartment project, Ridge Flats (Quale & Smith, 2017).

Mid-rise apartments are particularly interesting in promoting prefabrication as they disprove the idea that prefabrication lacks variability. Through either aesthetic or structural design choices, variability can be achieved. For example, prefabricated apartments built with modules can be assembled in interestingly stacked forms. Diversity can also be achieved within the apartments. By providing different unit typologies, lifestyle considerations, such as live-work units for those with home businesses, can be attained. Hence, integrating mid-rise apartments into existing neighborhoods can be made smoothly with the use of prefabricated technologies.

8.3.3 Communities Made Up of Prefabricated Houses

Given the challenges in the housing market due to the diversity of homebuyers, there is a growing need for customized dwellings that can satisfy each household's members. Some initiatives have applied the concept of customization to the scale of communities. Through prefabrication methods, an array of customizable dwellings can be produced, paying attention to occupants' socio-economic concerns, as well as environmental changes.

There are multiple forms of mass customization, each offering unique advantages. Pine II represents the most popular and easiest form; it is a customizable approach that allows for the integration of standard products and services. This method is most easily adaptable to conventional housing and is, therefore, less radical. Before delivery, customers are granted customization through selection from a catalog. For example, offering a variety of single-level homes, townhouses, and single-family residences as part of one integrated community. Certain prefabrication companies, such as LivingHomes and PostGreen Homes, have developed interactive, web-based interfaces that allow customers to be involved in the design process. Modifications and changes in costs are available to customers, rendering the whole construction process more accessible. Currently, Pine II approaches generally rely on standardized components, with various assembly options (2 Pine Design, n.d.).

Another form is the mass production of customizable end products, which is favorable in terms of maximizing the advantages associated with standardization. Under this system, a home's design has the flexibility to be customized by buyers even after its purchase through the selection of alternative end products, which are mass-produced to work with a universal plug-in system. Therefore, this approach is adaptable to changes over time. The model of mass customization is restricted to its business model; housing typology, design and production of technology, and marketing strategy dictate the level of customer intervention within the design process (Friedman, 2021). Thus, this method relies on end-products that are mass-produced.

The use of prefabrication enables design to account for specific and dynamic user needs. Applying this method to the scale of a community is significant because it can create a holistic community design. Therefore, while individual needs are accounted for, public and shared connection spaces are also considered. The result is dwelling units that are integrated into the community, producing a socio-ecological system. In an effort to optimize new technologies while satisfying rising demands, mass customization can be applied at both the unit and community scales. Most methods rely on the assumption that products are standardized and mass-produced which goes hand in hand with prefabrication.

8.3.4 *Prefabricated Components*

Finally, prefabricated components that shorten construction time represent another typology. Since these components are assembled in a controlled factory setting, they are protected from harmful weather conditions and tend to have a higher quality of workmanship, compared to site-assembled ones (Knaack et al., 2012). Moreover, the large-scale repetition of standardized building components significantly reduces manufacturing and installation costs. Overall, it is apparent that prefabrication can and should be applied to a variety of typologies; ranging from components to large communities, prefabrication is beneficial at various scales. While new typologies entirely based on prefabrication are compelling, this method does not need to be employed simply for new building types. Prefabrication is beneficial to all forms of construction and effectively makes any home more adaptive.

8.4 Avoiding "Wet Work"

Dry construction is presented as a method that simplifies the construction process, while ensuring safety, quality, and durability. Currently used in North America, Asia, and Europe, this alternative technique is quickly gaining popularity in various parts of the world (Friedman, 2021). Simply put, dry construction dispenses the use of water in all stages, avoiding mixtures and the use of mortar. This is achieved through manufacturing structures in industries and assembling them on-site – the principle of prefabrication. The possibility of assembling a home by clipping sections together, without the use of water, is revolutionary. This technique, therefore, involves lightweight construction of interior walls, ceilings, and floors, by using plastered and microfiber board.

There are different types of dry construction, varying according to the type of material and technique employed. Dry construction generally utilizes panels which can take the form of plaster boards, cementitious slabs, plaster block, EPS panels, or double concrete wall. While this approach appears new, examples of its use are found in ancient architecture, such as the Parthenon. Although the method has evolved over time, the general characteristics persist: the use of local materials, simple construction techniques, and making advanced connections. Some recent cases show typically wet practices being adapted to dry construction. In Thailand, for instance, Habitech International develops site-intensive low-tech packages to construction dry interlocking bricks, which do not require mortar. This system is growing popular as a solution to low-cost housing and has been used in 36 countries around the world (Quale & Smith, 2017). Dry construction is desirable as it is easily removable, as well as cost-efficient. This approach also allows construction to effectively respond to strict legislation on environmental sustainability, energy savings, and earthquake-proofing, all without compromising design. Beyond guaranteeing higher quality, safety, and efficiency, dry construction allows the precision of industrial production to be combined with freehand design. Beam, pillars, uprights, cross-pieces, walls, floors, roofs, and unique works can be repeated at a large scale. Each element can be inspected, replaced, or implemented over time, effectively avoiding raw materials for the production of new components. It also represents an economically advantageous approach as the risk of errors associated with execution is lowered.

8.5 Design-for-Disassembly

While prefabrication and dry construction represent effective tools in achieving sustainable construction, a holistic approach needs to be implemented in the design process to transform the building industry. Design-for-disassembly is the ultimate solution for a circular approach to construction (see Figure 8.4). It aims to make any given product easy to disassemble into all of its individual components (Friedman, 2021). In the case of housing, disassembly refers to the disconnection of individual components, including the wall cladding, non-structural wall panels, flooring, kitchens, and internal finishes (O'Grady et al., 2021). Design-for-disassembly is involved throughout

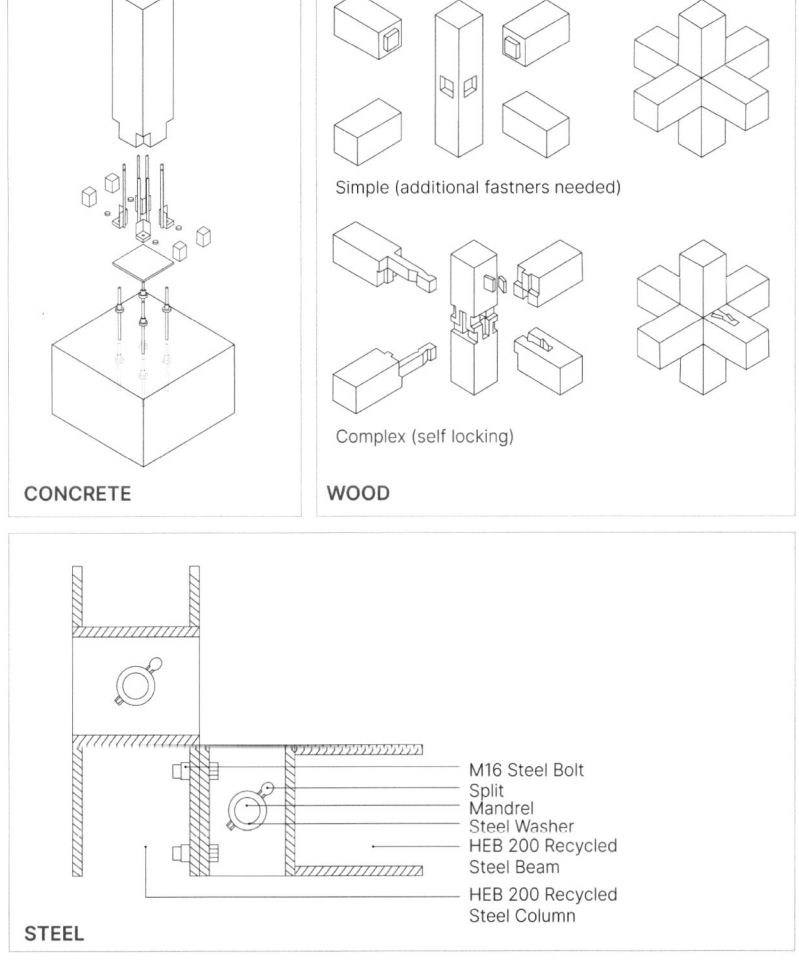

Figure 8.4 Design for Disassembly Detail Examples for Concrete (Mechanical Connection for Pre-Cast Concrete), Wood (Mortise and Tenon Connection), and Steel (Using Mandrel with Two Splits and Stabilizing Washers).

the entirety of the design process as it informs decisions and material choice and affects how components are joined and layered. The outcome of this implementation is construction that is accessible, reversible, and robust. Ultimately, the goal of design-for-disassembly is to eliminate waste with closed loops, by creating enduring and flexible buildings. Much like most prefabricated approaches, this approach offers financial and environmental incentives. If a product is made easier to assemble, then it is simpler and, therefore, less costly to produce. Easily disassembled materials are likely less contaminated, which allows them to conserve their characteristics when recycled (Vezzoli, 2018). Subsequently, this reduces its environmental footprint, as the product is easier to produce, repair, maintain, reuse, and recycle.

While there are various approaches, the key concept is to make the joint between two components reversible without damaging them. This is achieved by making joints visible, dissolvable, similar, and common. Thus, screws, splits, nuts, and bolts are favored over nails and glue. Presently, there are various examples of implementation of design-for-disassembly at various scales. For instance, the Quay Quarter Tower by 3XN Architects demonstrates how circularity principles can be applied to existing buildings at a significant scale. Located in Sydney, the 49-story high-rise building reuses substantial components of the existing structure. Rather than demolishing the original building, much of its core is reused (Nielsen, 2017). Through adopting design-for-disassembly principles, the design incorporates five volumes stacked together with a strong consideration of connection points. Beyond the financial and environmental benefits, this project reveals the social value of this approach, creating social cohesion while maintaining the possibility of reconfiguring space to better fit changing tenant and user needs.

Design-for-disassembly is appealing because it can be applied to any type of product, at any scale, and with any level of complexity. However, despite this, it currently is not being implemented at a large enough scale to promote a ubiquitous circular economy. Design-for-disassembly is key to a circular economy as it allows different components to fit into a close material cycle where they can be reused, reassembled, and recycled. Ultimately, design-for-disassembly has the potential to transform the building industry into a circular process. Once materials can be accessed in the future through disassembly with no loss of quality or value, then everything can be considered a material bank. One study demonstrated that design-for-disassembly in a variety of bio-based material constructions results in at least 10–50 percent decrease in greenhouse gas emissions compared to traditional construction (Keena et al., 2022).

8.6 The Role of Digitalization: BIM and Prefabrication

While prefabrication is fundamental in achieving sustainable construction, in its current state it cannot singlehandedly revolutionize design at a large scale. Digitalization represents the key to supporting prefabrication approaches, such as design-for-disassembly, benefitting all stages of the design process, particularly during the production and tracking of building components (see Figure 8.5).

During the construction and manufacturing stages, digitalization has transformed the production of building components. Fully automated production makes manufacturing

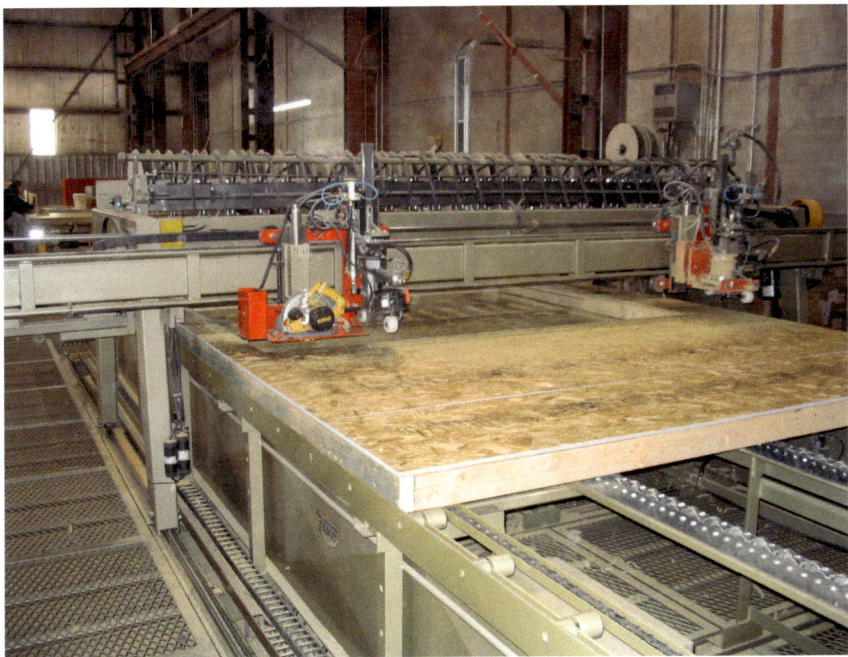

Figure 8.5 Fully Automated Panelized Prefabrication Process.

less expensive, and of higher quality. Various forms of automated manufacturing have emerged and have effectively renewed designers' interest in factory-built housing. For instance, panels can be produced using robotic arms for all aspects of fabrication, including cutting, nailing, and installing insulation. Another digitized production is 3D printing: the production of physical objects layer-by-layer, using automated computer-controlled machines (Merrild et al., 2016). CAD technologies are beginning to be employed during the production of physical models and prototypes. Through routing and milling, computer-aided manufacturing (CAM) and computer numerical control (CNC) milling both facilitate accurate and automatic translations of computer-generated design into built structures. These technologies shorten output times by effectively enabling the export of shop drawings and files for rapid prototyping machines (Dunn & ProQuest, 2012). This digitalized process is effective and precise in construction. Built in 2007, the Dragonfly in Los Angeles utilized CNC milling machines to inscribe and cut sheets. The sheets were then embedded into bands of assembly data for installation structure, including bending angles and cell position. This approach allowed the Dragonfly to be a bottom-up process, which did not require any conventional documentation. Thus, centralized materials, processes, and tools allow an increased speed and quality of production.

Digitalization has also transformed the life cycle of building components through innovative technology that can track materials throughout their use. Building information modeling (BIM) software allows three-dimensional design while promoting collaboration. BIM integrates and manages information during a building's entire life cycle and effectively allows for efficient coordination among stakeholders (Abdolmaleki et al., 2020).

BIM has the ability to visualize and track various components in three dimensions, rendering it uniquely capable of merging with factory production. One model has the ability to help extract material volumes, produce shop drawings for component fabrication, and test assembly scenarios. BIM can generate identification systems, allowing the direct transfer of coded information during fabrication, through barcodes or radio-frequency identification. This is widely beneficial to both assembly and disassembly. Hence, BIM allows a multiplicity of information to be gathered on a digital building model; from there, building material information can be extracted and integrated into detailed waste estimation and planning. As discussed in Chapter 4, the ability to track components use is fundamental to reusing and achieving circular construction. The prospect of creating digital twins for buildings and their subcomponents is revolutionary as it allows for greater planning, recovery, and managing, all in an effort to reduce waste.

Moreover, technologies such as BIM also render construction more accessible. User-friendly virtual interfaces for three-dimensional modelling programs allow users to custom design their homes and simulate walkthroughs before construction commences. Certain prefabrication companies, such as LivingHomes and PostGreen Homes, have developed interactive, web-based interfaces that engage customers in the design of their homes through a sequence of decision-making processes leading to customization (Friedman, 2021). This increases accessibility and allows customers to be involved in the design and choice of interior components, according to their own space needs and budget. These technological innovations represent breakthroughs for prefabrication and digitalization, as they simplify the manufacturing process, all the while expanding its possibilities. Digitalization optimizes prefabrication by reducing waste, through innovative fabrication and involvement of customers in the design and production stages. Innovative construction methods and digitalization converge to make building an accessible and efficient process. For instance, WikiHouse is an open-source construction system that was developed in 2014 (Granello et al., 2022). Freely downloadable, the system provides CNC machine-cut wood panels to build structures. Given that the designs use wedge and peg connections, users can simply download a kit of parts and assemble their homes without the need of any traditional construction skills or tools.

Overall, digitalization can effectively support prefabrication methods in achieving sustainable buildings. BIM, in particular, is key in construction as it enables computer-based reviews of the design and reduces construction waste generation by decreasing physical design changes (Merrild et al., 2016). BIM is essential in aiding platforms to enhance resource management and minimize human errors for on-site construction. The future of prefabrication and rapid construction relies on BIM software. One thing to consider, however, is that rehearsing assembly with digital tools yields unattainable precision. Moreover, miscalculations or material failures occurring in the factory can significantly disturb on-site processes. Therefore, error needs to be accounted for and construction planned accordingly.

Many studies show that using prefabrication and BIM can effectively reduce the amount of waste generated during construction, renovation and demolition activities (Merrild et al., 2016). Ultimately, BIM is critical to circular construction as it eases collaboration and efficiency in the recycling phase of a project. This is made even simpler when materials are prefabricated and easily separated.

8A

Project:
Maison Tropicale

Locations:
Niamey, Niger and Brazzaville,
Republic of Congo, Africa

Year:
1949

Team:
Jean Prouvé Workshops

**Mapping to Circular
Economy Framework:**

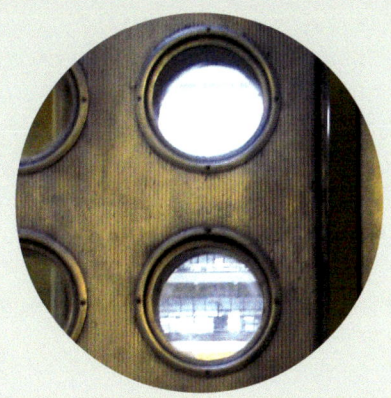

CIRCULAR ECONOMY PRACTICES

LIFE CYCLE PHASES

Recovery · Life Extension · Sharing Platforms · Service Models · Regenerate · Virtualize

Work of Geobiosphere

Sourcing

Manufacturing

Design & Construction

Use

End-of-Use

LAYERS + LIFESPAN
Structural Layers | Long Life
Skin, MEP Layers | Medium Life
Interior Layers | Short Life

Site 100+yr   Structure 50+yr
Exterior 25+yr   System 15+yr
Partition 10+yr   Stuff 1+yr

Maison Tropicale is a prototypical housing unit designed by French Architect and steel-worker Jean Prouvé in the mid-20th century (Figure 8.6). The units featured a large footprint with an aluminum façade lifted on concrete stilts (see Figure 8.6). This prototype, with a dark past of serving as housing for French colonialists working in several African colonies, is an early example of prefabrication in architectural design thinking (Etherington, 2008). Maison Tropicale was designed before digitalization occurred within the construction industry, through a lengthy and repetitive experimentation process with steel and aluminum components (see Figure 8.7) was first commissioned to deploy the dwelling in 1949 to provide housing for a French school director in Niamey, Niger. This pre-digitalization house was built through the development of a kit-of-parts that was lightweight and flat-packable to facilitate shipping to Niger via cargo plane, allowing for a minimal fabrication process by local labor. Two smaller units were designed for and shipped to Brazzaville, Congo, in the following years. The innovative application of prefabrication in Maison Tropicale resulted in a climate-responsive design and paved the way for efficient construction practices now facilitated by advancements in technology.

Jean Prouvé's plan, although designed and manufactured in France, was well suited for the tropical climates of Niger and Republic of Congo. Setting the house on concrete

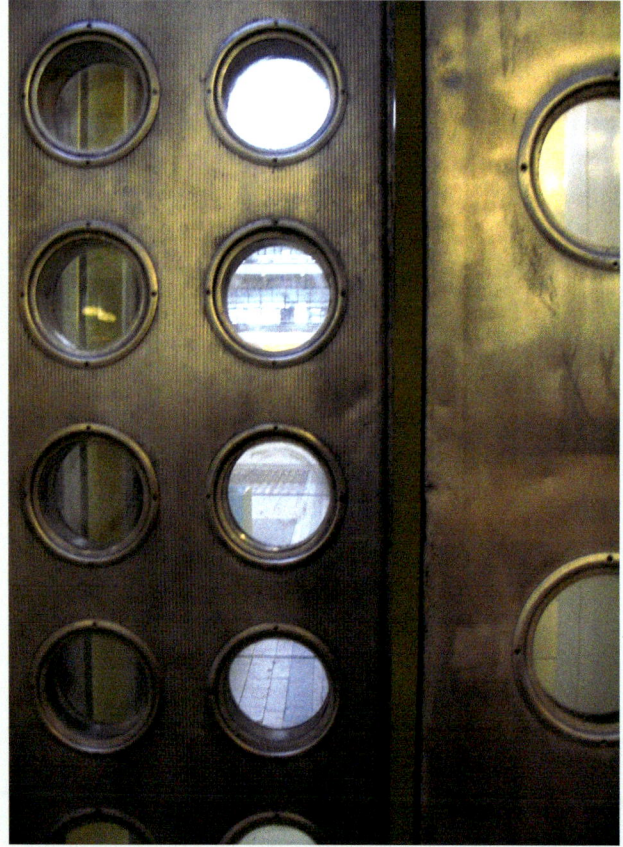

Figure 8.6 Materials Used in Maison Tropicale.

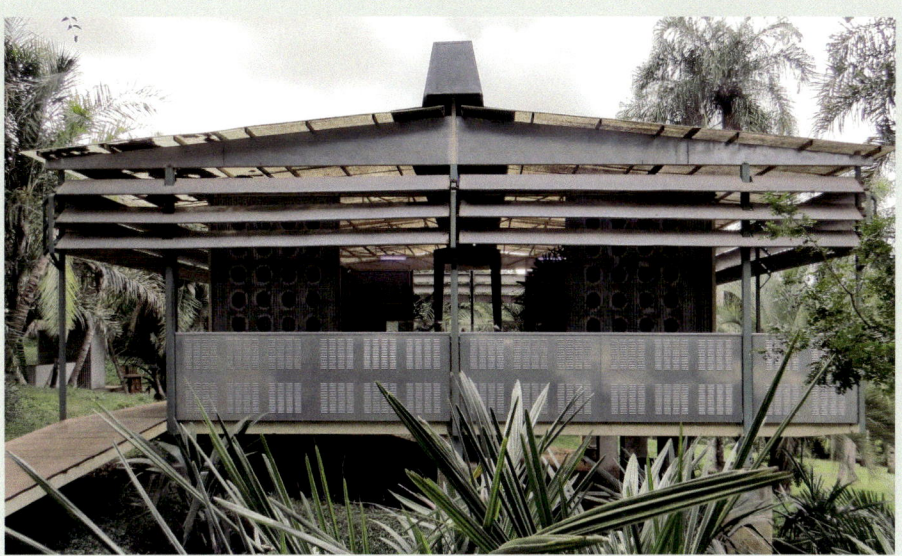

Figure 8.7 Façade of Maison Tropicale.

stilts allowed for a potentially sloping site, while encouraging natural ventilation, important in hot humid climates (Nelson, 2011). Natural ventilation is also achieved passively through a double-roof structure design. Heat on the roof draws fresh, cool air through openings in the walls and up toward the ceiling, creating constant airflow to decrease heat and humidity (see Figure 8.8; Etherington, 2008). A folded sheet steel frame held an aluminum panel façade, some fixed and some sliding to provide flexible opening and create a comfortable living space year-round. To provide insulation at a minimal weight to facilitate shipping, the panels were filled with crumpled aluminum insulation. The homes included wrapping verandas with an aluminum shading system; these outer panels provide a reflective skin to reduce heat gains and feature adjust-able-angle louvres. The home's iconic porthole windows are covered by a blue glass to minimize UV ray infiltration (Etherington, 2008). With his design, Prouvé illustrated that a site-sensitive design can be achieved through off-site construction techniques, improving a building's **lifespan** while achieving material and energy efficiency.

A kit-of-parts is designed to be shipped as a package and assembled on-site. These components were designed at widths under 4 m, which was the width of Prouvé's factory's rolling machine (Nelson, 2011). They were designed to be as flat as possible to be neatly packed into a cargo plane which would deliver them to the sites in Africa (*Maison Tropicale for Design Museum at Tate Modern*, 2008). Lightweight materials were chosen for shipping purposes, and so that they could be handled and assembled by two local construction workers. The parts were shipped to site and the houses were assembled in approximately two weeks, without heavy machinery. The construction techniques utilized can be considered an early version of the circular economy framework sharing platform, as they minimize material and energy waste through highly efficient and calculated design and manufacturing. Unfortunately, the project never really scaled up as planned and the home was instead exhibited in Paris as a pioneering attempt at prefabrication in architectural design (Figure 8.9).

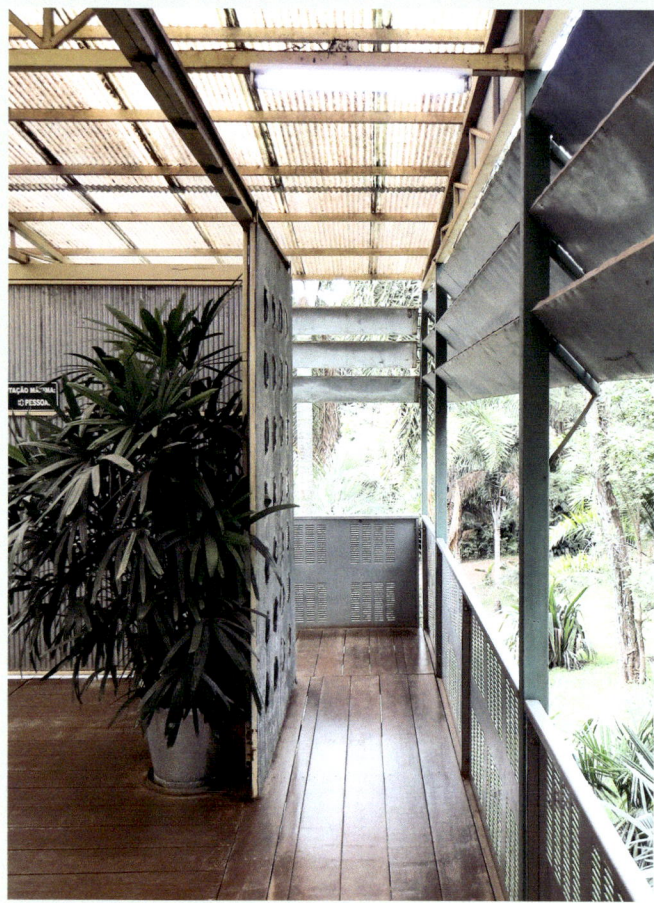

Figure 8.8 Interior of the Maison Tropicale.

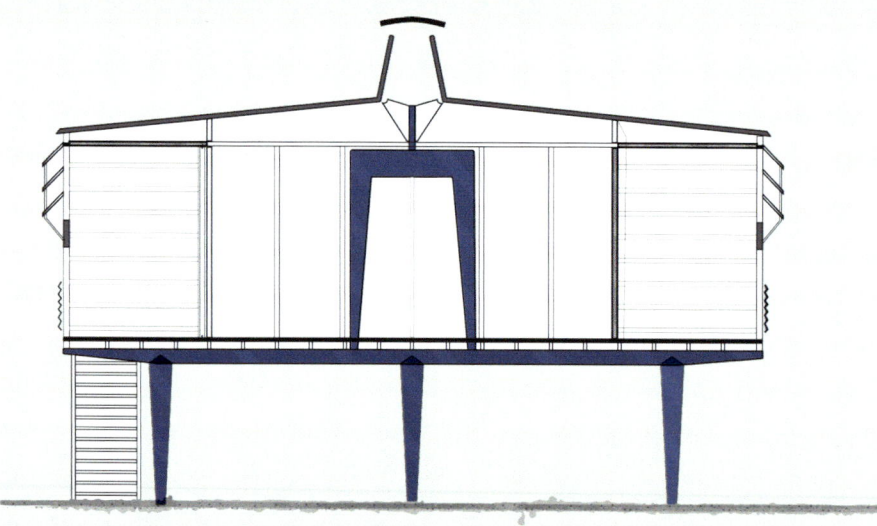

Figure 8.9 Cross Section of Maison Tropical.

8B

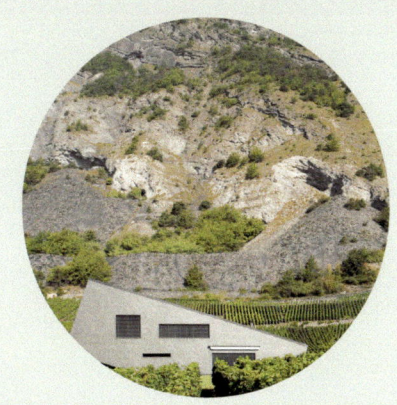

Project:
Zufferey House

Location:
Willis, Switzerland

Year:
2003

Team:
Nunatak Sàrl Architectes

**Mapping to Circular
Economy Framework:**

CIRCULAR ECONOMY PRACTICES

LIFE CYCLE PHASES

Recovery Life Extension Sharing Platforms Service Models Regenerate Virtualize

Work of Geobiosphere

Sourcing

Manufacturing

Design & Construction

Use

End-of-Use

LAYERS + LIFESPAN
Structural Layers | Long Life
Skin, MEP Layers | Medium Life
Interior Layers | Short Life

Site 100+yr Structure 50+yr
Exterior 25+yr System 15+yr
Partition 10+yr Stuff 1+yr

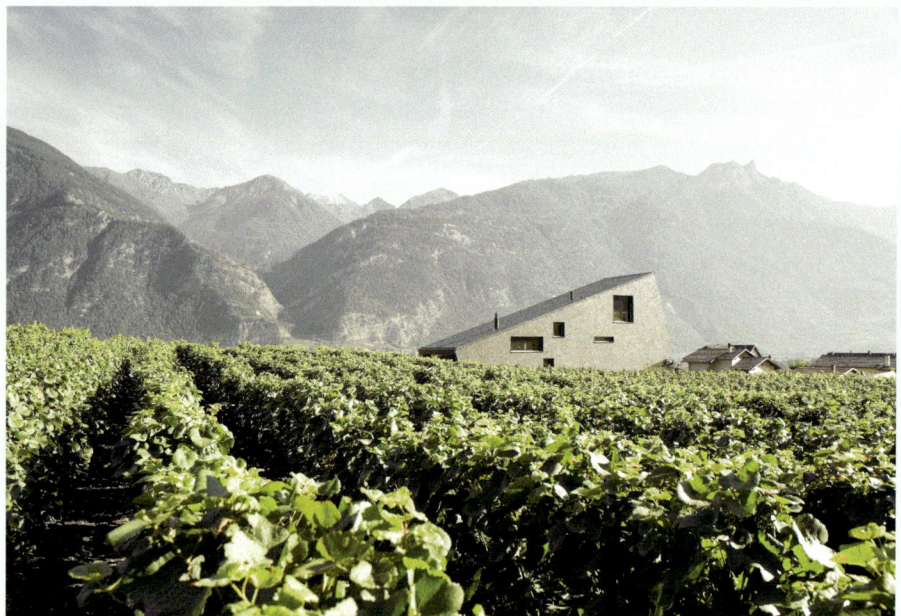

Figure 8.10 The House Appears as a Rock in the Landscape.

The Zufferey house, set against the rocky formations of the L'Ardévaz mountains in Willis, Switzerland (see Figure 8.10), sits as if teetering off-balance as both a complement and contrast to its environment. The uniquely tilted structure of the home earned the nickname "Angle" (Figure 8.11). The house mimics the slope of

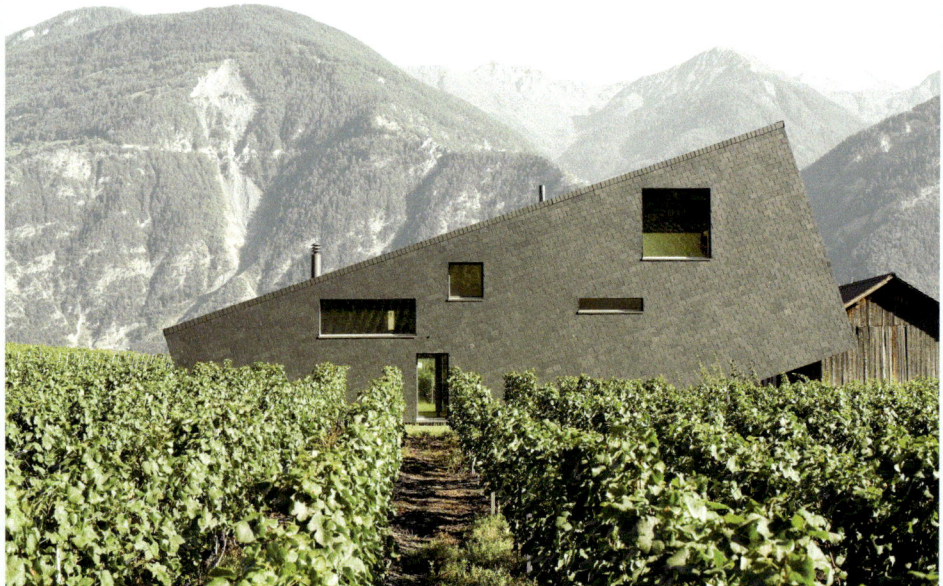

Figure 8.11 North Elevation of the Zufferey House.

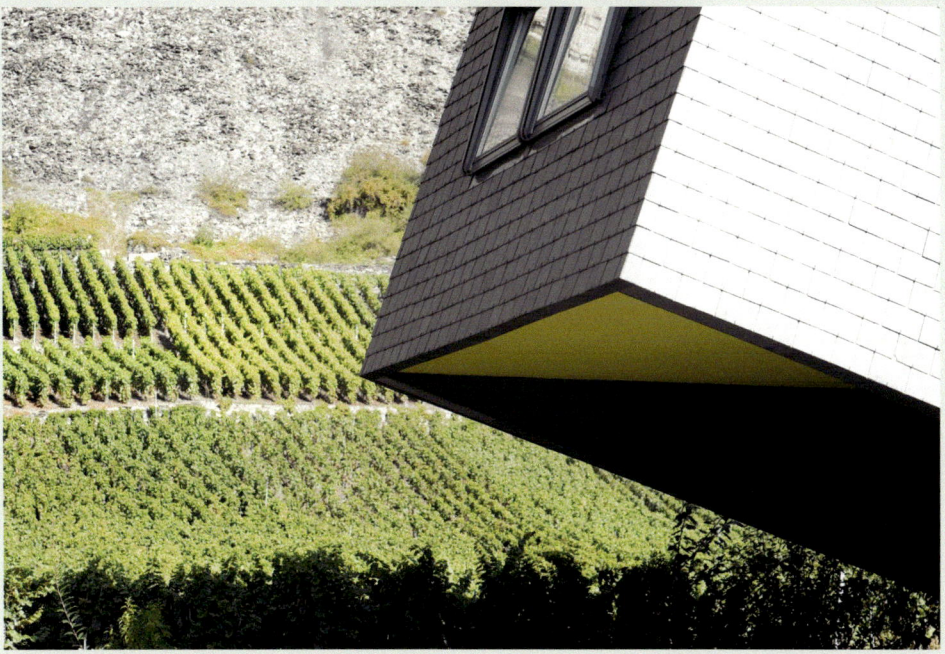

Figure 8.12 Detail of Cantilever and Grey Slate Cladding Which Mirrors from the Surrounding Mountainous Landscape.

nearby mountains in its cladding, with natural gray slate to fit into its natural sur-roundings (see Figure 8.12). The fully expressive architecture provides a comfort-able home, with 185 m^2 (1,990 sq. ft.) of floor area containing bedrooms and living areas on two levels (see Figure 8.13–8.15). Nunatak Sàrl Architectes incorporated eco-friendly building techniques such as the use of a prefabricated wood structural frame, passive heating techniques, and a connection to the building's surroundings. This project demonstrates that circular principles such as sharing platforms, prod-uct life extension, and regeneration can be achieved while creating unique forms and strong architectural expression.

The house features a playful combination of concrete slab flooring, wooden ceilings and trim, and spanning glass windows. The minimally decorated finishings employed in the house let these bare materials shine. The interior walls are covered by inex-pensive painted wood particle panels, and wood constitutes the building's structure. In an effort to decrease costs, Nunatak opted for a panelized prefabrication technique to make up the wood-frame structure (Saieh, 2009). Wall sections were manufactured and assembled as panels in a factory setting, then shipped to the hilly site for instal-lation. This prefabrication process is an example of the circular economy business model of **sharing platforms**, which uses shared materials and space as a resource. Because prefabrication occurs in a specialized factory, equipment and materials can be used more efficiently and be shared by multiple projects. In conventional, on-site construction, high quantities of material are wasted because of a higher degree of inaccuracy of measurements, and these wasted materials have no means of being used in other projects. A prefabrication facility uses **virtualized** models and drawings to maximize the use of materials, thus decreasing costs.

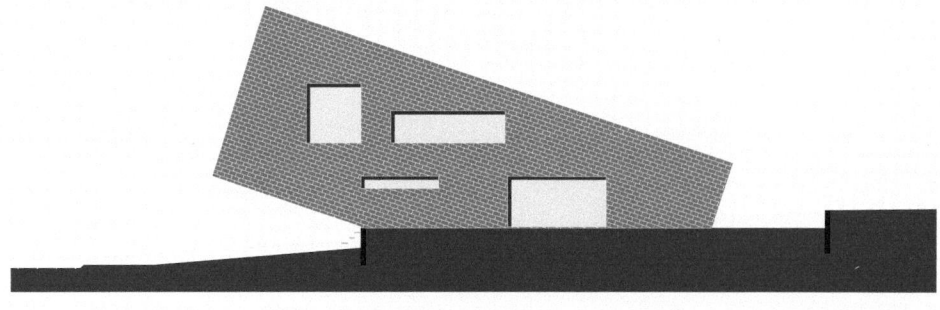

South Elevation

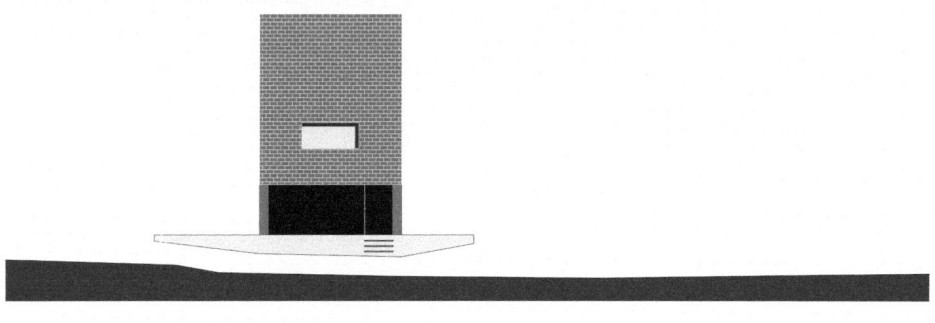

West Elevation

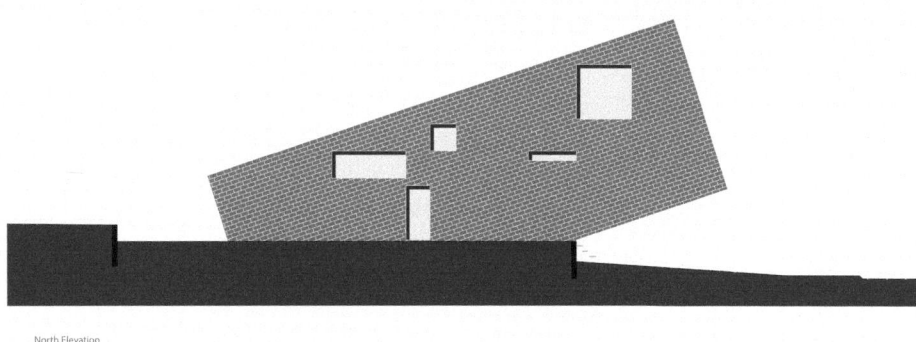

North Elevation

Figure 8.13 Elevations.

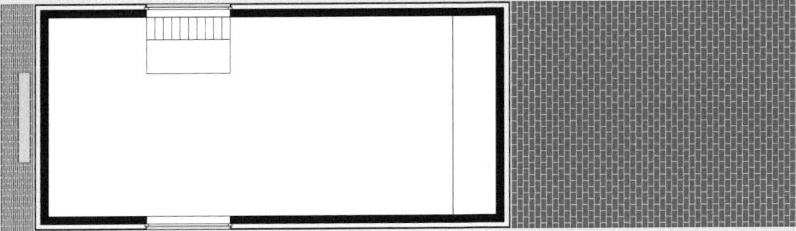

Second Floor

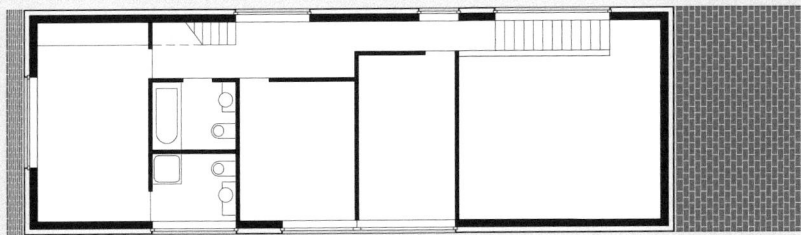

First Floor

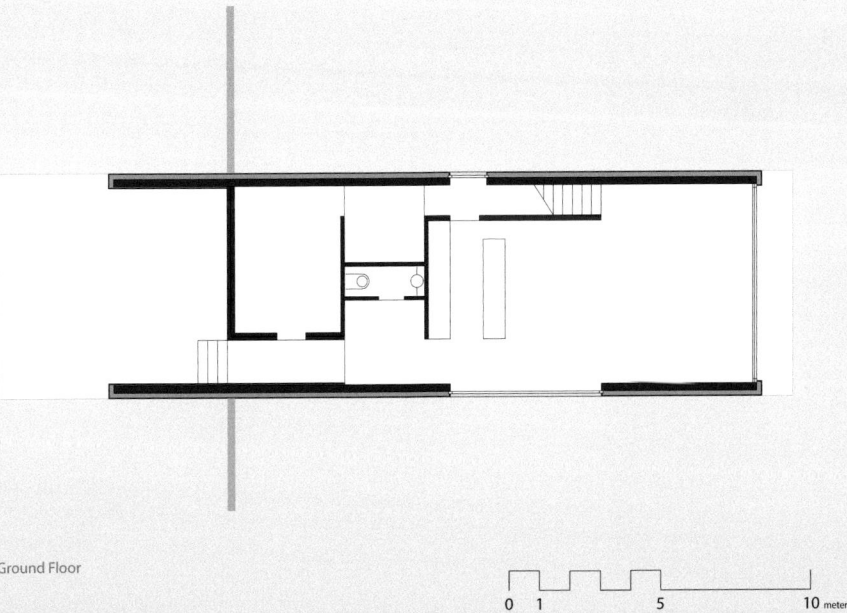

Ground Floor

0 1   5   10 meters

Figure 8.14 Floor Plans.

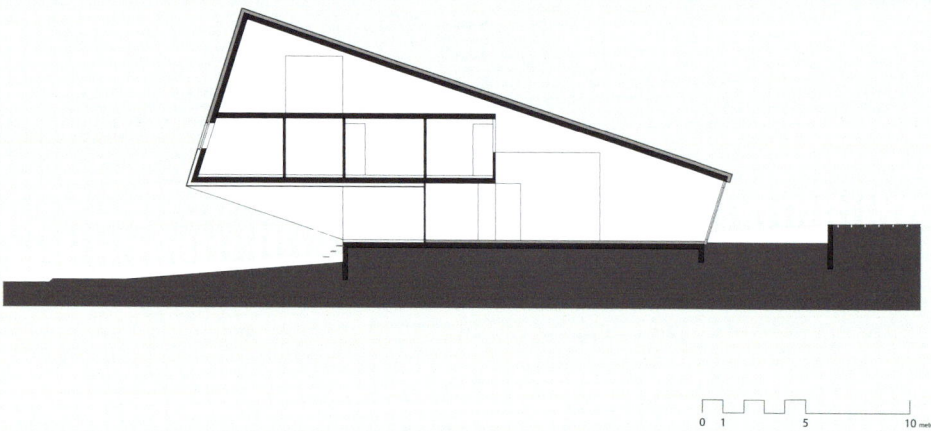

0 1   5   10 meters

Figure 8.15 Longitudinal Section of the Zufferey House.

The home, though striking and unusual, employs an air of sensitivity to its surroundings. Passive design techniques are incorporated with the design's form and envelope to adapt the home to its local climate and reduce reliance on the energy grid. Strategically placed window openings protect the building's occupants from excessive summer heat as well as wind coming from the western valley. The dwelling's tilted form also provides an overhang to shade and protects outdoor space at the entrance, creating additional living space even more immersed in nature (Chino, 2009; see Figure 8.16). These passive solar techniques, inherent to the building's

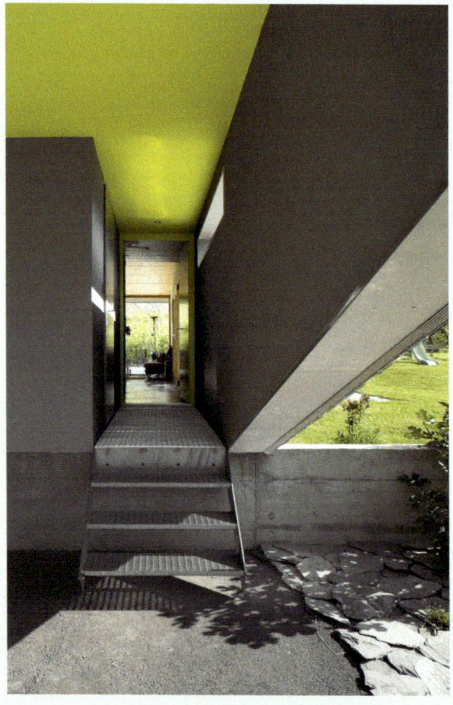

Figure 8.16 View of Covered Entrance Way.

form, are long-lasting and reliant when compared to a reliance on active cooling and lighting techniques. A common understanding of prefabrication techniques views them as short-lived, but when designed with attention to local climate, prefabrication can provide **longevity** and architectural appeal. Additionally, the use of natural slate as a cladding material, inspired by the landscape, provides a durable and resilient envelope made to last. Often, sourcing construction materials seen in a site's natural surroundings can be a great tool to find materials suited for its specific climate (see Figure 8.17). The use of wood as the primary material of the build promotes circular **regeneration**, as the biomaterial works to sequester carbon from the atmosphere for its lifetime. Wood buildings, at a large scale, can eliminate excess carbon dioxide from the atmosphere that results in global warming (Figures 8.16 and 8.17).

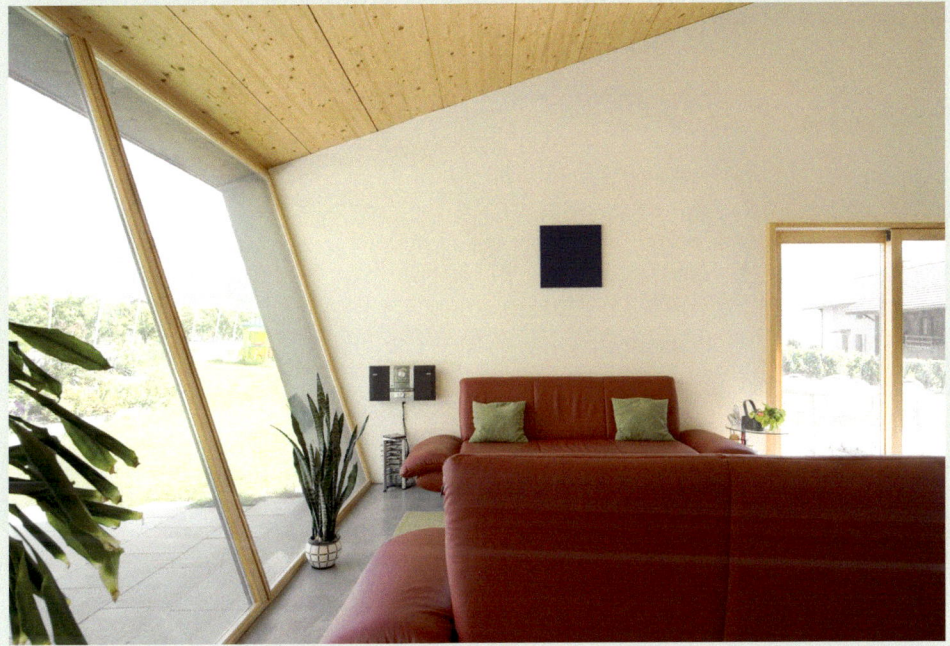

Figure 8.17 Interior View with Angled Window Which Frames the View of the Surrounding Landscape.

8.7 Conclusion

As current construction stands, occupants' dynamic and diverse needs are not satisfied. The adaptable housing concept is needed to bridge this gap and is achievable through flexible methods. A home is most adaptable if it can be designed to be easily reconfigured and taken apart. This is achieved through design-for-disassembly. In order for design-for-disassembly to be implemented, digitalization and prefabrication work must optimize planning, manufacturing, assembly, and disassembly. As observed through the various typologies, approaches, and examples, the principle of designing for disassembly can be applied to most situations. To reduce waste and achieve a circular economy, the building industry and its construction methods need to be reconfigured.

References

2 Pine Design. (n.d.). *About*. Retrieved January 25 from https://2pine.com/about

Abdolmaleki, G., Ghodrati, N., Babaeian Jelodar, M., & Naismith, N. (2020). *Improvement of off-site construction performance in construction waste reduction using building information modelling*. In Proceedings of the 6th New Zealand Built Environment Research Symposium (NZBERS 2020). Massey University, Auckland, New Zealand.

Brütting, J., Senatore, G., & Fivet, C. (2021). Design and fabrication of a reusable kit of parts for diverse structures. *Automation in Construction*, *125*, 103614. https://doi.org/10.1016/j.autcon.2021.103614

Burlinghouse, G. N., & Ebook Central – Business Ebook Subscription. (2009). *Green affordable housing*. Nova Science Publishers. https://catalogue.solent.ac.uk/openurl/44SSU_INST/44SSU_INST:VU1?u.ignore_date_coverage=true&rft.mms_id=9997176961104796

Chino, M. (2009). *Zufferey House by Nunatek Sarl Architectes*. Retrieved January 23, 2023 from https://inhabitat.com/prefab-home-inspired-by-rock-formation/prefabrock_7/

Dunn, N., & ProQuest. (2012). *Digital fabrication in architecture* (1st ed.). Laurence King Publishing. http://ebookcentral.proquest.com/lib/abdn/detail.action?docID=1876132

Etherington, R. (2008). *Jean Prouvé's Maison Tropicale in London*. Retrieved January 23, 2023 from https://www.dezeen.com/2008/01/28/jean-prouves-maison-tropicale-in-london/

Friedman, A. (2021). *Pre-fab living*. Thames and Hudson.

Granello, G., Reynolds, T., & Prest, C. (2022). Structural performance of composite WikiHouse beams from CNC-cut timber panels. *Engineering Structures*, *252*. https://doi.org/10.1016/j.engstruct.2021.113639

Hebel, D., Wisniewska, M. H., Heisel, F., & VleBooks. (2014). *Building from waste: Recovered materials in architecture and construction*. VLeBooks. https://www.semanticscholar.org/paper/Building-from-Waste%3A-Recovered-Materials-in-and-Hebel-Wisniewska/c49239bd9b89cac489b4bce5e5a414bb9b6c6e38

IRP. (2017). *Assessing global resource use: A systems approach to resource efficiency and pollution reduction*. In S. Bringezu, A. Ramaswami, H. Schandl, M. O'Brien, R. Pelton, J. Acquatella, E. Ayuk, A. Chiu, R. Flanegin, J. Fry, S. Giljum, S. Hashimoto, S. Hellweg, K. Hosking, Y. Hu, M. Lenzen, M. Lieber, S. Lutter, A. Miatto, ... R. Zivy. A Report of the International Resource Panel. United Nations Environment Programme. Nairobi, Kenya

Keena, N., Raugei, M., Lokko, M.-I, Aly Etman, M., Achnani, V., Reck, B. K., & Dyson, A. (2022). A life-cycle approach to investigate the potential of novel biobased construction materials toward a circular built environment. *Energies*, *15*(19), 7239. https://doi.org/10.3390/en15197239

Knaack, U., Chung-Klatte, S., Hasselbach, R., & DeGruyter. (2012). *Prefabricated systems: Principles of construction*. In *Principles of construction* (Version 1st ed., 2011). Birkhäuser. http://catalogue.londonmet.ac.uk/record=b2255620~S1

Maison Tropicale for Design Museum at Tate Modern. (2008). Retrieved January 23, 2023 from https://www.tate.org.uk/whats-on/tate-modern/maison-tropicale-design-museum-tate-modern

Merrild, H., Jensen, K. G., & Sommer, J. (2016). *Building a circular future*. GXN. http://issuu.com/3xnarchitects/docs/buildingacircularfuture/283?e=5740644/35968611

Nelson, M. I. (2011). *Re-imagining the Maison Tropicale: A 21st century prefabricated building system inspired by Jean Prouvé* [Massachusetts Institute of Technology].

Nielsen, K. H. (2017). Humanizing the high-rise. *CTBUH Journal*, *4*, 50–52. https://www.jstor.org/stable/90020911

O'Grady, T., Minunno, R., Chong, H.-Y., & Morrison, G. M. (2021). Design for disassembly, deconstruction and resilience: A circular economy index for the built environment. *Resources, Conservation and Recycling*, *175*, 105847. https://doi.org/10.1016/j.resconrec.2021.105847

Quale, J. D., Smith, R. E., & Bloomsbury. (2017). *Offsite architecture: Constructing the future*. Routledge. https://catalogue.solent.ac.uk/openurl/44SSU_INST/44SSU_INST:VU1?u.ignore_date_coverage=true&rft.mms_id=9997034747004796

Saieh, N. (2009). *Zufferey House/Nunatak Sàrl Architectes*. Retrieved January 23, 2023 from https://www.archdaily.com/28262/zufferey-house-nunatak-sarl-architectes/

US EPA. (2019). *Advanced sustainable material management 2017 fact sheet*. United States Environmental Protection Agency. https://www.epa.gov/sites/production/files/2019-11/documents/2017_facts_and_figures_fact_sheet_final.pdf

Vezzoli, C. (2018). *Design for environmental sustainability: Life cycle design of products* (2nd ed.). Springer. https://doi.org/10.1007/978-1-4471-7364-9

Wang, Y., Zhu, Y., Shen Geoffrey, Q. P., & Al-Hussein, M. (2018). *ICCREM 2018 sustainable construction and prefabrication*. American Society of Civil Engineers American Society of Civil Engineers. https://doi.org/doi:10.1061/9780784481738

Chapter 9

Clean Operational Energy

9.1 Introduction: Resource Efficacy and Climate Change

Greenhouse gas emissions from the building sector can come from multiple streams. The quantity of materials and resources used to make and operate the building throughout its life, the choice of materials used, where materials come from, and how they are made, all determine the level of greenhouse gas emissions from a building, and, thus, the amount of operational energy required to run a building (Keena et al., 2022). As of 2019, the operational energy use of buildings is responsible for 28 percent of the total global energy-related carbon dioxide emissions, its highest level yet, 17 percent of which comes from residential buildings (directly and indirectly) (United Nations Environment Programme & Global Alliance for Buildings and Construction, 2020). As the global population continues to grow and the rate of urbanization rises, low-carbon-emitting buildings become ever more essential. The World Bank estimates that about 300 million houses must be built to accommodate this growth by 2030 (The World Bank, 2016). Keena et al. (2022) argue that a bio-based economy that does away with linear extraction methods and non-renewable resources is a suitable pathway to a circular built environment.

Material and energy flow necessary for running a building, known as operational energy, is typically narrowly accounted for in the initial stages of architectural conceptual design, yet it has a huge impact on the levels of greenhouse gas and carbon emissions a building will produce throughout its lifetime. According to Lechner (2015), of the 48 percent of energy consumed by a building, 40 percent comes from its operation, and only 8 percent from construction (see Figure 9.1). Taking a life cycle perspective, in which the environmental impact of a building is assessed not at its inception or potential but throughout its useful life, how efficient and clean its energy sources are to run the building has an enormous impact on its operational carbon and greenhouse gas emissions. As Lechner (2015) writes, while renewable energy is an effective way to foster sustainable construction, the most effective, accessible, and least expensive way to reduce the embodied carbon emissions of a building throughout its life cycle is by reducing its operational energy. This chapter outlines two broad strategies for architects to lower operational energy emissions when designing and constructing a building. First and most impactful is the design of the building itself – this infers a climate-responsive approach in which the materials, design, and energy systems of a building are appropriate to its surrounding environment to achieve natural thermal comfort. Second, when a building does have to rely on energy sources to provide electricity, renewable energy sources must be prioritized. However, the nuances of this, and how energy efficacy should be accurately measured in a building, will be discussed. This leads to a discussion on energy rating systems, which sets targets for

DOI: 10.4324/9781003333975-12

FINAL ENERGY (EJ) BY USE

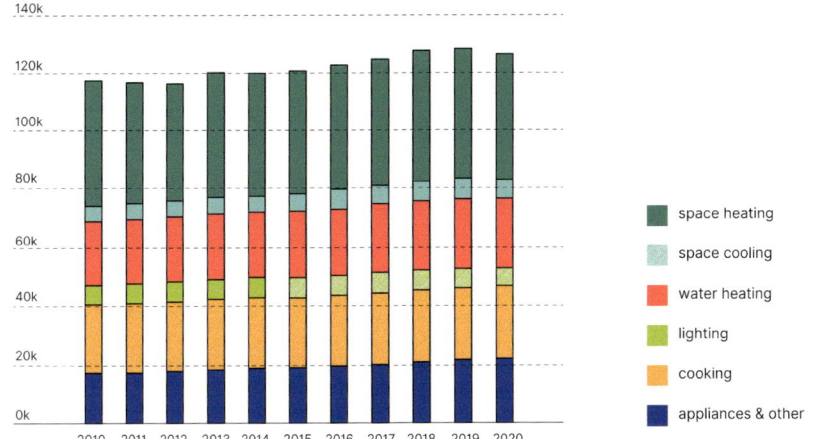

BUILDING SECTOR'S SHARE OF GLOBAL FINAL ENERGY

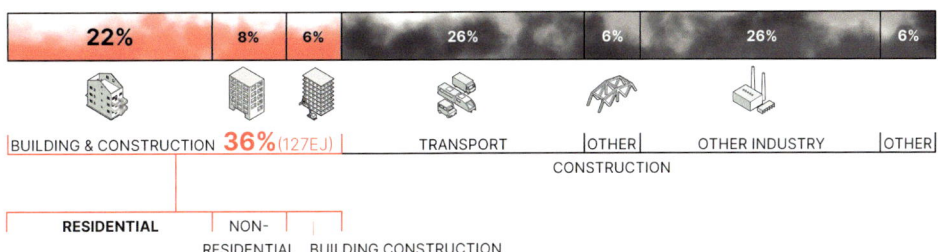

Figure 9.1 Global Share of Building and Construction Energy (Bottom) and By End Use (Top) in 2020.

architects to achieve operational sustainability goals and helps architects choose the most effective construction materials. Ideally, using strategies of bioclimatic design, renewable energy sources, and energy rating systems contributes to dematerializing a building and improving resource efficacy. The last section will discuss the cascading effects of implementing these techniques.

Note throughout this chapter "efficacy" is used to describe energy and resource use rather than "efficacy". This is intentional as it's not always about using "less". For example, if a house adds materials at the initial stage so that it performs better during the operational phase and hence lowers the energy demand during the life of the building – then it is achieving its goal of using resources in a useful and valuable manner. Similarly, if a material has more inputs during its manufacturing stage so that it produces a building component or product that can last many life cycles, then even if the initial use of materials may be seen as less "efficient", it ultimately creates an element with the desired result of an extended life; hence, avoiding both future waste and the need for new resources to manufacture something new. Hence, the most important aspect of smart circular design is to consider energy and material use across the entire proposed life cycle of a building.

This chapter will demonstrate that energy conservation or reduction is not the same as deprivation or discomfort. Rather, by designing buildings with a life cycle mentality, in which the very beginning and end of a building's life are factored in, buildings can be designed to accommodate environmental and climatic fluctuations, ensuring occupant comfort without a reliance on non-renewable energy-consumptive systems.

9.1.1 From Lechner's Three-Tier Approach to Sustainable Design to Frampton's Critical Regionalism

In his book *Heating, Cooling, and Lighting*, Norbert Lechner outlines a conceptualization of designing operationally sustainable buildings made up of three tiers, of which the first two are under the architect's responsibility (see Figure 9.2). The first tier is made up of all the decisions required when planning a building. If an architect considers approaches that respond to and leverage the climatic flows of the surrounding environment in every aspect of the building, they will be able to design a building that can achieve about 60 percent of heating, cooling, and lighting

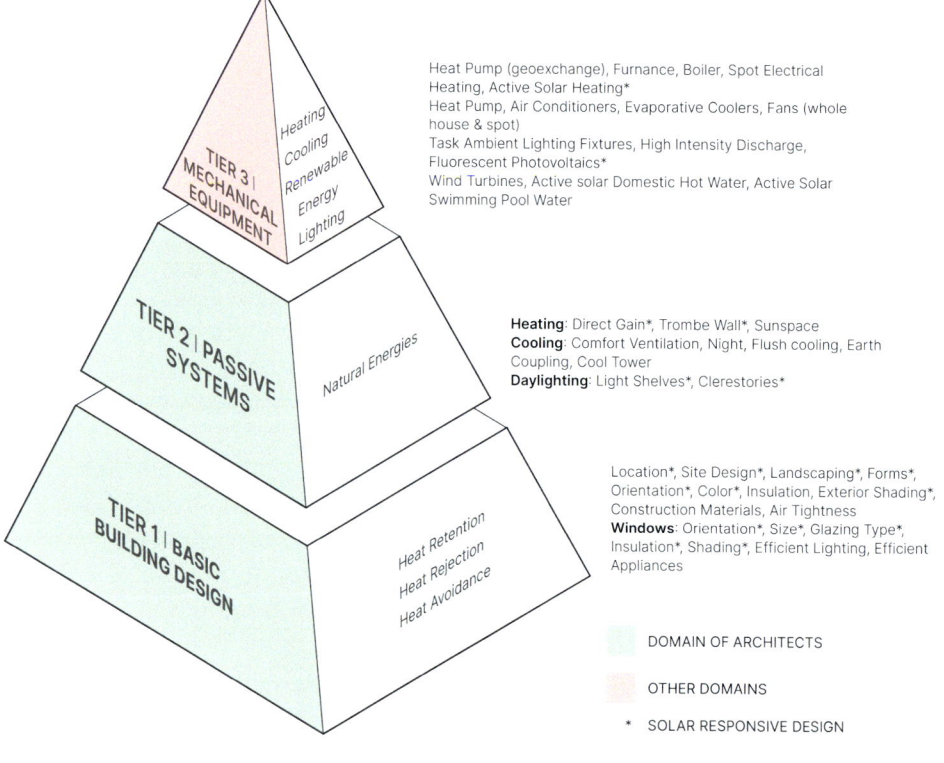

Source: Adapted from Norbert Lechner "Heating, Cooling, Lighting"

Figure 9.2 Lechner's Three-Tier Pyramid.

itself (Lechner, 2015). The second level involves employing natural energies such as passive heating and cooling strategies, and daylighting systems. For instance, night flush cooling is a type of passive cooling that capitalizes on the naturally cooler temperatures at night to regulate thermal comfort. In this strategy, the exterior of the building is well insulated during the day to keep the hot air outside and the interior cool. At night the building is opened to promote natural ventilation of the cool night air to lower temperatures in the building. Using strategies from the second tier can reduce energy consumption by an additional 20 percent. These techniques regulate thermal comfort without the need for the inclusion of mechanical systems. In the third tier, the mechanical and electrical equipment is made as effective as possible, reducing energy consumption by an additional 5 percent. Using this three-tier approach, the amount of energy a building would need to operate could be reduced by up to 85 percent (see Figure 9.3). For a low-carbon sustainable design, the final 15 percent should come from renewable sources. This implies, firstly, shifting all necessary mechanical systems for heating, cooling, and ventilation to electricity and making sure the electricity is coming from renewable sources.

Unfortunately, on a global scale, the emerging trends in conventional housing design are ignoring the first two tiers, with operational energy and indoor-environmental regulation seen as only within the realm of mechanical and electrical equipment and engineering. This can result in buildings that are inconsiderate of their natural surroundings resulting in a loss of national identity and vernacular design, and a global conformity in contemporary housing as described in Chapter 7. A climate-responsive approach to design can draw on what Kenneth Frampton termed "critical regionalism",

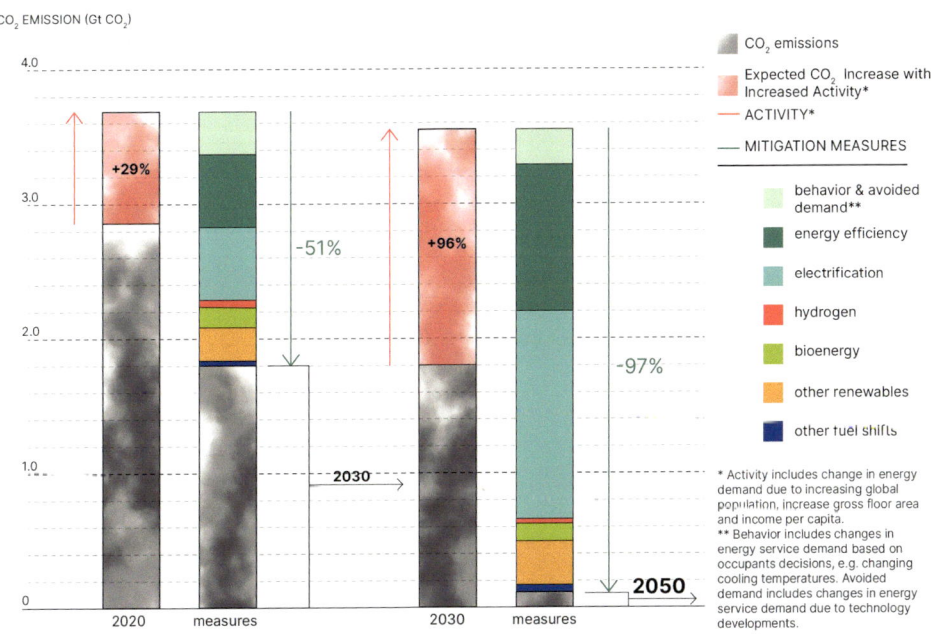

Figure 9.3 Global Direct Carbon Dioxide Emission Reductions by Mitigation in Building in the Net Zero Energy Scenario 2050.

an architecture that aims to counter the conformity, placelessness, and loss of identity associated with the international style (Frampton, 1993). This architectural approach is engrained in the modern tradition of a place but tied to its geographical and cultural context.

9.2 Climate-Responsive Bioclimatic Design Strategies

Bioclimatic design pays close attention to the building's location and its specific climate to achieve indoor comfort for the occupants (Olgyay et al., 2015). Bioclimatic design strategies have multiple dimensions. A building's morphology, the location of openings, its orientation, size, and massing, all contribute to how a building works within its environment. It determines the building's ability to harness local resources i.e., sun, wind, precipitation (rain, snow, etc.) (Keena et al., 2022). This allows for a building to provide thermal comfort by leveraging environmental resources rather than achieving it through energy-consumptive, and typically fossil-fuel-reliant, methods, such as mechanical heating, cooling, ventilation, and air conditioning (HVAC). Bioclimatic design is not a new concept; in fact, it was the natural approach to conditioning spaces prior to the advent of mechanical HVAC systems and the popularization of manmade architectural materials such as steel, concrete, and glass. Traditional local architecture is inherently bioclimatic, using materials that are sourced locally and with consideration of its environment. Because the building's materials and design are attentive to the local climate, these buildings typically are high-performing during their operational phase and often demonstrate circular material life cycles with low emissions and low embodied energy related to their production (Keena et al., 2022).

9.2.1 Biomaterials and the Operational Phase

Another potential opportunity to reduce both embodied and operational greenhouse gas emissions associated with buildings is by using biomaterials. Biomaterials affect multiple stages of a building's life cycle, from sourcing and production, operation and disposal. These materials are made from bio-based renewable resources rather than extracted mineral-based sources. Therefore, they are often biodegradable at the disposal phase; however, this can lead to the release of greenhouse gas emissions as they decompose. Choosing the right materials is an important contributing factor to the bioclimatic design, determining heat flow, time lag, and energy storage capacity (Keena et al., 2022). The energy transfer through a material or construction assembly is also dependent on the temperature and humidity conditions of the exterior environment in which the building is located. As is explored below, biomaterials which are local to their surroundings have very interesting properties in this respect as they've adapted over time to survive in their habitat. For example, in hot humid climates certain biomaterials have hygroscopic properties to readily absorb and retain moisture from the humid air. In addition, a mass timber panel, such as cross-laminated timber, has relatively a high heat capacity. This means it requires more heat energy to raise its temperature by 1°C. In other words, CLT can absorb and retain heat energy without experiencing significant change in temperature, making it an effective insulator with high thermal resistance. Additionally, many bio-based materials such as lumber or construction materials from agricultural waste by-products can be produced with low embodied energy, supporting many life cycles, instead of short-lived and energy-consumptive materials (Keena et al., 2022). This is discussed in detail in Chapter 7.

9.2.2 The Köppen-Geiger Approach: Designing with Climate as the Starting Point

In brief, a bioclimatic building combines human biology and climate – designing buildings for human occupants with local climate in mind (Watson, 2013). The aim of such an architectural approach is to provide passive comfort to occupants through knowledge of the microclimatic conditions of a building's location, providing daylighting, heating, and cooling (Watson, 2013). Thus, the Köppen-Geiger map is a helpful tool for climate-responsive architecture, categorizing the globe into five distinct climate zones: tropical (Zone A), arid/dry (Zone B), warm/mild temperate (Zone C), continental (Zone D), and polar (Zone E) (see Figure 9.4). Fun fact being that Köppen was a

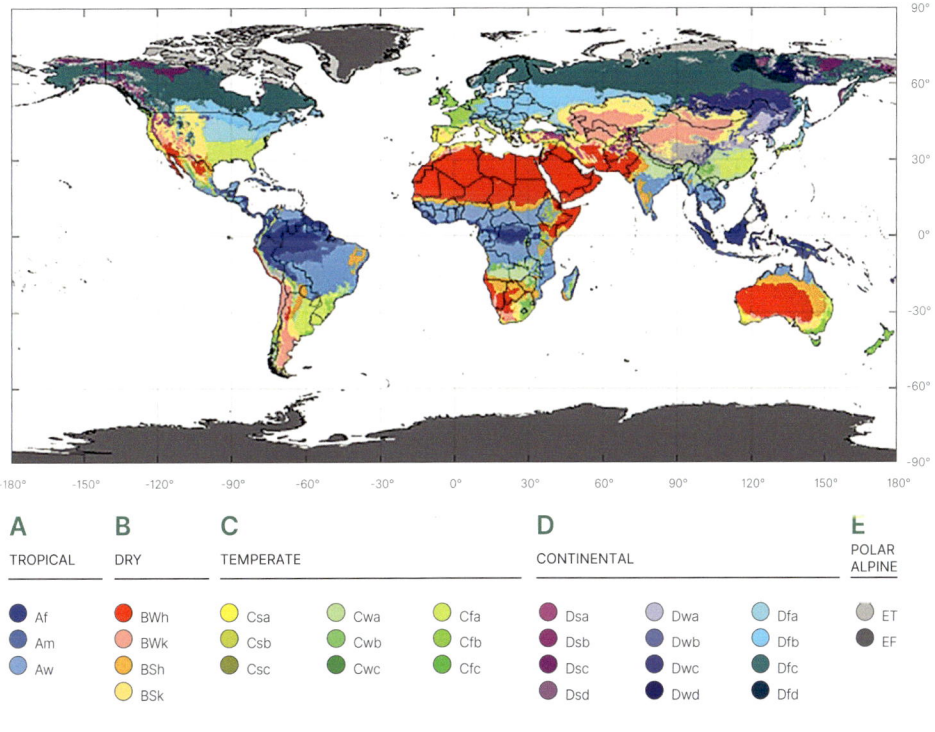

Source: Modified from Beck et al. 2018

Figure 9.4 Map of Köppen-Geiger Climate Classifications.

botanist, and hence, the main climate groups are based on the types of vegetation occurring in a given climate classification region. This means changes in vegetation types are helping scientists predict changing climates classifications due to climate change (Beck et al., 2018). Bioclimatic decisions are determined based on which climate zone a building is located within and thus the Köppen-Geiger map can be helpful in guiding designers to choose appropriate materials and design methods.

Zone A: Tropical

In a tropical zone, in which there are distinct wet and dry seasons and high humidity, lightweight and open design should be prioritized to ventilate the dwelling and account for such humidity (Keena et al., 2022). Wood, bamboo, agricultural waste combinations (e.g., coconut, rice, and straw) are all biomaterials that are native to tropical climates and perform well in humid conditions. Additionally, using materials that have natural desiccating properties, such as coconut coir, rice husk and cork, for insulation can prevent mold which is often a problem in moist environments. Thatched or attap roofing (roofing made with tropical palm) is similarly chosen for its low thermal capacity and insulating qualities. Designing for maximum ventilation and passive cooling is key, such as high ceilings to allow for high windows, and high gabled roofs without ceilings so the hottest air can rise and leave the interior. This can be seen in Figure 9.5 in the vernacular architecture of Sumatra, Indonesia,

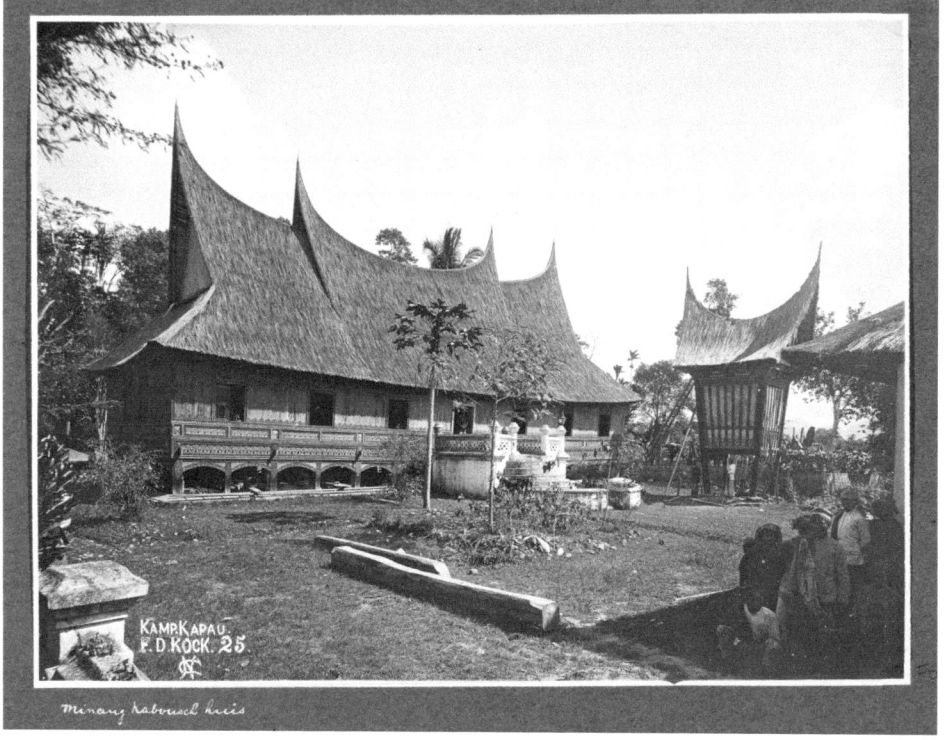

Figure 9.5 Sumatra, Indonesia, Architecture.

where buildings are constructed on silts with high roofs and open gables to increase air circulation (Lechner, 2015).

Zone B: Desert

In the dry climate Zone (B), designing a building that alleviates high temperatures indoors protects against the sun, utilizes evaporative cooling, and employs thermal mass to reduce diurnal temperature fluctuations are all important in providing thermal comfort (Keena et al., 2022). When a material has high thermal mass, it means that the material can absorb and store heat well. In a hot climate, walls benefit from thermal mass as they can absorb thermal energy when it is hot outside instead of transferring it to the inside of the building. When the temperature outside is cool in the evening, the trapped heat in the walls can keep the interior of the building warmer. Certain vernacular materials with high thermal mass are adobe and rammed earth, as well as bio-based concrete and clay brick. South Africa falls into Zone B. The country often uses clay brick for walling because of its thermal performance and supply access (GreenCape, 2014). Small windows are favorable over large ones to prevent solar heat from entering the interior yet still sufficiently lighting rooms (Lechner, 2015). An example of indigenous architecture is Montezuma Castle National Monument, in the dry desert climate of Camp Verde, Arizona. It was built by the Sinagua indigenous people, a pre-Columbian culture also related to the Hohokam indigenous peoples of the southwestern United States. Built approximately between 1100 and 1425 AD, it is believed that around the year 1400 AD people began leaving their homes there. Despite that, with cycles of care, over 500 years later, its walls were still largely intact – a fine example of the circular principle "building life extension". Native communities, who were consultants on its preservation, explained dwellings like this were meant to be recycled back to the earth after the people left. However, due to the sheltered alcove, that was cleverly chosen as the site, the homes remain to this day as illustrated in Figure 9.6.

Zone C and D: Temperate and Continental

Similar techniques outlined for Zone A should be applied to Zone C to mitigate high humidity. However, unlike Zone A, temperatures in temperate climates are often favorable most of the year, meaning that opening the building to the outdoors can be a useful strategy to cool the building and remove moisture. In some temperate areas such as the Pacific Northwest, where overcast weather is prominent, large open windows allow more of the light to come in (Lechner, 2015). Temperate climates, however, are some of the most difficult climates to design for, as architects must consider designing for distinct seasons, including extreme winters and summers. Continental climates (Zone D) similarly can have large seasonal temperature fluctuations. These zones typically have humid summers that can adopt similar techniques to Zone A, but cold and dry winters, which must also be accounted for.

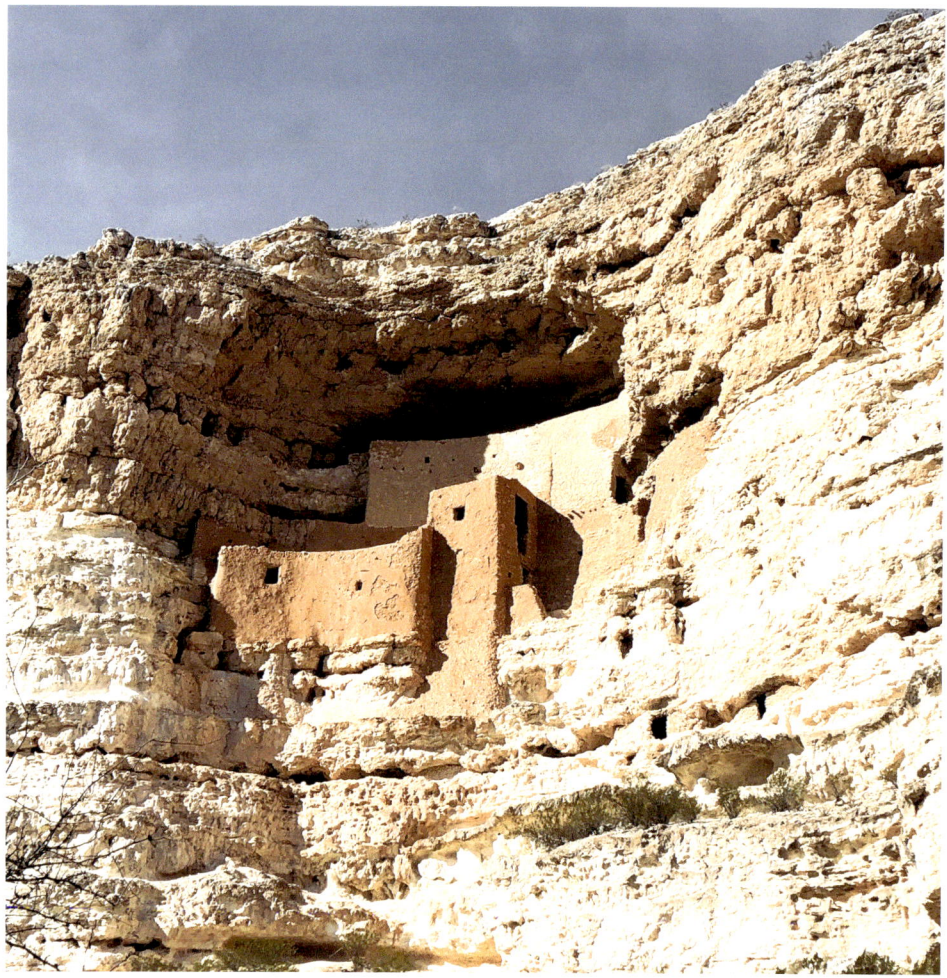

Figure 9.6 Montezuma Castle National Monument, in the Dry Desert Climate of Camp Verde Arizona Was Built by the Sinagua Indigenous People Approximately between 1100 and 1425 AD.

Zone E: Polar

In particularly cold climates, such as Zone E, thick walls, compact and small dwellings, and few windows are designed to conserve heat (Lechner, 2015). Unlike in hot climates, ceilings are often low to contain the warm air that rises, and materials with thermal resistance to the cold are preferred. Figure 9.7 shows an igloo. Igloos are a traditional home of the Inuit indigenous communities in the Arctic regions of Alaska, Canada, and Greenland. It is the most perfect example of a circular home. It uses locally available, renewable materials, that being snow. It is regenerative in that when it is no longer in use, in the summer months, it melts at the end-of-use phase. No carbon emissions result. In terms of operational energy, it relies solely on physics of energy, no mechanical system is needed. If built correctly, an igloo can create a difference of up to 40°C between its interior and the exterior environment

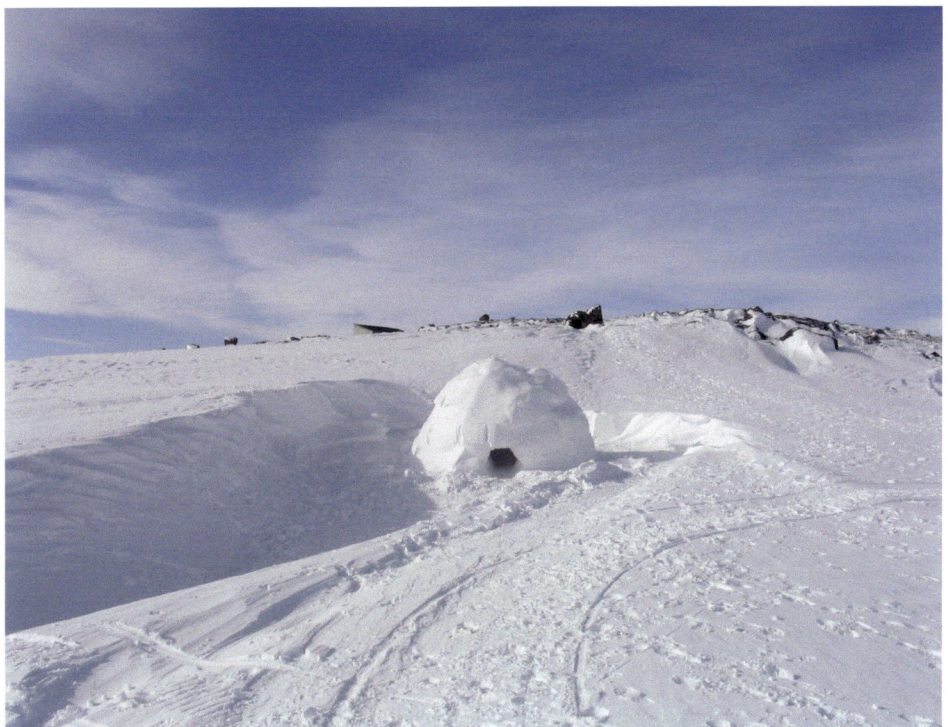

Figure 9.7 Igloo, an Exemplar Circular Home, in Nordic Regions of Canada.

just through the use of body heat. An igloo works to keep occupants warm by trapping body heat. It's made of compressed snow, which is almost 95 percent trapped air and hence a good insulator. This insulation prevents the loss of body heat, so occupants keep warm. The configuration and sectional layout are also important for heat retention. There is a small sunken tunnel at the entrance which acts as a cold sink, preventing snowstorms and cold winds from penetrating the interior. The igloo is divided into terraces. The main one is the upper platform for sleeping and the lower platform is for living. In one study it was found that inside an igloo, near the bodies of the people, the temperature was around 36°C. In the air surrounding the people, the temperature dropped to almost 16°C, and at the far end near the walls of the igloo, the temperature was around 1°C. The more people inside the Igloo, the warm it gets (Holihan et al., 2003).

These examples stress how in different climate zones, biomaterials available, qualities valued by materials, and architectural design differ drastically. Therefore, attention to a building's specific vegetation, climate, and vernacular architecture is required in designing for thermal comfort. Countries have been employing such vernacular building methods for centuries and have mastered how to build with such materials efficiently and effectively. Tapping into and reviving such knowledge by employing skilled local labor will be important.

This section boils down to two main ways to foster bioclimatic design. First, design for a building's specific climate. Creating passive heating or cooling methods through the size and orientation of a dwelling and ventilation methods allow buildings to respond to the environment and maintain thermal comfort rather than relying on energy-intensive mechanical equipment. Second, in a climate with extreme temperatures, choosing materials with low thermal capacity and conductivity is key. In addition, choosing materials that are locally sourced leads to low embodied energy and integrates the life cycle approach to the building. Sourcing materials, and especially bio-based materials, close to home reduces energy-intensive transportation and extractive mineral-based processes. Furthermore, bio-based materials can sequester and act as carbon sinks during their life cycle. At the end-of-life stage, these materials can often biodegrade and return to the earth, which means it will release the greenhouse gas emissions it was storing. Allowing it to biodegrade rather than burning it is the best option as it will slowly release the greenhouse gas emissions over time rather than in one roaring blaze. Although biomaterials hold much promise, their use must be governed by sustainable practices to reduce the risk of deforestation, land degradation, environmentally harmful land use patterns, and/or loss of biodiversity, among other impacts. While climate-responsive design strategies are extremely effective, the remaining temperature regulation of a dwelling can be achieved through renewable energy sources, the third tier in Figure 9.2, which the next section will detail.

9.3 Clean Operational Energy: Renewable and Non-Renewable Forms of Energy Used to Operate Housing

There are two kinds of operational energy that can power a building: non-renewable and renewable. Non-renewable energy comes from resources that cannot be replenished after use, such as crude oil, natural gas, and coal. While these resources are naturally produced, it takes millennia for them to form and replenish from the fossilized, buried remains of plants and animals, and they require extensive, energy-intensive extraction methods. Renewable energy, by contrast, comes from resources that replenish themselves through processes of the natural environment. Keena et al. (2016) found that, as expected, non-renewable sources such as natural gas to power a building's electricity have the highest unit emergy value (6.58E+05), which is the total amount of energy and material inputs needed to produce an output unit (see Chapter 2). As explained in Chapter 2, the unit emergy value is an interesting metric to consider forms of energy. Unlike other methods such as life cycle assessment, it includes the work of the geo-biosphere in producing the raw materials. In terms of energy sources, this is an important consideration because, as mentioned above, some of these resources relied on geo-biosphere processes over millennia to be produced. In general, the higher the unit emergy value, the more resources and processes need to produce that form of energy, and vice versa. Since non-renewable resources rely on external factors to provide energy, such as the biochemical methanogens process necessary to convert natural gas to electricity, their values are typically higher (Keena et al., 2016). Renewable resources tend to have lower UEVs because of their small reliance on external environmental support to produce energy. Referring to Lechner's Three Tiers, while 85 percent of operational energy should come from building design, passive systems, and a small amount from mechanical engineering, the remaining 15 percent of operational energy should be "clean" and "net zero carbon". Clean operational energy would, therefore, come from renewable resources, such as hydro, wind, or solar. A net zero energy building is a building in which all of its operational energy, or its energy required to perform the functions of the building, is generated by renewable energy.

9.3.1 Does a Switch to Renewable Energy Mean Less Electricity?

While it is evident that a shift to renewable energy is better for the environment, this does not mean a sacrifice in terms of energy usage in buildings. The concept of Energy Return on Investment (EROI) is a measure of whether a renewable energy technology results in net energy. Net energy, or energy surplus, is the sum of the energy produced by a facility and the energy needed to operate that facility. Both are required. Concerns have been raised that renewable electricity grids will not produce the level of EROIs that their non-renewable counterparts would, reducing the flow of net energy and affecting people's access to plentiful electricity. Murphy and Raugei (2020) find this to be false. In fact, an electricity grid in Chile that started relying on wind and photovoltaic power and pump hydro for storage, raised the EROI of the grid, meaning that the energy surplus increased (Raugei et al., 2018). Therefore, not only is renewable energy more environmentally friendly, but it has the potential to come with no sacrifices for the consumer.

9.3.2 Where Does Electricity in Buildings Come From?

To meet operational phase demands, there are two alternative electricity systems that a building can rely on (see Figure 9.8). The first is a municipal utility supply, which provides electricity under public control, to the entirety of an area. These electrical grids, depending on the location, can be powered by renewable sources, non-renewable, or a mix of both, to generate energy for a region. For instance, the hydro-Québec electricity transmission system applies to the whole province of Québec, Canada, and is powered entirely by hydroelectric energy, mainly from hydroelectric dams (Hydro Québec, n.d.). In these systems, electricity is generated at an external location and then distributed to buildings across a region via power lines and transformers. While in the case of Québec, all operational energy is renewable, in many cities, non-renewable sources, like natural gas, coal, and oil, are still heavily relied upon to generate electricity. Therefore, if an architect wants to build a net zero energy building in the context of a non-renewable or even a mixed grid (mixed renewable and non-renewable) municipal system, the second source of operational energy – onsite electricity production – is a favorable option.

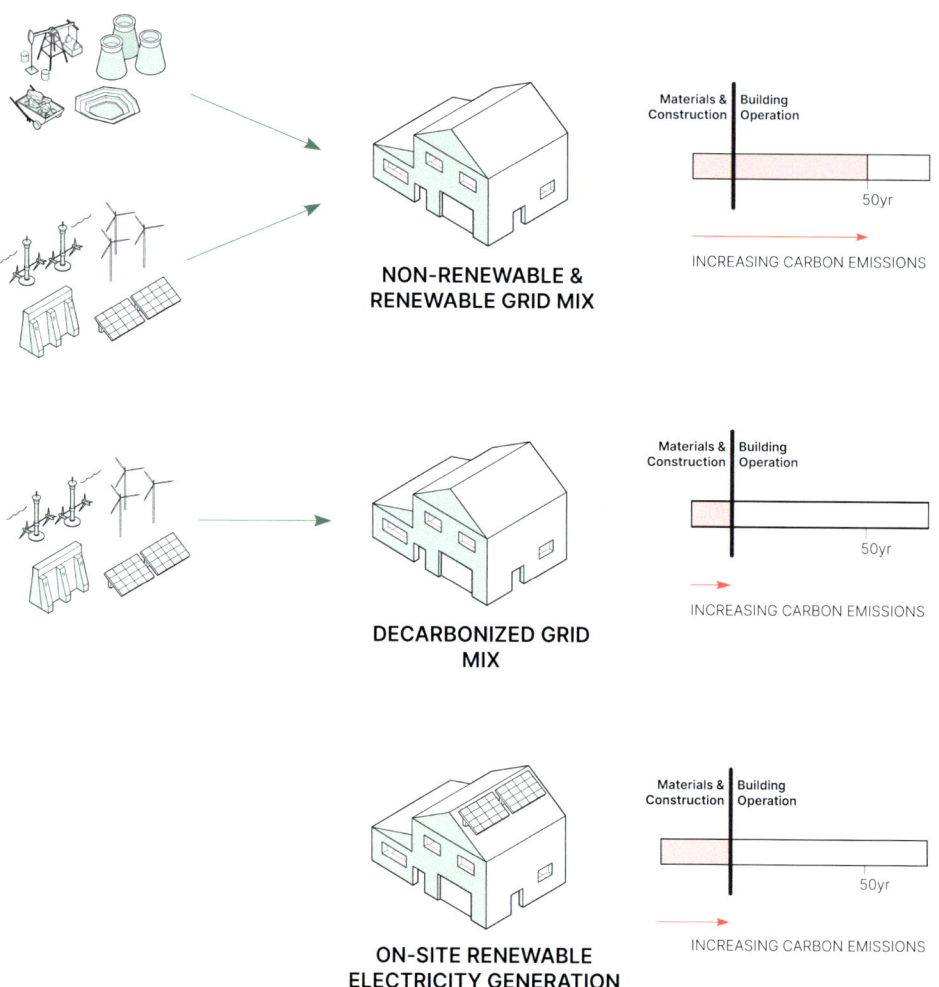

Figure 9.8 The Difference Between Municipal Utility Supply (Mixed Grid and Decarbonized) and Onsite Electricity Production.

Photovoltaic (PV) panels installed on building rooftops have become a common form of this operational electricity generation. Since PV panels regenerate power on site, they minimize a building's reliance on external factors, particularly when non-renewable sources are involved, increasing lifetime energy assurance (Raugei et al., 2021). In London, United States, for instance, a "Two Degrees" development plan is underway to decrease the city's carbon emissions through reducing greenhouse gas emissions by 80 percent by 2050 (Parliament of the United Kingdom, 2008). While their grid mix is trying to phase out coal- and gas-reliant steam turbines, there is still a significant reliance on nuclear energy, making the system vulnerable to the volatility of non-renewable primary resources and operational greenhouse gas emissions. Therefore, if an architect wants to build a net zero energy building today, onsite renewable energy generation would be encouraged. In terms of a circular economic logic, renewable forms of energy are circular as they can be replenished continuously. They are also regenerative as their use does not negatively impact the environment unlike non-renewable fossil fuels which emit carbon emissions.

9.3.3 Should Net Zero Energy Really Be the Measurement of Success?

Net zero energy is a good goal in theory but disregards important aspects of the life cycle of a building. This is because "net zero energy" focuses only on the operational energy of a building, not the embodied energy. Operational energy is the energy required to power a building and, as this chapter stresses, is a crucial aspect of building circular housing. However, to achieve "clean", or "net zero" operational, energy should not be done at the expense of embodied energy, or the energy used to construct a building and its materials. While achieving net zero operational energy is important, to properly assess the environmental impact of a building, operational energy is too narrow a focus. As discussed throughout this book, a life cycle approach needs to be fostered, meaning an assessment of all the environmental factors that go into producing, running, and ending the useful life of a building. For example, if on-site electricity is to be achieved via solar panels, then even if that home is fully operating on solar power, it is perhaps untrue to say this is "net zero energy" or definitely not "net zero carbon". The reason for this is that much energy and resources, and hence embodied energy and embodied carbon, went into producing the solar panels which are being used to achieve electricity. A home without solar panels will have less upfront embodied energy and carbon in its construction because it uses less materials. However, over the life of the building, it may accrue a lot more embodied energy and embodied carbon in its reliance on fossil fuels for operational energy than that needed to produce solar panels. Hence, a life cycle approach is key in understanding "net zero energy" and the only way available today to achieve "net zero carbon" is to not build anything. One of the broadest and most comprehensive analyses for a building is an emergy analysis, not a net zero energy analysis or even an embodied energy analysis. See Chapter 2 for more details on emergy analysis.

Consequently, this nuance in "net zero" energy homes is underscored in the discussion on photovoltaic panels. While a photovoltaic energy source is renewable, a life cycle assessment of environmental impact highlights that materiality, sourcing, and manufacturing of renewable energy technology are contributing factors to emissions and must be mitigated (Raugei et al., 2021). In the case of PV panels, while the environmental impact of solar cells is negligible, the materials chosen to design such PV panels and the manufacturing process can have a harmful environmental impact – producing net zero operational energy, but high embodied energy. Nonetheless, it can be argued that this could still lead to less overall emissions than a mixed grid that runs partly on fossil fuels. However, this is where context and time must be factored in. In the past 30 years, it has become clear that the reliance many countries have on non-renewable energy is not sustainable, resulting in a series of goals and targets to reduce greenhouse gas emissions. The United Nations Framework Convention on Climate Change (UNFCCC) created in 1992, led to the Kyoto Protocol in 1997, an international conference that set emission reduction targets for 37 countries (United Nations, 1998). The Paris Agreement, nearly ten years later, specified their target to a reduction of carbon emissions and to maintain global temperatures below 2°C (United Nations, 2015). States across the United States have put efforts into decreasing their greenhouse gas emissions. California set the target for 60 percent of its energy to be renewable by 2030; Vermont aims for 75 percent; and the District of Columbia, 100 percent (Council of the District of Columbia, 2019; Department of Public Service, 2019; Domonoske, 2018). New York state is putting efforts into integrating renewable energy, setting the goal of 70 percent of its electricity coming from renewable sources by 2030 (Murphy & Raugei, 2020). With these efforts toward decarbonizing the municipal grid underway in certain cities, combined with the environmental costs of installing PV panels for onsite energy, an emergy analysis would tell us that in the long term, maintaining a semi-net zero energy building on the municipal grid (that will eventually become completely "net zero") without building PV panels might be more sustainable in the long term than achieving net zero energy right away through onsite production (Raugei et al., 2021).

Therefore, when an architect is presented with the goal of clean operational energy, it is impossible to assess whether one renewable energy system is better than another. Rather, a specific focus on location, climate type (is there much sun or wind?) energy and decarbonization goals, and existing and projected grid structures, must be considered to choose the most appropriate renewable energy system for the life cycle of a building (Raugei et al., 2021).

9.4 Energy (Efficiency) Ratings

Nonetheless, the gold standard for sustainable building is still seen as a "net zero" building, which many energy rating measurements are built around. There are a range of energy efficiency ratings that measure sustainability differently. The main goal is to compare homes and to understand the operational energy use of a building. Scales like the Energy Rating Index (ERI), range from 0 to 100, where zero is a net zero energy home (RESNET, 2015). Each integer increase represents one percent of change in the total energy use of the building in relation to an ERI reference design. This index is popular in the United States, but other countries use different energy rating systems and values for measurement.

In Canada, the energy efficacy of a building is measured using the Canadian Standards Association (CSA) A440.2 standard (Government of Canada, 2022). Aspects like U-factor, solar heat gain coefficient (SHGC), Energy Rating (ER), R-value, Visible transmittance (VT), and center-of-glass rating, are all values used to measure different aspects of energy efficacy. For instance, U-factor measures the rate of heat transfer through a building element (wall, roof, floor, etc.) – the lower the number, the higher its resistance to heat flow and the more insulative it is (Government of Canada,

2022). The SHGC and the VT tend to go hand-in-hand, where the latter measures the ratio of visible light that can pass through an object – the higher the number, the more transmittance – and the former measures the amount of heat that is either rejected (i.e., reflected away from the building) or transmitted. When direct solar radiation is reflected away from the building, the heat goes into the neighboring buildings or ground, which can lead to an urban heat island effect in dense cities, raising the average temperature within a city compared to the surrounding rural areas. Energy Star certifications mark building materials such as doors, windows, and skylights as holding up to their energy efficiency standards (Government of Canada, 2022). An accredited laboratory in Canada can assess the ratings of these materials to issue a certification. The UK Energy Label is another certification that ranks appliances from A to G (see Figure 9.9) (West, 2021). In this rating system a QR code is provided that connects to the product's manufacturer's website, giving additional information on the given product (West, 2021).

Energy performance certificates (CPE), or energy passports, are another form of energy rating, reporting on the energy requirements of a new or existing building. This links back to the discussion on housing passports (HPs) in Chapter 4. The benefit of an energy rating is to help governments and cities understand the environmental impact of the building stock due to operational energy use.

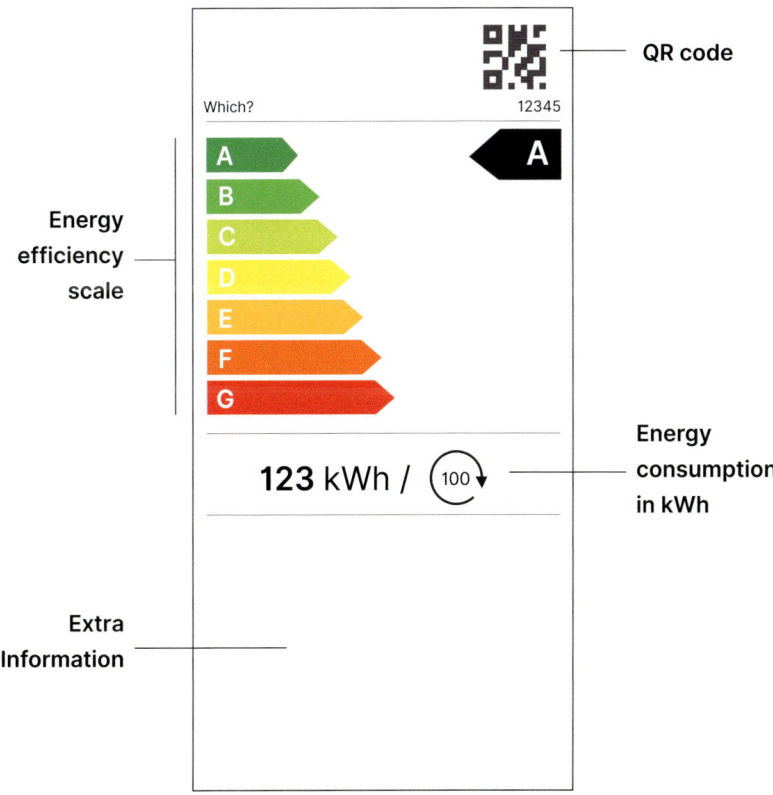

Figure 9.9 Example of an Energy Label.

The HP, like the UK Energy Label, standardizes residential building characteristics, including materials, to give information to the consumer and builder about the manufacturing of the product. An energy passport states the energy efficacy and performance of a building and can be easily compared to other buildings, encouraging architects to build for low energy consumption. Adding this level of transparency to each component of a building can help builders identify which products are not energy-efficient and replace them.

While energy rating systems can be helpful in setting benchmarks for a building's energy consumption, many shortcomings discussed earlier are repeated in these rating systems, namely, that a building's embodied energy is dismissed from consideration. Like the discussion on net zero energy buildings above, measuring a building's operational energy use only is not sufficient in accounting for life cycle energy use. Often energy rating systems do not link use and consumption to the material composition and construction assemblies of a building. While building materials are included in the rating system, the consideration only extends as far as the operational performance of the material, not the environmental impact of extracting and manufacturing said material.

For instance, as discussed with the Köppen-Geiger climate zones, different climate zones respond differently to building techniques and materials. In this vein, energy ratings measure the efficacy of a dwelling in unalike climatic zones differently. For instance, until 2020, Energy Star in Canada categorized products into one of three climate zones, with 1 being the mildest weather and 3 the coldest. Therefore, the conditions for a product to qualify as Energy Star certified in Zone 3 would follow the most rigorous criteria, conserving the most heat than in Zone 1. Setting energy efficacy standards based on climate zones is important to properly assess the energy efficacy of a product in that specific climatic condition. However, using the proper building materials is not enough for energy-efficient buildings to be achieved. Even if a builder chooses an Energy Star certified building material, a building cannot be energy inefficient if the building is not constructed properly, leading to a loss of thermal comfort. Therefore, while energy rating systems can be a convenient tool for comparing and benchmarking the operational energy use of a building, it needs to be paired with good bioclimatic design and an understanding of building physics as well as a measure of the building's embodied energy for an accurate assessment of the building's energy use across its life cycle.

9.5 Cascading Effects of Implementing a Systems-Wide Approach to a Circular Economy on Residential Operational Energy Demand

While bioclimatic building techniques and renewable energy sources are effective methods for increasing the operational energy efficacy of a building, dematerialization strategies – or the efficient use of materials and space – cannot be ignored when discussing pathways to circular energy use. Many of the concepts discussed in Chapters 5–8 offer important strategies for dematerialization and resource efficacy. Resource efficacy is a broad term that involves the shrewd use of water, materials, energy, and land (IRP, 2020). Creating built ecologies for production and consumption that can foster a resource-efficient economy. Dematerialization is one prominent strategy for fostering this resource efficacy, which involves reducing materials and energy use while achieving the same outcome and wellbeing (IRP, 2020). The International Resource Panel (2020) offers a slew of strategies to implement dematerialization at the onset of building to result in less operational energy use in the long term (see Figure 9.10). Many of these strategies are in line with the circular business models discussed in Chapter 3, including product life extension, recovery and recycling, reuse, and a more intensive use of space. Others include designing for less materials, substituting high-carbon-emitting materials with lighter materials, and planning for yield improvement through building information modeling. Indeed, implementing digital technologies helps avoid inefficient construction that leads to high energy consumption (see Chapter 8). These strategies can be roughly divided into two categories: build less from the start; and when a building is required, put

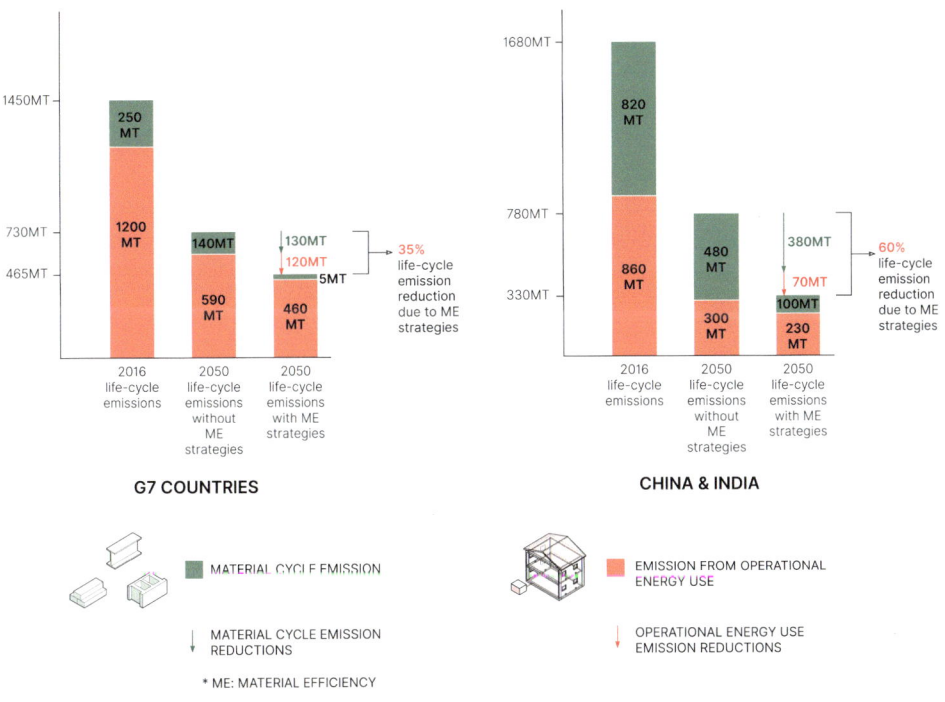

Source: Adapted from IRP 2020 "Resource Efficiency and Climate Change"

Figure 9.10 The Potential of Material Efficiency Strategies in Reducing Carbon Emissions from Operational Energy Use on a Global Scale.

efforts into reducing the materials used to make such a building. Reducing materials used in a building can lower greenhouse gas emissions from construction, demolition, and operation in G7 countries in 2050 by an additional 35–40 percent compared to improving energy efficiency (IRP, 2020). This is because reducing or making material use more efficient lowers the demand for virgin resources, brings secondary materials into the construction market, and increases the intensity of use which lowers operational energy emissions (IRP, 2020). This might seem self-evident – using less materials means using less energy – but it is integral that architects consider this before building as this is the clearest and more economical way to reduce operational greenhouse gas emissions.

9.5.1 Building Less from the Start

Building smaller and with multiple functions is a clear way to reduce material reliance in construction. According to the IRP, reducing floor space demand by up to 20 percent would decrease the need for new construction in G7 countries (2020). This can lower operational emissions by up to 70 percent in the G7 by 2050 (IRP, 2020). Some ways to increase the utilization rate of a building is by living in smaller units, so more people can live in a building, share homes through co-housing operations, and have different businesses or groups share space so the building is constantly in use (see Chapters 2 and 3). While it may seem that increasing the usage of a building could increase operational energy use, looking at energy use in the large scale reveals that intensive use of buildings reduces overall operational emissions for heating and cooling (IRP, 2020). If the overall floor space is reduced, so is the need to heat and cool such space, which could result in an estimated saving of 120–130 million metric tons of emissions in the G7 in 2050 (IRP, 2020).

9.5.2 Using Less Materials

When a building is required, using less and lighter materials may also reduce operational energy emissions. IRP (2020) recommends replacing materials like steel and cement with wood that has low life cycle emissions. Moreover, recycling building materials saves 15–20 percent of material cycle emissions in G7 countries (IRP, 2020). Smart design of a building to be dynamic rather than static is another effective way to reduce materials used in construction while maintaining thermal comfort. In other words, like the discussion in Chapter 6, designing buildings to adapt over time extends the life of a building while keeping the building in use for as long as possible. Just as buildings must adapt to the changing conditions of their inhabitants, it should also be able to adapt to the changing temperature of its environment. For instance, Lechner (2015) outlines the design for a retractable shading façade that extends to create shade in the sun and retracts in overcast conditions. Shade is a helpful tool for cooling, and exposure to the sun is, of course, a helpful tool to increase natural lighting when it is overcast, thus reducing the reliance on manmade cooling and lighting systems. Dynamic design employs technology to reduce the need to build additional structures, not only increasing the thermal efficacy of the dwelling but also avoiding additional materials used. Paul Rudolph's Walker House is a prime example of the concept of dynamic, adaptable design toward usability of space while offering thermal comfort to the inhabitants.

It is important to clarify, however, that using "light" material does not necessarily mean always choosing the lightest weight material upfront. As mentioned earlier, in hot arid climates, high thermal mass materials are the most energy-efficient and are also notably thick and heavy to retain heat. While the materials may weight more upfront, in the long term, they will reduce operational energy through passive heating and cooling abilities. Like retractable shading facades, this smart design avoids unnecessary additional construction in the future, thus making the overall material use of the building "lighter".

Technology like the HPs can help with this material efficacy, as it increases building information management to allow architects to plan ahead and choose the most efficient and lightweight use of each material where appropriate (see Chapter 4). It allows for the organization of data across the life cycle of a house rather than solely focusing on the operational phase.

While many of these ideas have been discussed in previous chapters, these decisions continue to have positive implications throughout the operational phase as well.

9A

Project:
Meme – Experimental House

Locations:
Taiki, Japan

Year:
2011

Team:
Kengo Kuma and Associates

Mapping to Circular Economy Framework:

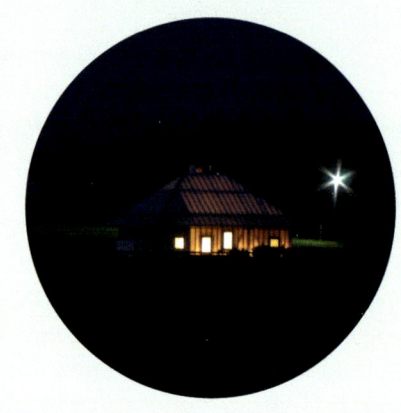

CIRCULAR ECONOMY PRACTICES

LIFE CYCLE PHASES

Recovery | Life Extension | Sharing Platforms | Service Models | Regenerate | Virtualize

Work of Geobiosphere

Sourcing

Manufacturing

Design & Construction

Use

End-of-Use

LAYERS + LIFESPAN
Structural Layers | Long Life
Skin, MEP Layers | Medium Life
Interior Layers | Short Life

Site 100+yr Structure 50+yr
Exterior 25+yr System 15+yr
Partition 10+yr Stuff 1+yr

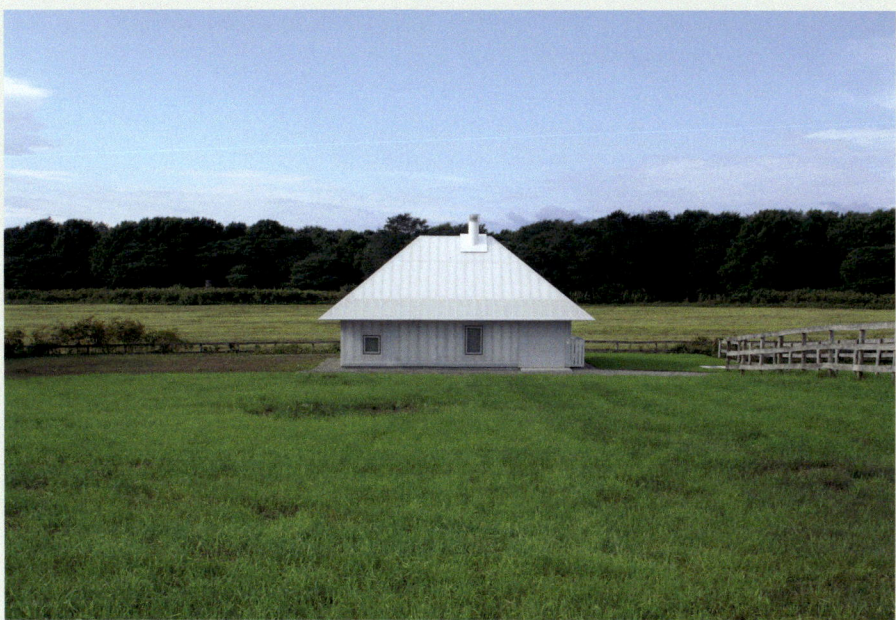

Figure 9.11 Landscape of Meme.

Meme is an experiment in housing design located on the 45-acre research facility called Meme Meadows, designed by architect Kengo Kuma (see Figures 9.11 and 9.12). The experimental house sought to explore design and material solutions to harsh, cold climates such as its location, Taiki, Japan. The designers applied vernacular inspiration to develop a housing prototype reliant on clean energy.

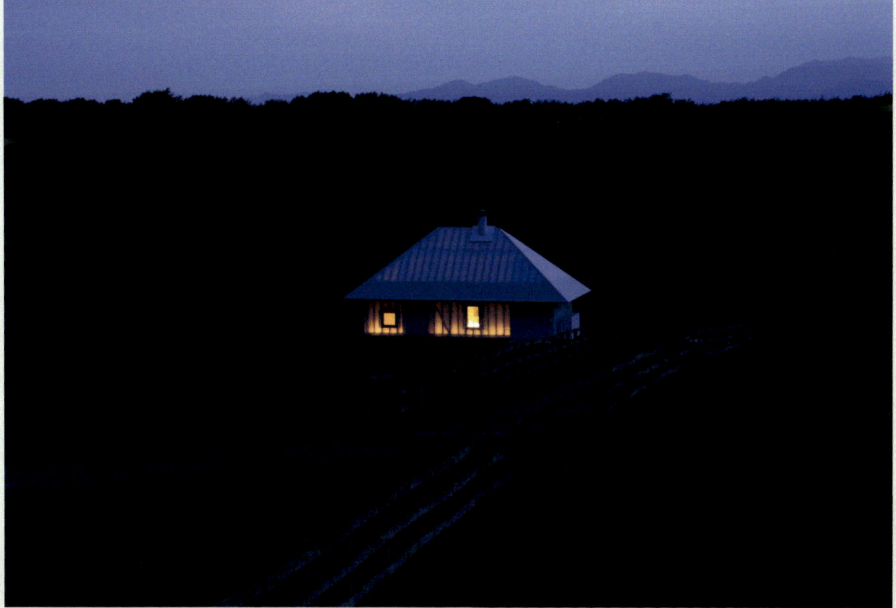

Figure 9.12 Meme at Night.

The experimental design approach, a whimsical approach to architecture, pushed circularity through "design for disassembly" and virtual monitors.

Many elements of the house take inspiration from a traditional home called a chise, used as a dwelling by the region's indigenous people, the Ainu (Jordana, 2013). A traditional chise has a rectangular plan and pitched roof and is thatched with straw. As an exterior material, straw has great insulating properties and provides a soft and slightly translucent façade. In taking inspiration from indigenous housing, Meme is a celebration of vernacular techniques that were adapted to the local climate based on generations of knowledge. Kuma and his team sought to replicate the transparency of the chise with modern and energy-efficient solutions, employing a membrane material as cladding and interior coverings (see Figure 9.13). A wood frame built from locally harvested larch trees was wrapped in the membrane material and then stuffed with polyester insulation made from recycled plastic bottles, a transparent insulating material (see Figure 9.14). The result is a home that is synchronized to the natural rising and setting of the sun, with daylight flooding the entire space. Another element inspired by the vernacular housing type is a geothermal floor heating system. Traditionally, Ainu people laid sleeping mats directly on the ground and used a burning fire to heat the earth through the night, which then released heat to the interior throughout the day (see Figure 9.15). A geothermal energy system is employed in this case along the same principles, harnessing the heat within the earth to heat the floors and, indirectly, the space. These design choices, inspired by the local vernacular architecture, promote circularity as they provide resilience to local weather conditions and reflect the local culture

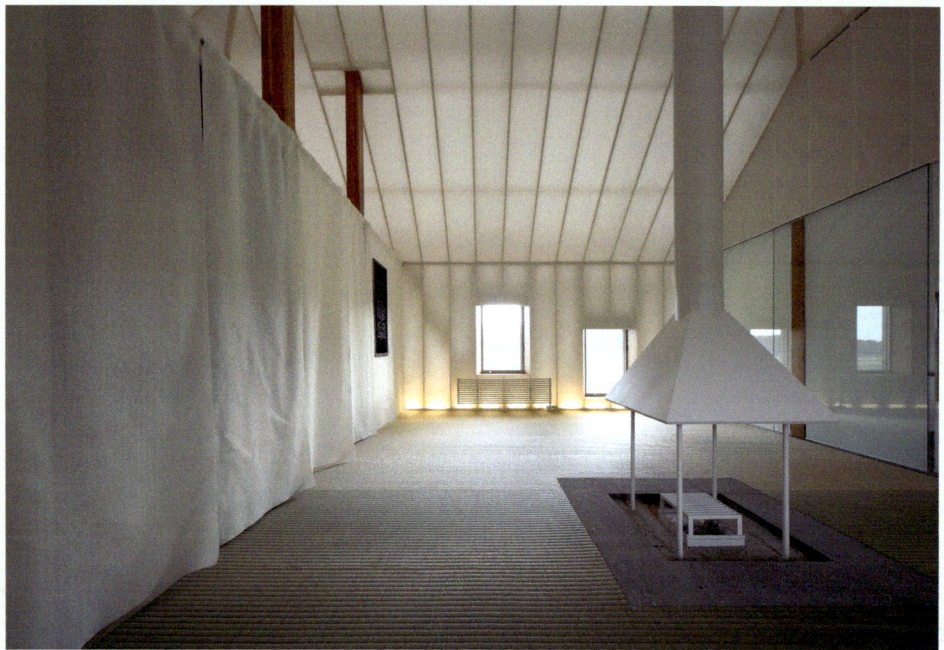

Figure 9.13 Interior of Meme.

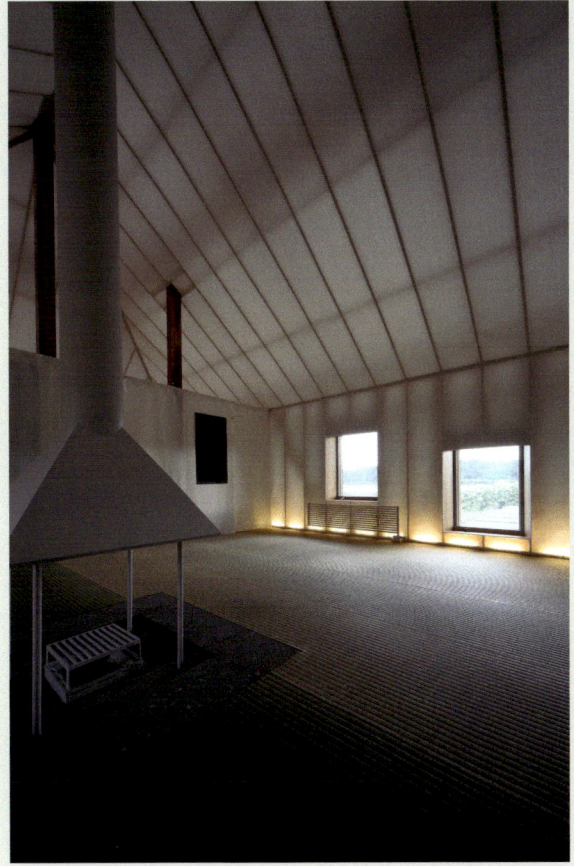

Figure 9.14 Ceiling of Meme.

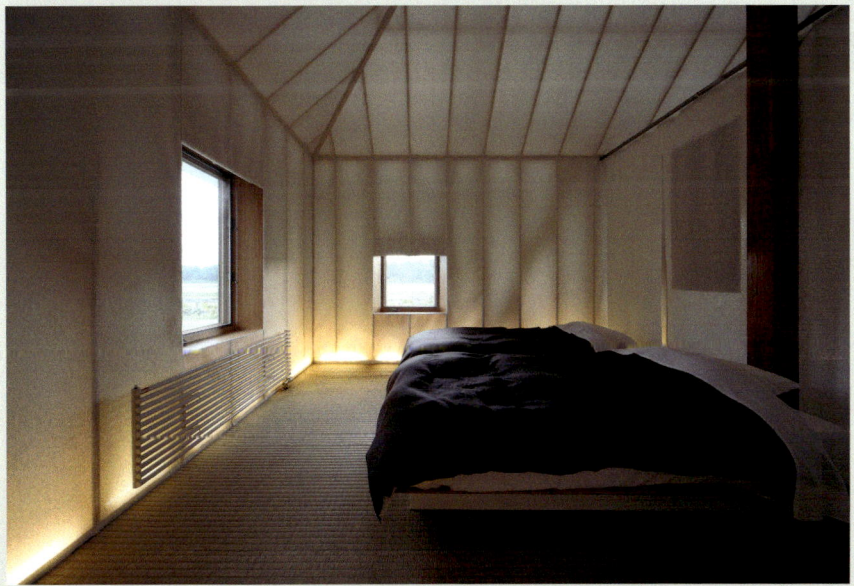

Figure 9.15 Bedroom of Meme.

(Dabaieh et al., 2021). Creating coherence with local traditions and climate **extends the life of a building** by minimizing maintenance and repair and prolonging the social relevance of the building that keeps them standing.

As the project was an experiment in material options in cold climates, Kengo Kuma and his team employed detachable elements to allow for testing of various materials. The interior wall coverings, made of a coated membrane material, are attached to the structure using only a Velcro-like "magic tape" (Yagi, 2012). This dry construction technique anticipates simple detachment that allows for the replacement of various wall-covering prototypes. Likewise, the windows are designed for disassembly. The structure is designed with openings that allow for the attachment of window frames to the exterior, allowing for quick and simple detachment that empowered the team to test different window frames. These systems, conceived in the building design, make renovations and replacements minimally invasive to the structure. This design-for-disassembly is another technique that can **extend the lifespan** of structures and products within a housing project, achieved by the firm in their goal of experimentation. The insulated window frames used in the project incorporate a device within the window sash to monitor exterior and interior climate conditions. This **virtual** tool aids the team in their tests by providing data on the conditions provided by different insulating and cladding materials, further driving the energy efficacy and climate responsiveness of the home.

The home's unique choice of materials pushes circularity while providing remarkable architecture. The transparent home appears magically illuminated at night and lets in diffused light from sunrise to sunset. Kuma sought to provide housing that, through transparency inspired by the vernacular, could allow residents to return to a dependence on natural light, waking with the slow rise of daylight. The experiment supports environmental sustainability through climate-specific passive techniques and alternative energy use and promotes cultural sustainability by celebrating local traditions and envisioning a space connected to the earth and to natural sun cycles.

9B

Project:
Deep Performance
Dwelling – Solar
Decathlon China

Locations:
Dezhou, China

Year:
2018

Team:
TeamMTL: McGill University
and Concordia University

**Mapping to Circular
Economy Framework:**

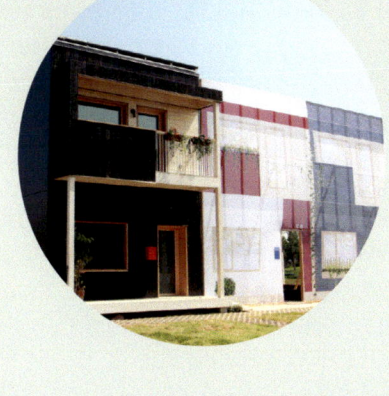

CIRCULAR ECONOMY PRACTICES

LIFE CYCLE PHASES — Recovery · Life Extension · Sharing Platforms · Service Models · Regenerate · Virtualize

LIFE CYCLE PHASES	Recovery	Life Extension	Sharing Platforms	Service Models	Regenerate	Virtualize
Work of Geobiosphere				●	●	
Sourcing	●					
Manufacturing	●					●
Design & Construction	●			●		●
Use	●	●	●	●		
End-of-Use						

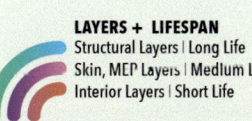

LAYERS + LIFESPAN
Structural Layers | Long Life
Skin, MEP Layers | Medium Life
Interior Layers | Short Life

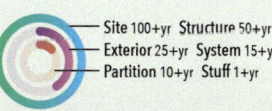

Site 100+yr Structure 50+yr
Exterior 25+yr System 15+yr
Partition 10+yr Stuff 1+yr

The Deep Performance Dwelling (DPD) is a single-family housing design that was developed by TeamMTL for the 2018 Solar Decathlon China, a global design competition to explore and advance sustainable housing solutions (see Figure 9.16). TeamMTL designed and constructed a prototype of a culturally responsive, net zero energy dwelling capable of operating in Montreal's harsh and varying climate with high-performance construction and a blend of passive and active systems (see Figure 9.17). The compact dwelling, inspired by typical Montreal row houses and the Chinese courtyard house, comfortably houses six people, with a flexible rear studio allowing for intergenerational living, live/work, or renting opportunities (see Figure 9.18; TeamMTL, 2018). The inclusion of a separate studio connected to a common courtyard allows for an extended useful life of the building while promoting community and collective living.

Material choices were considered to limit waste and stress on resources. Waste was reduced by sourcing **recycled** materials and manufacturing materials with high recycled content. For example, a central courtyard's wood cladding is 100 percent post-consumer recycled content, and the gypsum wall panels on the building's interior are composed of 90 percent post-consumer recycled content. The dwelling is constructed primarily from wood, a choice that encourages local tree planting and therefore carbon sequestration (see Figure 9.19). Another carbon negative material employed in the build is a cementless concrete made from industrial slag with

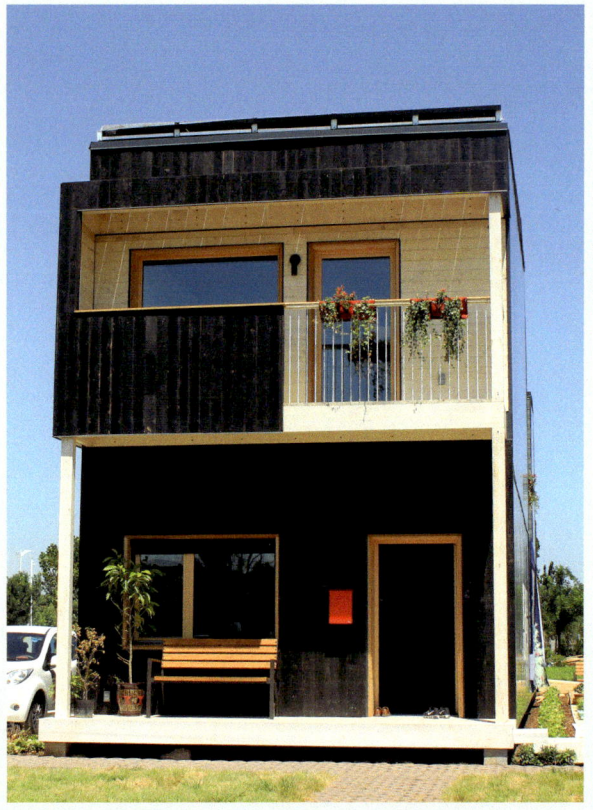

Figure 9.16 Front Façade of the Deep Performance Dwelling.

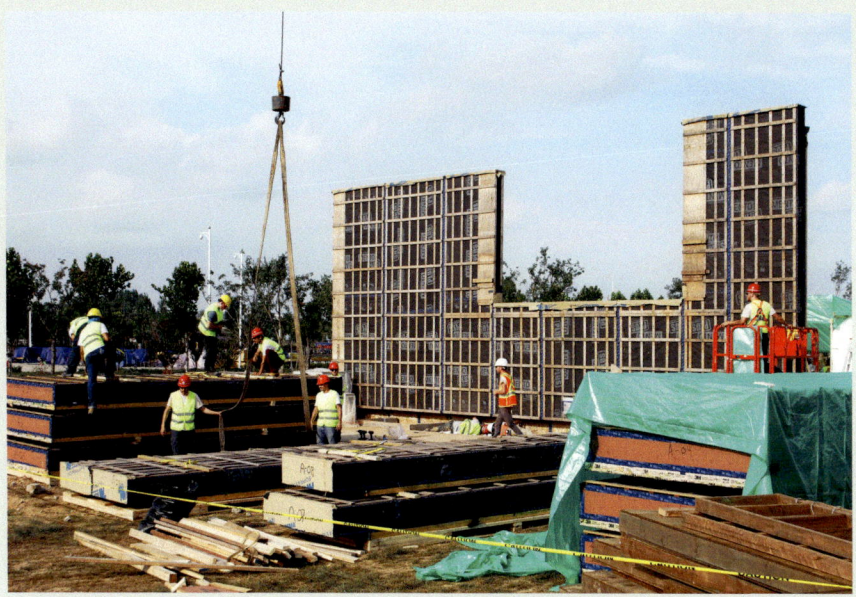

Figure 9.17 The Deep Performance Dwelling under Construction.

compressive strength coming from injected carbon dioxide which is permanently sequestered within the blocks; the two materials illustrate the possibility of **regeneration** of our geo-biosphere when building at a larger scale.

The DPD employs a super-efficient Passive House envelope constructed using panelized prefabrication made possible using a **digital** BIM model. A computerized

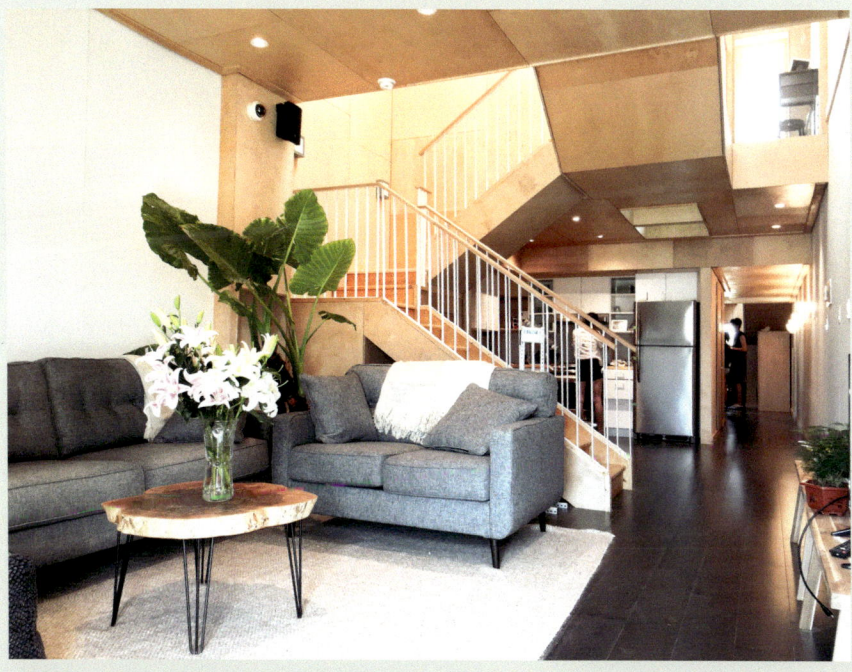

Figure 9.18 Interior of the Deep Performance Dwelling.

numerical control (CNC) machine was programmed according to the building's digital twin to cut the wood components of the thermal and structural frame, ensuring quality and performance of the envelope while reducing construction waste by 55 percent and carbon dioxide emissions by 43 percent (TeamMTL, 2018). This high-performing envelope was central to TeamMTL's design philosophy, as they aimed to reduce energy demand of the building through passive means before integrating active systems that can be costly and unpredictable. The Passive House principals applied to the construction of the envelope include superior airtightness, high levels of insulation, a mitigation of thermal bridging, and high-performance doors and windows. The bioclimatic strategies employed in the design include natural lighting and ventilation enhanced by the form the elevated courtyard space and careful placement of openings and shading devices to maximize winter solar gain and prevent overheating in summer.

These passive strategies are then coupled with efficient and architecturally integrated active systems to satisfy the energy demands of the dwelling and render it self-sufficient and resilient. Building integrated photovoltaic (BIPV) systems along with hidden maintenance areas are integrated with the form of the roof, which also facilitate rainwater collection in the courtyard used for irrigation and toilet flushing as illustrated in Figure 9.20. The DPD also features efficient ventilation and heating-cooling

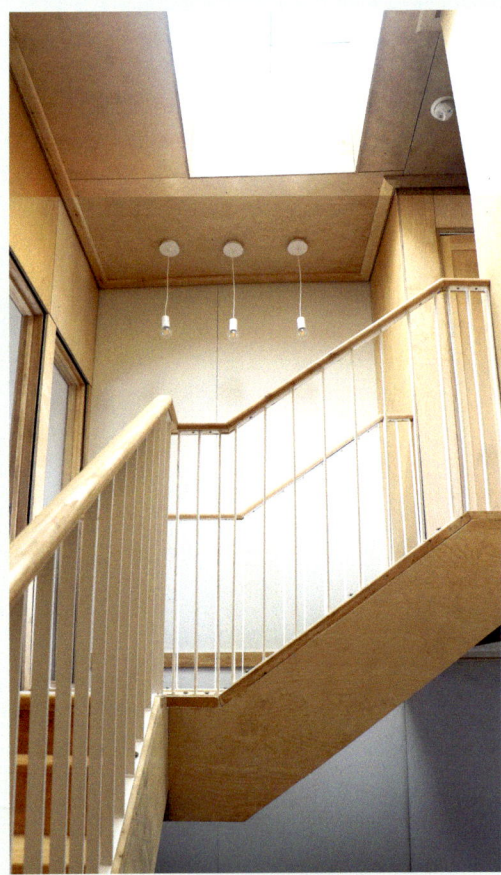

Figure 9.19 Stairway of the Deep Performance Dwelling.

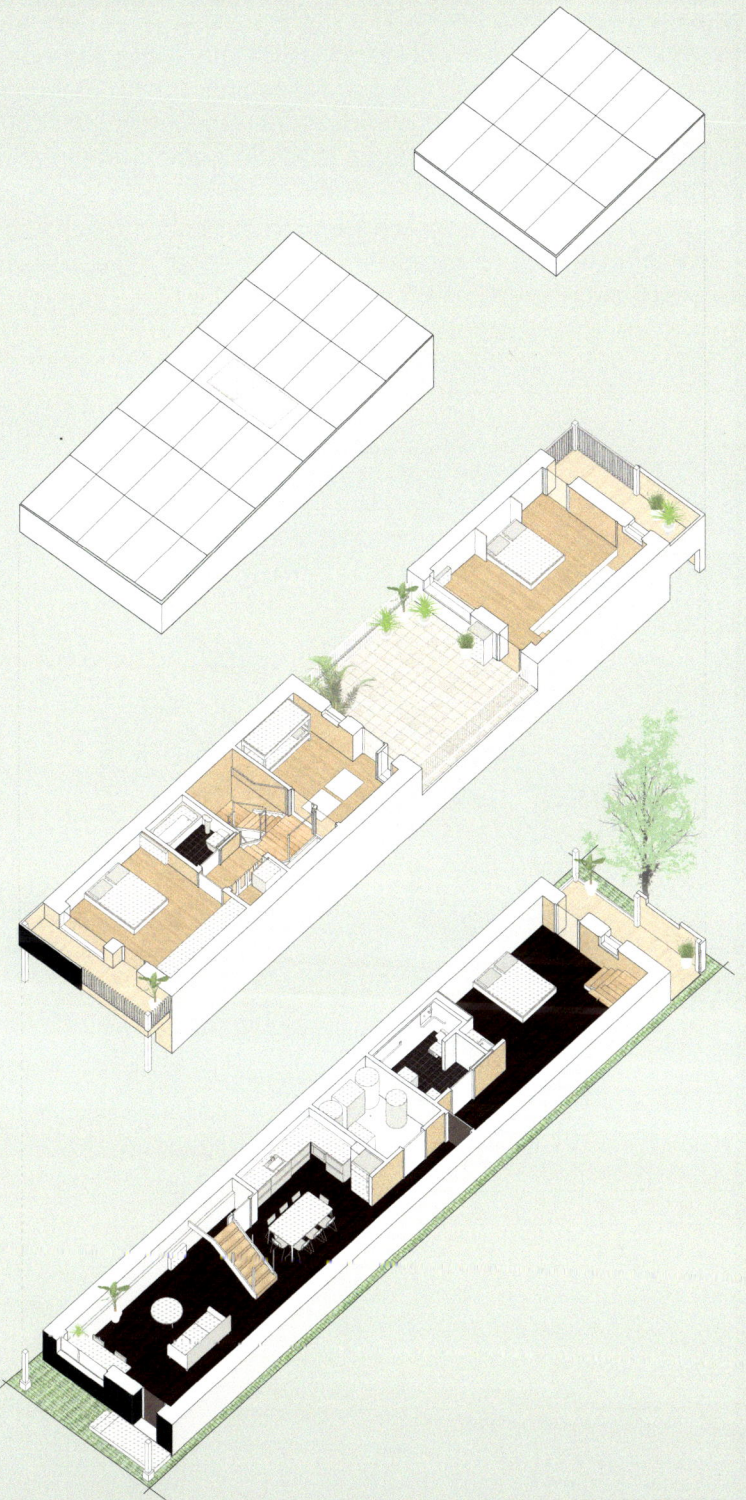

Figure 9.20 Schematic of the Building Integrated Photovoltaics (BIPV) Systems Installed on the Roof.

systems using energy recovery (TeamMTL, 2018). The net zero energy design is a result of the basic design, including material choice, construction techniques and form; passive energy systems; and mechanical equipment (Lechner, 2015). Together, these strategies result in a clean energy build that is capable of withstanding fluctuating temperatures and potential grid outages (see Figure 9.21). The design illustrates the potential of the circular economy **service model**, as the design has the potential to provide superfluous energy across the power grid to support surrounding buildings and assist with grid peak shaving. The team's concept of "deep-performance" speaks not only of the building's efficacy but also of its potential in form, flexibility, and resiliency to create community and the sharing of resources.

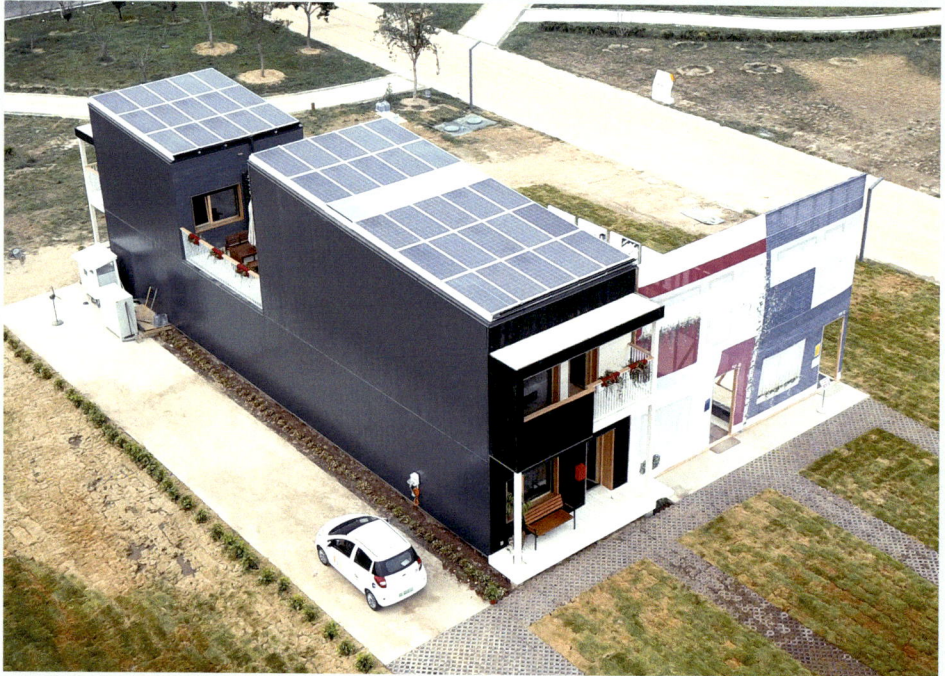

Figure 9.21 Ariel View Showing the Proposed Streetscape that the Deep Performance Dwelling Would Form within a Montreal Context.

9.6 Conclusion

This chapter examined circular operational energy use and found three main strategies that architects are encouraged to consider toward lowering operational emissions. First, using bioclimatic design strategies and vernacular-inspired design methods allows a new building to respond to its environment. Passive energy systems are designed in the building with special attention paid to the surrounding context of the building in order to regulate thermal comfort without superfluous mechanical systems. Second, when additional thermal, electrical, or lighting conditioning is required, renewable energy sources should be employed in most cases. However, just as the climatic context must be considered when designing a building, context must be considered when choosing where additional energy comes from. This context includes the embodied energy of the entire building, not just operational energy; decarbonization plans in place for the specific energy grid; and the degree of renewables and non-renewables in the composition of the current electricity grid mix. Nonetheless, choosing the right source of energy to power mechanical systems can significantly reduce operational emissions of a building. Indeed, while "net zero" homes are a commendable goal, the saturation of energy rating systems that value "clean" operational energy above all else is not always an accurate reflection of a building's genuine sustainability. Energy rating systems can serve as a helpful tool for comparing the operational energy use of buildings to each other, however, a more comprehensive measurement of energy is necessary. While climate-responsive design and renewable energy are valuable techniques, when new construction is underway, avoiding the use of more materials and construction is the most evident way to reduce operational energy use. This last strategy stresses dematerialization, referring to ideas discussed in previous chapters such as sharing space, designing for flexibility (see Chapter 8), and reducing the size of dwellings. The next chapter extends on technological tools and analysis, looking at data analysis, visualization, and computational tools to assess circularity in the building sector.

References

Beck, H. E., Zimmermann, N. E., McVicar, T. R., Vergopolan, N., Berg, A., & Wood, E. F. (2018). Present and future Köppen-Geiger climate classification maps at 1-km resolution. *Scientific Data*, 5(1), 180214. https://doi.org/10.1038/sdata.2018.214

Council of the District of Columbia. (2019). *D.C Act 22-583*. https://lims.dccouncil.us/downloads/LIMS/40667/Signed_Act/B22-0904-SignedAct.pdf

Dabaieh, M., Maguid, D., & El-Mahdy, D. (2021). Circularity in the new gravity—Re-thinking vernacular architecture and circularity. *Sustainability*, *14*(1), 328.

Department of Public Service. (2019). Report on Vermont renewable energy programs: A biennial report to the Vermont General Assembly. https://legislature.vermont.gov/assets/Legislative-Reports/2019-Renewable-Programs-Report-w-cover.pdf

Domonoske, C. (2018). California sets goal of 100 percent clean electric power by 2045. *National Public Radio*. https://www.npr.org/2018/09/10/646373423/california-sets-goal-of-100-percent-renewable-electric-power-by-2045#:~:text=California%20Gov.&text=The%20bill%20specifically%20requires%20that,%2C%20which%20is%20not%20renewable.

Frampton, K. (1993). Toward a critical regionalism: Six points for an architecture of resistance. In T. Docherty (Ed.), *Postmodernism: A reader* (pp. 268–280). Routledge.

Government of Canada. (2022). *Ratings and certification*. Government of Canada. Retrieved January 24 from https://www.nrcan.gc.ca/energy-efficiency/products/product-information/windows-doors-and-skylights/rating-criteria-and-standards/13978

GreenCape. (2014). *A catalogue of green building materials: A guide towards SANS 10400 XA compliance in the Western Cape*. Cape Town, South Africa. https://greencape.co.za/assets/Green-Building-Material-Catalogue-Final.pdf

Holihan, R., Keeley, D., Lee, D., Tu, P., & Yang, E. (2003). *How warm is an igloo*. BEE 453. https://ecommons.cornell.edu/bitstream/handle/1813/125/Igloo.pdf

Hydro Québec. (n.d.). *Power generation*. Retrieved January 24 from https://www.hydroquebec.com/generation/

IRP. (2020). *Resource efficiency and climate change: Material efficiency strategies for a low-carbon future*. International Resource Panel.

Jordana, S. (2013). *Même – experimental house/Kengo Kuma & Associates*. Retrieved January 23, 2023 from https://www.archdaily.com/322830/meme-experimental-house-kengo-kuma-associates

Keena, N., Duwyn, J., & Dyson, A. (2022). *Biomaterials supporting the transition to a circular built environment in the global south*. Yale Center for Ecosystems + Architecture and UN Environment Programme.

Keena, N., Aly Etman, M., Diniz, N., Rempel, A., & Dyson, A. (2016). *Towards a visualization framework to evaluate the emergy of built ecologies*. In Proceedings of the 9th Biennial Emergy Conference (pp. 127–142). Gainesville, FL: Center for Environmental Policy, University of Florida.

Lechner, N. (2015). *Heating, cooling, lighting: Sustainable design methods for architects* (4th ed.). John Wiley & Sons.

Murphy, D. J., & Raugei, M. (2020). The energy transition in New York: A greenhouse gas, net energy, and life-cycle energy analysis. *Energy Technology*, 8(11), 1901026. https://doi.org/10.1002/ente.201901026

Olgyay, V., Olgyay, A., Lyndon, D., Reynolds, J., & Yeang, K. (2015). *Design with climate*. Princeton University Press. http://www.jstor.org/stable/j.ctvc77kqb

Parliament of the United Kingdom. (2008). *Climate Change Act*. https://www.legislation.gov.uk/ukpga/2008/27/contents

Raugei, M., Keena, N., Novelli, N., Aly Etman, M., & Dyson, A. (2021). Life cycle assessment of an ecological living module equipped with conventional rooftop or integrated concentrating photovoltaics. *Journal of Industrial Ecology*, 25(5), 1207–1221. https://doi.org/10.1111/jiec.13129

Raugei, M., Leccisi, E., Fthenakis, V., Escobar Moragas, R., & Simsek, Y. (2018). Net energy analysis and life cycle energy assessment of electricity supply in Chile: Present status and future scenarios. *Energy*, 162, 659–668. https://doi.org/10.1016/j.energy.2018.08.051

RESNET. (2015). *Energy rating index performance path*. http://www.resnet.us/wp-content/uploads/archive/resblog/2014/06/EnergyRatings_FactSheet1_Final.pdf

TeamMTL. (2018). *A step-by-step guide to an energy efficient home in Canada: Requirements and how to achieve them*. https://www.teammtl.ca/

The World Bank. (2016). *Housing for all by 2030*. https://www.worldbank.org/en/news/
infographic/2016/05/13/housing-for-all-by-2030#:~:text=Providing%20people%20with%20
access%20to,scale%20investment%20in%20housing%20production

United Nations. (1998). *Kyoto protocol to the United Nations framework convention on
climate change.* https://unfccc.int/resource/docs/convkp/kpeng.pdf

United Nations. (2015). *Paris agreement*. https://unfccc.int/sites/default/files/english_paris_
agreement.pdf

United Nations Environment Programme & Global Alliance for Buildings and Construction.
(2020). *2020 global status report for buildings and construction: Towards a zero-
emission, efficient and resilient buildings and construction sector*. https://globalabc.org/
sites/default/files/inline-files/2020%20Buildings%20GSR_FULL%20REPORT.pdf

Watson, D. (2013). *Bioclimatic design* (pp. 1–30). Springer. https://doi.
org/10.1007/978-1-4614-5828-9_225

West, A. (2021). *What does the new energy label mean for you and your home? Which?*
Retrieved January 24 from https://www.which.co.uk/news/article/what-does-the-new-
energy-label-mean-for-you-and-your-home-aO4486G5DiYq

Yagi, Y. (2012). *Même – experimental house – même – experimental house*. Retrieved
January 23, 2023 from https://www.world-architects.com/en/architecture-news/reviews/
meme-experimental-house

PART 4

Fostering Circularity, Implementation Strategies and Tools

Chapter 10

Toward Circular Housing Knowledge

Virtualizing the Housing Life Cycle

10.1 Circularity in Housing Design Needs a New "Ten Books of Architecture": The Role of Virtualization in Circular Architecture

As climate pressures increase and material scarcity is imminent, innovation in systems thinking and whole-building life cycle approaches will be critical to helping ensure that built environments embrace a socio-ecological future. Transitioning to a future of low-carbon, circular housing requires the design of multi-beneficial design strategies that take a whole-building life cycle and a systems-thinking approach. Such an approach has the potential to enable multi-stakeholder engagement and cross-industry collaboration which are currently siloed in the building process. This process involves energy, material, and information flows at each of its phases from initial extraction of material to final dismantle and deconstruction. Virtualization (e.g., digital technologies and big data) has a role to play in helping to establish collaborative networks with efficient construction practices which track material, energy, and information flows across the building life cycle. However, managing interconnections between life cycle phases poses many challenges, including linking siloed streams of heterogeneous data, uniting various stakeholders, and necessitating intellectual agility to respond to societal, economic, and environmental shifts. And yet, the organization and communication of architectural knowledge are not a new concept. Vitruvius' "De architectura" (Ten Books on Architecture), c. 30–20 BC, did just that.

Long before the age of technology, visualization was prominent. Prior to the formalization of written language, pictures were used as a mechanism for communication. Even today, one of the most valuable means through which to comprehend data and make it more accessible is through data visualization. A picture can contain an abundance of information and can be processed much more quickly than words, independent of local languages. Leveraging this principle, in c. 30–20 BC Vitruvius' "De architectura", represents the first notable compilation of knowledge on the built environment. It covers a broad spectrum of knowledge ranging from the microscopic ingredients of concrete to connection details of masonry and timber structures, ventilation and heating systems, and the aesthetic configuration of pillars and columns to large-scale infrastructural artifacts, including roads, sewage and water systems and the layout of cities and defensive structures (Beetz, 2018; Rowland & Howe, 2001).

DOI: 10.4324/9781003333975-14

293

Vitruvius made manual copies, which accompanied information with illustrations and were widely propagated, thanks to printing technologies. He was able to convey his principles through a structured, rigorous, and standardized format. Through organization, documentation, and visualization, Vitruvius effectively generated knowledge of the built environment (see Figure 10.1).

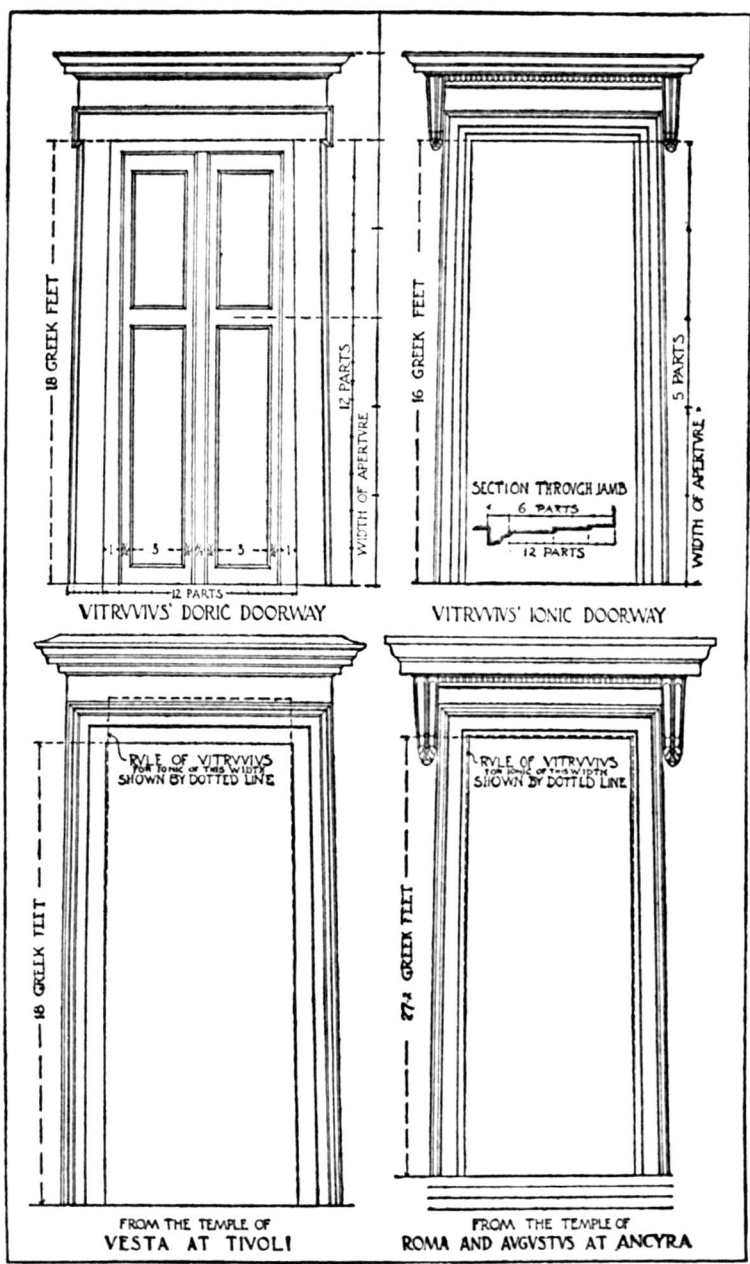

Figure 10.1 Vitruvius' Visualization and Rules for Doorways Compared with Two Examples, from De Architectura, c. 30–20 BC.

The system that Vitruvius employed to communicate concepts in his book has evolved and can be adapted to today's digital age to facilitate communication among housing industry stakeholders. This chapter will discuss the circular economy principle of "virtualization" and its role in organizing today's knowledge of our built environment while supporting the implementation of a more circular approach across the building life cycle.

10.2 Virtualization: A Key Principle of Circular Economy

The current building industry dynamic is highly fragmented. Buildings have long life cycles which rely on the interaction of various actors at various stages each of whom have different priorities and incentives. Adding to the complexity is the fact that due to these multiple actors and long lead times, there is rarely continuity of ownership and control. For example, an architecture firm that designs the building rarely has decision-making power at the end-of-use phase (Zimmerman et al., 2016). This complex building life span means fragmentation of building information is widespread within the building sector and acts as an inhibitor for innovation and major change. Previous chapters up to this point have stressed and proven the importance of a circular economy framework to reform the building industry toward environmental, social, and economic sustainability. A "life cycle approach" to design, for instance, conceptualizes and plans for the entire life cycle of a building at the onset, which requires stakeholders to have continuous communication and coordination along the supply chain to create a harmonious final design and ultimately a shared vision for a circular building. To achieve circularity thus requires stakeholders to have access to standardized in-depth building information, which currently does not exist. Indeed, unlike other large industries, the construction sector is made up of small, trade-based firms, as well as subcontractors. In Europe, for instance, less than one percent of all construction firms have more than 250 employees, yet these firms contribute to 21 percent of the industry's output (McKinsey Global Institute, 2017). This structure prevents firms from attaining the size required to achieve scale benefits and prevents coordination among different actors along the supply chain. The biggest culprit to this stunt in productivity, however, appears to be the construction sector's pointedly low levels of digitization. Over the past ten years, a sector's productivity growth and its level of digitization appear to be highly correlated, as depicted in Figure 10.2. According to a McKinsey Global Institute report of a digitization index, the construction industry is among the least digitized in the world, so it follows that it remains unproductive (McKinsey Global Institute, 2017). While there have been developments in robotics, three-dimensional printing, artificial intelligence, and biotechnology, construction companies continuously underinvest in technology that would allow productivity gains and lack synchronization among software platforms. Fragmentation of data limits productivity and causes major information asymmetries among actors. Thus, there is a need in the construction industry to employ virtualization to standardize housing data for increased material

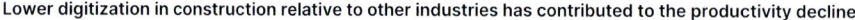

Lower digitization in construction relative to other industries has contributed to the productivity decline

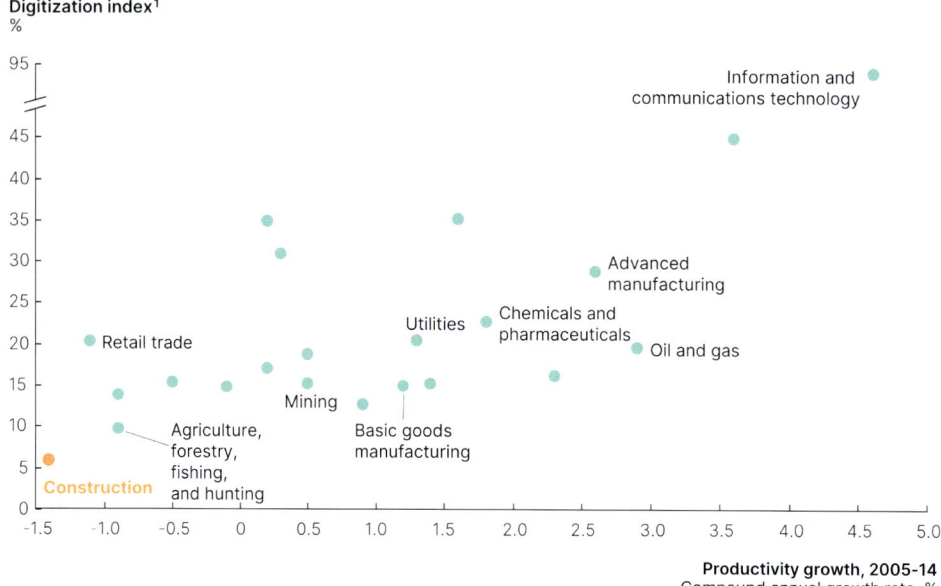

Figure 10.2 Correlation between Digitization and Productivity among Industries.

efficiencies and increased coordination, in order to plan for long-term circular sustainability (Issa & Olbina, 2015).

This chapter will flesh out the seventh tenet in our proposed circular economy framework from Chapter 3 – "Virtualize". Virtualize involves displacing resource use with virtual use. In the built environment, this can include replacing physical products and services with virtual ones. Replacing physical with virtual locations as well delivering services remotely (Zimmerman et al., 2016). Throughout this chapter we explain how virtualization can be achieved by leveraging advancements in digital technologies. First, there will be a description of how different digital tools function and how they can improve the construction sector. Particularly, virtualization can help aggregate data and foster communication which is needed for a life cycle approach to building. The next section goes through each phase of the building life cycle – design, sourcing, construction, operation, renewal, disassembly, and repurpose – and explains how virtualization can help achieve circularity at each phase, thus fostering a life cycle approach. While virtualization can help aggregate and organize data, the next step is transferring this knowledge to a range of relevant stakeholders who can then collaborate with one another to ensure a consistent circular economy approach is being done throughout a building's life cycle. This requires the creation of a so-called common language which uses semantics and web ontologies to categorize buildings and visualize data. The aim of this chapter is to highlight how virtualization can successfully be implemented in the building sector to achieve circular economy.

Circularity allows for connections throughout various stages of a building project. It brings stakeholders from various places and disciplines together, effectively replacing the industry's siloed approach to collaboration. However, many of these circular changes require virtualization. For instance, circularity of insights requires connecting digital tools – such as big data and smart algorithms – to the cloud, in order figure out innovative and effective solutions to highly complex design problems. Hence, circularity and virtualization go hand-in-hand and can help resolve the issue of fragmentation by making collaboration across diverse stakeholders easier.

10.3 Housing in the Cloud: Digitization and Virtualization Tools for a Digital Circular Marketplace

The lack of central procurement, standardized procurement tools, supply chain, logistics organization, and communication among relevant actors is detrimental to a circular economy in the building sector. Building information modeling (BIM), smart building materials, prefabrication, autonomous robotic three-dimensional printing, artificial intelligence, etc. – the development of technology shows the potential in transforming the construction industry in an effort to increase productivity and, ultimately, mitigate environmental impacts. By employing appropriate technology, companies can make construction more efficient, safe, and sustainable ensuring benefits across the value chain. Employing digital tools improves productivity by minimizing variability and waste. The specific tools and software are less relevant; the digitization of the building industry allows construction to be understood as a system, and therefore accessible for collaboration. Ultimately, virtualization supports visibility and transparency. In addition, given the long timespan of a building life cycle, virtualization can assist in providing knowledge about a building without the need for stakeholders to engage in order to retrieve that knowledge. In other words, in a building lifespan of 60 years, information about how that building was designed and constructed would be documented and not lost. Such knowledge can prove valuable during the use phase as well as at the end-of-use phase allowing a feedback loop in the building process and making the overall system more efficient and circular.

Digitization creates new opportunities by offering data relating to a product's condition, location, and availability (Antikainen et al., 2018). Digitization also enables new digital platforms and helps create new markets based on the virtualization of products and processes. Digital tools refer to tools that identify and create value. For instance, some of these tools can identify company spending by sorting historical data on invoices and material-cost indexes which allows industries to optimize their resource use and minimize profit lost. "Procure-to-pay" is another digital tool that employs quantities of order and invoicing data to create predictive order configurations and automatically identify potential suppliers, thus preventing leakages of value (McKinsey Global Institute, 2017). Virtual tools, such as 5D BIM, permit the "virtual twinning" of projects, which allow simulations of alternative conditions, allowing shared feedback among activities during a building's life cycle (Asdrubali & Desideri, 2019). Using light detection and ranging (LiDAR) laser scanners to create three-dimensional outputs has allowed near-perfect surveying and geolocation. Sensors and communication technology (such as the Internet of Things [IoT]) can track asset utilization and performance of construction assets and equipment (Hennemann Hilario da Silva & Sehnem, 2022). Moreover, digital and mobile collaboration embraces the involvement of consumers through intuitive and user-friendly applications that allow real-time collaboration and communication between producers and users. BIM is one example of an innovative digital tool. BIM allows for communication of information regarding all phases of a building. This is particularly useful as virtualization needs to be implemented throughout an entire life cycle in order to be effective (Antikainen et al., 2018). BIM – along with other digital tools that are explored in this chapter – promotes collaboration which, consequently, supports optimized designs and efficiency (Kensek & Noble, 2014). By making such tools accessible to all stakeholders along the supply chain, transparency in design, costing, and progress visualization are facilitated. When used effectively, digital trends have been shown to improve productivity by optimizing coordination and transparency.

Improving these digital tools incentivizes building more sophisticated procurement systems. In other words, just as digital tools help the organization and management of companies, as digital tools advance, computerized systems that companies may use for procurement processes need to match such innovation, which results in an overall improvement of a company or industry's management. Hence, advancements made in data processing technologies have led to systems which must ensure accessibility and transparency of building data acquired by such technologies. The question of procurement is key in a circular economy, as materials needed for a new building will come from secondary materials (reused, remanufactured, recycled, etc.). Consequently, the supply and demand model changes where the supply is not coming from extracted resources which have been produced into a new standardized building product. Hence, the tracking of secondary materials by companies for selling can be assisted via digital technologies which can also allow them to showcase their diverse inventory of secondary materials. This allows building management teams and architects to source the materials virtually and accordingly in a new circular marketplace. This will be discussed further in the next section regarding "sourcing" in a circular life cycle.

10.4 Designing the Housing Ecosystem: Circular Economy Design for Housing Involves Designing the Whole Housing Life Cycle

As discussed, in previous chapters, a life cycle approach is key to achieving a circular economy, meaning that each phase of a building life cycle must consider and achieve circularity principles for genuine sustainability to be met. Along these lines, to achieve circularity, interconnections among systems and stakeholders are required, which poses many challenges as this requires linking isolated heterogeneous data from various stakeholders and building phases. Virtualization of the built environment process (BEP), however, can facilitate this interdisciplinary collaboration in the building sector to achieve a life cycle approach to circularity. The circular economy framework, developed in Chapter 3, plays a significant role in achieving an ecosystem that distributes knowledge across life cycle phases (Keena et al., 2020). This collaboration across the building life cycle would enhance users' experiences of a building, since flexibility, interchangeability, and customization become easier when transparency of building data and construction characteristics are ensured (Wong & Yuen, 2011).

This life cycle virtual approach to the building process utilizes digital tools to bring opportunities to the whole value chain, from early design stages to end-of-use phases. This digital project model, which has been shown to be facilitated through blockchain technology and BIM, is a reliable tool to support the development and management of all phases of the construction process (Daniotti et al., 2020). Nonetheless, software that tracks a building's life cycle must be pre-planned and consider model content, level of detail, format, etc. so that this information can be used and understood by future stakeholders in the building value chain. Moreover, stakeholders need to continuously update data, accurately and comprehensively, all while coordinating with other stakeholders. As well, circular goals that relate to the end of the building's use need to be addressed at the very beginning of its design. For instance, optimizing disassembly and reuse from the beginning of the project will have implications on the operation, renewal, and repurposing of the building's components at the end (Crawford, 2011). If information on these circular goals, such as designs for disassembly, are not documented and shared for future end-of-use stakeholders to leverage, the building may easily be demolished without realization of the original design intent.

The circular economy framework, as outlined in Chapter 3, consists of a series of principles to be employed at various stages of a building's life cycle. It comprises the following tenets: *circular supply chain*, *recovery and recycling*, *product life extension*, *sharing platform*, *service model*, *regenerate*, and *virtualize*. These tenets reflect numerous goals and indicators of the 17 United Nations Sustainable Development Goals and discuss the role of data and technology, collaboration, climate action, economic growth, and health and well-being. *Virtualize* is inherently relevant to each life cycle stage; the incorporation of technology allows other tenets to be achieved. Displacing resource use with virtual use promotes circularity and should, thus, be aimed for in all stages of a building's life cycle. The following sections will go in depth on how virtualization can be implemented in each phase of the building process, and how this incorporation can improve productivity and efficacy to ensure a life cycle approach to construction.

10.4.1 Design

Designing a house goes beyond planning form, structure, and space. In order to reduce emissions, for instance, a building's operation and performance need to be carefully devised at its first stages. Energy-efficient principles, such as passive design (see Chapter 9), remodeling, reuse, and retrofitting abilities, must be designed at the beginning of a building process. Implementing certain circular economy framework models within a project's period of conception is key.

In order for the circular economy framework to be maintained throughout a building's life cycle, virtualization within this stage needs to be implemented. Using digital tools, mapping the design phases creates an archive of design decisions and analysis. Within a circular economy, open-source design may become standard practice, in which architects, engineers, and designers will share their designs and build on each other's work. This bank of knowledge facilitates project management through online platforms by integrating schematic design options, three-dimensional models, construction drawings, as well as site, climate, and performance analyses. Finally, most significantly, virtualizing the design phase allows for transparency within the team, allowing members to share data narratives or journeys with their clients and stakeholders. This open-source and transparent digital platform can help achieve other circular economy tenets such as *Regenerate* – the model focused on restoring natural capital – and *Product Life Extension* – the tenet focused on extending the lifespan of a building.

10.4.2 Sourcing

As discussed in Chapter 7, materials and their sourcing have become a rising issue in the construction industry. Given their carbon contents and emissions, the choice in building materials has serious environmental consequences. Currently, popular materials such as concrete, glass, and steel, and their extraction, are detrimental. Moreover, extracting materials is becoming more difficult as materials become scarce. Despite their associated issues, materials also have the potential to positively revolutionize the building industry and its environmental impact. There is a rising shift in the industry, as people opt for flexible, durable, and reusable components, as well as biomaterials. Therefore, the material sourcing stage of a project has a significant impact on subsequent stages and overall effect on the environment. Transforming the sourcing of building materials requires shifting from the extraction of raw materials, to using biomaterials, as well as modular and adaptable components. Virtualizing is required to produce such materials. For instance, concrete components could be transformed into new building modules, with the proper technology (Zimmerman et al., 2016). Moreover, digitizing sourcing through thorough documentation and tracking will enable design-for-disassembly.

Circular Supply Chain – the criteria focused on ensuring responsibility and sustainability – reforms the sourcing phase. As opposed to a linear approach, in which manufacturers are incentivized to extract virgin materials, value is made in a circular supply chain while avoiding the consumption of raw materials. This model intends for all aspects of a product to be reused or disassembled; thus, circularity is completed once a product's initial use is complete and enters into a new cycle. By implementing this criterion within the sourcing stage, houses would become true material banks – producing virtually no waste and maintaining a circular process. Virtualization can enable a circular supply chain through leveraging big data and embracing BIM for greater stakeholder engagement.

Open, accurate, and big data can support suppliers in accessing secondary materials as well as enhancing product life extension. The promise of big data is by leveraging access to a large volume of data organizations can gain valuable knowledge, all with minimal human intervention (Santos & Costa, 2020). Some examples of big data being employed in areas of manufacturing include demand forecasting for supply planning. While such demand forecasting systems are not in themselves new, there has been a significant shift due to the emergence of flexible, quick, autonomous, and scalable processes. This innovation allows suppliers to adapt to real-time changes in demand. Using such systems have shown increased performance in business and collecting and processing transactional data has resulted in more accurate and detailed facts. Hence, providing data analysis and rendering information more usable has resulted in superior management decisions. For example, the digitalization of the construction sector through the use of BIM technologies supports waste diversion, by monitoring and controlling material use, and alerting recycling and manufacturing companies in advance of the type and amount of construction renovation and deconstruction (waste) materials that will be transported to them (Baporikar, 2020; Chen et al., 2022). Assuming the construction and deconstruction processes are digitalized, using processes, such as demand forecasting, can assist suppliers in forecasting when local supplies will become available as part of an urban mining approach. Then in real time a supplier can track when the building is being deconstructed and the volume and types of materials available. Virtualization effectively transforms construction into a web of connections among teams, insights, outcomes, construction, assets, etc. (Casini, 2022). By connecting big data and smart algorithms to infinite computing power in the cloud, stakeholders are brought together, allowing them to collaboratively come up with innovative solutions and operate within a digital circular marketplace.

10.4.3 Construction

The construction phase involves multiple stakeholders making project management difficult. This phase is notorious for its slow pace and lack of productivity (McKinsey Global Institute, 2017). Within the context of a circular economy, the construction phase refers to the assembly of the building. Virtualization hold promise for the construction phase by promoting organization, effectively optimizing efficiency, and reducing waste via technology in the fabrication of buildings off-site in a controlled facility. In particular, digital mapping allows organization of construction teams. Web-based platforms allow the live footage of construction sites to be uploaded in order to promote on-site safety, site management, waste reduction, and carbon abatement. The result is a project with a more holistic organizational system. Digitalization in the construction process toward prefabrication and modular construction has also been proven to reduce waste be 23–100 percent (Chen et al., 2022; Jaillon et al., 2009; Lu & Yuan, 2013).

Virtualization overlaps many of the other circular economy framework tenets. For example, *Sharing Platform* – the principle focused on the sharing of space and/or services for a more efficient and socially sustainable environment – is useful in off-site construction where the use of controlled construction facilities and digital fabrication equipment can be shared among contractors and designers. Spaces known as "fab labs" (digital fabrication laboratory) are examples of this. The Fab Foundation is a network of fab labs worldwide with a creative community of fabricators, artists, scientists, engineers, educators, students, amateurs, and professionals alike, across more than 100 counties (The Fab Foundation, 2023). They range from community labs to advanced research centers. The goal is to democratize access to tools for technical innovation and the sharing platform principle is key to this. Figure 10.3 illustrates a robotic arm for digital fabrication in Autodesk's BUILD (Building, Innovation, Learning, Design) space in Boston which is a research and development fabrication facility focused on the future of the building industry.

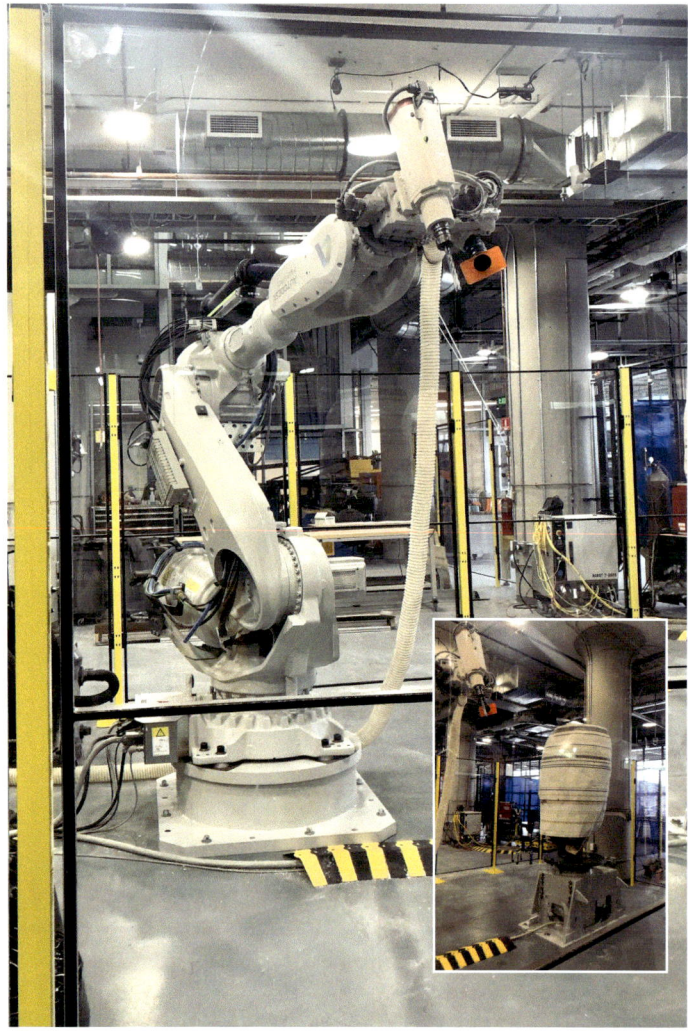

Figure 10.3 Digital Fabrication at the Autodesk BUILD Space in Boston, Massachusetts.

10.4.4 Operation

When a building is in use, its operation is critical regarding its effect on the environment (see Chapter 9). Ideally, buildings would be net producers of renewable energy that can meet the demands of the operational consumption. This may require on-site integrated building systems which capture and transform renewable energy into electricity or other usable means. It also requires the structure, systems, and components to be regularly managed using preventative maintenance techniques. In order to render housing operation more sustainable, circular models need to be implemented, which require the help of digital tools. Managing and mitigating the effects of a house's operational phase can be made possible by low-energy and low-cost sensor technology that helps reduce costs, minimize disruption, and maximize the useful life of the building and its fittings (Zimmerman et al., 2016).

The *Sharing Platform* tenet is pertinent for the operational use of a house, as it encourages treating space as a resource to converse. By making space co-livable or by converting a restaurant into a co-workspace by day and restaurant by night, for instance, the operational use can be shared. Intensive use of spaces is a circular economy principle and virtualization can assist in implementing this. For example, in many co-working environments the availability of spaces can be communicated via a web application so users can decide where they want to work from. The *Service Model* – which prioritizes careful consideration of resources and technology and can also be facilitated by a user-friendly virtual platform – relates to the operational phase of a house, as the use of space can be optimized and conserved. For instance, homes or rooms can be rented or shared, effectively considering energy. Energy consumption for lighting, heating, cooling can be connected to IoT and easily controlled and monitored from an occupant's smart phone (see Figure 10.4). Any on-site electricity generation can also be tracked and displayed using a data visual analytics environ-

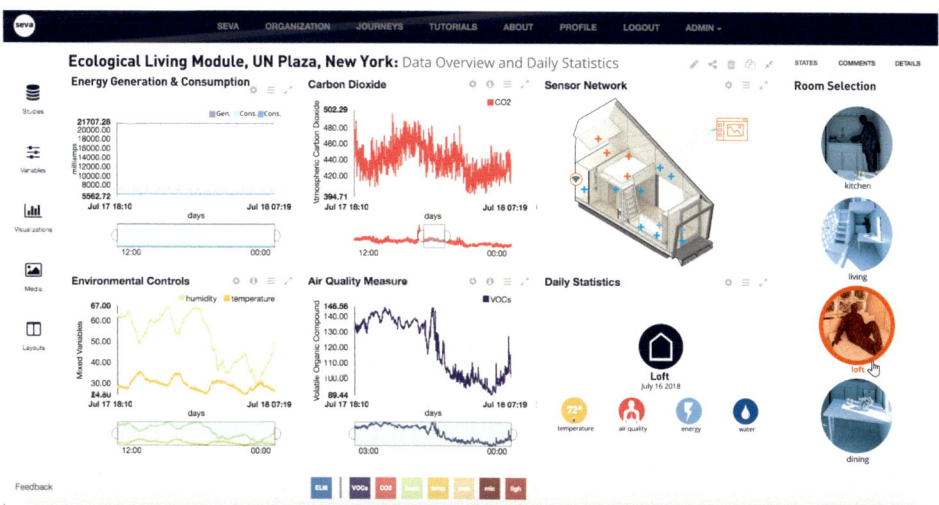

Figure 10.4 Tracking the Operational Phase of the Ecological Living Module Home with the Visual Analytics Environment SEVA.

mental similar to Socio-Ecological Visual Analytics (SEVA) illustrated in Figure 10.3, in order to compare the electricity being generated with that being consumed in an attempt to meet net zero energy demand. Any excess electricity generated which can be sent back to the utility grid can easily be tracked and visualized with the use of such technologies. Sensors and thermostats can regulate energy use and prevent its superfluous use. Additionally, employing sensors in products offers proactive maintenance which can ultimately support building life extension.

The *Regenerate* model is applicable to the operational phase as its consideration in the design phase aims to avoid the use of fossil fuels for heating and cooling needs that cause environmental overloading. Understanding the relationship between the natural, built, and social systems is key in determining how operation affects the environment. Many forms of virtualization can assist in achieving circularity in the operational phase.

10.4.5 Disassembly

The disassembly phase of a building represents a fundamental role, as it is capable of transforming buildings into material banks, which is a central goal of a circular economy. New construction details are emerging to allow for the easy dismantling of buildings. These are discussed in Chapter 8. Digital tools can help. For example, in many cases an intermediary piece (i.e., the sacrificial lamb of the detail) is needed which becomes the element that may end up in waste at the end-of-use but which serves to retain the value of the large component elements. Currently, in a linear model, many of these larger component elements and materials end up in landfill. These intermediary connection parts can often be 3D printed if a connection is particularly complex. Designing these details and documenting them can allow for knowledge sharing of how circular detail design is evolving in architectural and engineering practices. Although many of these practices, particularly in carpentry, have been perfected in Japanese construction for decades. Certain digital tools facilitate the extension and recovery of building components. Primarily, digital models allow stakeholders to easily model the dismantling of a building, and the redesign of its materials and component parts in a new build.

10.4.6 Repurpose

Finally, repurposing represents the final phase of the building process. The culmination of circular economy principles in the previous stages, along with large amounts of planning, allows for repurposing to be achieved. Digitization is essential to the repurposing of building materials in order for them to be tracked. BIM models coupled with visual analytics platforms can carefully track and record materials throughout a building's life cycle (see Figure 10.5) (Keena et al., 2020). By establishing value networks and second-use strategies ensures that all components are adequately used in additional industries. Technology minimizes the value lost and

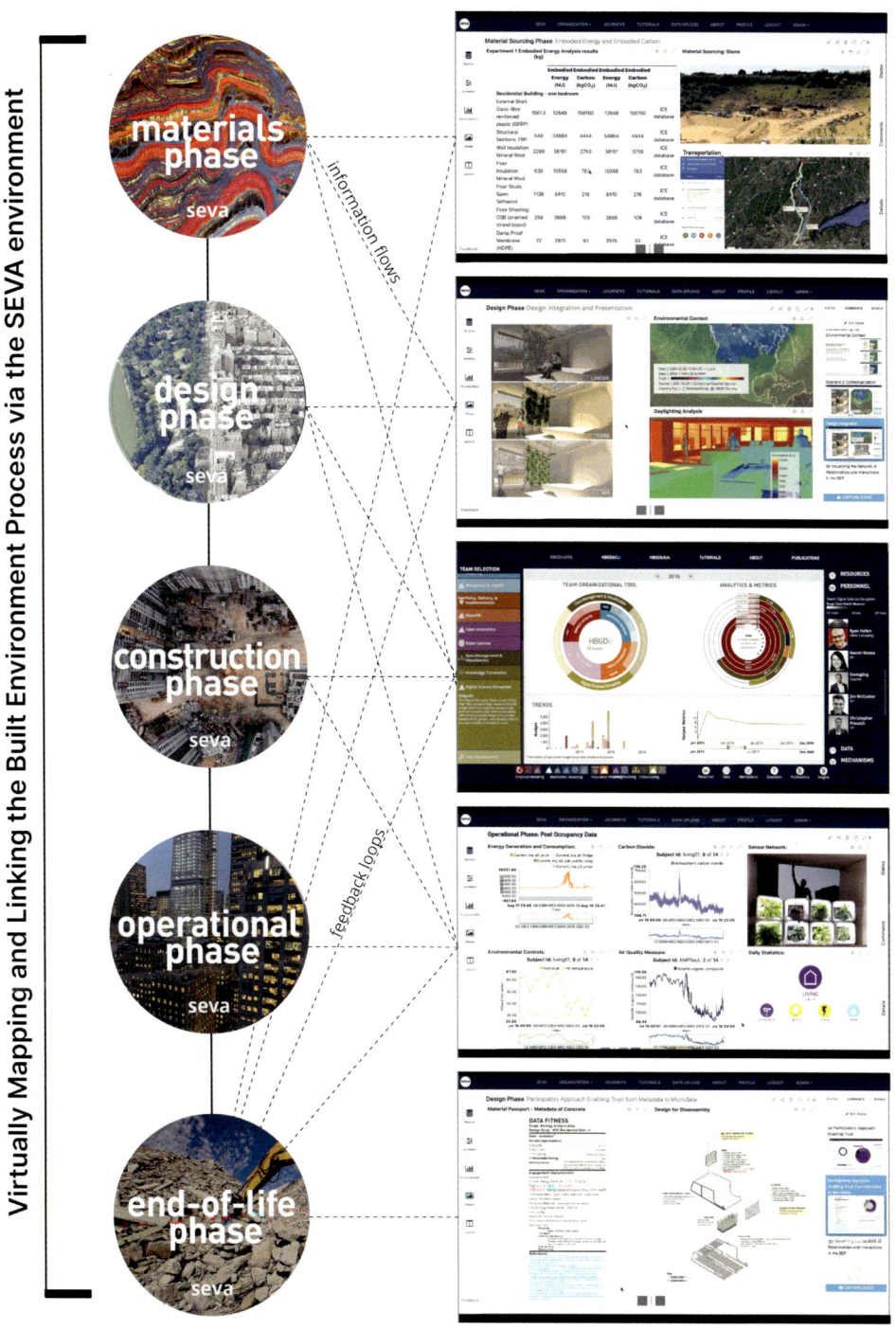

Figure 10.5 Visualizing the Whole Building Life Cycle with Virtualization Enabling a Digital Connection between All Phases and Its Stakeholders.

ensures numerous repurposing cycles (Baporikar, 2020). Recycled materials, combined with three-dimensional printing for example, enable the repurposing of waste (Sobh, 2008). Moreover, as stated in sourcing as we come full circle, digital models can be employed at the end-of-use phase to monitor the number of materials sent for reuse of recycling, which gives advanced notice to relevant companies, effectively allowing for planning of incoming stock.

The integration of all phases of the project's life cycle requires collaboration among all relevant actors and knowledge management. In order for circular principles to be effectively implemented in the housing sector, real-time connection is necessary between physical and digital layers. Beyond a building's life cycle, the circular model requires a building's construction to be integrated with the resource and reuse cycles of other industries. Hence, employing technologies allows for integration among all realms of building.

10.5 Speaking a Common Language: Breaking Down Siloes in the Building Industry via "Intelligent" Housing Semantics and Ontologies

As is depicted throughout this chapter, digital technologies can help housing stakeholders make smart decisions that enable a circular economy. Given the many stakeholders and disciplines in the housing industry, there is a challenge with sharing data. Interdisciplinary collaboration and the sharing of information among disciplines are vital for the participation in a circular building life cycle. The sharing of data across stakeholders generates large amounts of multivariate data, which can pose as an issue as it creates different understandings of possible relationships between variables and their relevance to problems. However, technology offers a means to assist in making information accessible and shareable. This calls for our communication methods to be reconsidered and digitalized, in order to yield a "common language".

Today, structured vocabularies are playing an increasingly important role. Intelligent functionalities in automation systems and interoperability in information exchange processes require machine-readable formalization of knowledge. Moreover, accounting for relevant data requires a dedicated ontology that is both human and machine readable. Within semantic data, ontologies provide structured formal names and definitions for the types, properties, and relationships of the entities expected within a particular knowledge domain.

10.5.1 Ontologies

In its classical philosophical meaning, ontology refers to a study of being and a discourse on "that which is" (Beetz, 2018). Ultimately, the intention behind creating an ontology of one's data is to document one's viewpoint and biases, making others aware of them when using the data. Within the realm of technology and information science, ontology refers to explicit specification of a conceptualization. It seeks the classification and explanation of entities by showing the properties and relations between a set of concepts and categories in a domain. Both classically and technically, ontology includes dictionaries and relates concepts to one another through logically defined relationships.

Ontology provides a representation of a subject area such as its properties and how they are related. It does this by defining a set of concepts and categories that represent that subject area. The representation of a single building component can be achieved through various categories (see Figure 10.6). For example, a column

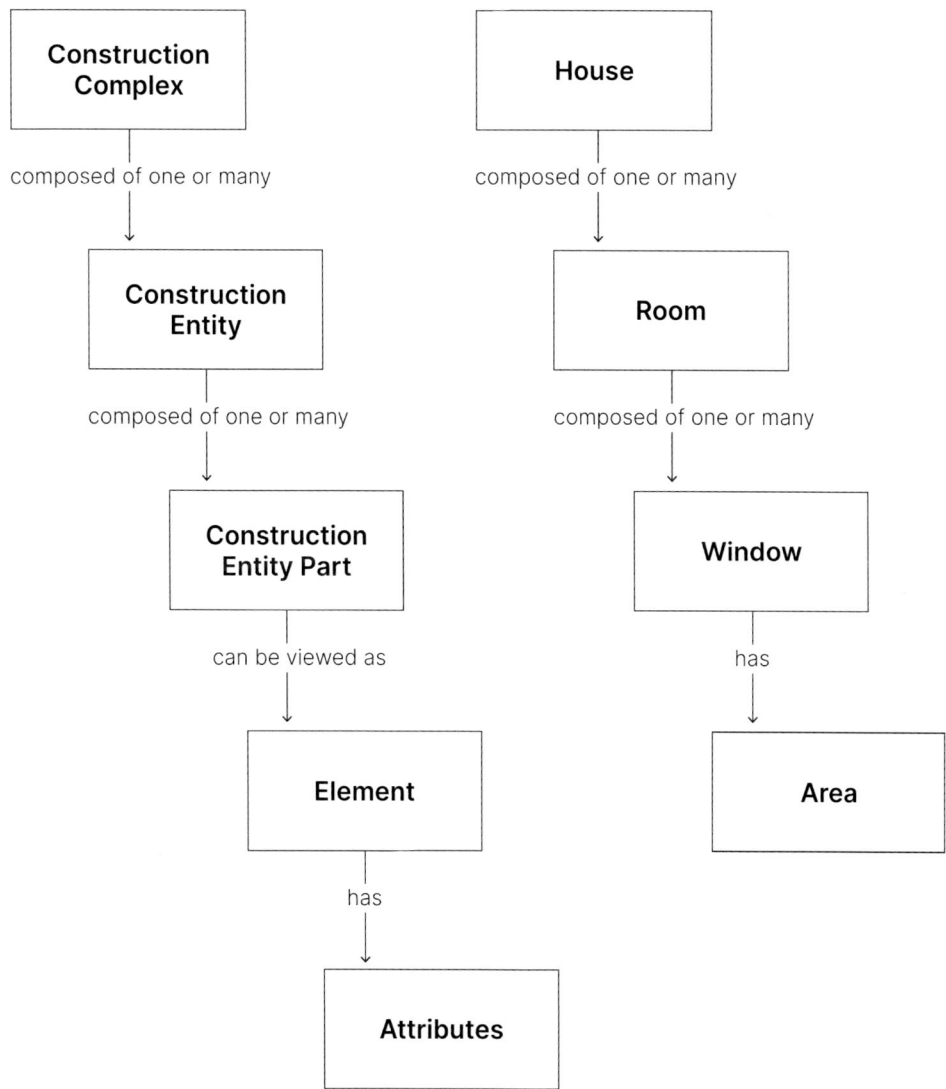

Figure 10.6 Illustrating the Semantic Linking and Meaning of Data and Metadata via Tree Structure of Classes and Their Subclasses Using a Housing Example.

can be defined as load bearing (according to function), cylindrical (form), vertical (orientation), concrete (material), or structural versus architectural (domain). The types of axes and discriminators are what determines a building's classification. The multiple connections made among nodes create a tree structure or a graph that can continuously grow and evolve as more properties (or nodes) about that subject emerge. In the 1950s, a classification of functions, elements, and processes in building was proposed by the Swedish committee for building matters and still remains as the basis for current classifications, such as OmniClass and UniClass (Beetz, 2018).

By understanding information through ontologies, aspects and relationship types can be represented using a common model. There are formal logic principles underlying ontologies. Thus, the benefit of using a standardized model to understand and classify information is that it can generate further connections and information (without human intervention) that is both human and machine readable. Ontologies can be checked for consistency using the underlying logic, allowing new facts to be inferred based on statements of facts (axioms). For example, "all buildings have walls", "a house is a building" "all houses have walls". Moreover, a multitude of formal logics and languages are available, which can generate knowledge models of varying complexity.

10.5.2 *Semantics*

There is a longstanding fundamental issue with structuring knowledge and information for automated processing regarding the heterogeneity of representations. Over time, various vocabularies, classification systems, conceptual models, and ontologies were created based on different modeling languages, data formats, and interfaces. This led to challenges, especially in the building industry, in terms of exchanging semantically unambiguous information. Recent attempts have aimed to combat this heterogeneity.

Web ontologies allow data and metadata to be aligned, integrated, and semantically annotated. A web ontology is a semantic web language aimed to represent complex knowledge about things, groups of things, and most importantly relations between things (McGuinness & Van Harmelen, 2004; OWL Working Group, 2012). Semantic web technologies enable combined acquisitions of data and metadata to manage, organize, semantically annotate, and link domain-related data and metadata into a knowledge graph. Knowledge graphs are used to support flexible representation, which can support improved understanding and data analysis in similar settings (Pinheiro et al., 2017, 2018). Metadata (data about data) is encoded to the data using semantic web technologies and this enhances the data by providing a rich collection of contextual knowledge.

The semantics (i.e., meaning) of a concept can be captured in layers of increasing complexity. For effective sharing along the value chain, data needs to be open and linked. Linked data is a semantic method of storing information and relating it to other data (Schiuma & Carlucci, 2018). Semantic data can be used to identify and detangle information by determining if it is the same or different from another piece of information. This is done by linking it to an established authority record. Elements within semantic data are referred to as entities as they represent "things" existing within the world. Each entity – including objects, persons, places, dates, events, and concepts – is established as being "unique" by assigning it to a unique resource identifier (URL). To achieve large-scale harvesting and analysis of data, not only do individual data sets need to be produced, but they must also be translated to linked data using a common descriptive language. Figure 10.7 illustrates this concept for the modernist iconic home Ville Savoye designed by renowned architect Le Corbusier and located in Poissy a suburb of Paris in 1931. The semantic representation of this house as subject shows its name, the architect, the location, the geolocation. This can continue to grow, where numerous heterogenous aspects of a house can be represented – its energy use, its carbon footprint, its materials, its construction, its owner(s), its sale price, its current value, its mortgage details, etc. Essentially, it is similar to a social network but instead of the information being about a person, it is about a house – a new societal network. This flexible means of gaining knowledge about a house can greatly enhance the possibility of a circular economy where information about the house can be used to extend its life, support regenerative approaches, and allow for recovery at end-of-use.

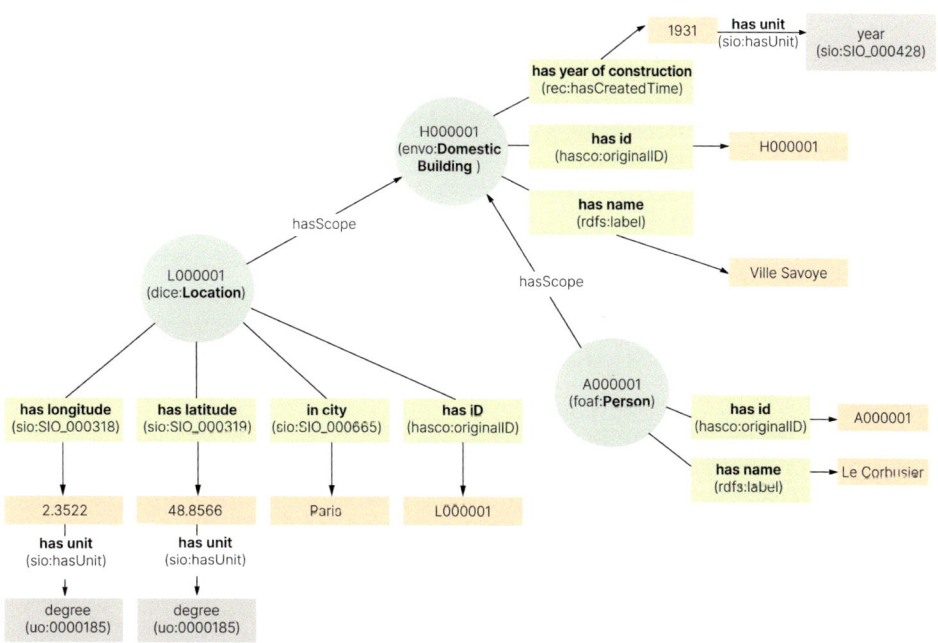

Figure 10.7 A Sample of a Knowledge Graph Representing Ville Savoye (1931) by Le Corbusier.

The main idea is for standardized, generic means of modeling and representing of information. This would facilitate uniform, decentralized, linking of resources in a global network. Some frameworks, such as the resource description framework (RDF), capture statements in any model, including a subject, predicate, and object. By identifying components with a uniform resource identifier (URI), they can be distributed and linked across internet network structures (Beetz, 2018). This allows for the reuse of concepts, properties, models, and data across domain boundaries, effectively promoting access and transparency.

10.5.3 Structuring Building Information in a Circular Economy

With the help of both ontologies and semantics, a "common language" can emerge that effectively allows building information to contribute to a circular economy. Ontology provides the vocabulary for a semantic web, and semantics provides a common framework that enables sharing data. There is a need to transition from an industrial economy into a knowledge-based one, which requires data-to-knowledge frameworks capable of decoding complexity. Mapping the BEP is achievable through knowledge frameworks that have been designed to link heterogeneous data. An example of a knowledge framework is the SEVA, which uses web ontology language and semantic web frameworks to generate a knowledge graph of the BEP (Keena et al., 2020).

SEVA's data knowledge framework maps the BEP from material extraction, all the way to the building's end of use (Keena & Dyson, 2017; Keena et al., 2020). Figure 10.4 conveys this life cycle perspective that SEVA takes on. SEVA effectively links heterogeneous data by enabling the comparison across a far greater range of heterogeneous data types and analysis techniques across multiple scientific and sociodemographic categories and scales – from metadata to microdata. Following the principle of semantic web, this framework provides a common toolkit to allow sharing and representing data across multiple types, formats, applications, and pre-existing frameworks (see Figure 10.8). Through an interactive dashboard, users can juxtapose and recombine the data and data analyses across diverse studies, variables, methods, and participants. Ultimately, the goal is to facilitate inquiries to provide answers to the Why, How, Who, and What questions by reconciling, integrating, and visualizing data, as well as facilitating interaction with data.

Overall, SEVA aims to facilitate the acquisition of unanticipated and disruptive insights and discoveries, by virtually connecting each BEP phase and associated stakeholder. The system acts as an overview tool, facilitating decision-making at each stage of the building's life cycle. SEVA proposes an environment in which multiple data streams allow for a comprehensive analysis of built ecologies, human systems, natural environments, technological environments, and human data (Aly Etman et al., 2020). SEVA demonstrates how the tenet of virtualization can be employed

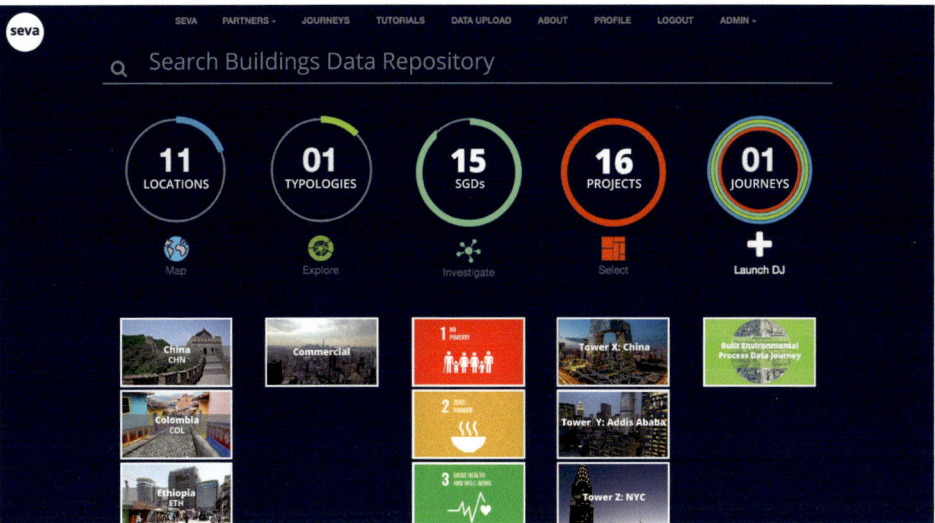

Figure 10.8 Visualizing and Querying the Buildings Data Repository in SEVA with a Range of Building Projects Filtered by a Variety of Factors.

throughout the life cycle of a building to foster transparency and efficiency between building stakeholders.

Ultimately, to achieve a circular economy, employing ontologies and semantics assists in classifying buildings. By utilizing digital tools to track carbon, energy, and material flows, for instance, the concept of the building is surpassed. Instead, the building is understood as a system which undergoes energy journeys and material transformation in its initial construction and future disassembly. Hence, by breaking a building down into data and linking datasets, our understanding of the building can transcend physical and local barriers. Concepts, such as the Housing Passport proposed in Chapter 4 of this book, require a building's information to be thoroughly shared and verified. A nesting structure is crucial for classifying data and requires proper managing of interconnections among systems. For a building's passport to be comprehensive, it needs to integrate separate disciplinary data, concepts, theories, and methods, to provide an interdisciplinary understanding of complexity. Moreover, sophisticated analytic systems are required for large-scale, interactivo, and insightful analyses. For all of this data and relationships to be digestible, they need to be visualized; visualization provides an ease in understanding that offers a quicker route for decision-making.

10A

Project:
Data Homebase

Location:
Montreal, Canada

Year:
2021

Team:
McGill University's Circular
Homebuilding

**Mapping to Circular
Economy Framework:**

CIRCULAR ECONOMY PRACTICES

LIFE CYCLE PHASES

Recovery · Life Extension · Sharing Platforms · Service Models · Regenerate · Virtualize

Work of Geobiosphere

Sourcing

Manufacturing

Design & Construction

Use

End-of-Use

LAYERS + LIFESPAN
Structural Layers | Long Life
Skin, MEP Layers | Medium Life
Interior Layers | Short Life

Site 100+yr   Structure 50+yr
Exterior 25+yr   System 15+yr
Partition 10+yr   Stuff 1+yr

Data Homebase is a web application to visualize Canada's Housing Passports. It started at McGill University's School of Architecture as part of the Circular Homebuilding team under the guidance of Professors Naomi Keena and Avi Friedman. This project utilizes the power of data technology and the **virtualization** pillar of the circular economy framework to detail circular economy characteristics of housing materials, components, products, and composition. Figure 10.9 shows multi-variant design layouts of Data Homebase. To achieve circularity and sustainability requires a combination of building choices to work in congruence with one another. It is not enough to merely choose recycled materials, renewable energy sources, or energy-efficient mechanical systems on its own to achieve sustainability. Rather, a detailed acknowledgment of every aspect of a building's construction, its ability to be easily disassembled, and contextual factors need to be addressed before the erection of a building. This becomes difficult with scattered data. By standardizing housing data, communicating exactly how a building was able to achieve its sustainability will help architects design sustainable buildings with a whole-building life cycle perspective in mind, as well as allow multiple stakeholders to compare levels of sustainability between projects.

The web-based prototype has five key sections accessed on the top navigation bar: Housing, Toolkit, Materials, Case Studies as shown in Figure 10.9. The Housing tab presents a housing map, showing the affordability measurement, energy performance, and embodied carbon of dwellings in a number of Canadian cities. The information is presented on an urban, neighborhood, and building scale; Figure 10.10 shows the

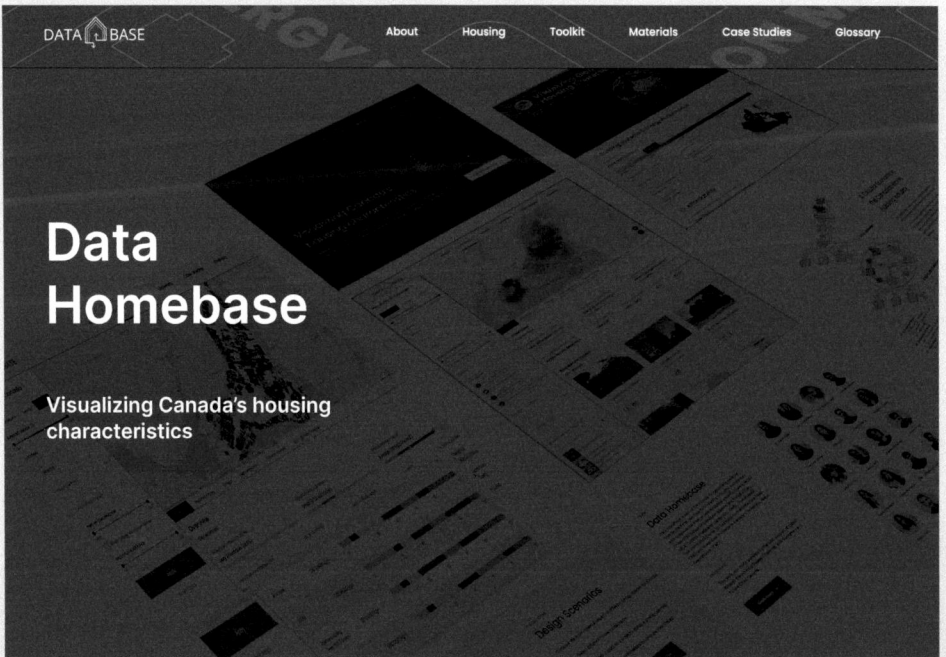

Figure 10.9 Data Homebase Aims to Visualize Canada's Housing Characteristics to Foster a Circular Economy in the Homebuilding Industry.

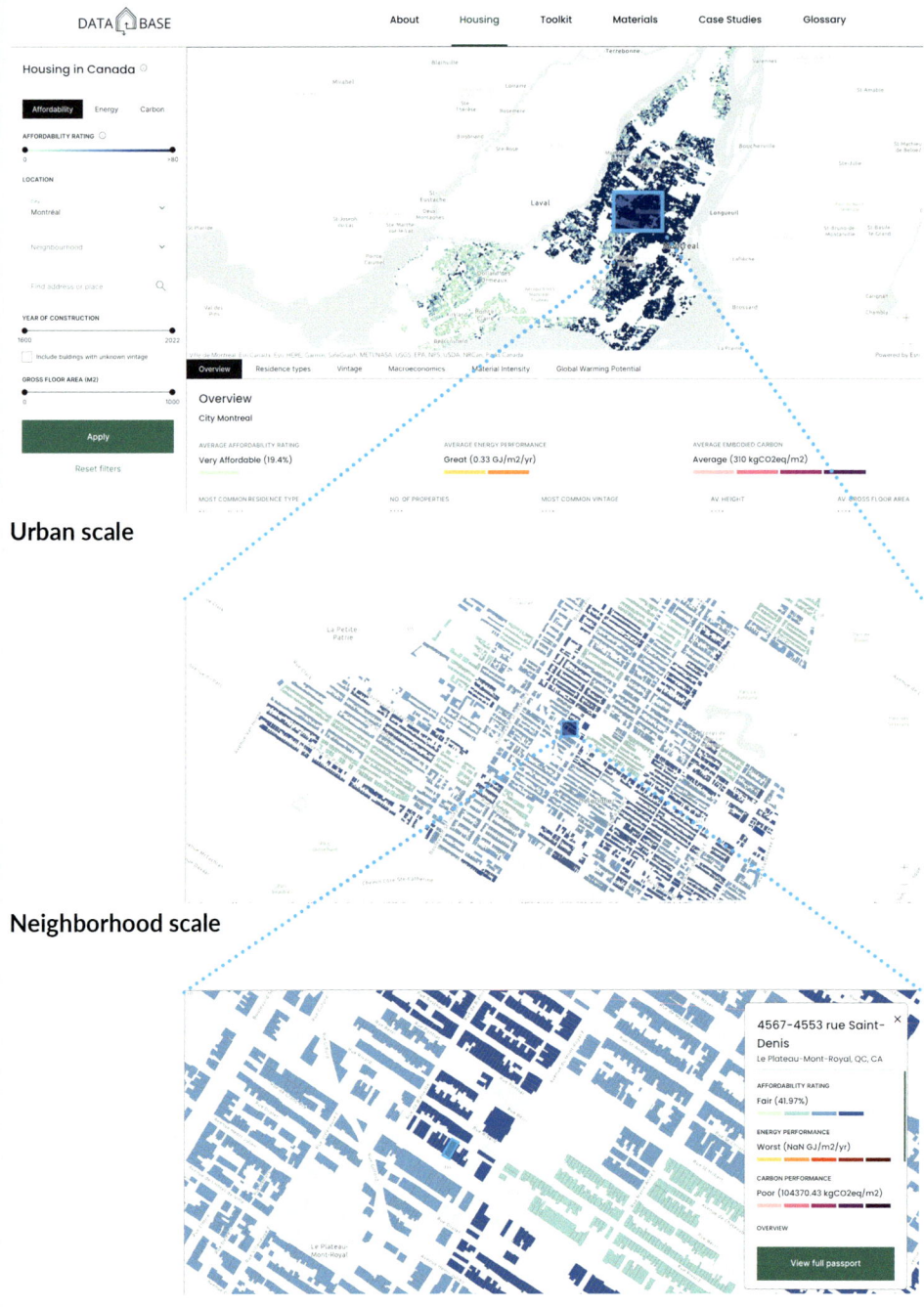

Urban scale

Neighborhood scale

Building scale

Figure 10.10 Visualizing a Multi-Scalar Approach: Affordability and Environmental Impacts of Housing Are Visualized at the City, Neighborhood, and Building Scale.

multi-scalar approach the housing map uses. Figure 10.11 illustrates housing maps for the city of Montreal that visualize affordability, energy performance, and embodied carbon. A heat map visualization changes color to indicate the variable being considered. Figure 10.11 also shows the overview panel which is found below the map and provides information on (in this case) the city-level values for housing affordability, energy performance, and embodied carbon. A view of the energy performance map at

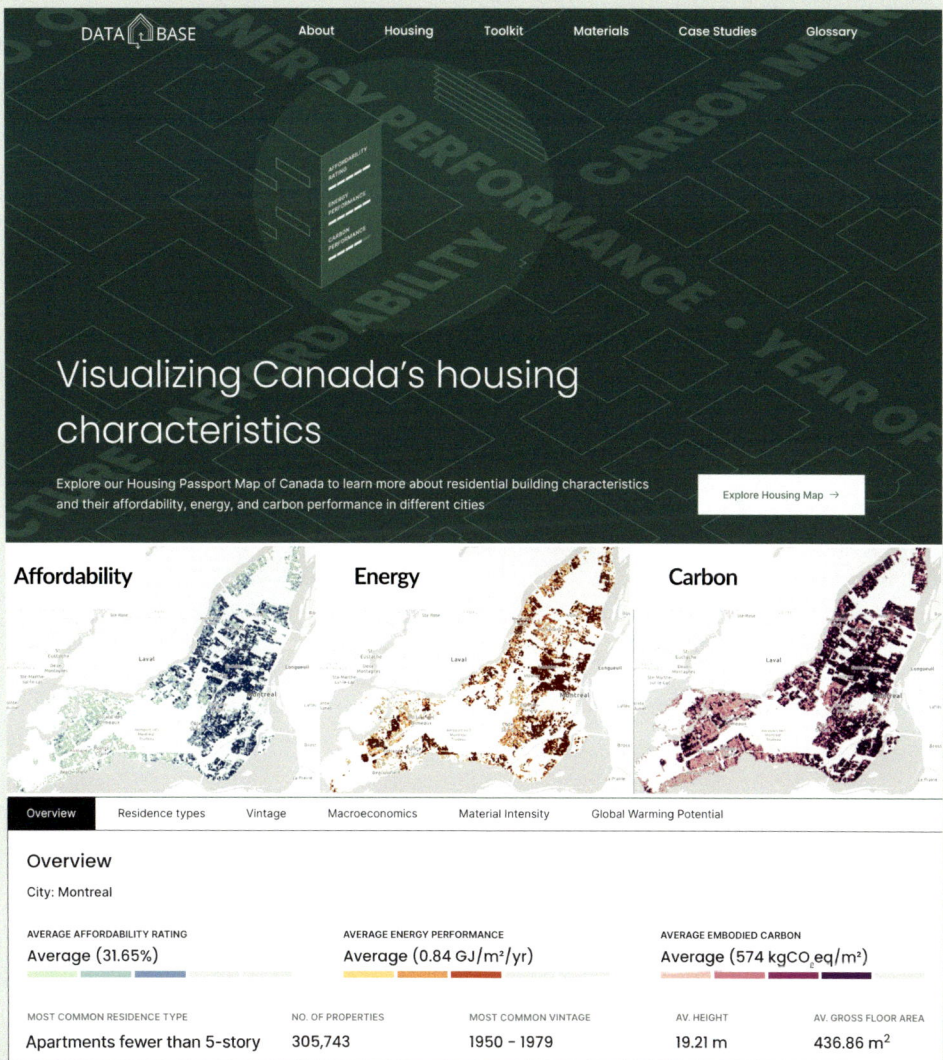

Figure 10.11 A View of Data Homebase Homepage (Top). Color Coded Scales Coordinate to the Data Displayed on the Map: Affordability Blue-Green Scale; Energy Red-Yellow Scale; Carbon Purple-Pink Scale (Bottom).

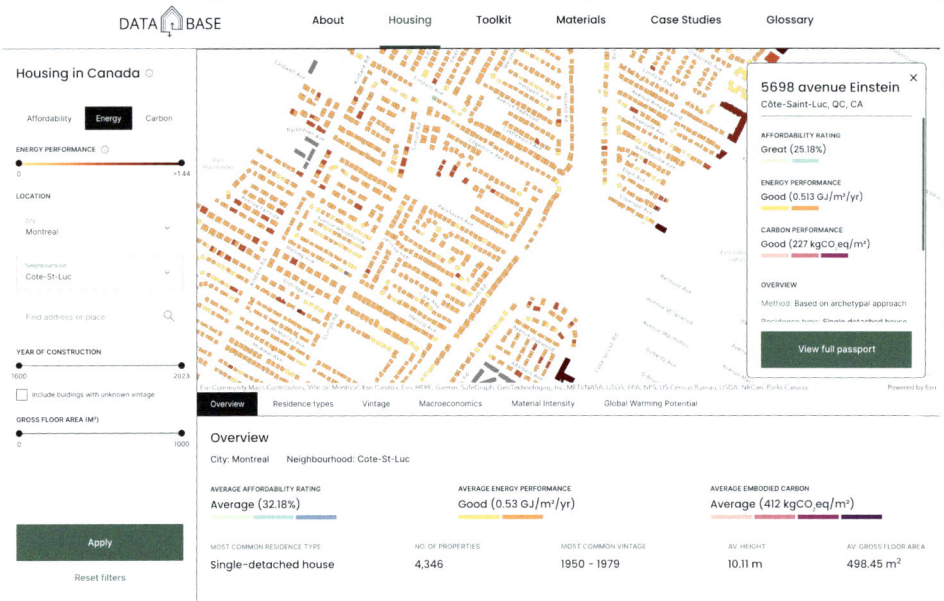

Figure 10.12 Energy Performance Map of the Data Homebase for Montreal, Quebec, Canada.

the neighborhood scale is shown in Figure 10.12, here the overview panel changes to show the data related to the neighborhood level. By clicking on a house on the map, a user gains access to a full housing passport as illustrated in Figure 10.13 for the selected residence.

The housing stock for different cities across Canada is defined in Data Homebase by archetypes. These archetypes, as illustrated in Figure 10.14, are based on Census Canada housing classifications (Statistics Canada, 2017). Each archetype is defined by different vintages. Existing houses are then mapped to the archetypical system using a geographic information system (GIS). Generated data from energy simulation and life cycle assessment along with existing datasets are also mapped to the existing housing used GIS in order to gain a clear understanding of Canadian housing. This data is then visualized using data-driven narratives so that the information is readily accessible and understandable to a diverse range of housing stakeholders as illustrated in Figure 10.15. The methodology for how the housing map is created is explained in more detail elsewhere (Keena et al., 2023). The ultimate goal of the housing map is to make housing passport data easily accessible to a wide variety of housing stakeholders.

In the Materials section of Data Homebase, individual materials and their associated impact on health, embodied carbon, operational energy, circularity, supply chain, the environment, ability to be disassembled (Design for Disassembly), and cost are outlined (see Figure 10.16). This becomes helpful for users to understand the life cycle impact of choosing one material over another. Under finance, economic and financial approaches to circular economy housing are explained, and the policy bar looks at circular economy policymaking case studies to encourage circular economy housing construction. Lastly, the Toolkit section allows users to create their own

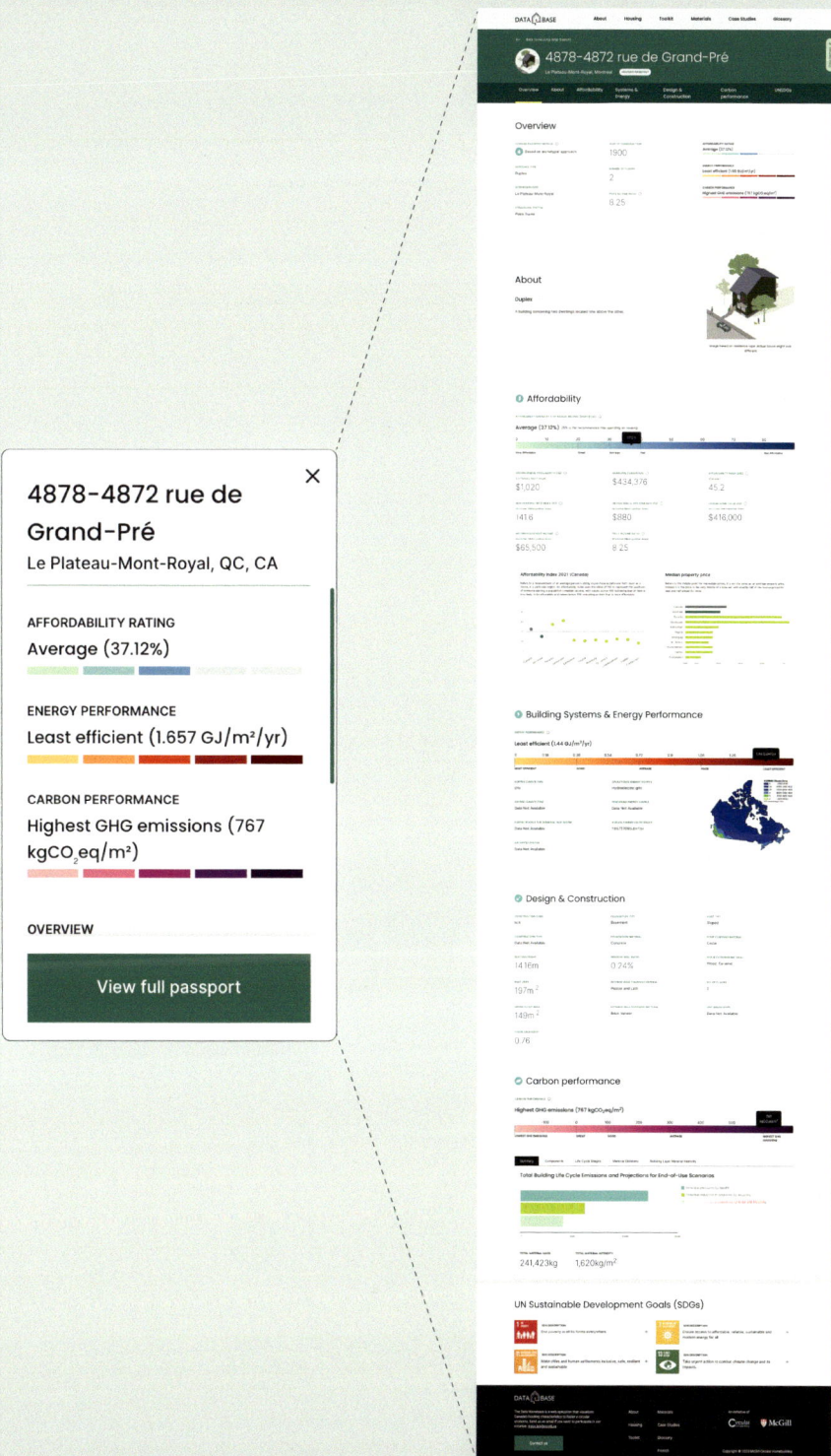

Figure 10.13 Housing Passport (HP) Digital Report: At the Scale of an Individual Residence, the Resultant HP Presents a Detailed Standardized Digital Description of a Home's Characteristics.

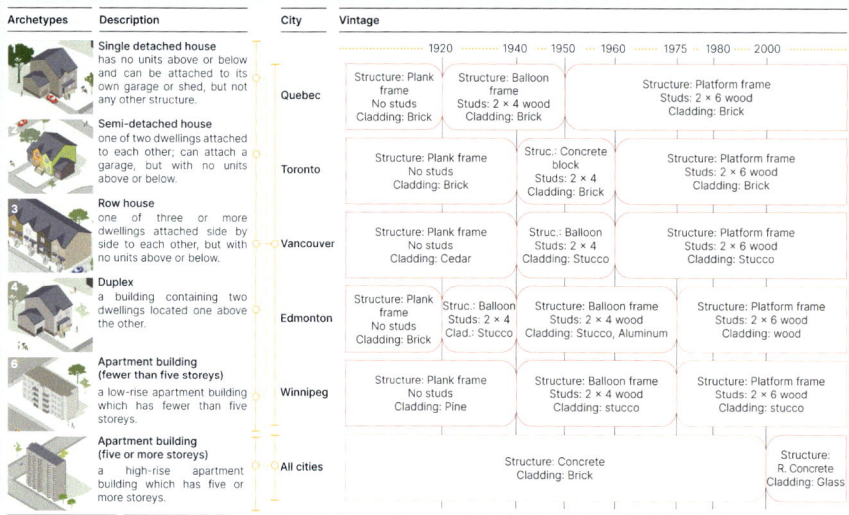

Archetypes	Description	City	Vintage

Single detached house
has no units above or below and can be attached to its own garage or shed, but not any other structure.

Semi-detached house
one of two dwellings attached to each other; can attach a garage, but with no units above or below.

Row house
one of three or more dwellings attached side by side to each other, but with no units above or below.

Duplex
a building containing two dwellings located one above the other.

Apartment building (fewer than five storeys)
a low-rise apartment building which has fewer than five storeys.

Apartment building (five or more storeys)
a high-rise apartment building which has five or more storeys.

Quebec — 1920: Structure: Plank frame, No studs, Cladding: Brick | 1940: Structure: Balloon frame, Studs: 2 × 4 wood, Cladding: Brick | 1975: Structure: Platform frame, Studs: 2 × 6 wood, Cladding: Brick

Toronto — Structure: Plank frame, No studs, Cladding: Brick | Struc.: Concrete block, Studs: 2 × 4, Cladding: Brick | Structure: Platform frame, Studs: 2 × 6 wood, Cladding: Brick

Vancouver — Structure: Plank frame, No studs, Cladding: Cedar | Struc.: Balloon, Studs: 2 × 4, Cladding: Stucco | Structure: Platform frame, Studs: 2 × 6 wood, Cladding: Stucco

Edmonton — Structure: Plank frame, No studs, Cladding: Brick | Struc.: Balloon, Studs: 2 × 4, Clad.: Stucco | Structure: Balloon frame, Studs: 2 × 4 wood, Cladding: Stucco, Aluminum | Structure: Platform frame, Studs: 2 × 6 wood, Cladding: wood

Winnipeg — Structure: Plank frame, No studs, Cladding: Pine | Structure: Balloon frame, Studs: 2 × 4 wood, Cladding: stucco | Structure: Platform frame, Studs: 2 × 6 wood, Cladding: stucco

All cities — Structure: Concrete, Cladding: Brick | Structure: R. Concrete, Cladding: Glass

Vintage timeline: 1920 · 1940 · 1950 · 1960 · 1975 · 1980 · 2000

Figure 10.14 Canadian Housing Archetypes – Their Definitions, and Vintages for Five Major Cities.

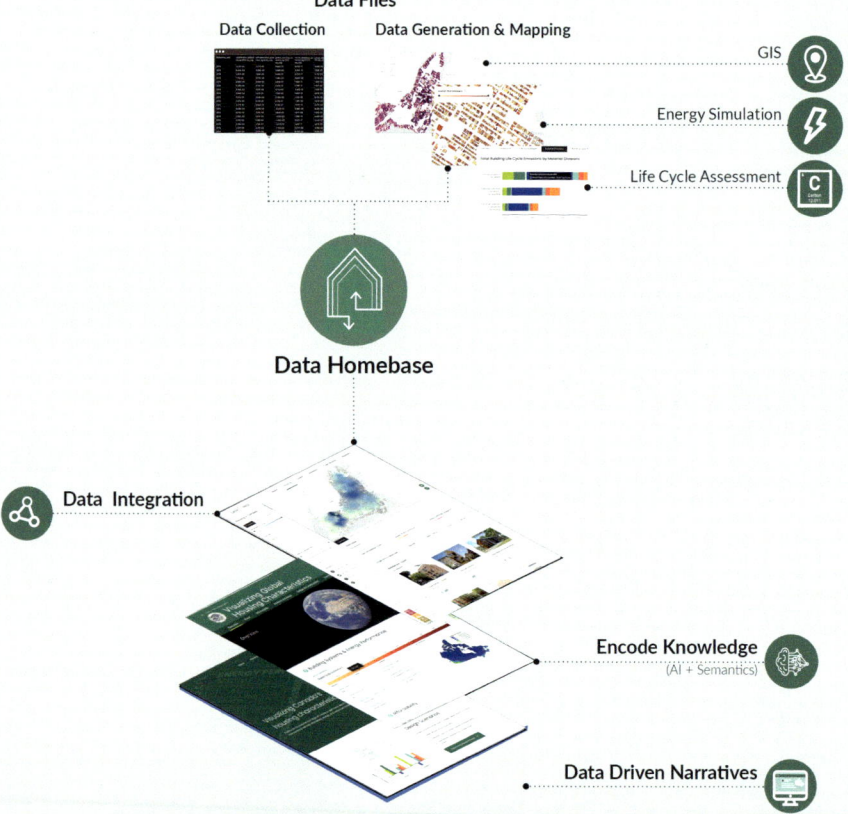

Figure 10.15 Designing Data-Driven Narratives to Tackle the Global Challenge of Sustainable Housing: Diagramming the Research Methodology in Developing the Data Homebase Web Application. Methods Include (1) Housing Data Collection; (2) Data Generation and Mapping (i.e., Generating GIS Maps, Building Energy Use Simulation, and Life Cycle Assessment for the Carbon Footprint of Housing); and (3) Visualizing via Data-Driven Narratives the Integrated Housing Passport Data for Easy Access by a Broad Range of Housing Stakeholders to Foster Circularity.

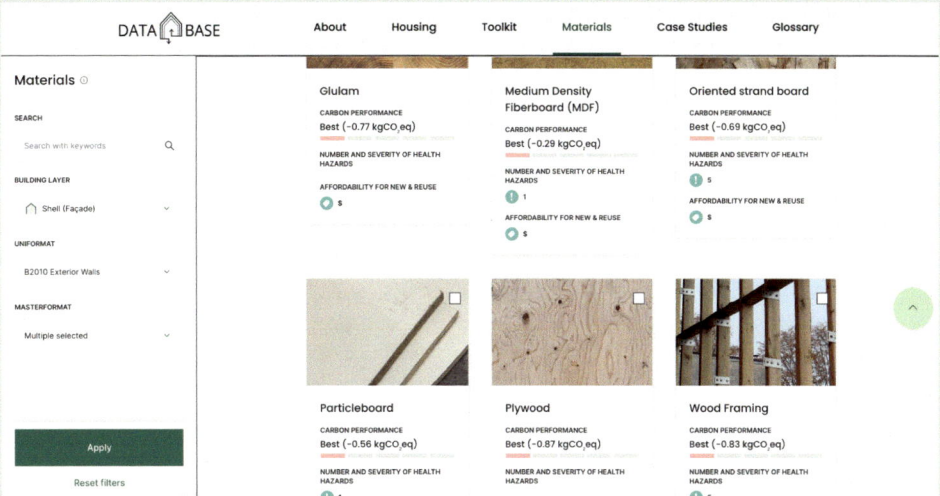

Figure 10.16 The Materials Page of the Data Homebase Provides Material Passports for Construction Materials Searchable by Building Layer, Uniformat and Masterformat. Employing These Standards Allows Design and Construction Professionals to Easily Filter the Data and Learn of the Materials Health Impacts, Cost, and Carbon Impact as Well as Its Potential for Design for Disassembly and Recovery at End of Use.

Housing Passport, understand the environmental and economic impacts of housing, gain circular economy insights, and understand which stakeholders are key in implementing circularity in their specific region and context. Figure 10.17 shows different design scenarios that a user can choose from in the Toolkit section. Environmental monitoring, Affordable and a Circular Financing Calculator, Design for Disassembly Recommendations, and Building Capacity and Circular Economy Implementations are all included in the Implementation section of Data Homebase.

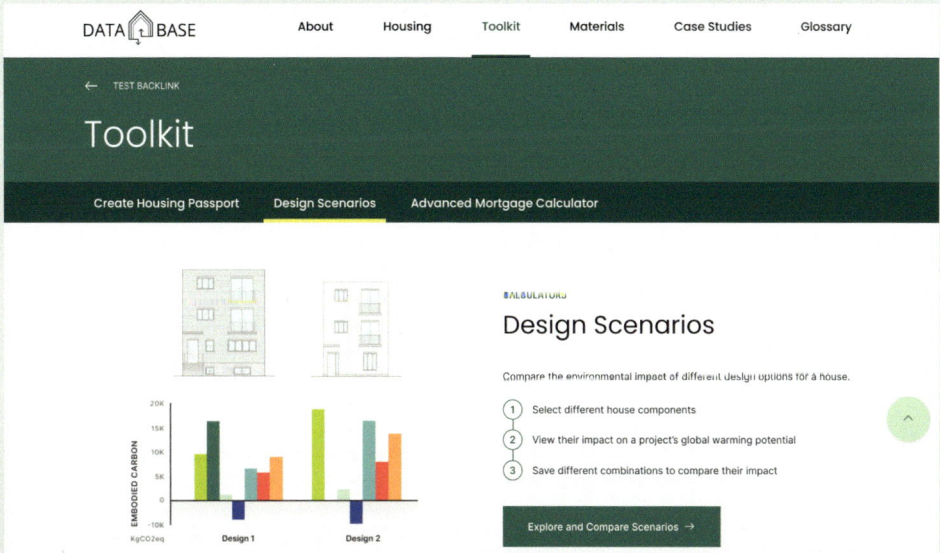

Figure 10.17 The Data Homebase Toolkit's Design Scenarios Allow Users to Compare the Environmental Impact of Different Design Options for a Number of Housing Archetypes.

Data Homebase is an effective example of how engaging with data analysis and virtualization can help achieve other tenets of the circular economy framework, such as product life extension and recycling and reuse. A wide range of stakeholders are involved in the building-making process and a wide variety of building decisions must be combined to genuinely result in life cycle sustainability. Not only does Data Homebase collect and standardize housing passports but does so in an easily accessible visual manner that a range of stakeholders can understand, from building and construction experts to policymakers and financial institutions, as well as homebuyers and users. This heightened communication and knowledge transfer could help guide financial institutions in green financing property assessments or aid in asset management of government housing for cities. Thus, providing clear, standardized, and comprehensive data about home-building projects and their materials through Housing Passports offers a digital space for a variety of stakeholders to consult at any time. This allows circular policies, construction, and financial decisions to be achieved simultaneously. It achieves this by combining GIS, energy simulation, and life cycle assessment with existing data to get a clear understanding of Canadian housing. This data is then visualized using data-driven narratives so that the information is clearly understandable to a wide variety of stakeholders as mentioned above (Figure 10.16). As outlined in the next chapter, a major barrier to productive sustainable development is the lack of knowledge about exactly how our housing stock was constructed, making it difficult to assess the most circular method for deep energy retrofits, material reuse, spatial reuse, and new construction techniques. Data Homebase standardizes scattered and unclear data about buildings, allowing for effective circular economy and future decision-making.

10B

Project:
VMD Prefabricated House

Location:
Mexico City, Mexico

Year:
2019

Team:
Taller Escape and Studioroca

Mapping to Circular Economy Framework:

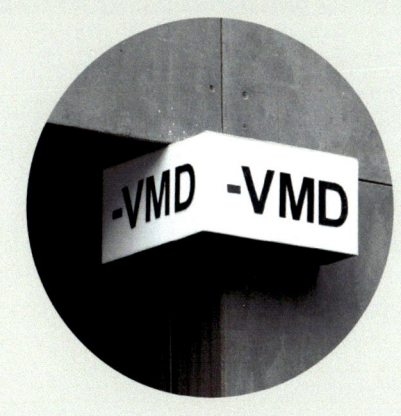

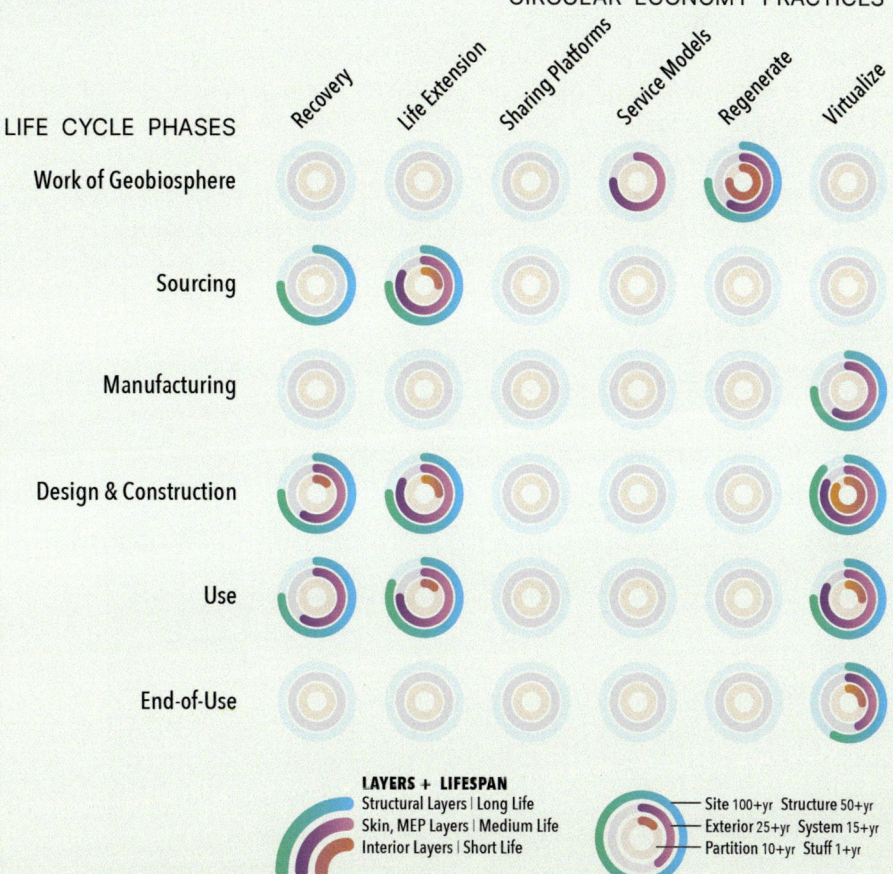

CIRCULAR ECONOMY PRACTICES

LIFE CYCLE PHASES

Recovery | Life Extension | Sharing Platforms | Service Models | Regenerate | Virtualize

Work of Geobiosphere

Sourcing

Manufacturing

Design & Construction

Use

End-of-Use

LAYERS + LIFESPAN
Structural Layers | Long Life
Skin, MEP Layers | Medium Life
Interior Layers | Short Life

Site 100+yr   Structure 50+yr
Exterior 25+yr   System 15+yr
Partition 10+yr   Stuff 1+yr

▲VMD

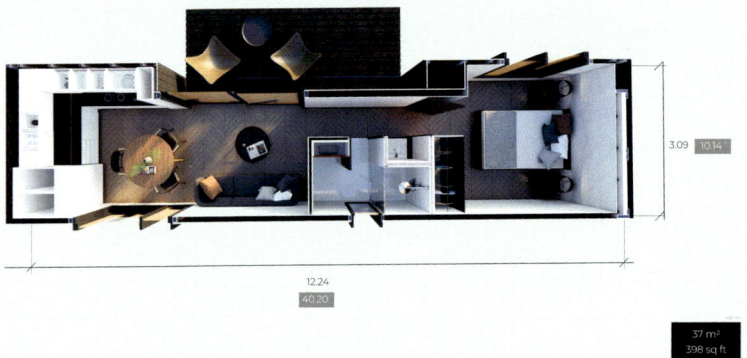

Figure 10.18 A Ready-to-Order Customizable Design that Can Be Purchased Online, the VMD Can Be Modified so the Client Can Choose the Model and Finishes They Wish.

The VMD (Vivienda Minima de Descanso – Minimum Rest Housing) Prefabricated House is a wonderful example of virtualization. Based in Mexico, this home can be ordered and customized online, prefabricated off-site in three-months, and shipped to a site where it is erected in one week (VMD, 2019). A user can customize the different layouts and fixtures and fittings via the VMD housing website before choosing their ideal version of the home. An example of a layout sold online is shown in Figure 10.18. There are six models to choose, each offers different spatial experiences, and some include an extra bedroom. The user can choose from a palette of materials and colors (e.g., pure oak vs dark oak for the floor or pure brown vs dark brown for the decking, medium gray steel façade vs black steel façade) (Archdaily, 2019). Views of the exterior and interior of the prefabricated, customizable, modular house can be seen in Figures 10.19–10.22.

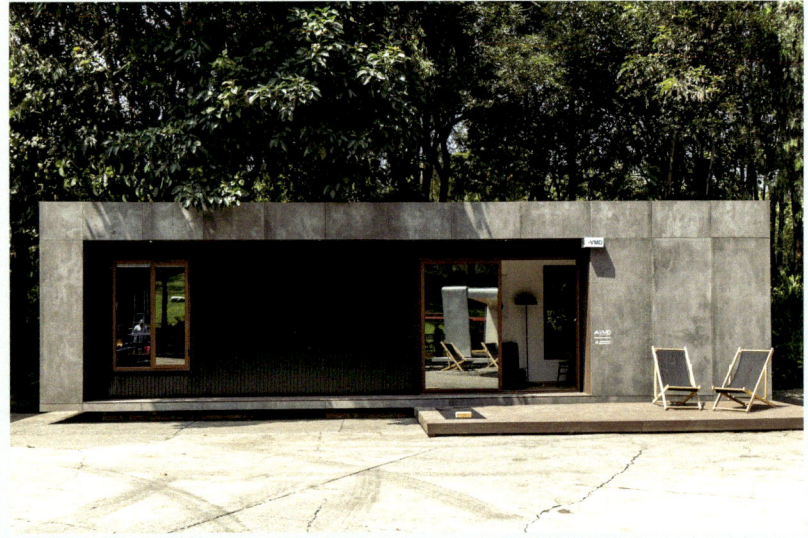

Figure 10.19 Exterior View of the VMD a Prefabricated Shipping Container with Modular Design.

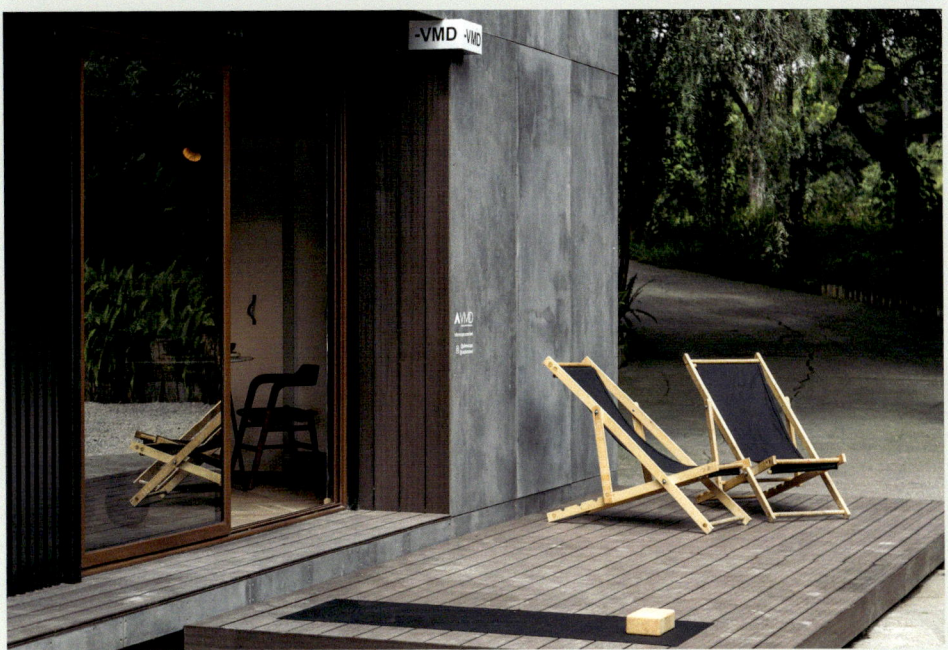

Figure 10.20 Detailed View of the Entrance. Once Ordered Online, the Home Is Prefabricated Off-Site in Three Months and Takes One Week to Be Finished On-Site.

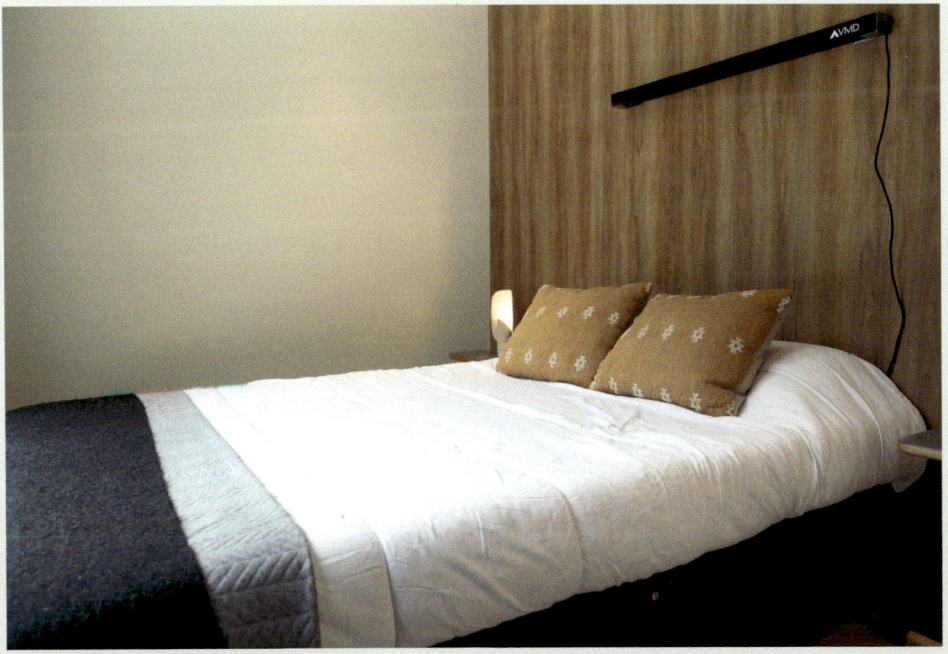

Figure 10.21 Interior View of the Bedroom.

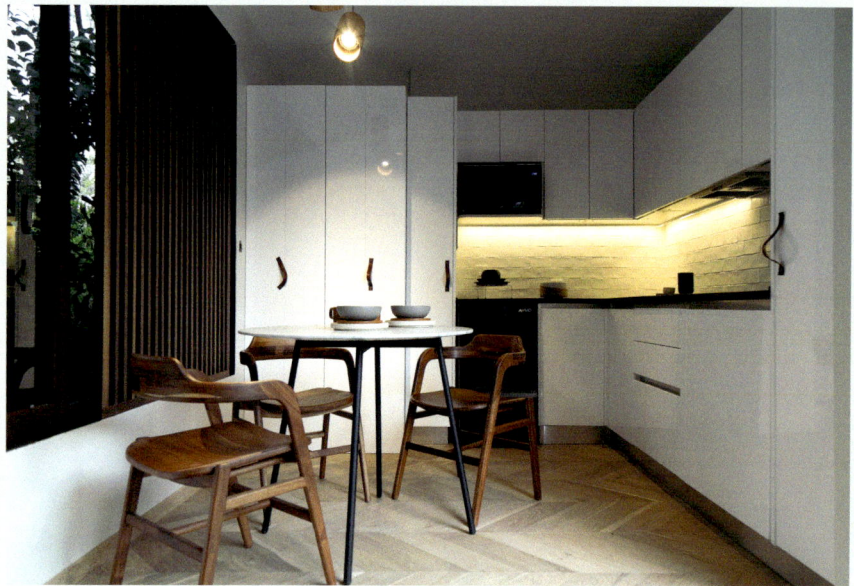

Figure 10.22 Interior View of the Kitchen and Dining Space.

Each model works around the same idea. They all have solar panels, solar heaters, and a rainwater collection system and the home runs entirely on electricity for heating, cooling, lighting, and equipment needs. There is an option to install a toilet incinerator and a treatment plant for wastewater. The interior walls and panels are fitted with acoustic and thermal insulation in order to stabilize the temperature of the home. The furniture comes as a package, and it is all designed by Studioroca and sourced from local Mexican furniture craftsmen (Wang, 2019) (Figure 10.23).

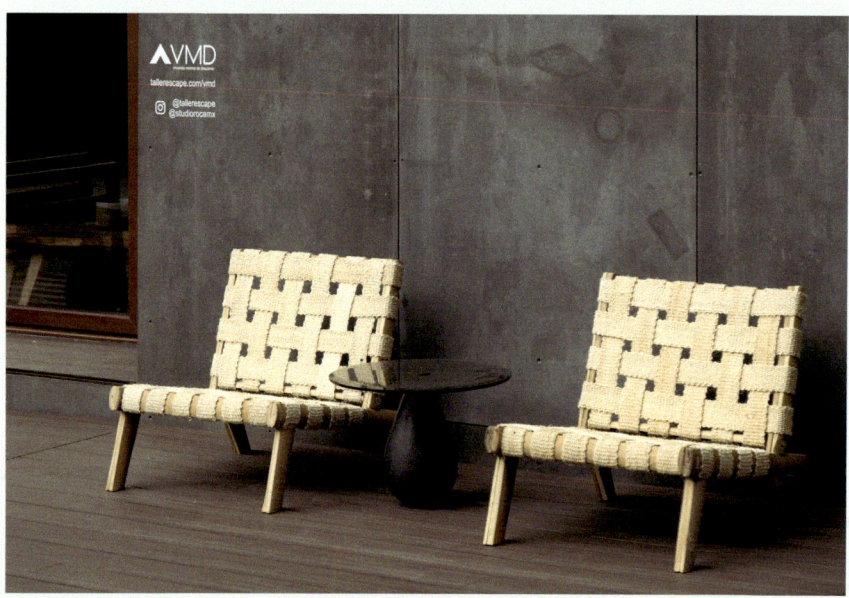

Figure 10.23 Much of the Fixtures, Finishes and Furniture Are Locally Sourced and Benefit from Mexican Craftsmanship.

All of the homes are made from reusing and adapting shipping containers. Hence, the homes follow the *recovery* principle of circularity. The homes are transported to site via a truck and placed on the desired site with the help of a crane. No foundation is needed. By minimizing the use of materials to only that which is needed, the architects aim to minimize the environmental impact of a new build (Borgobello, 2019). This highlights the regeneration principle as site and foundation work have a large impact on the ecosystem of a site. In this case it is somewhat avoided. One of the goals of the project is to provide clients with an eco-conscious retreat from urban life. Hence, the VMD is imagined as a second home to "escape" to the countryside. The architects felt this could be achieved by building with less (Archdaily, 2019). The aim was to not only limit material use but to also conserve space by providing a compact footprint, while reducing waste and cost. Additionally, given the simple robust design using a shipping container maintenance can be kept at a minimum.

10.6 Conclusion

To repair fragmentation in the building industry and, ultimately, promote circularity, housing knowledge needs to be virtualized. At each phase of a building's life cycle, virtualization can be employed to promote circular principles. While the advancement of technology and its increased employment in the construction industry is critical, it is pertinent to understand the building as a whole using human and machine-readable classifications. The ultimate goal is to have a comprehensive understanding of a building's entire life cycle and connect this information to the pertinent disciplines and stakeholders across the housing value chain. By so doing, they can make informed circular decisions. Transparency and accessibility are crucial for collaboration and therefore require a "common language". This entails unambiguous classifications, clear definitions and glossaries, and reliable specifications and rules. Ultimately, by employing data visualization tools and organizing complex-building information into technical terms, stakeholders can engage in collaboration and effectively promote a circular economy. This concept of stakeholder collaboration will be expanded in the next chapter, which will discuss stakeholder engagement and building capacities.

References

Aly Etman, M., Keena, N., & Dyson, A. (2020). Socio-ecological visual analytics environment "SEVA": A novel visual analytics environment for interdisciplinary decision-making linking human biometrics and environmental data. *IOP Conference Series: Earth and Environmental Science*, *588*, 032062. https://doi.org/10.1088/1755-1315/588/3/032062

Antikainen, M., Uusitalo, T., & Kivikytö-Reponen, P. (2018). Digitalisation as an enabler of circular economy. *Procedia CIRP*, *73*, 45–49. https://doi.org/10.1016/j.procir.2018.04.027

Archdaily. (2019). *VMD prefabricated house/taller escape + Studioroca.* Retrieved July 13 from https://www.archdaily.com/928375/vmd-prefabricated-house-taller-escape-plus-studioroca?ad_source=search&ad_medium=search_result_all

Asdrubali, F., & Desideri, U. (2019). *Handbook of energy efficiency in buildings: A life cycle approach.* Butterworth-Heinemann, an imprint of Elsevier. https://doi.org/10.1016/C2016-0-02638-4

Baporikar, N. (2020). *Handbook of research on entrepreneurship development and opportunities in circular economy.* Business Science Reference, an imprint of IGI Global. https://doi.org/10.4018/978-1-7998-5116-5

Beetz, J. (2018). *Structured vocabularies in construction: Classifications, taxonomies and ontologies.* Springer International Publishing.

Borgobello, B. (2019). *Off-the-grid container house in Mexico is move-in ready in 99 days.* New Atlas. Retrieved July 13 from https://newatlas.com/architecture/vmd-container-house-mexico/

Casini, M. (2022). *Construction 4.0 advanced technology, tools and materials for the digital transformation of the construction industry.* Woodhead Publishing.

Chen, Z., Feng, Q., Yue, R., Chen, Z., Moselhi, O., Soliman, A., Hammad, A., & An, C. (2022). Construction, renovation, and demolition waste in landfill: A review of waste characteristics, environmental impacts, and mitigation measures. *Environmental Science and Pollution Research International*, 29(31), 46509–46526. https://doi.org/10.1007/s11356-022-20479-5.

Crawford, R. (2011). *Life cycle assessment in the built environment*. Spon Press.

Daniotti, B., Gianinetto, M., & Della Torre, S. (2020). *Digital transformation of the design, construction and management processes of the built environment*. Springer Open. https://doi.org/10.1007/978-3-030-33570-0

Hennemann Hilario da Silva, T., & Sehnem, S. (2022). The circular economy and Industry 4.0: Synergies and challenges. *Revista de Gestão*, 29(3), 300–313. https://doi.org/10.1108/REGE-07-2021-0121

Issa, R., Olbina, S., American Society of Civil Engineers. Technical Council on, C., & Information, T. (2015). *Building information modeling: Applications and practices*. American Society of Civil Engineers. http://ascelibrary.org/doi/book/10.1061/9780784413982

Jaillon, L., Poon, C.-S., & Chiang, Y. H. (2009). Quantifying the waste reduction potential of using prefabrication in building construction in Hong Kong. *Waste Management*, 29(1), 309–320.

Keena, N., & Dyson, A. (2017). Qualifying the quantitative in the construction of built ecologies. In D. Benjamin (Ed.), *Embodied energy and design: Making architecture between metrics and narratives*. Columbia University GSAPP Lars Müller.

Keena, N., Dyson, A., & Etman, M. A. (2020). *Mapping the built environment process (BEP) ecosystem via a data to knowledge framework*. In AIA/ACSA intersections research conference: CARBON, Pennsylvania State University.

Keena, N., Friedman, A., Parsaee, M., & Klein, A. (2023). *Data visualization for a circular economy: Designing a web application for sustainable housing*. Technology | Architecture + Design, 7:2, 262–281, DOI: 10.1080/24751448.2023.2246803

Kensek, K. M., & Noble, D. (2014). *Building information modeling: BIM in current and future practice*. Wiley. https://doi.org/10.1002/9781119174752

Lu, W., & Yuan, H. (2013). Investigating waste reduction potential in the upstream processes of offshore prefabrication construction. *Renewable and Sustainable Energy Reviews*, 28, 804–811.

McGuinness, D. L., & Van Harmelen, F. (2004). OWL web ontology language overview. *W3C Recommendation* – World Wide Web Consortium. https://www.w3.org/TR/2004/REC-owl-features-20040210/

McKinsey Global Institute. (2017). *Reinventing construction: A route to higher productivity*. https://www.mckinsey.com/business-functions/operations/our-insights/reinventing-construction-through-a-productivity-revolution

OWL Working Group. (2012). *W3C web ontology language (OWL)*. Retrieved January 10 from https://www.w3.org/OWL/

Pinheiro, P., McGuinness, D. L., & Santos, H. (2017). Human-aware sensor network ontology: Semantic support for empirical data collection. *arXiv preprint arXiv:1704.01806*.

Pinheiro, P., Santos, H., Liang, Z., Liu, Y., Rashid, S. M., McGuinness, D. L., & Bax, M. P. (2018). HADatAc: A framework for scientific data integration using ontologies. In *International semantic web conference (P&D/Industry/BlueSky)*.

Rowland, I. D., & Howe, T. N. (2001). *Vitruvius: 'Ten books on architecture'*. Cambridge University Press.

Santos, M. Y., & Costa, C. (2020). *Big data: Concepts, warehousing, and analytics*. River Publishers.

Schiuma, G., & Carlucci, D. (2018). *Big data in the arts and humanities: Theory and practice.* CRC Press, Taylor & Francis Group.

Sobh, T. M. (2008). *Advances in computer and information sciences and engineering.* Springer. https://public.ebookcentral.proquest.com/choice/publicfullrecord.aspx?p=364599

Statistics Canada. (2017). *Structural type of dwelling and collectives reference guide, census of population, 2016.* Canada Minister of Industry.

The Fab Foundation. (2023). *Bridging the digital divide: Design, fabricate, share.* The Fab Foundation. Retrieved July 05 from https://fabfoundation.org/

VMD. (2019). *What are the advantages of a minimum rest house?* Retrieved July 13 from https://www.vmd.com.mx/en/index.php

Wang, L. (2019). *These new prefab shipping container homes can be built in just 99 days.* Dwell. Retrieved July 23 from https://www.dwell.com/article/vmd-shipping-container-home-studioroca-taller-escape-5d3af200

Wong, T.-C., Yuen, B. K. P. (Eds.). (2011). *Eco-city planning: Policies, practice and design* (1st ed.). Springer Dordrecht. https://doi.org/10.1007/978-94-007-0383-4

Zimmerman, R., O'Brien, H., Hargrave, J., & Morrell, M. (2016). *The circular economy in the built environment.* Arup. https://www.arup.com/perspectives/publications/research/section/circular-economy-in-the-built-environment

Chapter 11

Stakeholder Engagement and Building Capacities

11.1 Introduction: A Need for Change in the Delivery System

A circular economy approach aims at keeping buildings in use, reducing waste, and lowering the cost of new construction for a building's end-of-life. The previous chapters have displayed how the circular economy offers a promising opportunity to combat the housing supply challenge and meet important sustainability goals. As outlined by Canada's Circular Economy Coalition, a complete transition to a circular economy requires all stakeholders in the value chain to redefine their roles (Jagou, 2021). Multiple stakeholders of varying fields must actively work together, from government bodies to financial institutions to construction companies and architects, to address barriers to circularity that permeate throughout multiple stages of the building supply chain. Figures 11.1 and 11.2 show how the roles of stakeholders will change from a linear to a circular economy.

This chapter outlines the different roles of stakeholders in the homebuilding process. First, a discussion on the current housing delivery model will be conducted; then, how a new integrated design process can reshape stakeholders' roles; and lastly, some general changes that this integrated design approach will have on the overall construction process.

11.2 The Current Housing Delivery Model

Stakeholders from both the public and private sectors, from varying fields, but with interlocking goals, contribute and have the potential to contribute to a circular building process. This section will go through each of the actors involved in the building-making process. Stakeholders, as Friedman (2011) describes, can be categorized into three groups: controlling agencies, the supply process, and the demand Process.

11.2.1 Controlling Agencies

These stakeholders hold positions of authority and have the power to grant permission or credentials to other stakeholders. Two important controlling agencies in a housing supply context are governmental bodies and financial institutions.

DOI: 10.4324/9781003333975-15

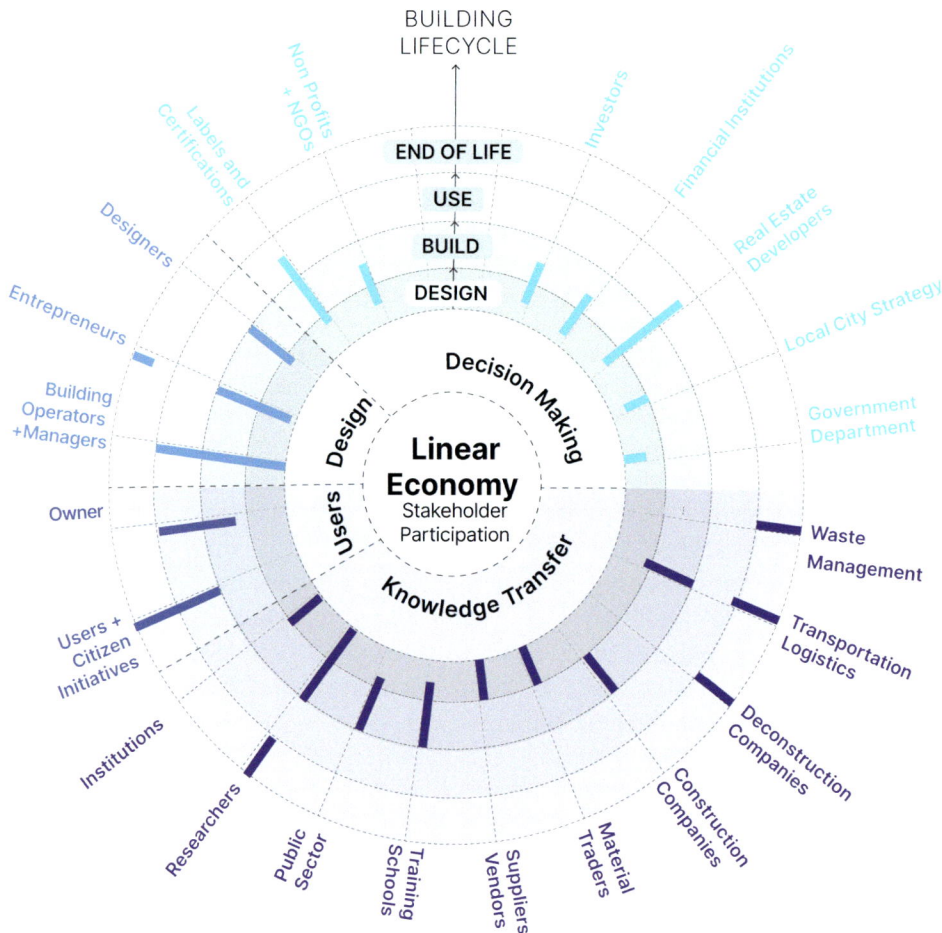

Figure 11.1 The Role of Stakeholders in a Linear Economy.

Government Departments (Federal, Provincial, or Municipal)

The government oversees, regulates, and promotes housing policies and safety. This can be done through financial incentives, codes, and standards (Friedman, 2011). The municipal government uses local legislation to turn its policies into a master plan, which includes a system of incentives and bylaws. North American governments intervene in the housing markets for two major reasons: elector pressure and pressure to stimulate the economy (Friedman, 2011). Indeed, the construction industry is a major player in the national economy, having generated about 13 percent of the world's gross domestic product (GDP) in 2018 and makings up about 7 percent of the world's labor population (RyFan, 2018). In Canada, the construction sector accounts for 7.5 percent of the country's GDP and employs 1.4 million people (Canadian Construction Association, n.d.). Therefore, the prominence of the residential construction industry has a profound effect on employment

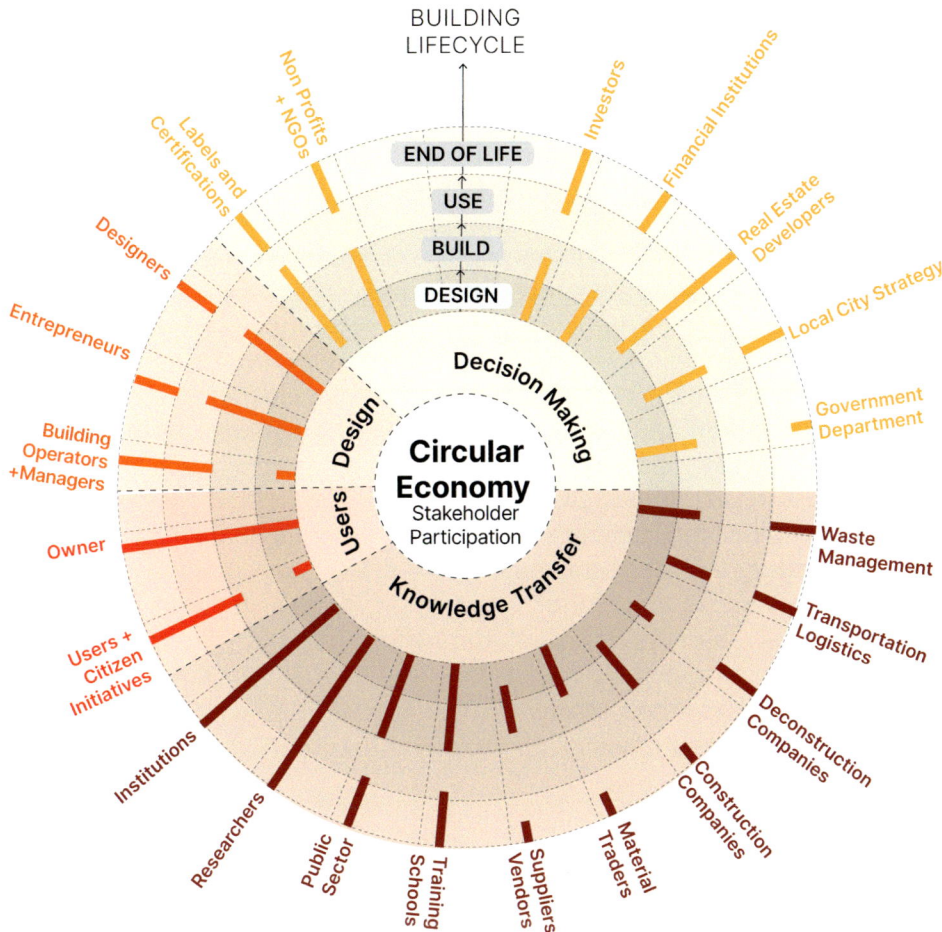

Figure 11.2 The Role of Stakeholders in a Circular Economy.

in fields related to construction and can be a large determinant of the economic health of a country. This incentivizes governments to get involved in the housing market. For example, the Canadian government, through the Canadian Mortgage and Housing Corporation (CMHC), makes political and legislative decisions to portion economic resources to housing (Friedman, 2011). Since the government's motivating factor to involve itself in the housing sector is economic, supporting flexible and sustainable design is unlikely to be supported if it is at the expense of finances.

Financial Institutions and Banks

Lending institutions such as banks or trust companies will lend finances needed to pursue a project or complete a purchase of a unit to a homebuyer. This gives banks substantial power over the builder and the buyer's decisions. Chartered banks provide the most funding for homes, followed by trust companies, credit unions, and then finance companies (Friedman, 2011). While lending institutions have control over whether a buyer can purchase a unit, they have minimal involvement in the actual building process. Banks are concerned about reducing risk and thus adopt conservative policies that disadvantage innovation that might not ensure maximum return on investment (Friedman, 2011). This acts as a barrier for flexible and innovative circular design that may require more financial risk or upfront cost but reap enormous long-term benefits. Some of the reasons financial institutions may resist circular design approaches is because these ideas may reduce residential mobility, which is a fruitful source of banking activities (e.g., mortgages) (Friedman, 2011). Second, circular economic design reduces unit cost through transferring finishing work to the user. Not only could this reduce the mortgage requested by the user, but it may become harder to sell a unit that is semi-finished (Friedman, 2011). Hence, the current system disincentives financial institutions from supporting innovative building strategies. However, worldwide, banks are unequivocal that climate change is the biggest emerging risk they face (EY & Institute of International Finance, 2021). Hence, due to pressures of global warming and the risks associated with changing weather patterns, many banks are offering lower mortgage rates for housing ("green mortgages") that can prove energy-efficient and associated with lower greenhouse gas emissions. Stakeholders believe it is in the best interest of banks to support clients' transition to a zero-carbon economy. With this new trend, circular housing has much to offer in providing housing which meets the requirements of lowering climate-related risk.

11.2.2 The Supply Process

Supply process stakeholders are those in charge of creating and providing goods (i.e., buildings) to users. This includes residential developers, architects, construction companies, and suppliers and vendors.

Residential Developers

Builders redevelop, construct, and refurbish buildings (Thelen et al., 2018). In the linear approach to building, buildings are seen as a short-term asset to invest in and profit from. They can act as a private or public entity. Builders are responsible for acquiring building permits and designing and planning the work as well as supervising construction (Friedman, 2011). Often, builders have small firms with little overhead, resulting in builders taking on more responsibilities than they are qualified for. They often decline the employment of in-house consultants with technical, managerial, and economic skills to save money, instead, relying on standardized routines to design and construct buildings to compensate for their lack of specialization (Friedman, 2011). This regimented system of building lends little opportunity to innovation.

Architects

The designer, which is often the architect or engineer, oversees the design of the building. Many design firms, however, do not participate in the residential housing sector because of the lack of control they have over their designs (Friedman, 2011). As a result, many residential units are planned by specialized house designers who are not registered architects, are charged below the recommended rates, and create a single plan that is copied several times in different settings (Friedman, 2011). Little-to-no project follow-ups are conducted, such as selection of materials, supervision of quality, advice to users, and no communication between the designer and the user. This prevents knowledge sharing and long-term maintenance of a design. While this approach has lower upfront costs, these designs lead to higher life cycle costs. In this scenario, there is communication and a contractual agreement between the architect and the builder, but no communication between the user and the architect, meaning that the design is not reflective of the user's needs.

Construction Companies

The project executor oversees the actual building of the project. Construction companies are usually at the command of the builder, meaning that the specialty contractor linked to the company is often at the end of the line when signing formal contracts. These firms are often small with little financial security. This, combined with a lack of certainty provided by the builder in terms of how execution will be done, puts the project executor in a place of vulnerability (Friedman, 2011).

Suppliers and Vendors

Vendors manufacture and supply materials for construction. Unlike other stakeholders, suppliers and vendors often have sufficient investments and overhead in terms of equipment and facilities. As a result, pressure for innovation often comes from this stakeholder. A supplier or sales representative is often the link between the manufacturer and the builder, communicating knowledge about the product to the architect and builder (Friedman, 2011).

11.2.3 The Demand Process

Stakeholders in the demand process are those who demand the goods or services given. In a housing context, the most common demand stakeholder is, of course, the user of the home.

Users

This stakeholder engages with the built product in its operational phase. The user is a unique stakeholder in that they are concerned primarily with the quality of the housing and are not typically active during the conceptualization phase of the building (Friedman, 2011). While economic decisions are important for the user, their concerns go beyond this. Little information is provided to the user about the physical structure of the home, materials used, and quality of the building (Friedman, 2011).

Each stakeholder functions in a specific way to help transition to a circular economy (see Figure 11.3). Their roles must change when moving from a linear to a circular economy by intervening or participating in new stages of the building process (Thelen et al., 2018). In a linear design process, each stakeholder performs their role in a sequential process, one after another (see Figures 11.1 and 11.4). The participants in the housing delivery process are a team, but composed on a short-term basis, which

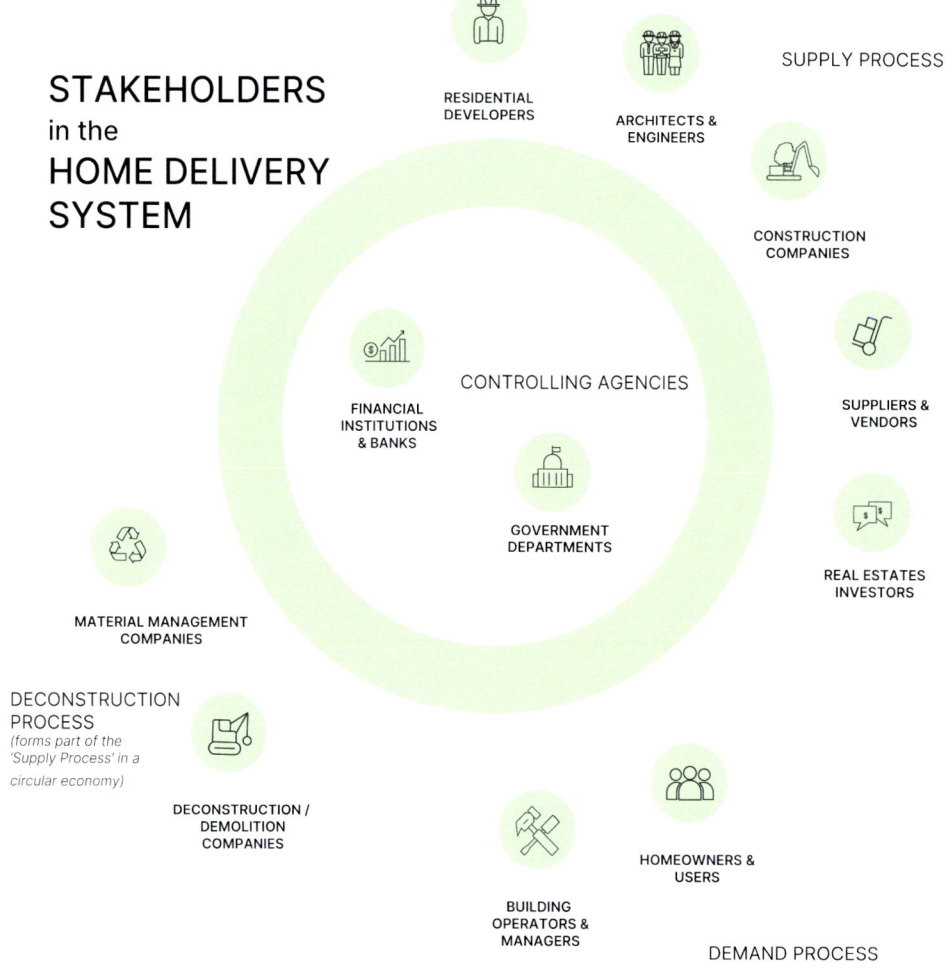

Figure 11.3 The Different Stakeholders in a Building Process.

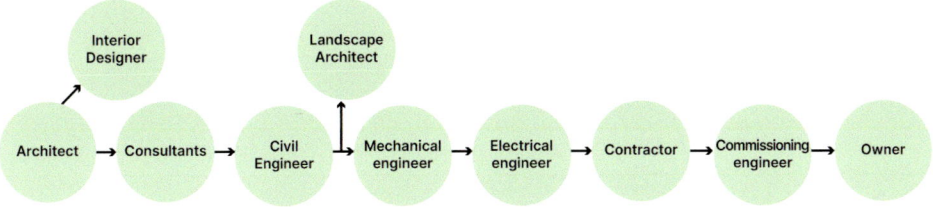

TRADITIONAL DESIGN PROCESS BY PROFESSIONS

Figure 11.4 The Traditional Linear Design Process by Building Sector Professions.

leads to conflicts (Friedman, 2011). This is because each team member is treated as independent, but their actions are, indeed, not independent and affect every other stakeholder's actions (Friedman, 2011). This is partly due to the way contracts are drawn up in the housing delivery process. There are three main contracts that are signed between stakeholders. First, a contract between the user and the builder; second, the financial lending institution and the building; and lastly, between the builder and the specialty contractor (Friedman, 2011). These contracts outline what each party is expected to deliver and receive. This sequential and simple process of each stakeholder performing a specific task and then passing on the torch to the next results in a seemingly efficient system. However, it inhibits collaboration or flexibility and fosters competition between stakeholders. For instance, Lechner (2015) provides an example of all-glass façades in buildings, which require an energy consumptive mechanical system. If an architect designs this façade at one of the initial steps of the building process, it is often too late by the time the building process gets to the mechanical equipment point to change the design, resulting in an excessively large mechanical system. The solution, therefore, is an integrated approach to design, which the next section describes in-depth.

11.3 A Circular Home Delivery Method: New Rolls and Methods of Communication

Clearly, there are a multitude of stakeholders involved in a building's life cycle that have the potential to influence a building's sustainability. As Lechner (2015) explains, buildings are too complex to rely on one realm of design and planning sustainable buildings comes with even more complexity. An integrated whole-building design process considers the needs of multiple systems at the beginning of the design process in order to foster collaboration and avoid scenarios outlined above from occurring. There are two general perspectives that the integrated design process considers. First, various functions (e.g., from aesthetics and structure to heating and lighting) are considered at the initial stage of the building process to ensure that the final design is harmonious, rather than prioritizing one need over another. This synergy of functions improves the performance and sustainability of a building.

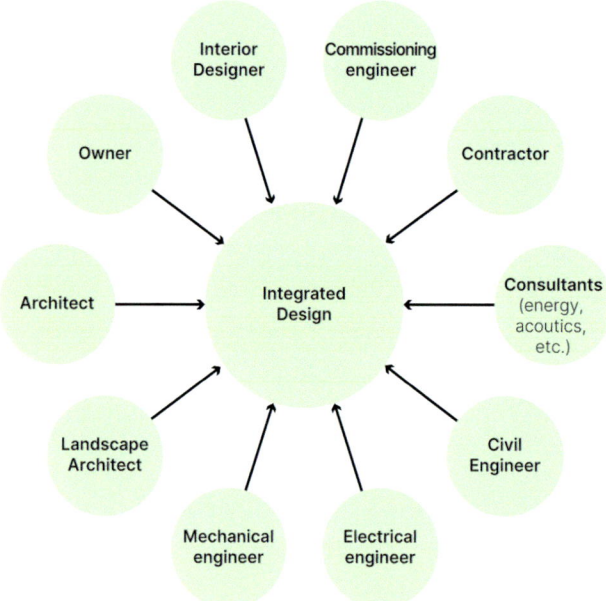

INTEGRATED DESIGN PROCESS BY PROFESSIONS

Figure 11.5 Integrated Design Process by Building Sector Professions.

Second, and most relevant to this chapter, the multiple stakeholders involved in the building process to achieve these various functions are involved from the beginning (see Figure 11.5). This allows the architect to create a whole-building design that meets the needs of each stakeholder.

Going back to the all-glass façade example, if multiple stakeholders were communicating at the initial phase of the design process, it would become clear that an all-glass façade would be overly consumptive and require an extensive mechanical system. This new integrated whole-building process asks stakeholders to reimagine their roles in relation to one another. The following will outline how the role of each stakeholder would change when incorporating a circular and integrated approach into the building process as illustrated in Figure 11.6. In this figure, the circular economy framework outlined in Chapter 3, which includes the circular business models, is overlapped against the architectural design process, and different stakeholder roles along the building life cycle.

11.3.1 Controlling Agencies

Government Departments (Federal, Provincial, Municipal)

Government departments have an important role to play in the implementation of a circular economy. First, governments should explain what circular economy is to the public and share the benefits of this shift to stimulate legislative measures.

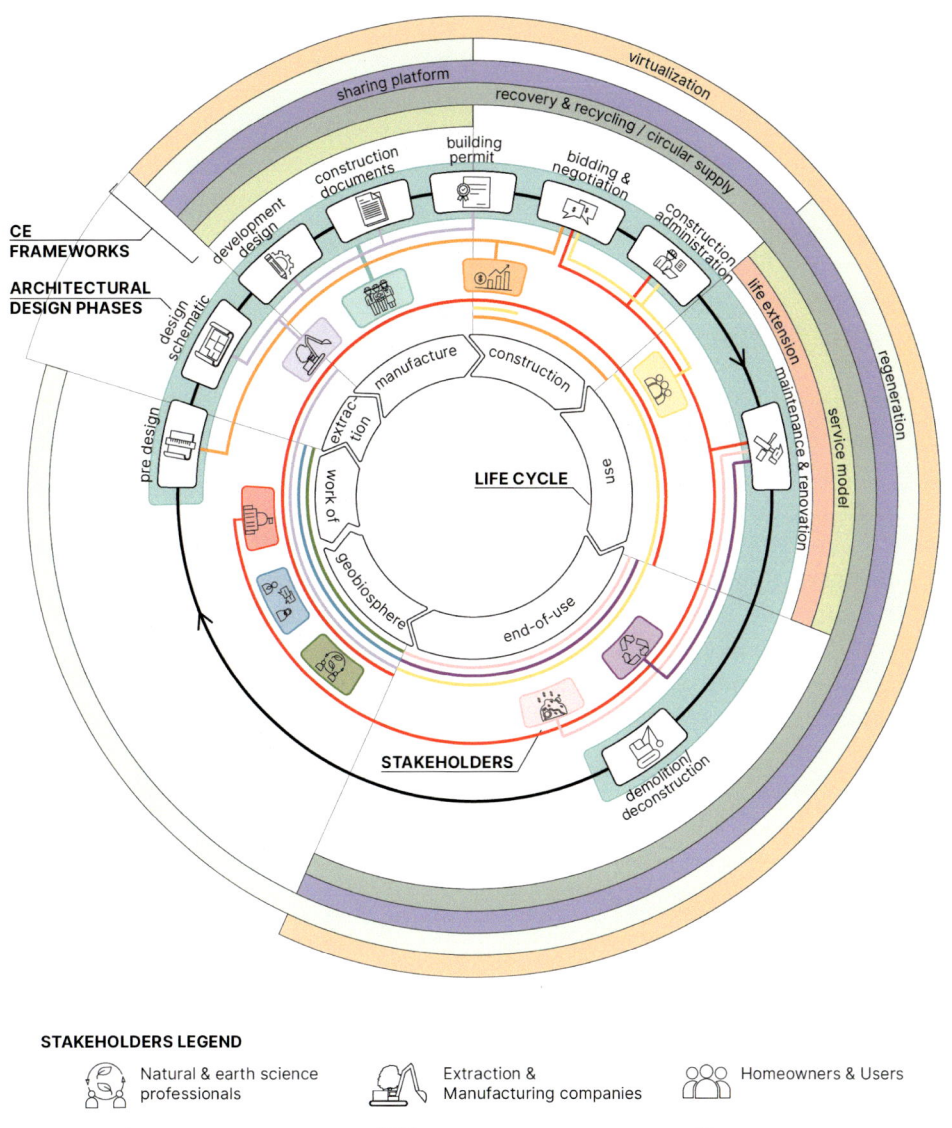

Figure 11.6 A View of How the Circular Economy Framework Overlaps with the Architectural Design Phases, Stakeholder Roles, and the Building Life Cycle.

Municipal actors should design city policies and agendas that encourage homeowners and local companies to choose circular solutions (Keena & Friedman, 2021). Second, policymakers should invest in developing a highly skilled workforce, creating a labor force that is able to apply innovative building practices and stay loyal to a project throughout the building-making process. For instance, Singapore developed the SkillsFuture program, which allowed workers to acquire new skills throughout their careers and accumulate credits in a "skill account". Governments should provide rebates for licensure, training, and certification programs to reduce fast turnover in the workforce. Lastly, governments could increase transparency between their knowledge and that of the contractor. Transparency between stakeholders will clarify what the cost of a building project is and hold stakeholders accountable for their performance goals (McKinsey Global Institute, 2017).

Financial Institutions and Banks

Banks can play a large role in implementing a circular economy by modifying their current business and funding models. Absorbing risk to support circular solutions and creating circular finance models for emerging companies will help with the establishment of a circular economy (Keena & Friedman, 2021). For instance, expanding financial tools to offer a more complex ownership model, providing consultancy services for new business models, and adjusting risk models to account for the risk of using secondary materials, complex approval procedures, and maintenance risk (Thelen et al., 2018). While the previous section outlined some reasons why a financial institution may resist the adoption of flexible design, there is a case for banks to support the introduction of flexibility systems. Lowering the cost of units can make the housing market more accessible for first-time buyers who may need financial services. Also, lowering the rates of residential mobility or easy adaptation of units for the next user may increase the value of a property (Friedman, 2011).

Intesa Sanpaolo, an Italian International banking group, has committed to applying a circular model to promote economic sustainability (Intesa Sanpaolo, 2022). Intesa Sanpaolo is the largest bank in Italy by total assets and spans to countries in Europe, the Middle East, the United States, China, and more. With this broad influence, the financial institution believes that a circular model will help with medium- to long-term competitiveness as well as positively impact communities. To achieve this, Intesa Sanpaolo has dedicated circular aids, such as The Plafond, a EUR 6 billion credit facility to support companies that are adopting circular economy principles, and the Circular Economy Lab, that helps corporations as well as small and medium-sized enterprises transition to a circular economy model through education and open innovation programs (Ellen Macarthur Foundation, 2020; Intesa Sanpaolo, 2020). To the bank, supporting a circular economy model has potential for value creation by expanding the investments that Intesa Sanpaolo will pursue, thus creating new business and increasing resilience against market risks such as climate change as described above (Ellen Macarthur Foundation, 2020). They found this to be true – between 2018, when The Plafond was founded, to June 2021, Intesa Sanpaolo funded 263 applications, valuing more than EUR 3.5 billion (Ellen Macarthur Foundation, 2020). In total, within this time period, they received 650 applications, underscoring that when the tools are in place, companies, including the construction sector, will adopt circular economy models.

11.3.2 The Supply Process

Real Estate and Residential Developers

Developers are instigators of the construction process and thus must support circularity by embracing new economic models (Keena & Friedman, 2021). In a circular approach, developers are collaborators for the user and construction phase (Thelen et al., 2018). Their roles must shift to develop networks of knowledge exchange, stimulate innovative practices, and raise building standards (Keena & Friedman, 2021). Using sharing platforms discussed in Chapter 3, developers can stimulate integrated design and reduce the operational carbon emissions of a building. Product as a service model is another business model that developers can promote. Supporting new business models in their buildings is one way to stimulate circularity, reshaping the role of short-term investors to a holistic developer. Adopting circular economy design, including designing for flexibility, for instance, can reap benefits for builders. For instance, allowing users to adapt the internal layout of their unit lowers the cost of labor, time, and material in unsold units (Friedman, 2011). As well, to market a company as "innovative" may increase sales of units (Friedman, 2011).

Architects

Architects, advisors, and engineers are in charge of planning, designing, calculating, and reviewing the construction of buildings in line with requirements in terms of budget and design (Thelen et al., 2018). However, in a circular design approach, designers must play a more holistic and collaborative role, working with clients, developers, contractors, and investors, with the life cycle perspective in mind. One way to do this is by designing with upcycled materials and collaborating with material upcyclers to incorporate resources that can be recovered after deconstruction. This collaborative perspective in the initial design phase not only changes the weight of the role of the architect but that of the supplier and building companies as well (Thelen et al., 2018). Architects must understand the new material solutions for sustainable and circular buildings, including how to use secondary materials and reusable materials (Thelen et al., 2018). The availability of existing materials must be calculated in the initial phases. Architects should participate in the sharing platform when planning their building, using such platforms as a database or market venue for reusable material to connect with material supply (Thelen et al., 2018). Lastly, when architects apply a life cycle approach, deconstruction of a building must also be planned. There are two central ways to expand an architect's role for flexibility and circularity: expanding the architect as an advisor to the user of the dwelling unit; and expanding the architect's role to that of a researcher developing new spatial archetypes, construction techniques, and organizational patterns that the homeowner and builder can use (Keena & Friedman, 2022). Architects must understand the user's specific needs. Studying and implementing the socio-economic characteristics of the user, applying a life cycle cost technique as well as an environmental life cycle assessment to the decision-making process, and familiarizing oneself with technical systems that allow for flexibility in multi-unit housing will be important. Figure 11.6 illustrates the architectural design phases and the potential for circular economy business models to be incorporated along the building life cycle. This can lead to a new circular design approach.

Construction Companies

Building companies are in charge of the construction of individual or multi-unit projects. While in a linear approach, these contractors may be the central decision makers for their buildings, in a circular approach, construction companies gain expertise from other venues (Thelen et al., 2018). They can expand their role from the construction phase to that of maintenance, operation, and deconstruction (Thelen et al., 2018). These companies view building materials as providing a service in a circular economy (Keena & Friedman, 2021). Design and construction best practices should be made in collaboration with designers and deconstruction companies. Furthermore, establishing the Product Life Extension model (see Chapter 3) will significantly impact the role of the construction contractor. Rather than a goal of building a large number of buildings and moving on, working on smaller refurbishment projects and extending the useful life of a building by overseeing multiple phases of a building's life will be more commonplace (Thelen et al., 2018).

Suppliers and Vendors

Suppliers and vendors can supply secondary resources, and even building materials as services. They can create bio-sources and provide renewable and recycled products as well as offer upcycled services (Keena & Friedman, 2022). In a linear model, suppliers and vendors' procurement of materials is cost-driven with little consideration of modifications or improvements (Thelen et al., 2018). Changing the construction documents can lead to capital risk and is thus avoided. In a circular economy, however, the supplier's role changes, offering not only sustainable and renewable materials but also services such as leasing and remanufacturing. Providing transparency about products contributes to effective communication between stakeholders. Standardizing information through such platforms as a material passport (see Chapter 4) is one way to do this. A product's circular details, quality, and sourcing would be provided in the passport and can be shared to meet clients' needs. Therefore, a notable change is required in the role of the supplier. Materials supplied should shift from virgin primary materials to renewable and recycled secondary materials. Innovative business models discussed in Chapter 3 should be incorporated as well, such as service-based models, which do not require the supplying of new materials but are based on resource recovery instead (Thelen et al., 2018). This also comes with a life cycle perspective of the materials provided – suppliers are expected to ensure the quality of their product, reducing waste, and encouraging refurbishment for long-term usage. Transparency is an important aspect of this, which can be achieved through sustainable performance labels, such as material passports, or life cycle assessments. Since suppliers often have a sizable amount of overhead and financial security, they are often the actors to push new technological innovation. Better communication between stakeholders will allow such innovation to progress throughout the building-making process.

11.3.3 The Demand Process

Homeowners and Users

Homeowners have an important role in implementing circularity in a way that is not necessarily charged by profit. Owners see a building as either a short- or long-term asset that should maintain the highest possible value throughout its life (Thelen et al., 2018). A homeowner typically has a unique relationship as they both own the asset and benefit from its functions until they sell. In a circular approach to building, the building has multiple contracts involved, changing the homeowner's role from the owner of a single asset to getting involved in data management, acting as contract managers and smart solution providers (Thelen et al., 2018).

Users typically see buildings as objects that fulfill a singular function for them, creating a direct relationship between the demand and the asset price. However, in a circular economy, this perspective needs to change, where users see buildings as part of a larger environment (Thelen et al., 2018). Asset prices should be influenced by the level of sustainability the building provides. Rather than a building servicing a singular use, it should act as a healthy and holistic environment for working and living (Thelen et al., 2018). This could result in the user then performing multiple different tasks and functions within a space, contributing to a sharing platform model (see Chapter 3). Moreover, educating the user on the sustainability of a building as a cog in a larger environment can help inform the user to establish sustainable behaviors and lower energy consumption. Furthermore, users hold owners and managers accountable and require transparency and communication. Instead of a top-down approach to building, sharing information allows users to be an active participant with experts to develop circular solutions (Keena & Friedman, 2021).

Building Operators and Managers

Building operators and managers are in charge of the operational phase of a building, such as contracting of lighting, IT facilities, and waste and utility management (Thelen et al., 2018). However, as stressed in Chapter 9, the operational use phase must not be seen in a vacuum. Buildings managers and operators should monitor the building's facilities and material quality throughout the building's life cycle to ensure maintenance needs are met. To increase collaboration and knowledge sharing, shared inventories should be created to allow other stakeholders to report issues and solutions for building maintenance and track the life cycle of building materials (Keena & Friedman, 2021). Managers can then predict problems and understand patterns to ensure maintenance needs are met, including the use of deconstruction techniques during maintenance to avoid waste and promote the recovery of secondary materials. Therefore, building operators and managers must gain data management skills. Collaboration is key as operators and managers oversee all contracts with companies and secondary material banks. Furthermore, as new contracts are incorporated into buildings to provide services and lease constructions, a building's operational role becomes more interconnected with other actors, stressing the need for collaboration and communication, making the manager's role more complex (Thelen et al., 2018).

11.3.4 The Deconstruction Process

Deconstruction replaces demolition in a circular economy. Hence, these roles are new and are often adopted by construction and demolition companies. In a circular economy, the stakeholders in the deconstruction process hold an integral role, acting as the link between one life cycle to the next. New stakeholders, such as deconstruction companies, become important to ensure materials are repurposed and reused.

Deconstruction Companies

Demolition companies are typically in charge of demolishing a building to go to bulk waste streams, while deconstruction companies carefully remove parts of a building for reuse in the future (Thelen et al., 2018). These companies recover resources to avoid complete demolition. From a circular perspective, they can help arrange the shift in ownership of materials from one building to another after deconstruction, using tools like material passports by suppliers and building managers. Demolition and recycling professionals can act as advisors for architects, on material lifespan. Therefore, rather than finishing the job at demolition, these companies expand their role to become suppliers of resources to reinforce circularity and take part in a sharing platform. This will require collaboration with architects and construction companies to find innovative ways to deconstruct buildings into elements of high value (Thelen et al., 2018). This brings in the concept of an integrated design process, breaking away from the sequential construction phases to one that transcends and interconnects.

Material Treatment Companies

Waste treatment companies typically either partially recycle or dispose of waste in landfills. These companies have the potential to amend their role to prioritize a reduction in downcycling and an increase in recycling and upcycling. Specialization in the reuse of materials will complement the work of deconstruction companies and traders, making it pertinent for these stakeholders to communicate and work together (Keena & Friedman, 2021). In addition, linking recycled and reused materials with relevant actors can close the loop of circularity. In this way, waste treatment companies will not be placed at the end of the linear value chain, as they will become providers of resources and are known as "material treatment companies".

11.4 Methods and Technology Knowledge Transfer and Education in the Industry

While specific changes in the role of each stakeholder have been outlined, this section will trace general changes that the building sector must adopt to achieve an integrated design approach, by encouraging productivity in the construction industry, communication, and knowledge transfer. As mentioned in previous chapters, the construction and building sector is notably behind other sectors in terms of productivity and efficiency. Despite making up one of the world economy's largest sectors, with about 10 trillion USD spent on building-related goods and services per year, there is an estimated 1.6 trillion dollar gap in productivity (McKinsey Global Institute, 2017). According to McKinsey's global study on productivity growth, less than 25 percent of construction firms match their overall economy's production growth over the past decade. One of the reasons for this lack of productivity is a lack of communication between stakeholders and transparency between actors along the value chain (Blanco et al., 2018; McKinsey Global Institute, 2017).

Applying an integrated design process is crucial to improving the productivity and efficiency of the building sector. Establishing an integrated design process can be accompanied by seven measures outlined by McKinsey (2017) to tackle the root causes of poor productivity in the building sector. Three of these measures – reshape regulation (for more flexibility), reskill the workforce, and infuse technology into the construction sector – are fundamental to improving productivity and reflective of an integrated design process. According to McKinsey (2017), productivity in the construction industry would improve by 50–60 percent by 2030 if these measures were in place. The remainder of this section will describe in detail these first three foundational measures and how their implementation can improve construction productivity for stakeholders.

11.4.1 Reshape Regulation and Raise Transparency

Government actors can support the reshaping of regulation to ensure that construction is organized, well-planned, and high-quality (McKinsey Global Institute, 2017). The International Construction Measurement Standard project is an example of this, providing global consistency when classifying construction costs from a small-scale individual level to an international scale. This allows for comparative analysis between countries.

One way that regulation can be reshaped is by increasing flexibility by replacing existing regulation with outcome- and risk-based approaches. Rigidity in the materials, equipment, and designs that construction companies can use tends to restrict how companies build, making it difficult to adopt new productive and innovative approaches. An outcome-based approach allows for flexibility. Unlike a prescriptive regulation, in which, for instance, specific spacing of wall studs is written into the building code, an outcome-based code will essentially require that the wall withstand a certain amount of vertical and horizontal force, giving room for new approaches to building to be discovered. The Eurocode in the European Union (EU) has started to adopt an outcome-based approach to building regulation for three main reasons. First, giving construction companies flexibility to build within the bounds of safe outcome requirements allows these firms to decide how to achieve the outcomes on their own, making it easier to transfer building methods between countries (McKinsey Global Institute, 2017). Second, knowledge sharing should be encouraged instead of regulating a percentage of the labor force to local supply. Third, 'performance-based' safety regulation is a form of outcome-based safety regulation that sets the pre-defined outcome but allows firms to seek their own means on how to achieve it. Countries that use this approach see, on average, a tenfold increase in health and safety (Bjerager, 2016).

Second, to encourage forward-thinking regulation, policymakers must incentivize and support productivity. This can come in the form of direct government funding for research and development. For instance, the German Federal Ministry of Transport, Building and Urban Development (now referred to as the Federal Ministry of Transport and Digital Infrastructure since 2013) has been sponsoring research for technical studies to advance building materials and make buildings more environmentally sustainable since the 1990s. Governments can further aid in the push for research and development by providing tax credits or mandating its use on public-procurement projects. In 2017, Belgium, for instance, used fiscal policy to aid in productive practices, awarding grants from a 10 million Euro fund to citizens for the purpose of home renovation if those homes installed energy-efficient appliances. This kind of support allows for productive and repeatable implementation of energy-efficient building practices. Governments can also arrange for a dedicated organization to review innovative materials like Singapore's Building Innovation Panel, which evaluates and approves innovative construction materials and methods (McKinsey Global Institute, 2017).

Increasing transparency and allowing for flexibility gives room for stakeholders to get involved in other stages of the building-making process that a linear approach would prevent. This will foster knowledge transfer between different professionals and give room for innovative design approaches to be experimented with.

11.4.2 Reskilling the Workforce

A major cause of low productivity in the construction sector is a lack of labor-force skills. Training and gaining appropriate workers fall within the realm of contractors, governments, and industry bodies (Thelen et al., 2018). According to the Associated

General Contractors of America, about 91 percent of construction firms are struggling to find workers to fill open positions (Associated General Contractors of America [AGC], 2022). Similarly, in 2015 the Federation of Master Builders found that about 67 percent of 8500 firms were forced to turn down work in the United Kingdom due to a lack of labor (Thelen et al., 2018). On top of an aging workforce that will soon retire, stakeholders must make a concerted effort to train and maintain the local labor force in order to ensure a productive construction sector. This can be done by developing apprenticeship models of circular construction techniques, investing in training frontline workers, and investing in knowledge management (Thelen et al., 2018). Building on this last point, there is a need for workers from different fields, such as engineering to trade peoples, to communicate with one another to solve problems, sharing best practices (Thelen et al., 2018). This form of knowledge sharing is important in an integrated design process – rather than compartmentalizing stakeholders and workers into their specific task, companies must create a culture of knowledge sharing between firms to allow efficiency improvements found in one firm to be transferred to another. Investing in knowledge management systems like software tools, libraries, or company intranets aids in this circulation and codification of best practices. Chapter 10 discusses in detail the role of digital technologies in knowledge sharing in the building sector.

It has become increasingly common for firms to rely on transient workers in the construction sector. This disincentivizes any form of permanent or long-term training programs and perpetuates a sort of low productivity in the construction sector. Construction firms must take on the role of reskilling the workforce, maintaining, at minimum, a small core group of highly skilled labor who can share their knowledge of best practices through knowledge sharing platforms (Thelen et al., 2018). This is reflective of a shift to an integrated building process – trades workers are not a transient entity that work only during the construction phase; rather, skilled labor should be valued by other stakeholders, and their knowledge should be appreciated and transferred to other stakeholders at different stages of the building life cycle. This long-term treatment of skilled labor requires an integration between multiple stakeholders and phases of the building life cycle and as a result will lead to a more productive and reliable workforce.

11.4.3 *Incorporate Virtualization and Digital Technology*

As mentioned in previous chapters, the construction sector is notable in its lack of adoption of digitization to help with productivity, and it has led to significant consequences in their productivity and communication with other stakeholders. One way that digital technologies can help with productivity is by digital collaboration. Having multiple stakeholders use apps that track productivity, and the construction process contributes to transparency and permits real-time collaboration between stakeholders (McKinsey Global Institute, 2017). For instance, Bechtel, the engineering company, has partnered with Rhumbix, a software company, that provides a cloud-based platform for the company to track, in real time, the location of the workforce as well as monitor on-site production, performance, and safety (Bechtel, 2015). Creating collaborative platforms like this is another form of integrative design as it allows a genuine level of transparency between stakeholders at any stage of the construction process, rather than a stakeholder being blind to the stage that does not directly pertain to their task. According to the MGI Construction Production survey, a major barrier to adopting technology like this into the building sector is a lack of internal communication pushing for such innovation. Therefore, it is important for contractors to dedicate the piloting of new construction technology, as Bechtel did with their 'future fund', an accumulation of resources that is made to support the invention and incorporation of new technology (Bechtel, 2015).

In order to successfully implement data technology and virtualization into the design process, a life cycle cost attitude must be valued to justify its adoption. Indeed, adopting new technology can have a large upfront cost, however looking at it through the lens of a long-term return on investment will give owners the fact-based foundation to rationalize such innovation (Blanco et al., 2018). Another way to implement the use of such innovation is by strengthening ties with stakeholders, namely suppliers and owners. Suppliers are often achieving innovation, and with the help of owners to amend industry standards for new methods and materials, contractors will be able to easily adopt such innovation into their projects. Collaboration between stakeholders can also redefine new standards for innovation, providing financial resources, grants, and subsidies to support pilot projects. Reducing risk aversion can be done by multiple stakeholders, like owners and contractors, co-investing in technology pilots so costs and rewards are shared, which would build confidence toward more ambitious projects (McKinsey Global Institute, 2017).

11.5 Conclusion

The building process requires several stakeholders who all have integral roles. In the current linear process of construction, each stakeholder is seen as independent, performing their individual roles in a sort of assembly line fashion. Communication, if done at all, is often with the stakeholder directly before or after them in the building-making process. There are notable consequences to this approach, including a lack of overall communication and long-term life cycle planning. Often stakeholders pursue the route of lowest cost, for their own personal ease and benefit. The integrated approach to construction, however, requires stakeholders to be involved in each step of the building-making process to some extent, fostering knowledge sharing, communication, and long-term life cycle planning. This chapter outlined some of the major stakeholders involved in this process, including different levels of government, financial institutions, real estate developers, architects and designers, project executors, suppliers and vendors, and users. A description of how each stakeholder's role might change when using an integrated approach is detailed. These changes boil down to three main themes: reshaping regulation and raising transparency, reskilling the workforce, and incorporating digital technological innovation.

While these changes have a benefit in terms of building long-term, high-quality housing and sustainable dwellings, this approach also has important impacts on the productivity of the construction sector. In order to achieve a circular economy, stakeholders must redefine their roles in the building process, which has proven to not only lead to environmental and social benefits but economic benefits as well.

References

Associated General Contractors of America (AGC). (2022). *Construction workforce shortages risk undermining infrastructure projects as most contractors struggle to fill open positions*. https://www.agc.org/news/2022/08/31/construction-workforce-shortages-risk-undermining-infrastructure-projects-most-contractors-struggle-0

Bechtel. (2015). *The Bechtel report*. https://www.bechtel.com/getmedia/c3458c29-4000-4b2d-9374-99b134a01eef/2015-bechtel-annual-report-ns.pdf?ext=.pdf

Bjerager, P. (2016). *Performance-based safety regulation*. National Academy of Sciences.

Blanco, J. L., Fuchs, S., Parsons, M., & Ribeirinho, M. J. (2018). *Artificial intelligence: Construction technology's next frontier| McKinsey* & Company. https://www.mckinsey.com/capabilities/operations/our-insights/artificial-intelligence-construction-technologys-next-frontier.

Canadian Construction Association. (n.d.). *The impact of the construction industry is everywhere*. https://www.cca-acc.com/about-us/value-of-industry/#:~:text=The%20impact%20of%20the%20construction,gross%20domestic%20product%20(GDP)

Ellen Macarthur Foundation. (2020). *Embracing the circular economy at Italy's largest bank: Intesa Sanpaolo*. https://www.ellenmacarthurfoundation.org/intesa-sanpaolo

EY, & Institute of International Finance. (2021). *11th annual EY/IIF global bank risk management survey. Resilient banking: capturing opportunities and managing risks over the long term* https://assets.ey.com/content/dam/ey-sites/ey-com/en_gl/topics/banking-and-capital-markets/ey-resilient-banking-capturing-opportunities-and-managing-risks-over-the-long-term.pdf

Friedman, A. (2011). *Decision making for flexibility in housing*. The Urban International Press.

Intesa Sanpaolo. (2020). *Intesa Sanpaolo extends the circular economy fund to the UBI network*. https://group.intesasanpaolo.com/content/dam/portalgroup/repository-documenti/newsroom/comunicati-stampa-en/2020/10/CS%20Estensione%20Plafond%20CE%20UBI_EN.pdf

Intesa Sanpaolo. (2022). A wealth management, protection & advisory leader zero-NPL, digital & fee-driven: Intesa Sanpaolo 2022-2025 business plan. Intesa Sanpaolo. https://group.intesasanpaolo.com/en/editorial-section/the-strength-of-the-group/our-strategy#:~:text=The%202022%2D2025%20Business%20Plan%20envisages%20for%20the%20Group%20strong,%2C%20Social%2C%20Governance)%20commitment

Jagou, S. (2021). *Transitioning to a circular economy, 2014-2020 learning from the Quebec experience*. https://www.quebeccirculaire.org/data/sources/users/5777/20210519201748-quebec-circulairecereportfinalmay192021tiny.pdf

Keena, N., & Friedman, A. (2021). *Circular economy and the housing supply change – Toward affordability and sustainability*. McGill University School of Architecture.

Keena, N., & Friedman, A. (2022). Circular economy in the built environment: Towards housing affordability and sustainability. In W. Leal Filho, A. M. Azul, F. Doni, & A. L. Salvia (Eds.), *Handbook of sustainability science in the future: Policies, technologies and education by 2050*. Springer International Publishing Cham.

Lechner, N. (2015). *Heating, cooling, lighting: Sustainable design methods for architects* (4 ed.). John Wiley & Sons.

McKinsey Global Institute. (2017). *Reinventing construction: A route to higher productivity*. https://www.mckinsey.com/business-functions/operations/our-insights/reinventing-construction-through-a-productivity-revolution

RyFan. (2018). *Construction conundrum*. https://www.ryfan.ca/company/construction-connundrum

Thelen, D., Van Acoleyen, M., Huurman, W., Tom, T., can Brunschot, C., Edgerton, B., & Ben, K. (2018). *Scaling the circular built environment: Pathways for business and government*. World Business Council for Sustainable Development & Circle Economy.

Chapter 12

Pathways Forward

12.1 Upcoming Challenges for the Construction Sector

A global housing affordability crisis, an ever-increasing aging population, and a looming climate crisis are pertinent urban problems that architects must address. Chapters 1–11 have outlined the current problems of the construction sector and argued that a shift to a circular building economy will help cities combat some of these issues.

12.1.1 Global Housing Affordability Crisis

To reiterate, the global housing affordability crisis stresses the unacceptability of the North American approach of expansive and energy-consumptive single detached housing (see Figure 12.1). By 2025, about half a billion households will have to resort to overcrowded and poor housing conditions as a result of the affordability crisis (Woetzel et al., 2014). The linear 'take-make-waste' approach to housing exacerbates this problem, incentivizing builders to maintain rigid building practices that block flexibility for affordability and promote the construction of larger, more expensive houses. In Canada, housing is qualified as "affordable" if the resident spends less than 30 percent of their household's before-tax income on housing (CMHC, 2019). This includes housing repairs, rent, or other expenses related to maintaining their dwelling's quality. This fraction of before-tax income is similarly agreed upon by the US Department of Housing and Urban Development (HUD, 2011). A switch to a circular economy can address many of the needs of renters and homeowners to combat affordability issues. For one, by switching to a circular model, value comes not from the quantity of houses sold or the highest price, but from the quality of housing, promoting product life extension, a sharing and service perspective, and designing for flexibility. As mentioned in Chapter 2, new economic models such as performance economy, loop, and lake economy underpin circular economy, offering new ways to make profit while ensuring long-term quality and maintenance. Furthermore, Chapter 6 described the circular economy's support for flexible design and construction, allowing one's dwelling to adapt to the spatial needs and financial circumstances of a person as they progress through life.

DOI: 10.4324/9781003333975-16

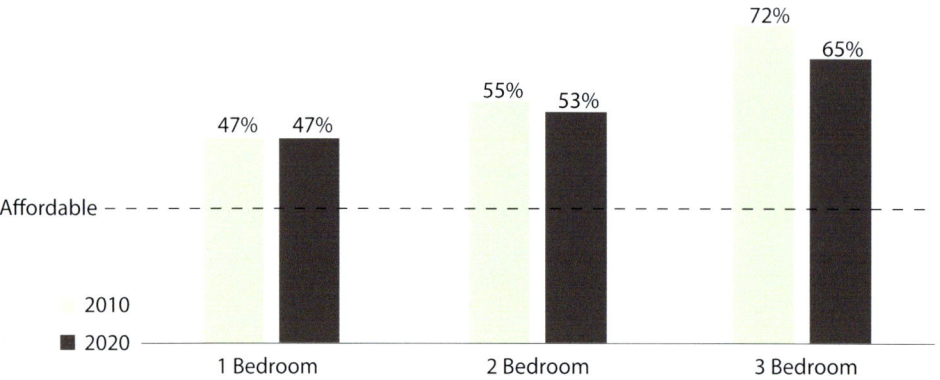

Figure 12.1 Amount That People Spent in Montreal Above the Recommended 30 Percent of Their Income on Housing.

12.1.2 The Need to Age in Place

An aging population is another challenge that the construction industry must seriously consider. As baby boomers age, people aged 55 or older have been rapidly increasing around the world. From 2019 to 2050 the number of citizens aged 65 or older is expected to double, from 703 million to a projected 1.5 billion (United Nations, 2019). "Aging in place" – the ability of older persons to remain in their home and community as they age in an independent, safe, and comfortable way – will be an important urban theme for two central reasons (CDC, 2009). First, the current infrastructure for old-age support is not large enough to deal with the expected number of older persons in cities; and second, autonomy over one's life and the ability to remain in contact with one's social connections have been found to be important factors for feelings of well-being for older adults (Mitzner et al., 2014). Therefore, flexible design that allows dwellings to accommodate limited physical or cognitive functions, as well as ensure high quality and affordability, will be important in the coming years (see Figure 12.2). Circular economy stresses design for disassembly (DFD), factoring in the disassembly and retrofitting processes at the beginning of a building's life cycle to make modifications for people's individual needs easy, affordable, and accessible. This will be important when retrofitting people's homes to accommodate aging and ensure aging in place be an option.

12.1.3 Environmental Damage

Most notably, the construction industry must address the growing environmental concerns posed by the current building-making process. The building sector contributes 50 percent of total raw material use and 36 percent of global final energy use (Norouzi et al., 2021). In the linear economy, the building-making process is treated as sequential, disregarding long-term stages of a building in early development phases. As a result, waste disposal after a building's useful life leads to enormous pollution, accounting for one-third of the total waste in the European Union (Norouzi

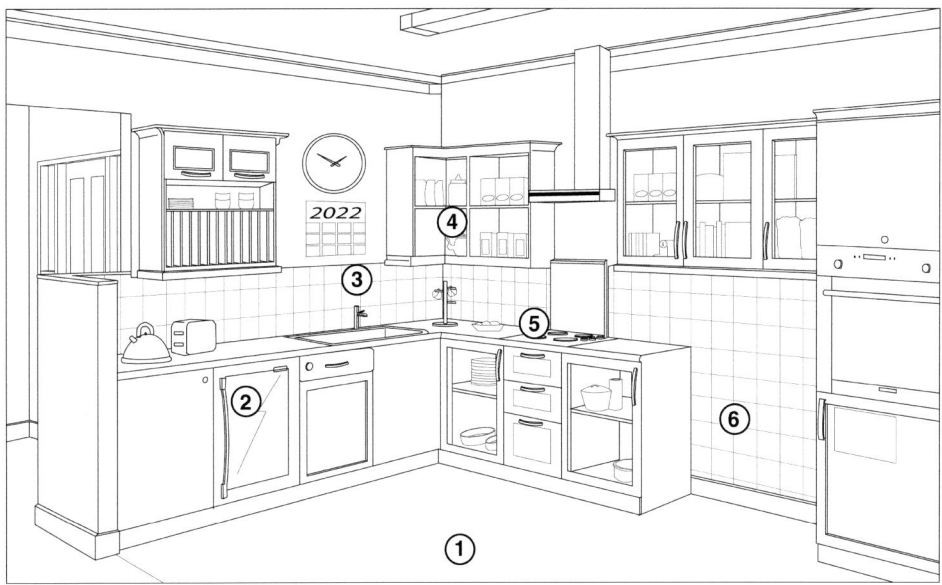

① Open and accessible floor plans for orientaiton

② Glass fronted fridge to show contents. If it is not possible a clear label is acceptable

③ Clocks and calendars for temporal orientation the rooms and a board for leaving

④ Open shelving which allows residents to easily see and use the items

⑤ Kitchen's cooked top is equipped with a "crash barrier"

⑥ Pastel colors in interior since reflections and repetitive pattern can cause fear

Figure 12.2 A Kitchen Designed for People with Dementia Who Age in Place.

et al., 2021). Of the roughly 100 billion metric tons of construction, renovation, and demolition waste generated annually, around 35 percent is sent to landfill on average (Chen et al., 2022). Despite the amount of waste that the linear construction process tends to generate, Yeheyis et al. (2013) find that about 75 percent of total waste generated by the industry had residual value and could have been recycled or reused. Choosing the wrong construction materials at the onset, and disregarding communication between stakeholders as to how to handle the chosen materials, makes it difficult to productively upcycle buildings at the end of life, which then leads to enormous demolition waste. As mentioned in Chapter 2, choosing biomaterials which can be returned to the biosphere after use is one example of a circular approach that aids in the regeneration tenet of the circular economy framework. As described in Chapters 4 and 11, direct and clear communication about the specific materials used in a building's construction, and knowledge sharing and transfer between stakeholders, ensures that methods of building work with one another in the most cost and environmentally efficient way.

Furthermore, operational energy consumption is another huge cost for the environment in the linear economy. Poor construction and material choices lead to inefficient energy use, requiring households to rely on mechanical systems to regulate household temperatures. In 2019, the United States saw 69 MMBtu per capita of average residential energy consumption (US Energy Information Administration, 2022). With rising global temperatures, air conditioners have become particularly prominent, with about 30 percent of households globally owning one, and about 90 percent in advanced economies (International Energy Agency, 2018). However, as discussed in Chapter 9, operational energy can be generated in a net-zero carbon way, by using renewable sources of energy as opposed to fossil fuel, and designing with passive heating, cooling, and lighting techniques that prevent the reliance on mechanical systems. This reliance on mechanical systems for heating, cooling, and ventilation can be avoided by proper planning of the home at the initial stage, where temperature regulation is designed into the building's morphology and orientation. With Lechner's three-tier approach to sustainable design, he outlines that a combination of bioclimatic design strategies, energy-efficient initial building design, and energy-efficient mechanical and electrical equipment can reduce about 85 percent of the operational energy needed for a building to run smoothly (Lechner, 2015). This requires an integrated design approach, planning operational energy methods in the beginning design phases, which circular economy accounts for. Chapter 9 outlines how a circular logic to operational energy design can reduce the superfluous use of energy to operate a building that is engrained in a linear paradigm.

12.2 Remaining Unresolved Questions: Taking Circular Economy from a Concept to Reality

A linear economy uses a "take-make-waste" model, while a circular one is restorative and regenerative, with a central goal of designing out waste, extending the usefulness of a product for as long as possible, and designing buildings which regenerate natural systems rather than harm them. While a circular economy approach to building provides stakeholders, particularly architects, with many of the tools to face pressing urban problems, there are, nonetheless, a number of unanswered questions regarding how to move the concept of circular economy from theory to reality. It is no surprise that this switch from a linear to a circular economy will change the construction sector's approach to building in fundamental ways that need to be addressed. Considering the practical implications of this shift may reveal some gaps that stakeholders should consider when going forward with a circular economy. Questions include how does the supply and demand model specifically change from a linear to a circular model? How do cities and policymakers market a shift to a circular economy so as to foster social acceptance? Who should pay for a switch to a circular economy approach? Should it be governments providing subsidies for homebuilders and homebuyers, or individual homebuilders who believe that buyers will be attracted to the more net-zero carbon home? What role (and power) do homebuyers have on influencing and establishing this shift from a linear to a circular construction industry? In the discussion on housing passports (HPs) in Chapter 4, unanswered questions include how these passports will be managed and by whom? Lastly, a timeline for a circular economy is still unclear, making it difficult to predict if these major urban challenges can genuinely be addressed through a circular economy change in a timely manner. Throughout the rest of this concluding chapter, these unanswered questions will be explored, some solutions may be offered or merely posed for future stakeholders to consider at the onset of their building-making process.

12.2.1 The Reality of the For-Profit Home Building Industry

One central critique of the current circular economy model is that circular economy tends to be somewhat vague and theoretical, making it hard to genuinely criticize but also hard to realistically implement (Kovacic et al., 2019). Circular economy is often framed as a "win-win" and while circularity in the construction sector will bring significant positive impacts to the field, outlining unanswered questions or realistic obstacles for implementation is necessary.

For instance, while recycling is notably better than waste disposal in landfills, having enough recyclable material is a practical obstacle. Back in 1996, Marcus and Kirsis predicted that global steel demand would rise and be dominated by electric arc furnace (EAF) steel (scrap steel; Broughton, 1996). While this is theoretically a good thing, the amount of steel scraps that can practically be recovered is unable to keep up with the demand – even with a demand in recycled goods, supply shortages prevent regeneration from occurring. Moreover, challenges when dealing with secondary resources include possible quality issues, contamination, legacy substances, and supply limitations, as well as price volatility, as Corvellec et al. (2021) explain. These uncertainties around secondary resources mean that although there can be a strong theoretical argument for using secondary materials, if there is a well-established value chain of primary resources, companies will likely still choose to go with the easiest option. This leads to another practical obstacle of circular economy implementation – even if policy is implemented to support circularity, without simultaneous policy to discourage or halt linear economy, circular economy may not be as impactful as theory would suggest (Corvellec et al., 2021). If linear structures are still in place on the market, circular innovations become more difficult to adopt and popularize (Brandão et al., 2020).

12.2.2 Marketability: Convincing the Industry and the Public

Homes are a large investment for a person or family to commit to. Location, personal taste, and size are just some of the considerations that are put into purchasing a particular home. The predicted resale value of a home is one of the major factors determining a house's mass-appeal (Friedman, 2007). Therefore, the question of whether a circular home will lead to high resale value, or higher resale value relative to a linear home, is an important question for homebuilders to consider.

The seven "Ps" of marketing are as follows: product, price, promotion, place, packaging, positioning, and people – all of which apply to circular homebuilding. For instance, 'packaging', or aesthetics, contributes to a homebuyer's decision to purchase a dwelling. Circular economy's flexible design approach will mean that a home may be left for owners to adapt and accommodate to fit their functional and aesthetic needs, avoiding the production of rigid identical homes to a variety of people (see Figure 12.3). A builder's ability to present a range of options for how a building can look and adapt can allow homebuyers to design their homes to align with their personal tastes (Friedman, 2007). Once again, it is the responsibility of other stakeholders, such as builders and the government, to convey that this freedom for customization is available, or else circular economy homes may appear somewhat unfinished to the uninformed eye.

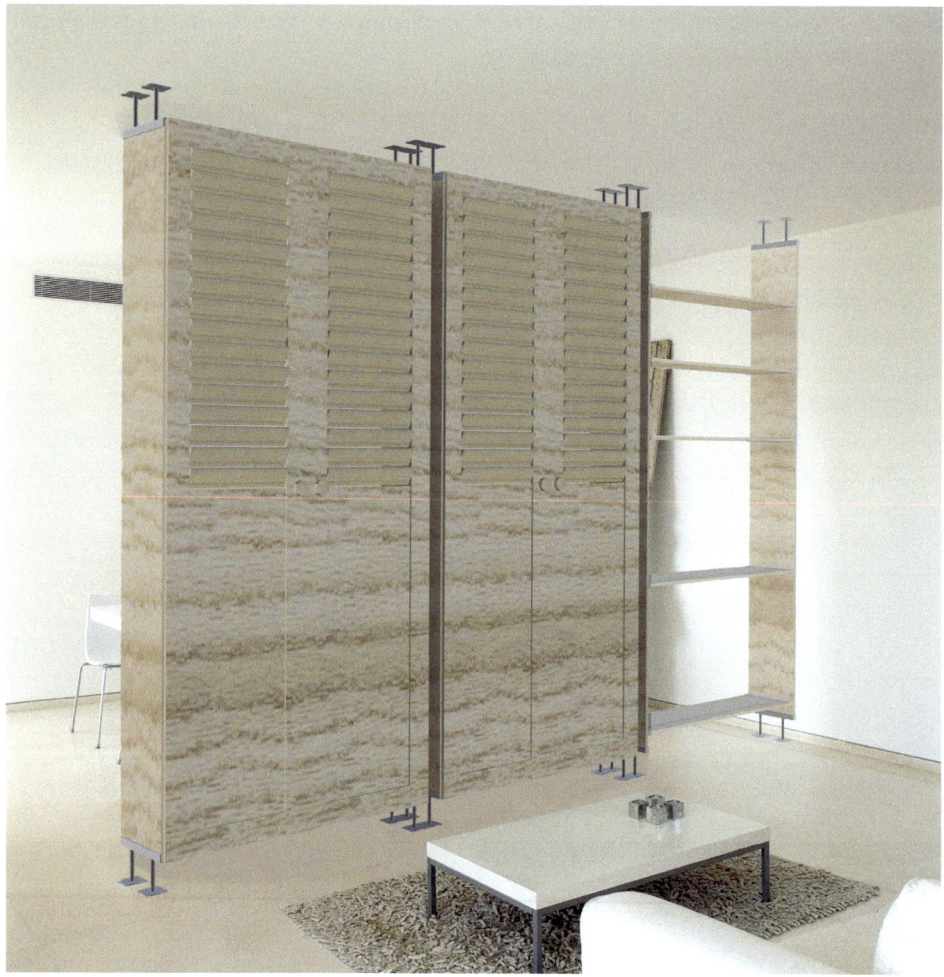

Figure 12.3 Instead of Permanent Partitions, Open Plan Configurations Can Use Furniture or Shelving to Offer More Flexibility.

In terms of price, as mentioned in Section 12.1, circular economy's ability to offer smaller homes and spaces that serve multiple functions (thus lowering cost per person) is an effective way of offering affordable housing for renters and profitable housing for owners. When looking through a life cycle perspective, circular economy building surely offers more affordable building options since its focus on durability and adaptive construction will lead to less costs on repairs down the line. When a building is made quickly or cheaply, there may be lower upfront costs, but less durable and lower quality materials will lead to frequent replacement and higher overall cost (Friedman, 2007). Although poor construction and insulation will lead to higher long-term costs, in order to justify the higher upfront cost required by circular economy, promotion and advertising of the benefits of adopting a circular economy approach must be done. Chapter 11 addressed the role of governments in explaining what circular economy is to the public to make potential buyers understand the long-term financial and social benefits of supporting a circular approach (Keena & Friedman, 2021).

However, a caveat to this assumption that a circular economy home is always more durable and higher quality than a non-circular economy home must be noted. While renewable materials are generally seen as more environmentally friendly than virgin resources, if untreated renewable materials require more energy to remain high quality, they may have a shorter useful life than an alternative product, making their environmental benefits marginal, potentially leading to higher costs for the user (Friedman, 2007). Establishing quality criteria for recycled products is a good solution to certify the final product as proficient quality and boost its marketability (Tam et al., 2018).

12.2.3 Cost Issues for Circular Economy Implementation

Another question related to circular economy implementation relates to what role stakeholders hold in terms of the cost attached to a circular economy shift. Which stakeholders should and could be responsible for the cost of this switch? While a long-term cost assessment may reveal that a circular home is less costly than a linear one, the higher upfront costs may be what separate someone from being able to buy versus rent. And if the buyer is unsure of how long they will live in the dwelling, the long-term payoff of a more environmentally sound and durable construction may not be justified (Friedman, 2007). A risk of the circular economy approach is it might price out homebuyers due to (often perceived) higher upfront costs. Therefore, the role of governments or lending institutions comes into the discussion, to possibly provide subsidies for building or purchasing a circular home. Although a circular home may be perceived to have higher upfront costs, it does not always have to be the case. The Circle House Demonstrator case study in Chapter 4 and the Resource Rows case study in Chapter 5 and are good examples of affordable circular housing.

Governments or banks can give out subsidies for companies or builders who choose circularity. Furthermore, they can provide subsidies or loans to help homeowners retrofit homes for energy efficiency to cover the initial added costs. Tax breaks can also financially incentive a circular economy shift. In Sweden, for instance, repairing consumer goods instead of tossing them to landfills is rewarded by tax breaks (Orange, 2016). Governments can provide grants, equity funding, loan guarantees, and leasing to finance private investment in circularity and research and development (R&D) (OECD, 2022). For instance, the European Investment Bank (EIB) provides medium- and long-term loans to large-scale circular economy projects and indirect financing for small-scale projects (European Investment Bank, 2020).

Moreover, along with financial incentives to encourage circular economy, there should be financial disadvantages to discourage continuing with linearity. Environmentally related taxes that increase the cost of raw material extraction, emissions, and waste demolition fees could be enforced. Moreover, Extended Producer Responsibility (EPR) policy instruments could be administered, putting the responsibility of a product's end-of-life stage onto the producer (OECD, 2022).

A switch to a circular economy will require additional costs before reaping the benefits. There are several ways for governments and financial institutions to incentive circular economy and disincentivize linearity. Each country must consider the myriad of options to determine how to realistically encourage and implement circularity in their specific country.

12.2.4 The Role of Homebuyers

While choosing a sustainable housing development may result in more upfront costs today, homebuyers have a role in this circular economy shift, by communicating to building companies that sustainability is what they value. Knowledge about how their home is built via HPs and the financial benefits of energy-efficient homes should push homebuyers to retrofit their homes for efficiency. Countries such as the United States and Canada have committed to funding retrofitting projects for aging building stock in order to improve energy efficiency, which is one way of making the housing stock more sustainable (Magwood et al., 2021). However, as stressed in Chapter 9, if these energy retrofits are ignoring material carbon emissions or fuel-source emissions associated with operational energy use, the energy retrofit will fail to address the accurate carbon use intensity and thus will not be significantly environmentally beneficial (IEA, 2021). Furthermore, failing to account for the embodied carbon levels linked to large-scale retrofits can pose a greater long-term environmental risk by increasing the demand for these materials (United Nation Environment Programme, 2007). This is particularly pertinent if circular principles are not considered in the initial design for retrofits. For example, new retrofit assemblies should be designed with DFD in mind if we are to avoid the problems of demolition and waste 60 years from now when these facades will need renovations. In brief, while government-supported retrofitting projects have the potential to have important environmental and financial effects, these must be deep energy retrofits that account for the whole building life cycle (United Nation Environment

Programme, 2007). Homeowners have the responsibility to seek out genuine environmental reform rather than surface-level shifts and advocate for their homes to be regenerative and restorative.

12.2.5 Housing Passport Management

Chapter 4 outlined the significance of HPs and Chapter 10 confirmed how data and technology can help bring the HP concept to reality. However, administrative questions about this concept are still unclear. For instance, which stakeholder will oversee the development and management of HPs? What will the actual process look like to collect the information on housing materials and quality for existing buildings? How will management of HPs work and by whom? These managerial questions are what will turn a concept like the HP into a functional reality.

12.2.6 A Circular Economy Timeline

While there can be significant benefits to transitioning to a circular economy and many governments are beginning to encourage and set goals for sustainability and circular economy, it is still unclear when circular economy will become socially accepted among users and stakeholders, when technological innovation in the construction sector will be fully developed and adopted, and when the linear economy's dominance will subside. In the past 30 years, global sustainability conferences have set global sustainability goals with years in mind. The Paris Agreement set the goal of maintaining global temperature to below 2°C (3.6°F) by cutting emissions by about 50 percent by 2030 (United Nations, 2015). The UN Sustainable Development Goals (SDGs) aim to be accomplished by 2030. However, these timelines are not necessarily realistic either. Recently, for instance, the Nationally Determined Contribution (NDC) Synthesis Report stresses that it is unlikely that the goals of the Paris Agreement will be achieved by 2030 (UN, 2021). The Council of Canadian Academies has recently published Turning Point, their official document on what a turn to a circular economy would entail for the country (Council of Canadian Academies, 2021). Documents like this are important, as it outlines different routes the country can take to establish circular economy policies, giving a regionally specific scenario of circular economy implementation and what the country would presumably look like if it did adopt different circularity approaches versus continuing as it has been in the linear realm. These visualizations and predictions are important to realistically understand when these benefits from circularity are expected. While setting goals is important, realistically accounting for current conditions and obstacles to visualize timelines can be helpful in sharing authentic information. More research should be done on creating realistic timelines of circular economy implementation in the coming years.

12A

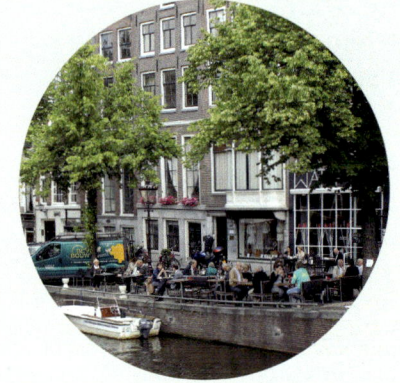

Project:
Amsterdam: An Innovative
Circular City

Location:
Amsterdam, the Netherlands

Year:
2020–2025

Team:
City of Amsterdam

**Mapping to Circular
Economy Framework:**

CIRCULAR ECONOMY PRACTICES

LIFE CYCLE PHASES

Recovery | Life Extension | Sharing Platforms | Service Models | Regenerate | Virtualize

Work of Geobiosphere

Sourcing

Manufacturing

Design & Construction

Use

End-of-Use

LAYERS + LIFESPAN
Structural Layers | Long Life
Skin, MEP Layers | Medium Life
Interior Layers | Short Life

Site 100+yr Structure 50+yr
Exterior 25+yr System 15+yr
Partition 10+yr Stuff 1+yr

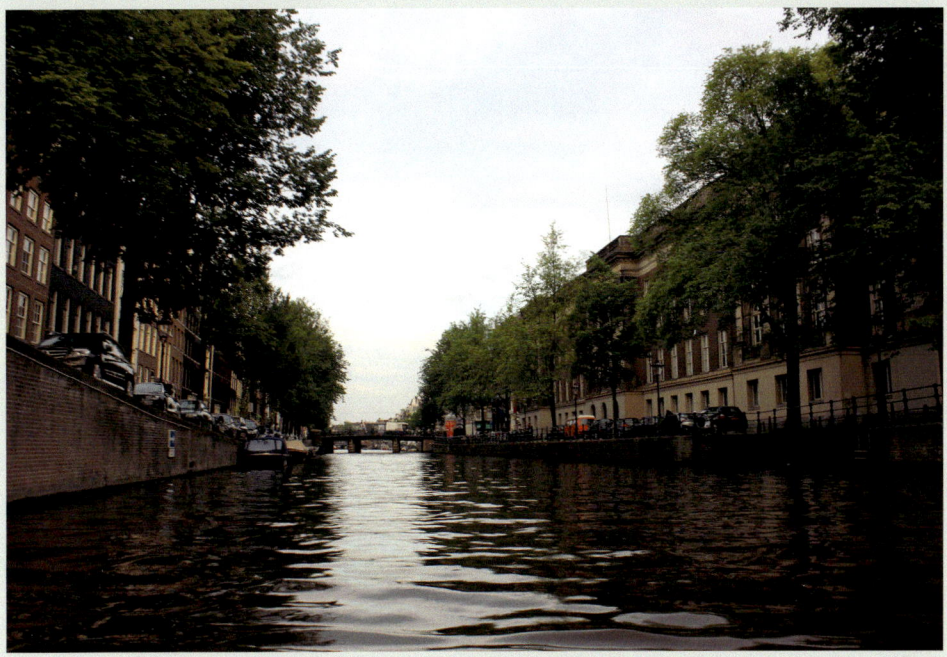

Figure 12.4 Amsterdam Is a City Taking the Lead on Urban Circularity.

In their 2019 report "Amsterdam Circular 2020-2025", the City of Amsterdam outlines pathways forward to a circular future, providing a rich example of a city that has taken the concept of circularity and is turning it into a reality(see Figure 12.4; City of Amsterdam et al., 2019). The report justifies how Amsterdam specifically will benefit from a circular turn, explaining their current state of circularity, and multiple different pathways that the city can go down to foster a circular economy in what Kate Raworth calls "doughnut economics". The city's goal is to be completely circular by 2025 and aims to cut primary raw material usage by 50 percent by 2030. To do this, a fundamental change is needed in terms of how Amsterdam conducts production and consumption. The city has prioritized three value chains for their shift to the circular economy: Construction, Biomass and Food, and Consumer Goods. Because of the sheer impact of these three value chains, starting with these reformations will have an enormous impact on Amsterdam's carbon footprint. However, rather than merely stating what they want to do, the city has come up with 17 directions that the city can pursue to achieve a holistic circular economy in these three realms, building off of existing policies and actions Amsterdam already has in place. For each direction, the city has run the ideas past external stakeholders and conducted tests in a participatory process of over 50 participants from Amsterdam. Questions that had to be answered to qualify the direction included "why is this circular strategy relevant to Amsterdam?", "what are the main impacts involved in a shift to a CE for Amsterdam?", "how close is Amsterdam to this circular direction regarding the policies and activities in place right now?", and "which stakeholders are most relevant to this strategy?". By asking these questions, the city can parse through potential

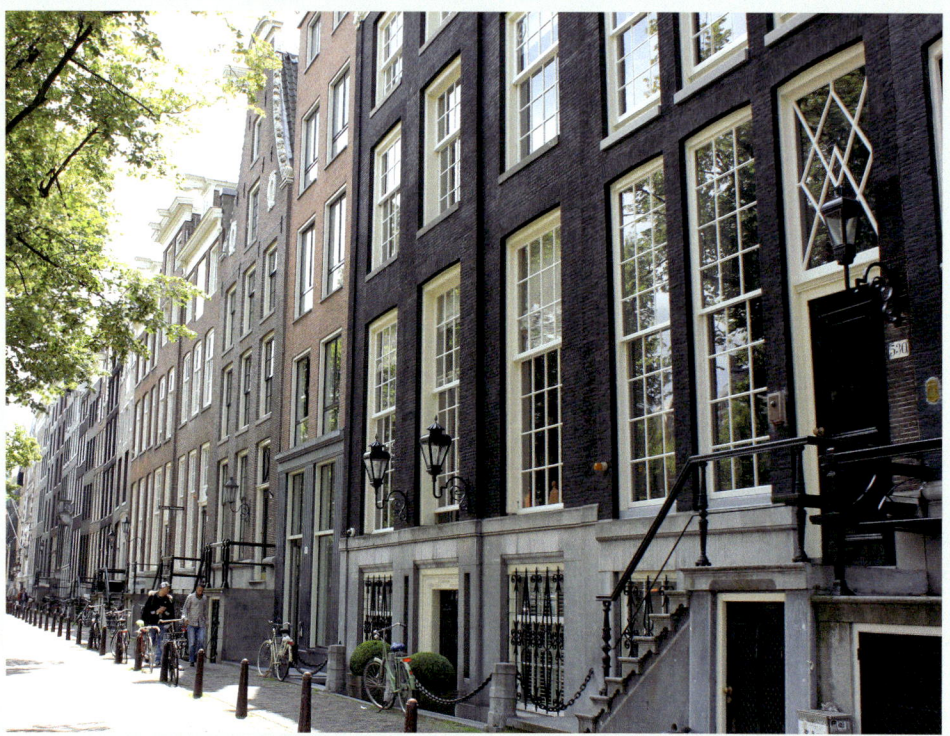

Figure 12.5 Amsterdam Rowhouses a Stable of Amsterdam's Housing Stock. The City's Circular Economy Roadmap for the Construction Sector Outlines Adaptable and Modular Buildings, a Switch to Secondary Materials, and Retrofitting Housing as Promising Pathways Forward in Considering the Circularity of Their Housing Stock.

circular economy actions that may be less impactful or less practical to their city, thus achieving a region-specific and pragmatic CE strategy.

In terms of the construction sector, there are six directions that the city of Amsterdam outlined: (1) foster flexible zoning, (2) incorporate circularity into land issuing, (3) make adaptable and modular buildings, (4) scale up mono-stream collection and circular dismantling, (5) switch to renewable and secondary materials, and (6) retrofit private and social housing (see Figure 12.5). Two of these actions will be described in more detail to understand how Amsterdam is personalizing these goals to their context.

Fostering flexible zoning will allow for circular activity 'hubs' that engage with climate adaptation and regenerative design. Flexible zoning also allows mixed uses in a neighborhood, allowing space to be more efficient, more walkable, and reduce negative environmental impacts of urban sprawl (see Figure 12.6). For Amsterdam specifically, this measure is compatible with past projects the city has conducted, such as Buiksloterham's Schoonschip – a small grass-roots neighborhood prototype – and Haven-Stad – a larger urban district that is being developed, prioritizing accessibility, identity, and sustainability. The Schoonschip is a circular economy community in Amsterdam with 46 floating homes as illustrated in Figure 12.7. Designed by Space and Matter architects along with the residences, the site at De Ceuvel was once a polluted post-industrial wasteland. The residential community now share solar electricity

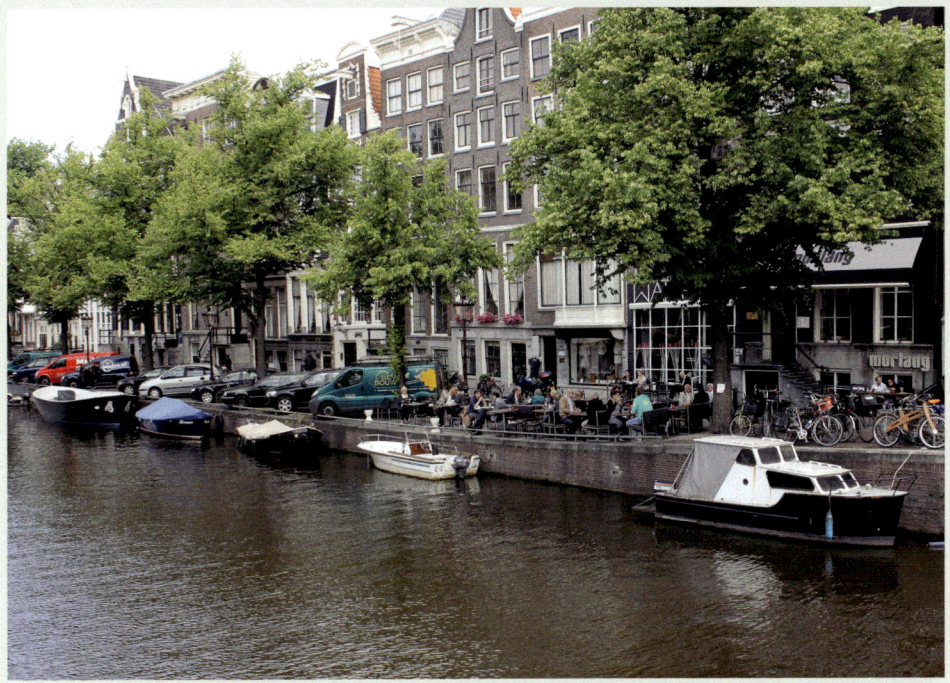

Figure 12.6 Along the Canals of Amsterdam Demonstrates Flexible Zoning where Mix Uses in a Neighborhood Are Promoted Thereby Reducing the Negative Environmental Impacts of Urban Sprawl.

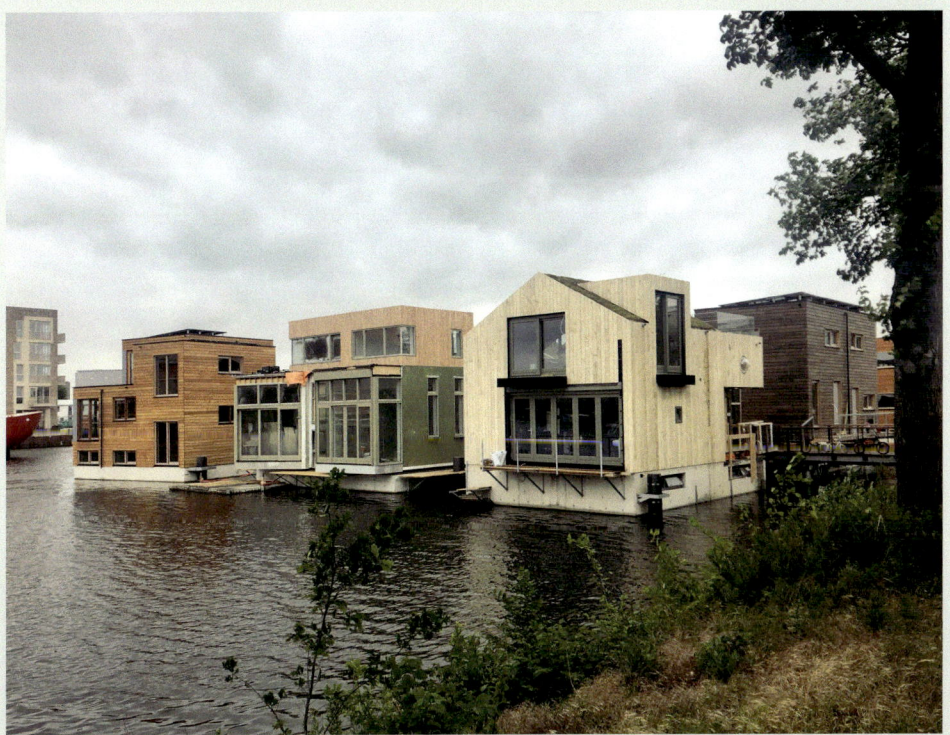

Figure 12.7 Floating Houses in the Schoonschip Circular Economy Community, Amsterdam.

361

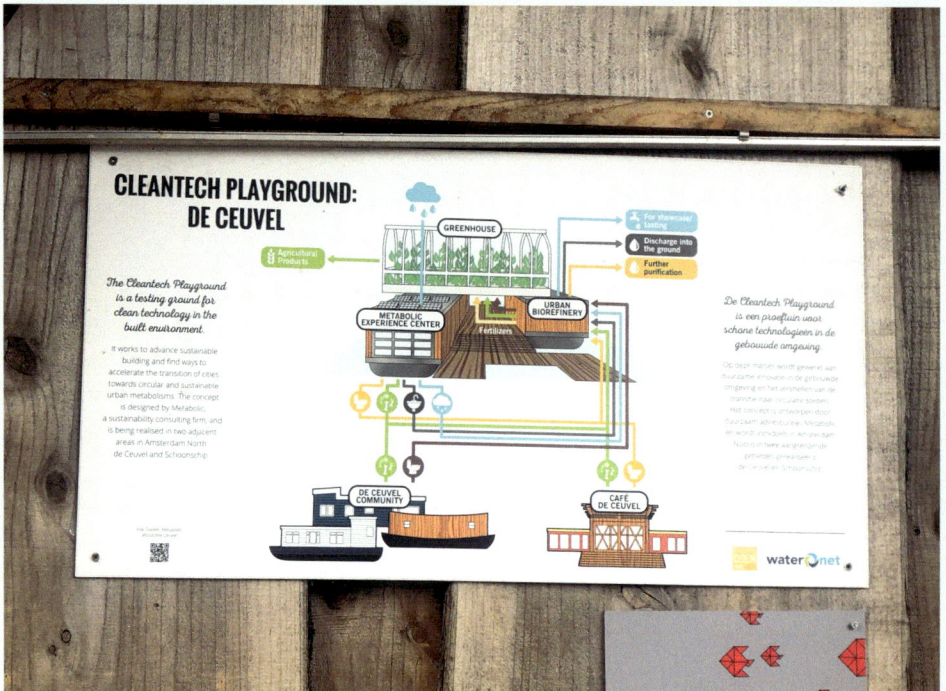

Figure 12.8 Throughout Schoonschip Education and Knowledge Transfer of Circular Economy Methods Are Shared Through On-Site Posters Which Clearly Explain the Circular Ecosystem at Play. This On-Site Poster Explains How Water Is Being Reused and Recycled for Use Throughout the Community.

through a blockchain smart-grid, recycle all waste including black water produced on-site, and have worked with Metabolic, a sustainability consulting firm, to restore and regenerate the water of the site via an urban scale biorefinery (Figure 12.8). The fact that mixed-use, environmentally sound neighborhoods have already been developed suggests that the city's residents and infrastructure are receptive to such a change. The report outlines exactly what regulations should be in place: adopt climate adaptative criteria and circular economy in land issuing and make spatial planning flexible. The report suggests platforms should be made to share knowledge and best practices in the fields of biomimicry and biophilic design. This should be shared between architecture and construction firms. On a more individual basis, stakeholders should research how flexible zoning can be applied through shorter leasehold periods. Similar to how Chapter 11 stresses that each stakeholder should have a role in the transition to a circular economy, this report goes into more detail, outlining the role of each stakeholder in making each circular direction become a reality. This includes different levels of governments, businesses, NGOs, public service providers, educational institutions, and the civil society.

Another circular construction direction includes a concept that has been suggested throughout this book – using renewable and secondary construction materials. However, rather than just explaining the benefits of using secondary material, Amsterdam outlines why such a change would work and benefit their city. In Amsterdam, the construction sector contributes a large part to the total carbon dioxide emissions, with most of these emissions coming from production of primary materials such as concrete. However, after assessing the practicality of using secondary materials for construction in Amsterdam, the city found that only about one quarter of newly built projects will be able to sufficiently use this material (Errami & Kootstra, 2018). Instead of relying completely on reused materials, the city is focused more on utilizing renewable bio-based materials such as wood, which can be sourced from neighboring areas. A caveat is stressed that while sourcing renewable materials can have a beneficial environmental impact, this must not be done at the cost of ethical sourcing practices which could lead to destructive land conversion on the local and global scale. This is a helpful example of a city assessing the life cycle of a product and determining that a method of circularity that could work in one location may not be as effective in this city. Ethically sourcing renewable material with low transportation emissions is the best scenario. Direct financial support to encourage secondary and renewable materials, providing training on new building methods and biomimicry education, lobbying for carbon taxation to encourage bio-based materials, and offering price incentives for private and corporate real estate owners who use renewable and reused materials, are all effective and clear actions that stakeholders can do to successfully implement this goal.

Using this sort of funnel framework, where the city recognizes a concept of circularity that could be helpful, and then slowly specifies that concept to become personal to their city, is a crucial process that cities need to conduct on their own. Looking at the current infrastructure and past projects that a city has achieved will help guide planners and architects as to what actions are most likely to succeed, what actions are most needed, and which stakeholders should and will be willing to be involved. Amsterdam effectively outlines possible circular economy actions, potential barriers to success, and the correlated solutions, thus creating a pragmatic strategy to achieve circularity. Cities should use Amsterdam's approach to a circular economy plan as a template for implementing circularity into their respective city.

12.3 Conclusion

Clearly, there are uncertainties and obstacles that must be addressed in more detail as the circular economy develops. Nonetheless, a circular economy approach to the building sector is a beneficial and necessary shift that stakeholders should seriously consider. This book acts as a guide for architects, as well as other building sector stakeholders, on the benefits, opportunities, and practicalities of implementing circular economy more generally in the building sector. Going forward, this chapter outlines specifications that need to be considered on a case-by-case basis. Regional timelines, consideration of specific recycling supply issues, and whether energy retrofits are whole life cycle renovations are just some of these specifications. A switch to a regenerative and restorative construction framework, however, is necessary in combating urgent urban and construction issues and is important in establishing social, economic, and environmental sustainability. Considering these potential obstacles is important for architects at the outset of planning to turn a circular economy into a reality.

References

Brandão, M., Lazarevic, D., & Finnveden, G. (2020). *Handbook of the circular economy*. Edward Elgar Publishing. https://doi.org/10.4337/9781788972727

Broughton, A. C. (1996). Scrap shortage: Fact or fiction. *Recycling Today*. https://www.recyclingtoday.com/article/scrap-shortage--fact-or-fiction/

CDC (2009). *Healthy places terminology*. Centers for Disease Control and Prevention.

Chen, Z. K., Feng, Q., Yue, R. Y., Chen, Z., Moselhi, O., Soliman, A., Hammad, A., & An, C. J. (2022). Construction, renovation, and demolition waste in landfill: A review of waste characteristics, environmental impacts, and mitigation measures. *Environmental Science and Pollution Research*, 29(31), 46509–46526. https://doi.org/10.1007/s11356-022-20479-5

City of Amsterdam, Circle Economy, & Kate, R. (2019). *Building blocks for the new strategy: Amsterdam circular 2020–2025*. https://assets.website-files.com/5d26d80e8836af2d12ed1269/5de954d913854755653be926_Building-blocks-Amsterdam-Circular-2019.pdf

CMHC. (2019). *Identifying core housing need*. Canadian Mortgage and Housing Corporation. Retrieved January 23 from https://www.cmhc-schl.gc.ca/en/professionals/housing-markets-data-and-research/housing-research/core-housing-need/identifying-core-housing-need

Corvellec, H., Stowell, A., & Johansson, N. (2021). Critiques of the circular economy. *Journal of Industrial Ecology*, 26, 1–12.

Council of Canadian Academies. (2021). Turning point. In *The expert panel on the circular economy in Canada*. Council of Canadian Academies.

Errami, S., & Kootstra, L. (2018). Quickscan Impact assessment (circulaire) bouwopgave MRA. Economisch Instituut voor de Bouw. https://www.eib.nl/pdf/Quickscan%20impact%20assessment%20(circulaire)%20bouwopgave%20MRA_web.pdf

European Investment Bank. (2020). The EIB circular economy guide : Supporting the circular transition. European Investment Bank. https://data.europa.eu/doi/10.2867/578286

Friedman, A. (2007). *Sustainable residential development: Planning and design for green neighborhoods*. McGraw-Hill.

HUD (2011). *Glossary of terms to affordable housing*. U.S. Department of Housing and Urban Development.

IEA. (2021). *World energy outlook 2021*. International Energy Agency. https://iea.blob.core.windows.net/assets/4ed140c1-c3f3-4fd9-acae-789a4e14a23c/WorldEnergyOutlook2021.pdf

International Energy Agency. (2018). *World Energy Outlook* 2018 (License: CC BY 4.0). IEA, Paris. https://www.iea.org/reports/world-energy-outlook-2018

Keena, N., & Friedman, A. (2021). *Circular economy and the housing supply change – Toward affordability and sustainability*. McGill University School of Architecture.

Kovacic, Z., Strand, R., & Völker, T. (2019). *The circular economy in Europe: Critical perspectives on policies and imaginaries* (1st ed.). Routledge. https://doi.org/10.4324/9780429061028

Lechner, N. (2015). *Heating, cooling, lighting: Sustainable design methods for architects* (4 ed.). John Wiley & Sons.

Magwood, C., Ahmed, J., Bowden, E., & Deva Racusin, J. (2021). *Achieving Real Net-Zero Emission Homes: Embodied carbon scenario analysis of the upper tiers of performance in the 2020 Canadian National Building Code*. https://www.buildersforclimateaction.org/uploads/1/5/9/3/15931000/bfca-enercan-report-web_08_21.pdf

Mitzner, T. L., Chen, T. L., & Kemp, C. C., & Rogers, W. A. (2014). Identifying the potential for robotics to assist older adults in different living environments. *International Journal of Social Robotics*, 6(2), 213–227. https://doi.org/10.1007/s12369-013-0218-7.

Norouzi, M., Chàfer, M., Cabeza, L. F., Jiménez, L., & Boer, D. (2021). Circular economy in the building and construction sector: A scientific evolution analysis. *Journal of Building Engineering*, 44, 102704. https://doi.org/10.1016/j.jobe.2021.102704

OECD. (2022). *The circular economy in Ireland*. OECD Publishing. https://doi.org/10.1787/7d25e0bb-en

Orange, R. (2016). *Waste not want not: Sweden to give tax breaks for repairs*. Retrieved January 23, 2023, from https://www.theguardian.com/world/2016/sep/19/waste-not-want-not-sweden-tax-breaks-repairs

Tam, V. W. Y., Soomro, M., & Evangelista, A. C. J. (2018). A review of recycled aggregate in concrete applications (2000–2017). *Construction and Building Materials*, 172, 272–292. https://doi.org/10.1016/j.conbuildmat.2018.03.240

UN. (2021). *Nationally determined contributions under the Paris Agreement* Conference of the Parties serving as the meeting of the Parties to the Paris Agreement, Glasgow, UK. https://unfccc.int/sites/default/files/resource/cma2021_08E.pdf

United Nations. (2015). *Paris agreement*. https://unfccc.int/sites/default/files/english_paris_agreement.pdf

United Nations. (2019). *World population ageing 2019: Highlights*. https://www.un.org/en/development/desa/population/publications/pdf/ageing/WorldPopulationAgeing2019-Highlights.pdf

United Nation Environment Programme. (2007). *Buildings and climate change: Current status, challenges and opportunities*. https://www.unep.org/resources/report/buildings-and-climate-change-status-challenges-and-opportunities

US Energy Information Administration. (2022). *How much energy does a person use in a year?* https://www.eia.gov/tools/faqs/faq.php?id=85&t=1#:~:text=In%202022%2C%20 total%20U.S.%20primary,per%20capita%20transportation%20energy%20use

Woetzel, J., Ram, S., Mischke, J., Garemo, N., & Sankhe, S. (2014). *A blueprint for addressing the global affordable housing challenge*. https://www.mckinsey.com/~/media/ mckinsey/featured%20insights/urbanization/tackling%20the%20worlds%20affordable%20 housing%20challenge/mgi_affordable_housing_full%20report_october%202014.ashx

Yeheyis, M., Hewage, K., Alam, M. S., Eskicioglu, C., & Sadiq, R. (2013). An overview of construction and demolition waste management in Canada: A lifecycle analysis approach to sustainability. *Clean Technologies and Environmental Policy*, *15*(1), 81–91. https://doi.org/10.1007/s10098-012-0481-6

Case Studies Teams

The following credits the teams who have provided information on the Case Study projects outlined in this book. We apologize for any omission, and we will make sure to include in future editions. Figures related to the following case studies were published with permission.

BAMB – Buildings as Material Banks
EU Horizon 2020 Project
https://www.bamb2020.eu/
Drawings: BAMB
Photos: BAMB

Benny Farm
L'OEUF and Saia Barbarese
    Topouzanov architects
Photos: Avi Friedman

Circle House Demonstrator
Lejerbo (Client), GXN Innovation,
    MT Højgaard, Danish Building
    Research Institute (SBi), The
    Danish Association for Responsible
    Construction.
GXN Copenhagen A/S,
Kanonbådsvej 8, 1427 Copenhagen K,
    Denmark
Drawings: GXN
Photos: Adam Mørk

Circular Multi-Family and Single-Family Housing (CMF and CSF)
McGill University's Circular
    Homebuilding Team
Montreal, Canada
Drawings: McGill University's Circular
    Homebuilding Team
Photos: McGill University's Circular
    Homebuilding Team

Data Homebase
McGill University's Circular
    Homebuilding Team
Montreal, Canada

Drawings: McGill University's Circular
    Homebuilding Team
Photos: McGill University's Circular
    Homebuilding Team

Deep Performance Dwelling – Solar Decathlon China
TeamMTL
McGill University + Concordia
    University
Montreal, QC, Canada
Drawings: TeamMTL
Photos: TeamMTL

Ecological Living Module
Yale Center for Ecosystems +
    Architecture and Gray Organschi
    Architecture in collaboration with UN
    Environment Programme and UN
    Habitat
New York City, USA
Drawings: Yale Center for Ecosystems +
    Architecture and Gray Organschi
    Architecture
Photos: David Sundberg/Esto; Naomi
    Keena

Hammarby Sjöstad
The City of Stockholm
Hammarby Sjöstad, Sweden
Photos: Avi Friedman

Loblolly House
Kieran Timberlake Architects
Maryland, USA
Photos: Peter Aaron/OTTO

Maison Tropicale
Jean Prouvé Workshops
Niamey, Niger and Brazzaville, Republic
of Congo, Africa
Drawings: Jean Prouvé Workshops

Même – Experimental House
Kengo Kuma and Associates
2 Chome-24-8 Minamiaoyama, Minato
City,
Tokyo 107-0062, Japan
https://kkaa.co.jp/en/
Photos: Kengo Kuma and Associates

Resource Rows
Lendager Group
Otto Busses Vej 27
2450 København S, Denmark
https://lendager.com/
Drawings: Lendager Group
Photos: Rasmus Hjortshøj

Reuse Made Easy and Opalis
Rotor
58 rue Prévinaire straat
1070 Brussels, Belgium
http://rotordb.org/en/projects/
rotor-dc-reuse-made-easy
http://rotordb.org/en/projects/opalis
Drawings: Rotor
Photos: Rotor

The Circular Building
Arup
Joachimsthaler Straße 41
10623 Berlin, Germany
https://www.arup.com/
Drawings: Arup
Photos: Daniel Imade

The House of Wood, Straw, and Cork
LCA Architetti
16, Via Carbonin
Varese, VA, Italy
www.lcarchitetti.com
Drawings: LCA Architetti
Photos: Simone Bossi

VMD Prefabricated House
Taller Escape and Studioroca
Del Carmen 9, Avandaro,
51200 Vale de Bravo, Mexico City,
Mexico
www.vmd.com.mx
Drawings: Taller Escape and Studioroca
Photos: @vmdhomes/www.vmd.com.mx

Zufferey House
Nunatak Architectes Sarl
Rue des Follatères 15, CH-1926 Fully,
Valais, Switzerland
https://www.nunatak.ch/portrait/nunatak/
Drawings: Nunatak Architectes Sarl
Photos: Dominique Marc Wehrli

Illustrations Credits

Figures not listed below are in the public domain or have been conceived, drawn, or photographed by the authors and members of their research and design teams. Their names are listed in the acknowledgements. Every effort has been made to list all contributors and sources. In case of omission, the author and the publisher will include appropriate acknowledgement or correction in any subsequent edition of this book.

Figure 1.2:	United Nations Sustainable Development Goals. Creative Commons Attribution-Share Alike 4.0 International license
Figure 2.12:	Photo by Polina Mukhamedova on Unsplash
Figure 2.13:	Photo by Zul Ahadi on Unsplash
Figure 2.14:	Photo by Michael Gaylard from Horsham, UK, CC BY 2.0, via Wikimedia Commons
Figure 2.15:	Photo by Fabio Fistarol on Unsplash
Figure 3.2:	Clockwise from top left: Low Angle Shot of a Cathedral's Dome by Lada Rezantseva CC; Old church dome in overcast weather by Rachel Claire CC; Black Wooden Dining Table In A Coffee Shop by Anna Tukhfatullina CC; Assorted Decors With Brown Rack Inside Store Creative Commons by Afta Putta Gunawan CC.
Figure 3.13:	Redrawn and adapted from Iyer-Raniga, U., & Huovila, P. (2020). Global state of play for circular built environment. A report on the state of play on circularity in the built environment across Africa, Asia, Europe, Gulf Cooperation Council countries, Latin America and the Caribbean, North America and Oceania.
Figure 3.22:	© Simon Kennedy
Figure 3.23:	© Daniel Imade_Arup
Figure 3.24:	© Daniel Imade_Arup
Figure 3.25:	Arup
Figure 3.26:	© David Sundberg/Esto
Figure 3.27:	Gray Organschi Architecture
Figure 3.28:	Yale Center for Ecosystems + Architecture
Figure 3.29:	Yale Center for Ecosystems + Architecture
Figure 3.30:	Naomi Keena
Figure 3.31:	Yale Center for Ecosystems + Architecture
Figure 3.32:	© David Sundberg/Esto
Figure 3.33:	Yale Center for Ecosystems + Architecture
Figure 3.34:	Gray Organschi Architecture
Figure 3.35:	Yale Center for Ecosystems + Architecture
Figure 3.36:	© David Sundberg/Esto
Figure 4.10:	BAMB – Buildings as Material Banks
Figure 4.11:	BAMB – Buildings as Material Banks

Figure 4.12:   BAMB – Buildings as Material Banks
Figure 4.13:   BAMB – Buildings as Material Banks
Figure 4.14:   BAMB – Buildings as Material Banks
Figure 4.15:   © Adam Mørk
Figure 4.16:   GXN
Figure 4.17:   © Adam Mørk
Figure 4.18:   © Adam Mørk
Figure 5.10:   Rotor 'Opalis' project at http://rotordb.org/en/projects/opalis
Figure 5.11:   Redrawn and adapted from L'OEUF and Saia Barbarese Topouzanov
                 architects
Figure 5.14:   © Rasmus Hjortshøj
Figure 5.15:   © Rasmus Hjortshøj
Figure 5.16:   Lendager Group
Figure 5.17:   © Rasmus Hjortshøj
Figure 5.18:   © Rasmus Hjortshøj
Figure 5.19:   © Rasmus Hjortshøj
Figure 5.20:   Rotor 'Opalis' project at http://rotordb.org/en/projects/opalis
Figure 5.21:   Rotor 'Reuse made easy' project at http://rotordb.org/en/projects/
                 rotor-dc-reuse-made-easy
Figure 5.22:   Rotor 'Opalis' project at http://rotordb.org/en/projects/opalis
Figure 5.23:   Rotor 'Reuse made easy' project at http://rotordb.org/en/projects/
                 rotor-dc-reuse-made-easy
Figure 5.24:   Rotor 'Reuse made easy' project at http://rotordb.org/en/projects/
                 rotor-dc-reuse-made-easy
Figure 7.1:   Data sourced from UNEP. (2021). 2021 Global Status Report for
                 Buildings and Construction.
Figure 7.4:   Redrawn and adapted from Lehne, J., & Preston, F. (2018).
                 Making Concrete Change: Innovation in Low-carbon Cement
                 and Concrete. Chatham House. Keena, N., Duwyn, J., & Dyson, A.
                 (2022). Biomaterials Supporting the Transition to a Circular Built
                 Environment in the Global South. Yale Center for Ecosystems +
                 Architecture and UN Environment Programme. Data sourced from
                 the Inventory of Carbon and Energy (ICE) databases. (Hammond
                 and Jones, 2008, 2011, 2019) and literature sources (Lawrence, 2015;
                 Yu, et al., 2011).
Figure 7.5:   Data sourced from United Nations. (2019). World Urbanization
                 Prospects: The 2018 Revision (ST/ESA/SER.A/420). https://
                 population.un.org/wup/publications/Files/WUP2018-Report.pdf.
                 OECD. (2019). Global Material Resources Outlook to 2060: Economic
                 Drivers and Environmental Consequences. OECD Publishing. https://
                 doi.org/10.1787/9789264307452-en
Figure 7.7:   Based on OMA/AMO 2014 Venice Biennale.
Figure 7.8:   Redrawn and adapted from Matos, G. R. (2022). Materials flow in the
                 United States—A global context, 1900–2020: U.S. Geological Survey
                 Data Report.

Figure 7.9:	Redrawn and adapted from H M Treasury. (2013). Infrastructure carbon review. London: HM Treasury. World Green Building Council. (2019). Bringing embodied carbon upfront: Coordinated action for the building and construction sector to tackle embodied carbon.
Figure 7.10:	Redrawn and adapted from IRP. (2020). Resource Efficiency and Climate Change: Material Efficiency Strategies for a Low-Carbon Future. E. Hertwich, Lifset, R., Pauliuk, S., Heeren, N. A report of the International Resource Panel. United Nations Environment Programme.
Figure 7.15:	Redrawn and adapted from Matos, G. R. (2022). Materials flow in the United States—A global context, 1900–2020: U.S. Geological Survey Data Report.
Figure 8.4:	Redrawn and adapted from Merrild, H., Jensen, K. G., & Sommer, J. (2016). Building a circular future. GXN. Ozzi, L. E. (2019). Design for Disassembly with Structural Timber Connections. Faculty of Architecture & the Built Environment, Delft University of Technology. https://repository.tudelft.nl/islandora/object/uuid:c8b85050-cd11-45eb-b3ac-c3624259654f/datastream/OBJ/download
Figure 7.18:	© Simone Bossi
Figure 7.19:	© Simone Bossi
Figure 7.20:	© Simone Bossi
Figure 7.21:	© Simone Bossi
Figure 7.22:	© Simone Bossi
Figure 7.23:	LCA Architetti
Figure 7.24:	LCA Architetti
Figure 7.25:	LCA Architetti
Figure 7.26:	© Peter Aaron/OTTO
Figure 7.27:	© Peter Aaron/OTTO
Figure 7.28:	© Peter Aaron/OTTO
Figure 7.29:	© Peter Aaron/OTTO
Figure 7.30:	© Peter Aaron/OTTO
Figure 8.6:	Photo by Patrick Charpiat, Creative Commons Attribution 3.0 Unported License
Figure 8.7:	Photo by Gabriel Fernandes, Creative Commons Attribution 2.0 Share-Alike Generic License
Figure 8.8:	Photo by Gabriel Fernandes, Creative Commons Attribution 2.0 Share-Alike Generic License
Figure 8.9:	Redrawn from Jean Prouvé Workshops
Figure 8.10:	© Dominique Marc Wehrli
Figure 8.11:	© Dominique Marc Wehrli
Figure 8.12:	© Dominique Marc Wehrli
Figure 8.13:	Nunatak Architectes Sarl
Figure 8.14:	Nunatak Architectes Sarl
Figure 8.15:	Nunatak Architectes Sarl
Figure 8.16:	© Dominique Marc Wehrli

Figure 8.17:   © Dominique Marc Wehrli

Figure 9.1:   Redrawn and adapted from United Nations Environment Programme (2021). 2021 Global Status Report for Buildings and Construction: Towards a Zero-emission, Efficient and Resilient Buildings and Construction Sector. Nairobi.

Figure 9.2:   Redrawn and adapted from Lechner, N. (2015). Heating, Cooling, Lighting: Sustainable Design Methods for Architects (4 ed.). John Wiley & Sons.

Figure 9.3:   Based on IEA (2021), *World Energy Outlook 2021*, IEA, Paris https://www.iea.org/reports/world-energy-outlook-2021, License: CC BY 4.0

Figure 9.4:   Redrawn and adapted from Beck, H. E., Zimmermann, N. E., McVicar, T. R., Vergopolan, N., Berg, A., & Wood, E. F. (2018). Present and future Köppen-Geiger climate classification maps at 1-km resolution. *Scientific Data*, 5(1), 180214. https://doi.org/10.1038/sdata.2018.214

Figure 9.5:   Photo by Christiaan Benjamin Nieuwenhuis, CC0, via Wikimedia Commons

Figure 9.10:   Redrawn and adapted from IRP. (2020). Resource Efficiency and Climate Change: Material Efficiency Strategies for a Low-Carbon Future. In: International Resource Panel.

Figure 9.12:   © Kengo Kuma and Associates

Figure 9.13:   © Kengo Kuma and Associates

Figure 9.14:   © Kengo Kuma and Associates

Figure 9.15:   © Kengo Kuma and Associates

Figure 9.16:   TeamMTL

Figure 9.17:   TeamMTL

Figure 9.18:   TeamMTL

Figure 9.19:   TeamMTL

Figure 9.20:   TeamMTL

Figure 9.21:   TeamMTL

Figure 10.1:   Text available under the Creative Commons Attribution-ShareAlike License

Figure 10.2:   Redrawn and adapted from McKinsey Global Institute. (2017). *Reinventing Construction: A Route to Higher Productivity*. By Barbosa, Filipe, Jonathan Woetzel, and Jan Mischke. McKinsey Global Institute.

Figure 10.19:   @vmdhomes/ www.vmd.com.mx

Figure 10.20:   @vmdhomes/ www.vmd.com.mx

Figure 10.21:   @vmdhomes/ www.vmd.com.mx

Figure 10.22:   @vmdhomes/ www.vmd.com.mx

Figure 10.23:   @vmdhomes/ www.vmd.com.mx

Figure 10.24:   @vmdhomes/ www.vmd.com.mx

Index

Note: Page references in *italics* denote figures.

Civil Society Organizations and the Global Response to HIV/AIDS

Why has the response to HIV/AIDS been unique? How did civil society organizations gain access to global decision-making forums to demand exceptional attention and resources for HIV/AIDS? This book seeks to answer these questions, among others, through a critical international relations approach that enquires into the role of civil society in global health governance. It documents how civil society forged the initial response to HIV/AIDS within a rights-based paradigm, and built international networks. It analyses why civil society was able to gain the right to participate in global health institutions and assesses what influence civil society representatives have within these institutions, particularly focusing on outcomes related to institutional legitimacy and downward accountability. It then discusses changes in the broader political economy of global health and how HIV/AIDS organizations have, or have not, adapted to these shifts. Finally the book tells the story of the many struggles civil society organizations have engaged in to advance a rights-based response to HIV/AIDS, the transformations achieved and the resistance experienced.

Julia Smith is Postdoctoral Fellow at Simon Fraser University, Canada, and a Research Fellow at the Health Economics and HIV/AIDS Research Division in South Africa.

Global Health

Series Editor: Nana Poku

The benefits of globalization are potentially enormous, as a result of the increased sharing of ideas, cultures, life-saving technologies and efficient production processes. Yet globalization is under trial, partly because these benefits are not yet reaching hundreds of millions of the world's poor and partly because globalization has introduced new kinds of international problems and conflicts. Turmoil in one part of the world now spreads rapidly to others, through terrorism, armed conflict, environmental degradation or disease.

This timely series provides a robust and multi-disciplinary assessment of the asymmetrical nature of globalization. Books in the series encompass a variety of areas, including global health and the politics of governance, poverty and insecurity, gender and health and the implications of global pandemics.

Most recent titles

Civil Society Organizations and the Global Response to HIV/AIDS

Julia Smith

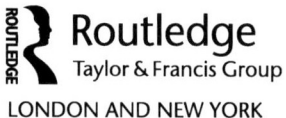
Routledge
Taylor & Francis Group

LONDON AND NEW YORK

First published 2017
by Routledge
2 Park Square, Milton Park, Abingdon, Oxon OX14 4RN

and by Routledge
605 Third Avenue, New York, NY 10017

First issued in paperback 2021

Routledge is an imprint of the Taylor & Francis Group, an informa business

© 2017 Julia Smith

Publisher's Note
The publisher has gone to great lengths to ensure the quality of this reprint but points out that some imperfections in the original copies may be apparent.

British Library Cataloguing in Publication Data
A catalogue record for this book is available from the British Library

Library of Congress Cataloging in Publication Data
A catalog record for this book has been requested

ISBN 13: 978-1-03-224233-0 (pbk)
ISBN 13: 978-1-138-22045-4 (hbk)

DOI: 10.4324/9781315412771

Typeset in Times New Roman
by Taylor & Francis Books

Contents

Acknowledgements

I am deeply grateful to the Global Health series editor, Nana Poku, for his invaluable support, guidance and encouragement over the years. I would like to thank Owen Greene, for his constructive criticism during the process of writing the thesis on which this book is based, as well as the examiners of the thesis – Neil Cooper and Colin McInnes – for their helpful feedback. I am further indebted to Véronique Dimier, Jim Whitman and Tom Woodhouse for their advice and kind encouragement. Finally, I would like to thank Kelley Lee for her remarkable mentorship as I brave the world of academia.

I could not have completed this project without the support of my family: my parents for supporting all my adventures (academic and otherwise); Carolyn and Kory for sharing their home; and Maggie for being a calming influence. Thank you Robin – for providing the support and encouragement that keeps me motivated.

Abbreviations

AIDS	Acquired Immune Deficiency Syndrome
ARASA	AIDS and Rights Alliance of Southern Africa
ART	Anti-Retroviral Therapy
ASO	AIDS Service Organization
CBO	Community-Based Organization
CSO	Civil Society Organization
CSS	Community System Strengthening
DALYs	Disability Adjusted Life Years
DTF	Dual Track Financing
EECA	Eastern Europe and Central Asia
FBO	Faith-Based Organization
FPM	Fund Portfolio Manager
GAVI	The Vaccine Alliance
GFAN	Global Fund Advocates Network
GFMSM	Global Fund for Men Who Have Sex with Men
GHI	Global Health Institution
GHG	Global Health Governance
GIPWA	Greater Involvement of People with HIV/AIDS
Global Fund	Global Fund to Fight AIDS, Tuberculosis and Malaria
GNP+	Global Network of People Living with HIV/AIDS
GPA	Global Program on AIDS
HIV	Human Immunodeficiency Virus
IAS	International AIDS Society
ICAD	Interagency Coalition on AIDS and Development
ICASO	International Coalition of AIDS Service Organizations
ICSS	International Civil Society Support
ICW	International Community of Women with HIV/AIDS
IMF	International Monetary Fund
INGO	International Non-Governmental Organization
INPUD	International Network of People Who Use Drugs
IR	International Relations
MAP	Multi-Country AIDS Program
MARP	Most at Risk Populations

MDG	Millennium Development Goals
MERG	Monitoring and Evaluation Reference Group
MSM	Men who have Sex with Men
NAC	National AIDS Council
NFM	New Funding Model
NGO	Non-Governmental Organization
OIG	Office of Inspector General
PCB	Program Coordinating Board
PEPFAR	President's Emergency Plan for AIDS Relief
PR	Principal Recipient
PWA	People/Person Living with HIV/AIDS
PWID	People/Person Who Injects Drugs
SDG	Sustainable Development Goal
TB	Tuberculosis
TRP	Technical Review Panel
UN	United Nations
UNAIDS	United Nations Joint Program on HIV/AIDS
UNESCO	United Nations Education, Scientific and Cultural Organization
UNICEF	United Nations Children's Fund
UNODC	United Nations Office on Drugs and Crimes
UNPF	United Nations Population Fund
USAID	United States Agency for International Development
WHO	World Health Organization

1   Introduction

The AIDS movement didn't do a good job of including people with AIDS; the AIDS movement is those people, and that is how the AIDS movement started. It wasn't like some outside force created a movement and said hey we should include these folks. People with AIDS started this and, everything else built around us – the entire global response.

(CSO Representative 2013)

In the early 1980s, a mysterious and fatal illness was identified as spreading among otherwise healthy young men in North America and Western Europe. In 1983, the Human Immunodeficiency Virus (HIV) was identified as the cause of Acquired Immune Deficiency Syndrome (AIDS). The modes of transmission, most often sex and sharing of needles, and lack of a cure or vaccine generated widespread panic. By the end of the 1980s it was clear that the virus was present in every region of the world and was particularly rampant in Sub-Saharan Africa. Between 1980 and 1996 (when treatment was introduced), over 6.4 million people worldwide died of AIDS related illnesses.

Both states and international institutions failed to respond quickly and proactively to the early epidemic. Within this governance gap, alliances of people living with HIV/AIDS (PWAs), medical professionals and human rights activists created their own response. By the time states and institutions recognized HIV/AIDS as a global threat, in the late 1990s, CSOs were already engaged in activism and service delivery. Drawing on their lived experience with and responding to the epidemic, they demanded the right to lead the global response. Their participation gained political acceptance with the signing of the Greater Involvement of People Living with HIV/AIDS (GIPWA) principle, at the Paris AIDS Summit in 1994, which committed the 42 states leading the global response to "support a greater involvement of people living with HIV at all levels" (UNAIDS 2007).

The exceptional role of CSOs in the global response to HIV/AIDS has been widely celebrated. The response has been credited with contributing to participatory transformations in global health governance (GHG) and ushering in an era of more legitimate and accountable global health institutions (GHIs) (Nay 2009). Sidibe et al. argue that HIV/AIDS CSO activism has created a

precedent in GHG: "the many governance innovations offered by the AIDS response, mainly driven by people living with or affected by HIV, that have remade the playing field for tackling other global challenges" (2010, 3). Similarly, the editor of *The Lancet* argues:

> AIDS occupies a unique place in the history of health and, in many ways, the AIDS response has "created" the concept and practice of global health – mainly due to the fact that AIDS forged the greatest civil society movement of the past half century.
>
> (quoted in UNAIDS PCB 2013)

As the global health community now orientates itself around the Sustainable Development Goals (SDGs) and new health challenges, there are calls to replicate and learn from these examples of inclusive governance (Buse et al. 2012). The President of the World Bank wrote a commentary titled *Want to Build a Social Movement? Learn from AIDS Activists*, in which he argued that those engaged with other issue areas should copy the activism HIV/AIDS CSOs (Yong Kim 2014). Health and human rights champion Paul Farmer (2014) wrote that those wishing to address Hepatitis C infections in lower income countries should learn from the successful mobilization around HIV/AIDS. When the Ebola epidemic broke out in Western Africa in 2014 there were immediate calls to mimic the anti-stigmatization campaigns of the AIDS response (Partridge 2014).

Despite widespread recognition that CSOs have fulfilled a unique role in HIV/AIDS governance, there is little reflexive analysis of how and why these governance arrangements emerged, or of what their outcomes have been. Instead there is an assumption that CSO participation is inherently beneficial, as an outcome in itself. There are few sustained analyses of the opportunities and limits CSOs engage with, their motivations, and the results of their efforts. Doyle and Patel (2008) note that though it is assumed that HIV/AIDS CSOs have positive impacts on the legitimacy of global health institutions (GHIs), there is little empirical research to support this claim. Lee writes that "there is a particular need for systematic analysis of the functions CSOs perform in global health governance" (2010, 2). There is a contradiction within the literature and commentary on CSOs and GHG: on the one hand there is acknowledgement of the prominent role CSOs fill in the global HIV/AIDS response; on the other, there is little analysis of the outcomes of their participation.

What this book is about

This book poses, and aims to answer, critical questions about the role of CSOs in the global AIDS response; asking if CSO participation has influenced how the HIV/AIDS epidemic is framed, how GHIs operate, and how GHG impacts those most affected by the epidemic. In short, it asks not only why and how CSOs became engaged in the global governance of AIDS, but what the

outcomes of their participation are. It aims to test assumptions about the role of CSOs in global governance in general, and the HIV/AIDS response in particular, while empirically documenting the results of CSO engagement.

The geographic focus of this book is broad. The term "global" in "global AIDS response" does not necessarily indicate transnational or trans-regional. Instead it refers to those processes that happen beyond the borders of the nation state. Most often these global processes, and the actors who have power within them, are located in the global north. Institutional headquarters, meetings and staff are most often based in northern locations, and much of the resources are generated in the north and then distributed elsewhere, based on the dynamics of the global political economy. Global responses usually, but not always, "happen" in the north and are imposed on other regions – but these regions also react to, respond to and reinterpret these processes, influencing them in turn. So while the majority of this analysis focuses on activity in centres such as Geneva and New York, it also analyses interactions with other levels of governance in various geographic regions.

Following Chapter 2, which presents a brief history of the early HIV/AIDS response, the majority of original research and analysis in this book focuses on developments between 2008 and 2015. The selection of 2008 as a starting point for primary analysis is due to the fact that it marks a crucial juncture in the HIV/AIDS response. Notable changes during this period include: the emerging backlash against AIDS exceptionalism; the economic recession in donor countries and consequent stagnation of overseas development assistance; and general shifts within GHG towards more integrated programmes (Whiteside & Smith 2009). It is hoped that analysis of this time period will contribute to illuminating the dynamics of recent developments in GHG. For example, the book accounts for a number of processes that have been neglected or not yet addressed in global health literature, such as the role of the civil society delegations on the UNAIDS and Global Fund boards; the involvement of CSOs in resource governance, particularly around the Global Fund's New Funding Model; and the shift from a human rights to key populations framing of the epidemic.

One of main themes of this book is the role of CSOs in creating and advancing the human rights-based responses to the epidemic. This is not a new narrative; others (Hein et al. 2007; Ford et al. 2011; Parker 2011) have written to the same effect. What is added here is that as opposed to focusing on rights outcomes related to treatment access (which the above authors do), the focus is on rights related to sexuality, access to harm reduction, the rights of sex workers, and women's sexual and reproductive health. Implicit to all of these rights campaigns is the need for social and economic rights, as well as legal and political rights. This expands the literature on HIV/AIDS and human rights beyond the narrow focus on treatment access.

This contribution is important because while the right to treatment is correctly viewed as a major achievement for those most affected by the epidemic, the outcomes of these other rights campaigns are arguably just as important,

but much more difficult to decipher (which may explain the gap in academic and policy literature). For example, it is more difficult to measure women's ability to make choices about family planning, than how many women have access to pre and postnatal ART to prevent vertical transmission. Despite this challenge, and while not attempting to quantify outcomes, this book aims to present a unique analytical discussion on efforts to advance comprehensive rights related to the global HIV/AIDS movement.

The daily lives (and deaths) of PWAs, and those at risk of and affected by HIV/AIDS, must be kept in mind throughout the reading of this book. Though the death rate from AIDS has declined rapidly over the past decade, due to the introduction of ART and effective prevention methods, in 2014, 1.2 million people still died of AIDS related causes, and there were 2 million new infections (UNAIDS 2015). HIV spreads through a complex mix of biological and social determinants. Those who are most vulnerable socially, economically and politically are also at greater risk of HIV infection. Globally, young women have an infection rate that is twice that of young men (UNAIDS 2013). Men who have sex with men (MSM), sex workers and people who inject drugs (PWID) are also at high risk of infection, partly because of biological determinants and behaviours, but largely because of poor access to health care, discrimination and social marginalization.

Access to prevention services, support, treatment and care is shaped by social, political and economic contexts. Only a little over half of those in need have access to life prolonging treatment, and the vast majority of People Living with HIV/AIDS (PWAs) without access live in low-income countries and rural locations. The majority of PWID still do not have access to harm reduction methods – the only proven HIV prevention method among this population group. Women in Sub-Saharan Africa continue to provide the majority of HIV/AIDS care work voluntarily, unsupported by the state or private actors.

Though such experiences are not the primary topic under investigation here, they are the impetus for it. Recognition that lived experiences of the epidemic are shaped by global systems of disease and political choices that shape the response necessitates critical reflection on whether the global response is relevant and responsive to those most at risk of and affected by the HIV/AIDS epidemic, and how it can better serve them.

Framework of analysis

This book aims to situate the HIV/AIDS response within the global political economy of global health, aid and development. While many international relations (IR) approaches to global governance focus on the global political economy of international trade, markets and development, this book falls into a specific grouping that focuses on institutions and social movements that attempt to bring about alternatives to not only economic systems, but also health, education and other social sectors. Other IR scholars and political economists who have pursued this line of inquiry include Bakker (2007) who

introduces the concept of social reproduction, such as care work, into political economy frameworks, and Petchansky (2003) who analyses global intersections between health, gender and development. O'Manique's (2004) work is most closely related to this study as she examines how neoliberal policies shaped the early response to HIV/AIDS. Building on this tradition, I particularly draw on frameworks that fall into the broad field of critical IR, which roots analysis in historical-materialist approaches; and has explicitly normative goals in that it aims to expose contradictions in order to illuminate how transformations to a more equitable world system might come about (Murphy 2005, 13). This critical IR approach is defined loosely recognizing that, as Cox writes:

> The problem facing anyone who seeks to define the "problematic" of the contemporary world is to draw upon and in so far as possible integrate modes of understanding from different sources so as to yield a result that both explains adequately and orients action. That is the only valid test, not whether you follow correctly some pre-established model.
>
> (1981, 129)

Therefore, some aspects of the analysis borrow from social constructivism (such as Chapter 2 on the framing of the response, and Chapter 5); others draw from institutionalism (as is apparent in Chapters 3 and 4 on the role of CSOs in GHIs), and historically grounded political economic analysis is weaved throughout.

Due to the gendered nature of the epidemic (over half of those living with HIV/AIDS are female), a critical feminist perspective is incorporated. This approach adopts Tickner's conception of feminist IR, which aims to "fundamentally challenge the often unseen androcentric or masculine biases in the way that knowledge has traditionally been constructed in all the disciplines" (2005, 3). While the topic under investigation (CSOs in the global HIV/AIDS response) may not appear to be explicitly gendered, feminist theory is woven into the analysis, and issues related to women's rights, sexuality and gender equality are highlighted throughout in order to ensure reflection on whether, and how, the HIV/AIDS response represents and responds to the group most affected by the epidemic. In line with other critical approaches, including feminist theory, emphasis is placed on documenting resistance, especially examples of resistance that have caused change, and explorations of how and why change has occurred or not (Tallis 2012; Murphy 2005).

Global health governance

The role of CSOs in the global AIDS response takes place within the broader historical context of global health and GHG. Up until the 1990s health was identified as a transnational issue, but was not substantially discussed within IR literature until relatively recently (Lee and Smith 2016). This began to change as processes of globalization increased awareness of the trans-boundary

nature of health threats and the need for global cooperation in addressing them, drawing the attention of IR scholars interested in the role of civil society, the impacts of international trade regimes and issues of human security, among others. This interest in health coincided with a general broadening of the IR field, following the end of the Cold War, characterized by the emergence of critical studies and constructivism (Davies 2000, 1170).

Interest in global health issues from politicians, policy-makers and public health professionals developed in response to recognition of how accelerated processes of globalization influenced health threats and outcomes. Lee defines globalization as:

> a set of processes that are changing the nature of how humans interact across three types of boundaries – spatial, temporal and cognitive … the changes they are creating are "global", in the sense that, familiar boundaries separating us as individuals and societies have become increasingly eroded.
>
> (2003, 5)

Transnational health threats and international responses to health issues were not necessarily the inventions of globalization (for example, the bubonic plague of the middle ages represents one example of an international health threat that was responded to cooperatively through international containment strategies). What was new was that, as globalization processes increased international travel and information sharing, health vulnerabilities and risks were no longer perceived as solely local and domestic issues. Lee writes:

> The health implications of global spatial change are wide-ranging. The most direct effect is how patterns of health and disease are altering according to new forms of social organization … in short, new spatial configurations of health and disease are emerging as consequences of globalization.
>
> (2003, 6)

While globalization, and its impacts on health, remains a debated concept (Brown & Labonté 2011), it is evident that as individuals, groups and states became increasingly aware of global interconnections, how disease was experienced, understood, spread and contained also shifted. This awareness generated various demands, which both competed and converged with each other, to generate systems of GHG.

Human rights activists and public health professionals recognized that globalization was exacerbating inequalities through the negative impacts of global capitalism on the health of the poor and marginalized – for example, that transnational corporations in South Africa drew impoverished men away from their homes by the promise of employment, which also exposed them to increased risk of TB, HIV and injury, which then impacted their families' well-being through loss of income and the spreading of disease (Msimang 2003). However, public health and human rights organizations also recognized that

globalization created opportunities to respond to such threats through new technologies, shared information and intensified international networks (Buse et al. 2009, 2). Arguing from this public health perspective, Owen and Roberts write, "In summary, the challenge is how to make globalization work for health and to use health to foster better forms of globalization" (2005, 5). Concerned public health professionals, policy-makers and activists collaborated to advance norms around health as a human right and as a social justice issue through global campaigns (such as for anti-retroviral treatment), and international organizations (such as Medicines Sans Frontiers). Harman writes, "It is awareness and a compulsion to address this [health] inequality that has precipitated the emergence of a broad and complex system of global health governance" (2012, 2). From this perspective, systems of GHG were conceived to counter the negative health impacts of globalization, and utilize global interconnections to advance health agendas.

Taking a more realist approach, Fidler attributes increased political interest in global health issues to awareness by states that, due to globalization, they could not respond effectively to health threats without international cooperation:

> Globalization exposed vulnerabilities of countries to public health threats that were previously non-existent, latent or ignored. Governments faced mounting public health threats with the realization that globalization constrained policy control over many determinants of health, limiting options to the detriment of population and individual health.
>
> (2006, 52)

States realized that health threats from other regions could easily cross borders, and national policy responses could only mitigate a certain amount of risk. A report by the US Institute of Medicine, in 1997, stated: "Distinctions between domestic and international health problems are losing their usefulness and are often misleading" (quoted in Frenk & Gomes Dantes 2002, 95). In particular, developed countries became increasingly concerned with communicable diseases from less developed countries, where it was feared the government did not have the capacity to contain epidemics. This fear was exacerbated by the SARS crisis of 2002–03 (Elbe 2010). Recognition that health threats emerged both within and from outside of the nation state led to demands for shared responsibility, international systems of response, and international intervention when necessary. Within this framework, health became increasingly linked to issues of security.

Calls for global cooperation in response to health threats reflected an emerging global public goods paradigm. Global public goods are defined "as outcomes (or intermediate products) that tend towards universality in the sense that they benefit all countries, population groups and generations" (Kaul et al. 1999, 11). Health fitted into this paradigm as, due to the interconnections of globalization, health outcomes in one region or population group were recognized as having the potential to impact others through the

biological, social and economic relationships that span the globe. Chen et al. wrote: "Globalization is not simply accelerating long-term trends but is ushering in contextual changes that are qualitatively and quantitatively different in disease risk, health vulnerability and policy response" (1999, 289). Recognition of health as a global public good created demand for a global architecture, or arrangement, to manage risk, govern responses and coordinate actors.

Linked to this understanding of health was increasing acknowledgement of the connections between health and development. The 1993 World Development Report, produced by the World Bank and the World Health Organization (WHO), described the economic costs of ill health and introduced the concept of Disability Adjusted Life Years (DALYs). In 2000, the WHO implemented a Macroeconomic Commission on Health mandated to demonstrate the economic impacts of ill health and well-being. Such initiatives gained attention and resources to address health issues; they also shifted how health issues were conceptualized, and therefore responded to. The economic perspective positioned health not only as an issue of public and individual welfare, but also as a commodity with an economic value (Kay & Williams 2009b, 6). This rationalization justified the increased involvement of actors outside the public realm, including private businesses and non-governmental organizations. At a time when many developing country public health systems were struggling due to the impacts of structural adjustment policies, these private actors filled gaps left by states, intensifying a shift from public to private health care. The linking of health and economic development reflected and contributed to dominant neoliberal approaches to addressing global threats, evidenced by the increasing role of the World Bank in health governance (Harman 2009).

For the WHO (the international organization created in 1948 to respond to global health threats) the shift away from a primarily biomedical and public health approach threatened its leadership role – as the state-based organization worked solely with health ministries and was primarily responsible for providing technical assistance. Due to a convergence of internal (such as leadership difficulties) and external (such as lack of support from the American administration) factors, WHO's stature did not rise with the increasing attention to global health issues. If anything it was crowded out by the new approaches and actors in the field (Harman 2012, 2). Hein et al. write, "The rising importance of transnational interactions compared to relations between nation-states leads to a very complex pattern of global health governance, which makes it difficult if not impossible for international governmental organizations to maintain their dominance in this policy field" (2007, 227). As competing conceptions of global health issues and approaches struggled for space and dominance, the WHO became one of many actors, representing one of numerous approaches.

Without specific leadership, and despite efforts to advance a shared global health agenda, the global health field became, and remains, fragmented. While a similar trend can be identified in other global governance arenas, GHG remains particularly disjointed. Severino and Ray suggest that global health is

an extreme case of their theory of hyper-collective action (referring to the double trend of proliferation and fragmentation of international cooperation) pointing out that more than 100 major organizations are involved in global health (2010, 6). Bartsch and Kolmorgen note that there are over 3000 CSOs involved in health governance (2007, 92). A British Department for International Development (DfID) review found that the health sector faces coordination and harmonization challenges at the global level, with more than 40 bilateral donors, 26 UN agencies, 20 global and regional funds, and 90 global health initiatives (Nay 2009, 16). GHG suffers from an acute case of fragmentation, with numerous actors (and types of actor), and little coordination between them. Lee writes that, "there is a sense that the emerging system of GHG is characterized by a considerable degree of dysfunction" (2007, 2). Fidler notes, "Efforts to address these and other global health problems often acknowledge that existing institutions, rules, and processes are insufficient to support collective action" (2010, 1).

The numerous approaches, actors and processes in global health have not necessarily resulted in efficient or effective global governance – in fact the opposite may be true. Despite advancements in some regions on issues related to access to medicines and child mortality, in the areas with the worst health outcomes the situation remains largely unchanged. The health related millennium development goals targets were not met in most Sub-Saharan African countries (English et al. 2015). Furthermore, the factors that gave rise to GHG – recognition of links between global processes and local outcomes, the impacts of international trade and security on health and vice versa, and global health inequalities – have not been resolved; if anything they have intensified. Fidler, writing specifically about women's health, refers to a "health paradox": the global level activity around health issues has not had corresponding outcomes at the local level (2008b, 148). In describing the persistent challenges of global health, Kay and Williams write, "the defining mood of contemporary analysis of GHG is one of failure; failure in GHG to meet the challenges posed by the scale and variety of problems that constitute the global system of disease" (2009b, 2).

IR scholars have developed multiple approaches to understanding and describing the rise, fragmentation and (to some) decline of GHG. Fidler introduces the concept of open source anarchy, through which he conceptualizes governance as "a normative 'source code' that states, international organizations, and non-state actors apply in addressing global health problems" (2007, 1). He argues that GHG is composed of overlapping and sometimes competing regime clusters that form a GHG complex in which states, intergovernmental organizations, and non-state actors apply old and new institutions, rules, and processes to strengthen collective action against health threats (Fidler 2010). Hein et al. (2007) suggest understanding GHG through nodes and interface – referring to critical points of interaction or linkages between different fields or levels of order. Buse et al. (2009) write that global health partnerships are like a "mosh pits" of governance – less structured, non-hierarchic forums where

multiple actors with different interests and ideas come together and "thrash-out" global health issues. While academics present various metaphors and terminology for describing GHG, they agree that it is complex and fragmented.

However, such conceptualizations fail to critically analyse power relationships within these multifaceted dynamics. For example, Fidler's (2008a) theory of open source anarchy has adapted realist concepts, which do not deconstruct hierarchies within governance arenas. Similarly, the concept of GHG as a mosh pit perpetuates conceptions of chaos, in which no one has control (i.e. power), and in which actors are free from the influences of historical processes. Recognizing these limits in GHG literature, Walt et al. (2009) argue that most analyses of GHG prioritize structure and form, neglecting agency. The conception of GHG as a "mess" (however it is illustrated) obscures questions about whose interest this complexity serves, and what power dynamics are played out within it.

McInnes and Lee note that GHG literature has been characterized by "weak theorizing", and propose greater analysis of how normative frameworks have defined the conceptualization and practice of GHG (2012, 101). They argue that recognition of the influence of ideas on historical forces raises critical questions such as: why do certain approaches to global health issues become dominant while others do not? And how do dominant and shifting ideas reflect and shape authority in GHG? Such questions have been investigated by scholars such as Rushton (2010), McInnes et al. (2012), Shiffman (2009), and Kay and Williams (2009a), who have begun exploring issue framing within GHG. Shiffman defines frames as: "the way in which an issue is understood and portrayed publicly" (2009, 609).

McInnes and Lee (2012) document how four frames shape GHG: biomedicine, economics, security and human rights. Kay and Williams note that among these various frames, there is a hierarchy that is "increasingly driven and structured by processes of commodification and liberalization in global health" (2009b, 2). They demonstrate that:

> key features of economic globalization also have concrete institutional and policy manifestations with regard to health, and interact with an enduring ideational alliance of neoliberalism and the biomedical model to intensify the scope and scale of the global system of disease.
>
> (2009, 2)

Though competing efforts to frame global health are apparent, frames related to biomedical and neoliberal approaches are dominant.

These frames, which can be termed biomedical neoliberalism, combine medical discourse and the interests of global capital. Biomedical neoliberalism includes an understanding of ill health as primarily an issue of resources, and/or of physical causes, such as infection or injury; a belief that solutions are predominantly scientific, technical and market-based; and a preference for

responses that are framed in evidenced-based, economic and security terms. Expressions of biomedical neoliberalism include, but are not limited to, the World Bank's concept of DALYs, which quantifies the value of life years lost to illness and injury (1993), and the WHO Commission on Macroeconomics and Health, which links health with poverty reduction and socio-economic development. Similarly, the announcement at the 2014 World Economic Forum by Bill Gates of a Commission on Global Health positioned economic growth as a dominant solution to poor health outcomes by asserting that "the international community can best support convergence by funding the development and delivery of new health technologies" (quoted in Jamison et al. 2013, 1898). While global financial institutions and public-private partnerships particularly promote biomedical neoliberalism, it is pervasive throughout GHG. While there are contestations within and around biomedical neoliberalism, it continues to dominate GHG. Alternative frames can operate within or against it, but cannot ignore it.

McInnes et al. note that analysis of ideas, or frames, within GHG "does not mean that the material world is of no concern, but rather that the material and ideational interact with each other" (2012, S84). The material work of raising and distributing resources, building coalitions, power struggles amongst the many actors in global health, all occur within the context of biomedical neoliberalism, and therefore either reinforce it or challenge it by posing alternatives. GHG is, as Murphy describes global governance in a general, "a site, one of many sites, in which struggles over wealth, power, and knowledge are taking place" (2000, 799). Such struggles are the source of change in that through them actors resist, challenge or strengthen existing structures.

These dynamics are often played out within and around global institutions. As described above, there has been a rapid increase in the number of GHIs over the past three decades. Previous forms of multilateralism that dominated the post-war institutional period have been upset by the increasing role of private actors and civil society (Walker 2011). Such changes require constant re-evaluation of the roles and outcomes of GHIs. As Murphy writes:

> We need for example to look for proposed institutional innovations that would have served the interests of the powerful just as well as those that came into being, yet, at the same time, would have better served the interests of the marginalized. What prevented those that better served the marginalized to be chosen? Conversely, have there been proposed institutions that would have served the marginalized less well than those selected? What allowed the better institutions to be chosen?
>
> (2005, 12)

In other words there is need for analysis of the power relationships within institutions, for questions about whether and how institutions serve the needs of those most affected by global health challenges, and how they either support or challenge dominant ideas within GHG.

Civil society organizations

The key type of actor that this book focuses on is CSOs. The UN definition of civil society is "a social sphere separate from both the state and the market. The increasingly accepted understanding of the term civil society organizations (CSOs) is that of non-state, not-for-profit, voluntary organizations formed by people in that social sphere" (WHO 2014). CSOs do not include profit-making activity (the private sector) or public sector governance arrangements. CSO networks are also referred to as social movements. Here the term civil society is preferred because it implies a diversity of actors, who may be orientated around different causes, but come together around a single issue (in this case HIV/AIDS) where and when those causes overlap. These actors might interact at varying levels of governance (local, national, regional and global), and might represent great differences, as well as similarities. For example both the Catholic Church and feminist organizations are civil society actors that participate in the HIV/AIDS response, though they disagree on related issues of reproductive rights. In the case of the HIV/AIDS response, CSOs involved include: AIDS service organizations (ASOs), various NGOs, associations of PWAs, women's rights groups, religious organizations, gay men's rights groups, youth groups, medical organizations, associations of particular races and ethnicities, and many others. As there are uncountable CSOs involved in the response to HIV/AIDS, the research here is directed towards the participation of global and regional networks, as well as associations of key populations and those CSOs that most frequently engage in global governance processes.

The concept of civil society has changed with how it has been applied over time. The Italian philosopher Gramsci saw state forces and civil society to be mutually constitutive, formed in relation to historical and structural forces. He was interested in how counter-hegemonic movements might promote social and revolutionary change, and saw CSOs as potential, but not predetermined, actors in such movements. He understood civil society as including both top-down forces of economic, cultural and political forces; and bottom-up processes lead by those marginalized by the current order attempting to develop counter-hegemonic projects (Bebbington et al. 2008, 18; Gramsci 1971). Gramsci recognized CSOs as potential agents of change, but did not assume they would necessarily be so, noting the influence of dominant states, corporations and other actors on what constitutes civil society, and the limits and opportunities within existing world orders. More recently, Cox writes that as states become increasingly responsive to market forces, citizens become disengaged and look to other avenues of engagement – one of which is through CSOs (2000). CSOs can create opportunities for direct engagement/confrontation with global governance forums (for example, the intellectual property regime which determines the price of HIV/AIDS treatment) when states do not. As a result, the involvement of civil society has expanded in global forums.

The participation of CSOs in global governance has been presented as having the potential to include those otherwise excluded. CSOs, it is suggested, can act as a discursive interface between global governance forums and actors, and as a "global citizenry" by monitoring policy-making, bringing citizens' concerns into deliberations, and empowering marginalized groups so that they can participate effectively in global politics (Nanz & Steffek 2004, 315). Assumptions about the ability of CSOs of fulfill this role in global governance, as well as demand from CSOs for such opportunities, has ensured that their participation has become something of a norm. Scholte notes that, "Most global governance agencies have now devised mechanisms of one kind or another to engage (at least to some extent) with these initiatives from civil society associations" (2004, 215).

However, while CSO participation has become accepted practice, the outcomes of this involvement remain debated by scholars. Proponents argue that:

> only civil society ... can add critical, alternative perspectives. The task of transnational civil society is to enable stakeholders of global governance to make informed judgments and choices. Civil society can (and should) give voice to citizens affected by regulations made at the global level.
> (Nanz & Steffek 2004, 333)

In particular, cosmopolitan scholars view CSOs as able to represent global citizens through their campaigns for human rights and poverty eradication, which seek to change dominate attitudes and approaches (Yanacopulos & Baillie Smith 2008). Such arguments rely on a number of assumptions: such as that the conditions for effective participation – defined as ensuring appropriate access to documents and meetings; incorporating all relevant concerns of civil society into agendas; openness of CSOs to citizen input and adoption on issues concerning marginalized populations (Nanz & Steffek 2004) – can exist despite the unequal power relationships. They further assume that CSOs that have access to decision-making forums will advocate responses that meet the needs and interests of those without access. In particular, cosmopolitan perspectives on the role of CSOs in global governance have been critiqued for failing to recognize that the majority of CSOs that have access to global forums are based in high-income countries, and for assuming these organizations can represent the interests of others. Such idealist conceptualizations also assume that CSOs function autonomously from government, and rarely consider that they can represent distinctly non-cosmopolitan interests, such as those based on fascism and racism (Lencucha et al. 2010, 75).

Recognizing these assumptions, academics from across theoretical perspectives have increasingly questioned expectations that CSOs are essentially "good" and representative of those otherwise marginalized. Scholte (2004) notes that the activities of CSOs involved in global governance should not be taken as necessarily democratic and benign, as such movements also reflect dominant power structures, claim authority without representation, and can have both

emancipatory and oppressive agendas. The 2002 Human Development Report similarly noted that the role of CSOs was not entirely unproblematic: "When such groups spring from agendas or use tactics that are contrary to democratic values, they can be both civil and uncivil. The rise of such groups poses challenges for truly democratic political engagement" (UNDP 2002, 19). The rise of racist groups and organizations linked to terrorism has forced theorists to recognize that CSOs represent a full spectrum of beliefs and aims.

Critical questions have also emerged about exactly who, or what groups, CSOs represent in global governance forums. Scholte notes that civil society networks:

> often lack clearly established procedures to formulate and execute joint positions, so that collective decision-taking among the participating groups can be cumbersome and confused. Moreover, members of a civil society network invariably have to negotiate differences – sometimes quite considerable divergences – regarding priorities, analyses, strategies and tactics.
>
> (2004, 225)

When such networks are negotiated, more powerful CSOs may exclude actors and groups that challenge their beliefs or approaches, raising questions as to whose alternatives gain greater visibility in global governance processes. Bebbington et al. (2008) argue that those CSOs that represent hegemonic interests, as opposed to presenting alternatives, have greatest influence within global governance forums.

Academics from southern contexts have critiqued the concept of global civil society. Cheru writes:

> The fashionable notion of transnational civil society also masks many contradictions. While Northern and Southern non-governmental organizations are collaborating together to lobby governments through the United Nations system on issues of human rights, ecology, poverty and other social issues of global dimensions, or in co financing of community development projects, their strength and capacity to conduct human-centered transitional foreign policy, independent of states, are exaggerated.
>
> (1997, 167)

Similarly, Chandhoke argues that civil society has become a "hurrah word" and "flattened out": "Witness the tragedy that has visited proponents of the concept: people struggling against authoritarian regimes demanded civil society, what they got were NGOs" (2001, 56). The assumption that civil society, and especially northern NGO involvement, is a global democratizing force that fulfills desires for more accountable global governance is increasingly challenged by such analysis.

Nuanced analyses further note that even those CSOs with "good intentions", or that are representative of marginalized community groups, have material

restraints on what ideals they can represent and achieve. In particular, because many CSOs receive state resources, need to attain funds can influence priorities to the detriment of constituent interests (Scholte 2004, 224). Flinders (2005) notes that in such cases truncated lines of accountability often result in mixed partnerships that are legally independent from government and yet spend public funds. Similarly, Bebbington et al. note that NGOs involved in international development often provide few options that differ from their states' bilateral priorities (2008, 2). Others argue that NGOs have become vehicles of neoliberal governmentality, by providing services for international financial institutions and governments (Townsend et al. 2004). It is argued that as NGOs become agents of governmentality, or service delivery options for states, their role as advocates for the poor declines.

In reviewing debates about the role of CSOs in global governance Benner et al. write that "neither naive optimism nor full-blown pessimism are helpful. Rather, we should aim at a realistic assessment of the conditions under which new forms of networked governance can provide value added by improving global governance" (2004, 192). The difficulty in achieving this critical assessment, according to Benner et al. (2004), is the lack of empirical research on the role of civil society in global governance. Bebbington et al. note that, in relation to the literature on the role of NGOs:

> What has perhaps been most remarkable of late is the extent to which these critical concerns have been allowed to pass by in the academic literature with very little evidence that they have been seriously addressed ... We are arguably no clearer now concerning questions of effectiveness, accountability and successful routes to scaling-up than we were when these questions were raised over a decade ago.
>
> (2008, 35)

In other words, while the theoretical debates about civil society have continued, there has not been a corresponding increase in research to inform these discussions. As an antidote to this lack of analysis, they advocate more studies that approach the concept of civil society "carefully, historically, conceptually and relationally" (Bebbington et al. 2008, 16).

CSO functions within GHG

Bartsch and Kohlmorgen (2007) present an analysis of CSO functions in GHG as including: participating in conferences, establish consultative relationships, participating in decision-making bodies, as well as implementing health projects and fulfilling "self-empowerment functions", such as representing the marginalized. Similarly, Lee (2010) draws on Haas' governance framework to map CSO contributions to specific governance functions within various GHG processes. Her study highlights the watchdog role CSOs play in global governance, and their influence in formulating policy agendas. Both studies

note that CSOs play a prominent role in framing policy debates by contributing expertise and building coalitions. However, both studies further note that CSOs in GHG act as both allies and watchdogs to states and GHIs, suggesting that CSOs' political functions are characterized by a dualism of cooperation and conflict.

CSO participation in GHG is often justified with claims that they represent affected and marginalized populations in decision-making. Influence in decision-making is conceptualized as the ability to both directly and indirectly shape policies, processes and resolutions. This influence is shaped by historical and bureaucratic structures. Bøås and McNeill argue that CSO influence in global institutions is shaped by institutions' "point of origin" (2003, 3). CSOs have greater influence where they share a history with the institution, which shapes how both CSOs and the institutions understand the issue at hand. CSOs, at least initially, are most likely to have influence when they reflect and advance the already dominant institutional approach. This constrains CSO influence within the institutional worldview, but facilitates participation within it. Also considering structural determinants of CSO participation in GHIs, Seckinelgin argues that bureaucracy restricts CSO participation (2009, 214). Because rules and institutional processes generally serve the interests of powerful actors and bureaucrats, they impose limits on CSO participation.

However, CSOs can exercise agency within these confines, and/or challenge them. Research on global environmental movements demonstrates that CSOs have influenced decision-making in international arrangements through knowledge production, modelling themselves as experts to be consulted (Jasanoff 1997; Betsill & Corell 2001; Humphreys 2004). Lencucha et al. document, in analysing the role of NGOs in producing the Convention on Tobacco Control, how CSOs assert knowledge and normative claims to exercise influence (2010, 411). They argue that CSOs exercised discursive influence (the ability to change arguments) and emotive force (communicating positions through morality frames). In this case, CSO influence contributed to a policy-making environment that reflected sensitivity to the priorities of poor countries rather than only the self-interest of high-income countries (Lencucha et al. 2011). CSOs also used networks to consolidate influence where issue areas and interests overlapped, and to shape policies and practice at multiple governance levels. Such analyses demonstrate that CSO influence is multifaceted; it shifts in response to the relationships between the types of agency CSOs employ and the structures they engage with (Lencucha et al. 2010).

CSOs are also credited with strengthening the legitimacy of GHG processes (Doyle and Patel 2008). The global governance literature on legitimacy conceptualizes it as having two forms: input and output. Input legitimacy relates to whether processes result in representation, transparency and accountability; output legitimacy is determined by the effectiveness of governance systems (Bäckstrand 2006). CSOs are positioned as able to strengthen input legitimacy by representing constituents, and as by contributing to output legitimacy through contributions of expertise and knowledge. Research on CSO participation in

global governance recognizes that the relationship between input and output legitimacy can be tenuous:

> To engage in the discourse of global health diplomacy, NGO diplomats ... are immediately presented with two challenges: conveying the interests of larger publics, including the most marginalized; and contributing to inter-state negotiations in a predominantly state-centric system of governance.
>
> (Lencucha et al. 2011, 406)

Similarly, Flinders (2005) warns that transnational civil society networks must make trade-offs between managerialist notions (such as efficiency) and democratic notions (such as accountability). These analyses suggest that assumptions that CSO involvement inherently strengthens the legitimacy of GHG processes need to be critically analysed.

The degree of input legitimacy an institution generates relates to its downward accountability to those it aims to serve. By claiming to represent constituencies, CSOs demand accountability from institutions through mechanism on actors, processes and outcomes (Benner et al. 2004, 193). In turn, CSOs must respond to accountability claims from constituents and peer networks. Yet, constructing accountable global governance systems is complicated by the hybrid nature of GHIs, which often lack democratic and hierarchical authorities (Bäckstrand 2006, 292). As opposed to resulting in an accountability deficit the plurality of relationships within GHG results in numerous accountability claims. As Keohane writes, "organizations are therefore anything but 'out of control bureaucracies,' accountable to nobody. ... These organizations are subject to accountability claims from almost everybody" (2002, 19). The multiple and complex accountability claims on international institutions requires "more imagination in conceptualizing, and more emphasis on operationalizing, different types of accountability" (ibid.). Because accountability within global governance relationships is multifaceted and complex, it is based less on representation (i.e. assumptions that a person from a particular community ensures accountability to that community) than on transparency, redress and reputation.

There is much debate about the role of CSOs in GHG processes. Questions persist about whether CSOs are parties to dominant approaches and therefore supportive of current power structures, or whether they are activists for a more just and responsive order. The most nuanced analyses caution against any such generalizations, pointing out the diversity within civil society. In order to understand CSO contributions to GHG there is need for empirically grounded research that asks if, and how, CSOs have shaped how global health issues are understood. Considering the urgent need for reform within GHG, as discussed above, it is worth reflecting on if and how CSOs have posed alternatives or maintained current structures, and to what effect.

Methodology

This book is informed by historical and personal accounts of the HIV/AIDS response, academic literature and the records of CSOs engaged in the response. Board and meeting minutes from GHIs were analysed, as were documents from their CSO affiliates. For example, the NGO Delegation to the UNAIDS Program Coordinating Board (PCB) publishes all UNAIDS board meeting documents online, as well as transcripts of interventions by CSOs. These were analysed for content and to verify accounts from key informants. Similarly, the Global Fund makes most of its documents available online, providing opportunities to analyse internal and external evaluations and reports. CSOs, such as Aidspan, provide further substantial databases of information on both CSO and GHI activities.

Interviews were conducted with 39 informants, including representatives of CSOs (19), staff from GHIs (18) and states (2). Participants were purposively selected, with resulting snowball sampling. Efforts were made to ensure that both men and women were included, as well as PWAs and representatives from key populations. The purpose of criteria around regional and key populations was not to ensure representation of these groups/regions in general (as the sampling would be much too thin), but of the much smaller populations from those groups/regions that participate in global governance processes. There was also an attempt to interview individuals from and living in various global regions, though a high percentage ended up being based in the global north because that is where staff of GHIs are most often located.

Interviews were semi-structured, revolving around three or four themes and related key questions, and then follow-up questions that emerged during the conversation. Interviews were conducted between February 2013 and April 2014, and were analysed using thematic analysis. Initial themes were derived conceptually, based on research questions and concepts emerging from the literature review (such as accountability, gender equality, etc.). Substantive codes (such as "key populations") were further derived inductively from the research process, and revised at regular intervals. Contradictions and conflicting information was situated within the broader context, and in relationship to other data, in order to be validated. In addition, a number of governance events were observed, such as the 32nd PCB meeting of UNAIDS (June 2013), a Global Fund replenishment meeting in Brussels (May 2013), and CSO consultation processes related to both events. Information from interviews and observations was triangulated with analysis of primary documents, such as meeting minutes and reports, as well as the existing literature.

Structure of the book

Following this introduction, Chapter 2 documents how CSOs around the world used the failure of biomedical responses to the early HIV/AIDS epidemic to advance human rights frames, which shaped the response and justified their own participation in GHG. Both the human rights framing of the epidemic

and CSO participation contributed to the concept of AIDS exceptionalism, at times conflicting and other times converging within biomedical and neoliberal approaches to global health, creating space for multiple understandings of HIV/AIDS. CSOs worked within these processes to advance their right to participate in global-level processes, and to continue to advocate rights-based approaches to HIV/AIDS in these forums.

Chapters 3 and 4 analyse governance outcomes of CSO participation in GHIs, asking if civil society actors promote greater attention to human rights within these spaces. In Chapter 3, UNAIDS is chosen as a case study as it was the first GHI to include CSOs in its global governance structure, the Program Coordination Board (PCB), and fulfills a leadership function in framing the global response. The focus is on governance outcomes related to CSO influence in decision-making, legitimacy and downward accountability.

Chapter 4 applies a similar analysis to the Global Fund, considering how the civil society delegations to the board, and those engaged with the Secretariat and through the Partnership Forum, influence decision-making, legitimacy and downward accountability. The Global Fund is selected as a second case study as it is the largest multilateral donor organization in the global HIV/AIDS response, and the first to include CSOs as equal decision-makers on its board. Due to the primarily financial function of the fund, a section analysing CSO participation in resources governance is included, which questions whether CSOs engaged in the Fund's governance have been able to direct greater resources to human rights-based responses.

Chapter 5 considers how recent changes in GHG have affected CSO participation in the HIV/AIDS response, and how CSOs have attempted to continue to advance a rights-based response to the epidemic. It finds that in the post-exceptionalism context HIV/AIDS CSOs have struggled to assert leadership, as is demonstrated by their efforts to influence the SDG process. However, they have been able to use the concept of key populations to justify their continued participation in GHG and the need for a rights-based response. Examples are included of how CSOs have used the key populations frame to advance access to GHG spaces and promote the rights of people who inject drugs, men who have sex with men, sex workers and women – and outcomes, or lack thereof, of these processes on regional, national and local processes are noted.

Chapter 6, the conclusion, reviews findings and insights that have emerged throughout the book, as well as implications for further research and policy discussions on CSO participation in GHG. It argues that there are lessons, relevant to other GHG processes, to be learned from CSO participation in the global HIV/AIDS response, and stresses the significance of the rights-based approach fostered by HIV/AIDS CSOs.

A personal note

I have worked with CSOs engaged in the HIV/AIDS response for over 10 years. Though the majority of my experience has been at the community,

not global, level, it is this local-level experience that prompted my interest in the role of CSOs in the global governance of the HIV/AIDS response. As a community advocate, working in Kenya, Canada and South Africa, I was constantly motivated and inspired by my peers working in the HIV/AIDS response. I worked with pastors who fought stigma in their local communities, PWID who challenged their government in order to keep one of the only supervised injection sites in the world open, sex workers who bravely shared their stories in United Nations (UN) forums. I was overwhelmed by the diversity of people and groups involved in the HIV/AIDS response, and how they organized to influence all levels of governance.

However, I also felt that the organizations I worked with were constantly coming up against barriers imposed from above: international guidelines that were disconnected from local realities, government ideologies that neglected those most in need and, increasingly, a declining interest in the HIV/AIDS response. Of course opportunities were also present, but these seemed more often than not shaped by donor preferences for current trends in public health and development than by the experiences of PWAs and those affected by the epidemic. I saw organizations struggle to find adequate support for care work, and the failure of social protection campaigns. As my frustration at the aspects of the HIV/AIDS response that were beyond the control of those on the front lines mounted, I wanted to understand what was happening "out there", where catchphrases like "an AIDS free generation" were created by people in board rooms who were also paradoxically reducing funding. I recognized that while my colleagues and peers struggled to engage with these macro level processes, it was difficult (except in a few cases) to identify clear outcomes. Instead it seemed a continual case of two steps forward, one step back – or vice versa. And so, while most of my previous research experience is at the local level, I decided to seize the opportunity of a PhD project (on which this book is based) to come to grips with global governance processes, how civil society has tried to influence them, and to what effect.

My background, no doubt, influences the analysis that follows. In particular I am an unapologetic advocate for a human rights-based response to HIV/AIDS. I also recognize the expertise, experience and moral force that CSOs often bring to governance forums. That said, I am not romantic about CSO involvement. Among many inspiring examples I have also witnessed questionable tactics and motivations: "experts" making a living off the ill and briefcase NGOs. I have been party to northern-based CSOs imposing their definition of human rights on to southern contexts, and have witnessed the power relationships fought out between different regional and key population groups.

Still, my own experience with CSOs necessarily shapes my perspective of their roles in global governance, and likely shaped my interactions with key informants. When asked about my own history I readily explained my background working with local CSOs, and this identified me as an ally in the response by CSO informants, and may have made other informants more cautious in communicating with me. In turn, my own assumptions that a

rights-based response is essential, and CSO participation ought to be a beneficial force, influenced how I interpreted data.

As opposed to a limitation, I see my subjectivity as an opportunity. Not only has it motivated me throughout the research and writing processes, it has also allowed me to connect with the subject matter, by requiring me to evaluate my own, and therefore others', assumptions. I believe my commitment to the HIV/AIDS response has made me perhaps more critical than I otherwise would have been. On the one hand, I want to share a remarkable narrative of CSOs taking on international institutions, powerful governments and big business; on the other, I know there is a need to reflect critically on what has been achieved because, despite all the effort, there is still so much to do. I do agree with those who argue that there is something to be learned from the history of the HIV/AIDS response, for HIV/AIDS advocates as well as other health and human rights campaigns, but this is not necessarily an unqualified success story.

References

Bäckstrand, K. (2006), "Multi-stakeholder Partnerships for Sustainable Development: Rethinking Legitimacy, Accountability and Effectiveness", *European Environment*, Vol. 16 No. 5, pp. 290–306.

Bakker, I. (2007), "Social Reproduction and the Constitution of a Gendered Political Economy", *New Political Economy*, Vol. 12 No. 4, pp. 541–556.

Bartsch, S. and Kohlmorgen, L. (2007), "The Role of Civil Society Organizations in Global Health Governance", in Hein, W., Bartsch, S. and Kohlmorgen, L. (Eds), *Global Health Governance and the Fight Against HIV/AIDS*, Palgrave Macmillan, New York, pp. 92–118.

Bebbington, A., Hickey, S. and Mitlin, D. (Eds) (2008), *Can NGOs Make a Difference? The Challenge of Development Alternatives*, Zed Books, London.

Benner, T., Reinicke, W.H. and Witte, J.M. (2004), "Multisectoral Networks in Global Governance: Towards a Pluralistic System of Accountability", *Government and Opposition*, Vol. 39 No. 2, pp. 191–210.

Betsill, M.M. and Corell, E. (2001), "NGO Influence in International Environmental Negotiations: A Framework for Analysis", *Global Environmental Politics*, Vol. 1 No. 4, pp. 65–85.

Bøås, M. and McNeill, D. (2003), *Multilateral Institutions: A Critical Introduction*, Pluto Press, London.

Brown, G.W. and Labonté, R. (2011), "Globalization and its Methodological Discontents: Contextualizing Globalization through the Study of HIV/AIDS", *Globalization and Health*, Vol. 7 No. 29, pp. 2–12.

Buse, K., Blackshaw, R. and Ndayisaba, M.G. (2012), "Zeroing in on AIDS and Global Health Post-2015", *Globalization and Health*, Vol. 8 No. 1, p. 42.

Buse, K., Hein, W. and Drager, N. (Eds) (2009), *Making Sense of Global Health Governance: A Policy Perspective*, Palgrave Macmillan, New York.

Chandhoke, N. (2001), "The Limits of Global Civil Society", in Glasius, M., Kaldor, M. and Anheier, H. (Eds), *Global Civil Society*, Oxford University Press, Oxford, pp. 35–53.

Chen, L., Evans, T. and Cash, R. (1999), "Health as a Global Public Good", in Kaul, I., Isabelle, G. and Stern, M. (Eds), *Global Public Goods: International Co-operation in the 21st Century*, United Nations Development Program, New York, pp. 284–305.

Cheru, F. (1997), "The Silent Revolution and the Weapons of the Weak: Transformation and Innovation from Below", in Gill, S. and Mittelman, J.H. (Eds), *Innovation and Transformation in International Studies*, Cambridge University Press, Cambridge, pp. 153–169.

Cox, R. (1981), "Social Forces, States and World Orders: Beyond International Relations Theory", *Millennium Journal of International Studies*, Vol. 10 No. 2, pp. 126–155.

Cox, R.W. (2000), "Thinking about Civilizations", *Review of International Studies*, Vol. 26, pp. 217–234.

Davies, S. (2000), "What Contribution can International Relations Make to the Evolving Global Health Agenda?", *International Affairs*, Vol. 5, pp. 1167–1190.

Doyle, C. and Patel, P. (2008), "Civil Society Organisations and Global Health Initiatives: Problems of Legitimacy", *Social Science & Medicine*, Vol. 66 No. 9, pp. 1928–1938.

Elbe, S. (2010), *Security and Global Health*, Polity Press, Cambridge.

English, M., English, R. and English, A. (2015), "Millennium Development Goals Progress: A Perspective from Sub-Saharan Africa", *Archives of Disease in Childhood*, Vol. 100 Suppl. 1, pp. S57–S58.

Farmer, P. (2014), *To Fight Hepatitis C, Look to HIV*, Partners in Health, Boston, available at: http://www.pih.org/blog/paul-farmer-to-fight-hepatitis-c-look-to-hiv (accessed 15 December 2015).

Fidler, D. (2006), "Health as Foreign Policy: Harnessing Globalization for Health", *Health Promotion International*, Vol. 21 Suppl. 1, pp. 51–58.

Fidler, D. (2007), "Architecture amidst Anarchy: Global Health's Quest for Governance", *Global Health Governance*, Vol. 1 No. 1, pp. 1–17.

Fidler, D. (2008a), "A Theory of Open-Source Anarchy", *Indiana Journal of Global Legal Studies*, Vol. 15 No. 1, pp. 259–284.

Fidler, D. (2008b), "Gender Politics, Gender Paradox: Establishing and Implementing Global Standards for The Promotion And Protection Of Women's Health", *Emory International Law Review*, Vol. 22, pp. 147–158.

Fidler, D. (2010), *The Challenges of Global Health Governance: Working Paper*, Council for Foreign Relations, New York.

Flinders, M. (2005), "The Politics of Public–Private Partnerships", *The British Journal of Politics*, Vol. 7 No. 2, pp. 215–239.

Ford, N., Calmy, A. and Mills, E.J. (2011), "The First Decade of Antiretroviral Therapy in Africa", *Globalization and Health*, Vol. 7 No. 1, p. 33.

Frenk, J. and Gomes-Dantes, O. (2002), "Globalisation and the Challenges to Health Systems", *British Medical Journal*, Vol. 325, pp. 95–96.

Friedrichs, J. (2009), "Global Governance as Liberal Hegemony", in Whitman, J. (Ed.), *Palgrave Advances in Global Governance*, Palgrave Macmillan, New York, pp. 1–120.

Gill, S. and Mittelman, J.H. (Eds) (1997), *Innovation and Transformation in International Studies*, Cambridge University Press, Cambridge.

Glasius, M. (Ed.) (2002), *Global Civil Society*, Oxford University Press, Oxford.

Gramsci, A. (1971), *Selections from the Prison Notebooks*, translated by Quintin Hoare and Geoffrey Nowell Smith, International Publishers, New York.

Harman, S. (2009), "Fighting HIV and AIDS: Reconfiguring the State?", *Review of African Political Economy*, Vol. 36 No. 121, pp. 353–367.

Harman, S. (2012), *Global Health Governance*, Routledge, New York.

Hein, W., Bartsch, S. and Kohlmorgen, L. (Eds) (2007), *Global Health Governance and the Fight against HIV/AIDS*, Palgrave Macmillan, New York.

Humphreys, D. (2004), "Redefining the Issues: NGO Influence on International Forest Negotiations", *Global Environmental Politics*, Vol. 4 No. 2, pp. 51–74.

Jamison, D. et al. (2013), "Global Health 2035: A World Converging within a Generation", *The Lancet*, Vol. 382, pp. 1898–1955.

Jasanoff, S. (1997), "NGOs and the Environment: From Knowledge to Action", *Third World Quarterly*, Vol. 18 No. 3, pp. 579–594.

Kaul, I., Isabelle, G. and Stern, M. (Eds) (1999), *Global Public Goods: International Co-operation in the 21st Century*, United Nations Development Program, New York.

Kay, A. and Williams, O.D. (Eds) (2009a), *Global Health Governance: Crisis, Institutions, and Political Economy*, International Political Economy series, Palgrave Macmillan, Basingstoke.

Kay, A. and Williams, O.D. (2009b), "Introduction: The International Political Economy of Global Health Governance", in Kay, A. and Williams, O.D. (Eds), *Global Health Governance: Crisis, Institutions, and Political Economy*, International Political Economy series, Palgrave Macmillan, Basingstoke, pp. 1–24.

Keohane, R.O. (2002), *Power and Governance in a Partially Globalized World*, Routledge, London.

Lee, K. (2003), *Health Impacts of Globalization: Towards Global Governance*, Palgrave Macmillan, New York.

Lee, K. (2007), *The Role of CSOs in Intergovernmental Health Organisations: Contributions to Global Health Governance*, Wall Summer Institute, 25–28 June, Vancouver.

Lee, K. (2010), "Civil Society Organizations and the Functions of Global Health Governance: What Role within Intergovernmental Organizations?", *Global Health Governance*, Vol. 3 No. 2, pp. 1–20.

Lee, K. and Smith, J. (2016), "International Organization and Health/Disease", in *International Studies Compendium Project*, International Studies Association.

Lencucha, R., Kothari, A. and Labonté, R. (2011), "The Role of Non-governmental Organizations in Global Health Diplomacy: Negotiating the Framework Convention on Tobacco Control", *Health Policy and Planning*, Vol. 26 No. 5, pp. 405–412.

Lencucha, R., Labonté, R. and Rouse, M.J. (2010), "Beyond Idealism and Realism: Canadian NGO/Government Relations during the Negotiation of the FCTC", *Journal of Public Health Policy*, Vol. 31 No. 1, pp. 74–87.

McInnes, C., Kamradt-Scott, A., Lee, K., Reubi, D., Roemer-Mahler, A., Rushton, S., Williams, O.D. and Woodling, M. (2012), "Framing Global Health: The Governance Challenge", *Global Public Health*, Vol. 7 Suppl. 2, pp. S83–S94.

McInnes, C. and Lee, K. (2012), "Framing and Global Health Governance: Key Findings", *Global Public Health*, Vol. 7 Suppl. 2, pp. S191–S198.

Msimang, S. (2003), "HIV/AIDS, Globalisation and the International Women's Movement", *Gender and Development*, Vol. 11 No. 1, pp. 109–113.

Murphy, C. (2000), "Global Governance: Poorly Done and Poorly Understood", *International Affairs*, Vol. 76 No. 4, pp. 189–803.

Murphy, C. (2005), *Global Institutions, Marginalization, and Development*, Routledge, London.

Nanz, P. and Steffek, J. (2004), "Global Governance, Participation and the Public Sphere", *Government and Opposition*, Vol. 39 No. 2, pp. 314–335.

Nay, O. (2009), *What Drives Reforms in International Organizations? External Pressure and Bureaucratic Entrepreneurs in the UN Response to AIDS*, University of Lille, Lille.

O'Manique, C. (2004), *Neoliberalism and AIDS Crisis in Sub Saharan Africa: Globalization's Pandemic*, Palgrave Macmillan, New York.

Owen, J. and Roberts, O. (2005), "Globalisation, Health and Foreign Policy: Emerging Linkages and Interests", *Globalization and Health*, Vol. 1 No. 1, p. 12.

Parker, R. (2011), "Grassroots Activism, Civil Society Mobilization, and the Politics of the Global HIV/ AIDS Epidemic", *Brown Journal of World Affairs*, Vol. 21 No. 2, pp. 2–37.

Partridge, N. (2014), *The Horror of the Ebola Virus: Learning Lessons from the HIV and AIDS Response of the 1980s and 90s*, Action Aid, London, available at: https://www.actionaid.org.uk/blog/news/2014/10/20/the-horror-of-the-ebola-virus-learning-lessons-from-the-hiv-and-aids-response (accessed 31 December 2015).

Petchansky, R. (2003), *Global Prescriptions: Gendering Health and Human Rights*, Zed Books, New York.

Rushton, S. (2010), "Framing AIDS: Securitization, Development-ization, Rights-ization", *Global Health Governance*, Vol. 4 No. 1, pp. 1–17.

Scholte, J. (2004), "Civil Society and Democratically Accountable Global Governance", *Government and Opposition*, Vol. 39 No. 2, pp. 211–233.

Seckinelgin, H. (2009), "Global Social Policy and International Organizations: Linking Social Exclusion to Durable Inequality", *Global Social Policy*, Vol. 9 No. 2, pp. 205–227.

Severino, J. and Ray, O. (2010), *The End of ODA (II): The Birth of Hypercollective Action: Working Paper 218*, Center for Global Development, Washington, D.C.

Shiffman, J. (2009), "A Social Explanation for the Rise and Fall of Global Health Issues", *Bulletin of the World Health Organization*, Vol. 87 No. 8, pp. 608–613.

Shiffman, J., Berland, D. and Hafner, T. (2009), "Has Aid for AIDS Raised All Health Funding Boats?", *Journal of AIDS*, Vol. 52 No. 1, pp. S45–S48.

Sidibe, M., Tanaka, S. and Buse, K. (2010), "People, Passion & Politics: Looking Back and Moving Forward in the Governance of the AIDS Response", *Global Health Governance*, Vol. 4 No. 1, pp. 1–17.

Smith, J.H. and Whiteside, A. (2010), "The History of AIDS Exceptionalism", *Journal of the International AIDS Society*, Vol. 13 No. 1, p. 47.

Tallis, V. (2012), *Feminisms, HIV, and AIDS: Subverting Power, Reducing Vulnerability*, Palgrave Macmillan, New York.

Tickner, J.A. (2005), "What is Your Research Program? Some Feminist Answers to International Relations Methodological Qu estions", *International Studies Quarterly*, Vol. 49 No. 1, pp. 1–21.

Townsend, J.P., Porter, G. and Mawdsley, E. (2004), "Creating Spaces of Resistance: Development NGOs and their Clients in Ghana, India and Mexico", *Antipode*, Vol. 36, pp. 871–889.

UNAIDS (2007), *Policy Brief: The Greater Involvement of People Living with HIV/ AIDS*, Geneva, available at: http://www.unaids.org/en/resources/presscentre/featurestories/2007/march/20070330gipapolicybrief (accessed 15 December 2015).

UNAIDS (2013), *AIDS by the Numbers*, Geneva, available at: http://www.unaids.org/en/resources/documents/2013 (accessed 15 December 2015).

UNAIDS (2015), *Fact Sheet 2015*, Geneva, available at: http://www.unaids.org/en/resources/campaigns/HowAIDSchangedeverything/factsheet (accessed 15 December 2015).

UNAIDS PCB (2013), *Agenda item 1.2 Report of the 31st Meeting of the Programme Coordinating Board*, Geneva.

UNDP (2002), *Human Development Report 2002: Deepening Democracy in a Fragmented World*, Geneva.

Walker, L. (2011), *Healing Power: The Global Fund, Disrupted Multilateralism and Mediated Country Ownership*, University of Warwick, Warwick.

Walt, G., Spicer, N. and Buse, K. (2009), "Mapping the Global Health Architecture", in Buse, K., Hein, W. and Drager, N. (Eds), *Making Sense of Global Health Governance: A Policy Perspective*, Palgrave Macmillan, New York, pp. 47–71.

Whiteside, A. and Smith, J. (2009), "Exceptional Epidemics: AIDS Still Deserves a Global Response", *Globalization and Health*, Vol. 5 No. 1, p. 15.

Whitman, J. (Ed.) (2009), *Palgrave Advances in Global Governance*, Palgrave Macmillan, New York.

WHO (2014), Civil Society Definition, available at: http://www.who.int/trade/glossary/story006/en/ (accessed 7 August 2014).

World Bank (1993), *World Development Report 1993: Investing in Health*, Oxford University Press, Oxford.

Yanacopulos, H. and Baillie Smith, M. (2008), "The Ambivalent Cosmopolitanism of International NGOs", in Bebbington, A., Hickey, S. and Mitlin, D. (Eds), *Can NGOs Make a Difference? The Challenge of Development Alternatives*, Zed Books, London, pp. 298–315.

Yong Kim, J. (2014), *Want to Build a Movement? Learn from AIDS Activists*, World Bank, Washington D.C.

2 Framing an alternative

Human rights pioneers

The early HIV/AIDS epidemic, in the 1980s, challenged established public health methods (such as containment, treatment and vaccines) of addressing infectious disease. The fact that the virus spread most rapidly among already marginalized groups further raised controversial questions about social norms around sexuality, race and discrimination. As established biomedical neoliberal frames failed to explain, prevent or develop an adequate response to what was a terrifying epidemic, space was created for alternative approaches – space CSOs occupied to demand a unique rights-based response.

This chapter documents the early CSO response to the epidemic, exploring how CSOs contributed to the framing of the emerging global response, in which they established themselves as key actors and experts. It considers who CSOs worked with and how they challenged global health processes to advance a rights-based response to the epidemic, up until 2008, when the prioritization of the AIDS response within GHG was increasingly questioned. This brief historical account sets the stage for the analysis in subsequent chapters.

The early AIDS response

In the early 1980s, a mysterious cause of death among young men in North America and Western Europe resulted in hysteria and fear. The originally inexplicable nature of the disease, unknown cause, and lethal result caused panic: "[HIV/AIDS] seemed to resurrect the true meaning of epidemic: a disease that spreads like wildfire, consumes lives, and then burns out, leaving devastation in its wake" (Fee 1995, 1478). As it was mostly young homosexual men who were inflicted, terms such as Gay Related Immune Disease linked sexuality with disease, feeding conservative discourses about punishment for "sinful lifestyles".

Once HIV was identified, in 1983, it was believed that both the deaths and the stigma would be short lived. Margaret Heckler, US Secretary of Health and Human Services, stated, regarding the discovery of HIV, "Today's discovery represents the triumph of science over a dreadful disease" (quoted in Behrman 2004, 14). WHO had recently eradicated smallpox, and faith in scientific ability to beat illness was high. Now the cause of AIDS was identified, it was assumed

that biomedical solutions, such as treatment and a vaccine, would quickly follow. In the meantime, technological public health practices (e.g. testing and quarantine) would contain the epidemic (Fee 1995, 1478). Politicians and policy-makers focused on supporting biomedical approaches of containment and cure, continuing to neglect and often stigmatizing those already infected.

However, HIV/AIDS presented particularly acute challenges to this techno-cratic response. On a scientific level, HIV proved difficult (and remains so) to develop a vaccine against, and effective treatment was not available until over 10 years into the epidemic. At a political level, technical prevention measures, such as condom and clean needle provision, were opposed by right-wing political parties and religious groups (Fee 1995, 1479). At a public health level, the fact that someone could live with HIV for years without having symptoms made testing and quarantine difficult to implement. At a moral level, questions arose about the purpose of testing when there was no treatment or vaccine, as testing exposed the individual to considerable social risk, due to stigma and discrimination, while offering no medical benefit (Fee 1995, 1478).

The lack of a quick biomedical solution resulted in public health programmes that focused on individual behaviour change through education as prevention (Söderholm 1997, 122). The effectiveness of this traditional public health approach was limited by the modes of transmission of HIV: sexual behaviour and drug use are not rational activities that are highly susceptible to change through access to education and information (Fineberg 1989, 593). Techno-cratic behaviour change approaches further lacked appreciation for the social and political context of the epidemic:

> In these campaigns, emphasis is placed on informed individuals taking responsibility for not engaging in such behaviours. HIV/AIDS was seen, in this context, as a disease of poor technical capacity, clinical practice or personal knowledge, and less a disease of broader structural features.
> (Gamson 1988, 25)

This individualist approach did not acknowledge the broader context of social marginalization and homophobia that HIV was spreading within.

As technological approaches failed to develop a vaccine or treatment, and as public health approaches placed emphasis on behaviour change, often bordering on blaming individuals for their positive status, PWAs and their allies developed an alternative response. The Gay Men's Health Crisis, founded in 1981 in New York City, was the first formal PWA support group, and throughout the 1980s similar ASOs developed across North America, Western Europe and Latin America (Knight 2008, 12). These were some of the first disease-specific organizations formed by patients (Söderholm 1997, 78). Membership largely consisted of middle class white men who were well educated, articulate and professional. They rejected state sponsored campaigns that characterized them as statistical risk groups and as popula-tions of disease carriers (Fee 1995, 1478). Instead, they argued that it was

not their sexual orientation or behaviours that were the problem, but the homophobia, stigma and discrimination that forced individuals to engage in risky activities, and avoid information and medical care (Bayer & Fairchild 2006).

In 1983, American ASOs met in Denver and produced what became known as the Denver Declaration. It condemned attempts to label PWAs as victims, and recognized the central role of these individuals in prevention (Merson et al. 2008, 479). A pillar of this approach was a rejection of the unequal and patronizing relationship between doctors and patients (Söderholm 1997, 78). This resistance to biomedical authority had its roots in the gay rights movements; activists had battled over the conception of homosexuality as an illness in previous decades and so had a history of questioning the medical establishment. They applied similar strategies as they had used to counter homophobia to address stigma and discrimination. Altman writes that, "The creation of the 'person with AIDS' as a specific identity clearly drew on earlier gay models of 'coming out' and has been a significant factor in breaking down the medical dominance of the epidemic" (2001, 74). By asserting expertise in addressing the social aspects of the epidemic, ASOs demanded an equal relationship with the medical establishment. In the context of HIV/AIDS, biomedical authority was challenged due to its inability to provide treatment or a cure, while PWAs claimed authority based on the experience of living with the virus. At the heart of this claim was the argument that the individual human rights of the infected individual trumped medical prescriptions for healthy behaviours, risk groups and testing. PWAs rejected the positioning of HIV/AIDS as purely biomedical and individual, and instead framed it as a social and collective experience.

The forces of the gay rights movement combined with that of health professionals, frustrated by watching their patients die, and human rights activists opposed to discrimination. This "exceptional alliance" included the gay community, liberal and left-wing parties, and the healthcare and psychosocial professions (Rosenbrock et al. 2000). Also termed, "t-shirts, white coats and suits", these groups advocated a response that recognized that HIV/AIDS was an exceptional health issue that required the empowerment of those most affected in order for prevention, at this point the only solution, to be effective (Gordenker et al. 1995, 65). In the absence of viable biomedical alternatives, public health programmes increasingly adopted this human rights frame, which took societal-based vulnerability into consideration and worked with those most affected (Mann & Tarantola 1998). In many respects, the rights based approach was successful; new infections in the United States fell from 130,000 in 1984 to 60,000 in 1991 (El-Sadre et al. 2010).

A global movement

Much of the documented history of the early HIV/AIDS movement focuses on the role of CSOs in North America and Western Europe, and there is little literature on the early response in other parts of the world. However, in the

region most affected, Sub-Saharan Africa, civil society was also responding to the epidemic by developing alternative responses. In the context of poor to non-existent health services, and a generalized heterosexual epidemic, the issues facing PWAs were different than in Western contexts. However, the stigma and discrimination that developed towards a disease that was related to sexual behaviour, and for which there was no treatment or cure, was similar. In response to this stigma, as well as near complete neglect by what state health systems existed, Ugandan Noerine Kaleeba founded The AIDS Support Organization (TASO), in 1987, after having nursed her husband until his death. TASO focused on supporting families who had to care for HIV/AIDS positive members, and on addressing stigma and discrimination (Hampton 1991). TASO challenged prevalent frames of blame and stigma by coining the phrase, "Living Positively", which would become the unofficial slogan of the global PWA rights movement. Kaleeba remembers:

> At that time the public health messages were saying "Beware of AIDS, AIDS kills." ... There were no messages for people who were already infected. What was implied was that people who were already infected should die and get it over with. We adopted the slogan of "living positively with AIDS" in direct defiance of that perception. We emphasized living rather than dying with AIDS. For us it was the quality rather than the quantity of life which was important.
>
> (quoted in Knight 2008, 12)

Over the next decade similar responses developed in Western and Southern Africa. Responses in African communities focused on the rights of the patient to live free of discrimination, and on the collective experience of the community as the primary care provider. Despite the different context and epidemic, this approach was similar to that of the exceptional alliance in North America and Western Europe in its rejection of purely technocratic public health approaches, focus on addressing stigma and discrimination, and framing of HIV/AIDS as a collective social and political, as well as individual medical issue. With increasing support from Western NGOs, these programmes adopted similar approaches to other HIV/AIDS CSOs by focusing on developing a sense of community among people with HIV/AIDS, and providing peer support and counselling (Nguyen 2010).

In Latin America a variety of actors became involved in the response – ranging from gay rights groups to the Catholic liberation theology movement. In Brazil, the first ASO, the AIDS Prevention and Support Group of San Paulo, was founded in 1985, followed by a host of similar organizations across the continent over the next three to five years (Parker 2011, 23). These organizations linked HIV/AIDS with activist movements challenging social and economic inequality, and poor health services.

In Asia, groups already engaged in struggles for the rights of sex workers and transgender populations became involved in the HIV/AIDS response. In

Thailand, EMPOWER (Education Means Empowerment of Women Engaged in Recreation), created in 1985, began to develop AIDS-related projects and programmes by 1988, mobilizing Thai women involved in the entertainment industry and in sex work (Parker 2011, 24). In 1994, the Asia Pacific Network of People Living with HIV/AIDS was formed to bring together various ASOs and related organizations from across the region.

Processes of globalization facilitated opportunities for CSOs to share information and experiences. A first truly global effort to bring HIV/AIDS CSOs together was attempted in 1989, when Canadian activists organized a five-day pre-meeting prior to the International AIDS Society (IAS) Conference in Montreal. Representatives of over 100 HIV/AIDS CSOs from around the world came together to discuss common issues. One participant remembers:

> You know probably half the people in the room had AIDS, and a large number of the other half, including me, my partner had AIDS. So most of us, if we didn't have AIDS ourselves, were involved with AIDS because of you know husband, wives, partners, children. So for all of the differences, and not just Salvation Army versus sex workers, but Zambian versus Canadian ... for all the differences, we had AIDS in common, and we all agreed that our governments were failing us, and we all agreed that the international system was failing us. So we had anger in common. So there was a lot of anger, but there was a lot of energy and a lot of excitement in discovering common bounds across such diverse people.
>
> (GHI Representative 2013 #3)

The unfortunately universal experiences of stigma and discrimination, and of death (due to lack of medical solutions), united CSOs. Diverse but shared reflections on mourning and loss were able to create common bonds between "the experiences of AIDS in inner-city San Fransciso and Newark with that of Kenyan and Zambian villages" (Altman 2001, 83). Similarly, the common experience of government neglect (as in almost all cases CSOs had established HIV/AIDS interventions before official government programmes were put in place) motivated CSOs to combine forces to demand a global response that would pressure states to act (Parker 2011, 24). Emerging CSO networks not only spanned countries, but also communities and worldviews.

Over 300 activists from the USA and Canada stayed on after the meeting to protest at the IAS Conference, which was primarily a medical research event. The activists occupied the opening ceremony stage and seats reserved for VIPs, demanding more robust state responses, PWA participation in all HIV/AIDS related processes, and recognition of the human rights aspects of the epidemic. A newspaper headline the following day read, "The International AIDS Conference will never be the same," which proved prophetic (IAS 2013). Every IAS conference since has included a mix of scientists and activists, policy-makers and CSOs, making the IAS conference "like no other medical meeting in the world". The editor of *The Lancet* goes on to explain: "It brings

together people living with HIV and their partners, scientists and health workers, activists and politicians, policy-makers and the private sector. The messages at the meeting are also like no other messages you will see at traditional medical conferences" (Horton 2012, 324). The claim put forward at the 1989 IAS conference, and reiterated at every conference since, is that PWAs and their allies must be involved in order to ensure an effective rights-based response to the epidemic. The demand for CSO participation transformed IAS conferences from a purely biomedical affair into a unique multidisciplinary, multi-actor event, including alternative messages, as well as biomedical frames.

It would be a gross over-simplification to assume that one, homogenous, human rights approach developed across the global network of CSOs engaged in the HIV/AIDS response. Western approaches of disclosure and peer support were adapted to local contexts around the world, and local systems of coping developed based on resource availability and understandings of disease. At times these differences resulted in divisions in the global movement.

At the following IAS Conference, which was boycotted by some CSOs (due to American refusal to provide visas to PWAs) but not others, tensions remained high during attempts to create a formal international HIV/AIDS organization, with differing interpretations of rights and concepts of sexuality fracturing an already diverse movement:

> Representatives of organised sex workers … were angered, because they believed that they were being treated as a problem, not as a group that suffered from discrimination. From groups of male homosexuals, some of which confronted the conference with strident, largely sexual demonstration came similar complaints. … The women's caucus voted to exclude men from its meetings. … the African caucus voted to exclude white Europeans from its meetings.
>
> (Gordenker et al. 1995, 97)

However, a certain level of agreement also prevailed as most groups advocated greater financing and political commitment to HIV/AIDS, as well as the participation of PWAs and their allies in global forums.

Over the next few years these commonalities continued to bring CSOs together, despite differences between them, and umbrella CSOs were created to represent the global movement. In 1993, the International Council of AIDS Service Organizations (ICASO) was formed. In 1994, the HIV/AIDS Alliance was established in response to the perceived failure of WHO to mobilize a global rights-based response (GHI Representative 2013 #3). The Global Network of People Living with HIV (GNP+) was formed to represent PWAs in 1992, and the International Community of Women Living with HIV/AIDS (ICW) was formed the same year. Regional and faith-based networks also continued to develop over the next decade.

In 1994, these networks promoted the Greater Involvement of People with HIV/AIDS (GIPWA) principle at the Paris AIDS Summit. As a result,

42 countries agreed to "support a greater involvement of people living with HIV at all ... levels ... and to ... stimulate the creation of supportive political, legal and social environments" (UNAIDS 2007, 1). PWAs, and their allies, ensured that the framing of HIV/AIDS as a human rights issue reached the global arena, and the rights of PWAs to participate in global discussions were widely recognized.

CSOs and allied epistemic communities, including some early activists who found themselves working in international institutions or with governments, promoted the human rights frame. One former activist was asked to work in the UN system because he was seen giving a speech at a demonstration, and appeared more knowledgeable about the issues than most bureaucrats (GHI Representative 2013 #12). Another began to lobby the WHO when his partner fell ill and went on to work for numerous UN agencies (GHI Representative 2013 #3). Many other activists found work in UNAIDS and the Global Fund, when they were formed in 1994 and 2001 respectively, as both established policies of employing PWAs and developed a culture of recruiting from CSOs (GHI Representative 2013 #24; GHI Representative 2013 #16). These individuals promoted the human rights approach to HIV/AIDS from inside institutions, while CSOs advocated externally.

The result was near universal rhetorical commitment to the human rights approach to the epidemic by GHIs. For example, the UNAIDS preamble states that its work must be based on "human rights and gender equality" (2013); the Global Fund "is committed to protecting and promoting human rights" (GFATM 2013); the World Bank argues HIV/AIDS interventions need to protect the rights of vulnerable groups (2008). Epistemic communities that grew out of civil society movements ensured human rights language became a staple of HIV/AIDS programming and policy.

Within the global governance to HIV/AIDS, the right to health and the right of affected communities to participate in all levels of the response to the epidemic became intrinsically linked. Sandoval and Cáceres note that "the 'success' of PWA organizations in becoming a global movement was related to local histories of gay activism, combined with worldwide mobilization to confront a pandemic, and the emergence of a health rights discourse" (2013, 5). Human rights claims provided HIV/AIDS CSOs with credibility as experts – with their authority derived from experiences of human rights violations, and from being among the first to propose viable responses when biomedical approaches failed. The demand for empowerment of those most at risk added a further justification for HIV/AIDS CSO involvement – participation (conceived of as an empowerment activity) addressed a cause of the epidemic (marginalization). The relationship between rights and participation was cyclical: "This gives rise to another complexity: effective participation is dependent upon the enjoyment of other human rights, such as freedom of expression, and the rights to information, assembly and association" (Potts 2008, 2). The human rights approach to HIV/AIDS, created and advanced by HIV/AIDS CSOs, expanded space for their participation in GHG, which in turned allowed them

to reassert the rights response. While other actors, such as some states and the emerging GHIs, also played a role in advancing the human rights frame, HIV/AIDS CSOs pioneered it, nurtured it and ensured its continued presence in GHG, justifying their own continued inclusion.

AIDS exceptionalism

Human rights and HIV/AIDS CSO participation fit into the broader discourse of AIDS exceptionalism – the idea that the HIV/AIDS epidemic demands a response above and beyond the norm in GHG because of the particular features and impacts of the epidemic. Exceptionalism was partially the result of the framing of the epidemic within the language of securitization and globalization – HIV/AIDS was viewed as a global emergency with implications for those directly and indirectly affected. It was argued – by policy-makers, activists and academics – that because HIV/AIDS had widespread impacts (largely due to its projected demographic effects) it could weaken state systems and reverse development gains in hyper-endemic countries, both of which could have global impacts (Barnett 2006).

This rhetoric justified a response above and beyond other health issues – resulting in a dramatic increase in resources for and attention towards HIV/AIDS (Smith et al. 2011). This occurred within a broader trend of heightened attention to global health issues and resulting resources from donor states. The Institute for Health Metrics and Evaluation argues that development assistance for health underwent a rapid-growth phase between 2001 and 2010 when funding almost tripled, climbing to US$28.2 billion in 2010 (IHME 2012). This was due to the increased attention to the potential economic, political and security implications of global health, and a period of relative economic prosperity in donor countries (Fidler 2009).

Resources for HIV/AIDS not only made up the largest share of this funding, but also increased at the fastest pace. While separating HIV/AIDS-specific resources from other global health funding is challenging due to inconsistent access to and formats of donor records, it is agreed that HIV/AIDS took up an increasing portion of the global health resource pie from the turn of the millennium until 2010 (Oomman et al. 2007, 8). Shiffman et al. suggest that HIV/AIDS resources rose from just five per cent of health and population international aid commitments in 1998, to 47 per cent of all commitments in 2007 (2009, 2). Oomman et al. find that annual funding for HIV/AIDS to low and middle-income countries increased 30 times between 1996 and 2006 (2007, 8). Annual donor support grew from US$1.6 billion in 2002 to US$8.7 billion in 2008.

With these increased resources, HIV/AIDS programmes in many highly affected countries expanded exponentially, creating new opportunities for CSOs in both service delivery and governance (Ingram 2012, 3). For example, in 2000 the World Bank introduced the Multi-Country AIDS Program, the first pro-gramme to offer African countries long-term funding for national HIV/AIDS

programmes. In order to qualify for funding states had to form National AIDS Councils (NACs), which were required to include CSOs and had to distribute 40 to 60 per cent of resources to CSOs (Lancet 2008, 1724; Harman 2007, 486). Greater resources and access to governance spaces in turn generated opportunities for CSOs to advocate and implement rights-based responses.

Exceptionalism facilitated the continued, and growing, influence of HIV/AIDS CSOs in GHG. Their involvement was justified based on agreement that such innovations were required to address the unique threat of HIV/AIDS. For example, as noted in the next chapter, the NGO Delegation was included in UNAIDS' governance structure because of recognition that HIV/AIDS was exceptional, and under the condition that the unique arrangement would not set a precedent in the UN system. CSOs were able to negotiate a role in global HIV/AIDS governance because HIV/AIDS was deemed different from other health issues, requiring a unique configuration of actors to address it.

Human rights became one of the key frames within AIDS exceptionalism – along with development and security (Rushton 2010). Though human rights claims conflicted with biomedical neoliberalism, these struggles were tolerated because of (near) consensus on the exceptional nature of the response:

> This framing of HIV/AIDS as an exceptional humanitarian emergency with security implications is highly significant in the context of struggles over neoliberal globalization because it enabled the argument that HIV/AIDS should be excepted from the actually existing neoliberal regime for dealing with infectious disease.
>
> (Ingram 2012, 6)

Because HIV/AIDS was different, alternatives that promoted greater resource transfers to support rights and empowerment interventions were tolerated, and even supported, as a necessary anomaly to curb a global crisis.

The emergency rhetoric of HIV/AIDS exceptionalism also overcame political uneasiness and differences around human rights language. While some powerful states, such as the USA, were unwilling to recognize health as a human right (due, for example, to domestic debates over national health insurance), the need to respond to what was conceived as a global emergency in innovative ways overcame the more contentious political debates. As a result, HIV/AIDS interventions took on a humanitarian language that obscured the political elements related to universal health rights, instead focusing on the need to rapidly deliver services (Ingram 2009, 98). The emergency rhetoric around the epidemic neutralized the inherently political nature of rights claims.

Furthermore, exceptionalism favoured the promotion of liberal human rights frames advanced by northern-based NGOs in the global HIV/AIDS response. O'Manique notes that many CSOs continued to frame empowerment as an issue of individual agency, divorced from social and global inequalities: "Yet the institutional response to AIDS in Sub-Saharan Africa remains

focused on the autonomous individual who is to be empowered to protect herself or himself from infection" (2004, 4). European and North American CSOs travelled to other contexts to promote peer support and care programmes based on Western experiences of coming out with HIV (Nguyen 2010). Campaigns focused on access to technologies, such as condoms and treatment, which supported the expansion of these markets, as opposed to addressing the social, economic and political challenges people at risk of or living with HIV/AIDS faced in applying these technologies to increase their wellbeing. For example, Seckinelgin (2012) notes how treatment access programmes in Burundi focused on medical provision, neglecting issues related to food security – also essential for treatment to be effective. While HIV/AIDS CSOs promoted the diffusions of human rights frames, these were primarily advanced through liberal conceptions of rights as related to individual access to technical resources.

As a result, while CSOs often struggled against biomedical neoliberal health rationales (Chapman 2009), they also increasingly participated in their promotion. For example, CSOs often advocated private, as opposed to public, responses to health care, in order to bypass state systems run by governments that did not abide by human rights standards. Altman wrote, "Successful AIDS work implies both the strengthening and weakening of the state, as 'the new public health' approach demands the empowerment of non-state actors and forces recognition of unpopular groups and behaviours" (2001, 84). The UN General Assembly Declaration on HIV/AIDS (2001) noted that while the leadership of governments is "essential", "their efforts should be complemented by the full and active participation of civil society, the business community and the private sector." The private–public partnerships that flourished within HIV/AIDS exceptionalism, created space for CSOs, private foundations and corporations in health care, contributing to greater private interests in GHG, most of which reflected a dominant biomedical neoliberal ethos (Ingram 2012, 3). CSO participation in HIV/AIDS governance both posed alternatives to biomedical neoliberalism and worked with it.

Within the space created by exceptionalism, the coalition of CSOs, states, private foundations, corporations, financial institutions and GHIs achieved remarkable gains. The UNAIDS 2008 World AIDS Report noted that the annual number of AIDS deaths was finally declining – falling from 2.2 million in 2005 to 2.0 million in 2007 – largely due to the roll out of treatment in Sub-Saharan Africa. Meanwhile, the number of new infections in many high prevalence countries stabilized as prevention efforts began to take root. The exceptional coalition, which brought unprecedented resources and attention to the HIV/AIDS response, was beginning to turn the tide on the epidemic.

However, since around 2007, both the privileged space for CSO participation and the prominence of human rights frames have been challenged by shifts within GHG away from AIDS exceptionalism. These shifts were indicated in key publications questioning the exceptional claims of the HIV/AIDS response. In 2007, Epstein published *The Invisible Cure: Africa, the West, and the Fight*

Against AIDS, arguing that exceptionalist research around HIV/AIDS failed to address the main cause of the epidemic – multiple concurrent partnerships – because it was not politically correct to discuss African sexuality in such terms. It was suggested that the politicization of the epidemic negatively impacted the response. Along similar lines, Pisani published *The Wisdom of Whores*, in 2008, arguing that the linking of HIV/AIDS with poverty and inequality obscured the basic biology of HIV transmission, over-complicating the response and allowing highly paid experts to create an "AIDS mafia" (205). It was argued that the "AIDS lobby" had garnered an "unfair" amount of resources, and was wasting them on socially dubious expenditures (Garrett 2007). The most strident, and perhaps effective, attacks were made by England who, in a series of editorials in the British Medical Journal (2007a, 2007b, 2008), openly called for an end to AIDS exceptionalism, arguing that the vertical prioritization of HIV/AIDS detracted resources from other, often more pressing, health issues.

Arguments against HIV/AIDS exceptionalism received a robust response. Nattrass and Gonsalves took on the economists who said that HIV/AIDS funding detracted from other health issues: "the balance of evidence suggests that AIDS funding has not been excessive nor at the cost of other health programs. ... AIDS spending thus did not 'crowd out' other health-related spending in any absolute sense" (2009, 5). Whiteside and Smith (2009) argued that HIV/AIDS exceptionalism remained relevant in high prevalence states that require foreign assistance to meet prevention and treatment needs. Forman (2011) wrote that AIDS exceptionalism should be seen as an important corrective in global health: that HIV/AIDS had set a standard, in terms of garnering financial support, which other health issues should aspire to.

These academic and policy debates were influenced by a number of shifts in knowledge around and material experiences of the HIV/AIDS epidemic. Improved evidence was replacing fears of a global generalized epidemic. For example, in 2007, UNAIDS reconfigured their epidemiological statistics downward from 39.5 million in 2006 to 33.2 million. UNAIDS explained this revision was due mainly to improved methodology, better surveillance by countries and changes in the key epidemiological assumptions used to calculate the estimates. The downward adjustment created the sense that the epidemic was not as bad as feared. Similarly, arguments that HIV/AIDS would contribute to state collapse were questioned by research that demonstrated a weak correlation between state security and the epidemic (Barnett & Prins 2006). These factors contributed to a further dynamic – the fading out of emergency rhetoric. Emergencies are generally conceived of as short-lived, and HIV/AIDS had been framed as an emergency for a quarter of a century. This rationale declined along with decreased fears of insecurity and mass death. As treatment programmes were rolled-out, deaths began to decline, and prevention was buttressed by evidence that people on ART were less likely to pass on the virus. While treatment required increased resources, it decreased the urgency of the response.

The rights-based framing, promoted by HIV/AIDS CSOs, also contributed to the end of AIDS exceptionalism: "the right to health brought groups together but then returned as a boomerang in a way. If health is a human right then surely there is no justification for prioritizing one disease" (CSO Representative 2013 #10). For example, access to ART spurred a general access for medicines campaign (Morin 2011). While this extended human rights to health arguments, it also recognized that HIV/AIDS was but one of many diseases (such as asthma and diabetes) that were chronic health concerns in high-income countries, and fatal elsewhere. Concurrently, the roll out of ART increased awareness about the dire need for stronger health systems and greater human resources for health in hyper-endemic contexts.

Some HIV/AIDS activists and CSOs began calling for an expansion of the rights-based response beyond vertical interventions. Vertical programmes, it was argued, contradictorily drew resources away from health systems in order to fund ART, which required strong health systems in order to be distributed. Sachs and Pronyk (2009) suggested that the Global Fund become a Global Health Fund, in order to provide resources for the health systems essential to disease-specific and general health programmes. Such proposals caused conflict among HIV/AIDS CSOs – with some arguing for continued prioritization of HIV/AIDS and others for integration (CSO Representative 2013 #10; Parker 2011). As the right to HIV/AIDS treatment and care grew to encompass greater health rights goals, arguments for AIDS exceptionalism were weakened by lack of consensus.

Concurrently, trends in funding for the HIV/AIDS response began to shift in response to broader changes in the political economy of global health. The economic recession in North America and Western Europe resulted in austerity measures, which contributed to the stagnation of overseas development assistance. For example, Italy, Ireland and Spain stopped contributing to the Global Fund when their economies were hit by the recession in 2008, and Denmark and the Netherlands also reduced their commitments (International HIV/AIDS Alliance 2012, A13). In 2010, the American government reduced financial targets for the scale-up of PEPFAR (Collins 2013). Resources for HIV/AIDS stagnated for the first time in 2010.

The backlash against AIDS exceptionalism caused HIV/AIDS donors to shift resources to health system strengthening. The Global Fund's New Funding Model (discussed further in Chapter 4) includes a funding stream particularly for health system strengthening. Similarly, bilateral donors, such as the Netherlands, have increased the portion of resources going to health systems, and the European Commission shifted its focus from HIV/AIDS, Malaria and TB to global health more generally in 2010 (MSF 2010). While such shifts create opportunities for more integrated and hopefully effective global health aid delivery, in the absence of additional resources, such changes also limit opportunities to scale-up the HIV/AIDS response.

The backlash against HIV/AIDS exceptionalism and economic crisis resulted in substantial fears of a decrease in funding with dire predictions from

UNAIDS and advocacy groups, such as the International HIV/AIDS Alliance (2012), and in the media (IRIN 2011).

CSO recipients of international aid speak of "fighting for survival" and "intense competition for resources" (CSO Representative 2013 #26). They note the context of resource scarcity impedes their work and ability to build partnerships with other CSOs, with whom they have to compete for the same funding (CSO Representative 2013 #26). Changes in HIV/AIDS resources have created a tense environment for HIV/AIDS CSOs to operate in.

Despite persistent fears, funding for HIV/AIDS has not actually declined, but has plateaued since 2010 (ONE 2012). This reflects the general trend in development assistance for health. The Institute for Health Metrics notes that, "Rather than falling sharply as expected, over the past two years development assistance for health has been sustained at levels of spending that would have been inconceivable a decade ago" (2012, 7). Research from the Kaiser Family Foundation and UNAIDS shows that donor funding for HIV/AIDS has remained largely flat over the past two years, levelling off after a decade of significant growth. As Fidler (2009) notes, the privileged position of global health, within development assistance, has not so much declined but stabilized.

Within this more established GHG regime, the position of HIV/AIDS as exceptional was questioned. By 2009, it was clear that acceptance of AIDS exceptionalism was declining, and a renegotiation of the positioning of HIV/AIDS within global health was in process. DfID reassigned a portion of its HIV/AIDS funds to maternal and child mortality programmes and health systems strengthening. The Netherlands cut its HIV/AIDS spending by US $70 million (MSF 2010). Most crucially, in 2011 the Global Fund announced that it was cancelling new funding rounds until 2014 due to governance challenges and lack of donor commitments (discussed more in Chapter 4). Continued arguments for a more integrated approach to GHG and backlashes against disease-specific interventions speed the end of AIDS exceptionalism.

Chapter conclusion

The failure of the medical establishment and governments to respond effectively to the early HIV/AIDS epidemic created space for HIV/AIDS CSOs to promote an alternative human rights frame. Despite vast differences among CSOs engaged in the HIV/AIDS response around the world, a global network emerged that shared an understanding of disease and response that conceived of vulnerability and experiences of ill health as directly related to rights. An effective response was therefore understood as one that not only asserts the rights of those affected, but also assures their right to participate in health governance. In this way the global HIV/AIDS CSO movement demanded both a rights-based response to the epidemic and CSO participation in GHG. CSOs created their own terms of participation in the global governance of the HIV/AIDS response through the human rights frame.

The frame of human rights and norm of CSO participation became incorporated into biomedical neoliberal approaches to HIV/AIDS, at the same time as promoting alternative frames. Struggles to frame the HIV/AIDS response did not unfold only as polarized conflicts: at times CSOs worked with states, institutions and other interests; they used economic and medical arguments to advance their cause, just as other actors at times used rights arguments. CSOs became engaged in building public–private partnership responses to the epidemic and disseminating liberal human rights ideals. They also continued to demand more responsive institutions and to challenge restrictive biomedical responses. These dynamics demonstrate and entwining of interests, and therefore frames, to shape the global HIV/AIDS response.

The role of CSOs, and the rights frame they promoted, flourished during the period of AIDS exceptionalism, which allowed for both a prioritization of HIV/AIDS, and space to pose alternatives and participatory innovations in GHG. However, rights framing also expanded to promote health as a human right in general, challenging the concept of AIDS exceptionalism. Such arguments combined with political-economic developments, and shifts within GHG, to raise questions about the prioritization of HIV/AIDS in GHG. As subsequent chapters will demonstrate, this questioning has greatly impacted the role of CSOs within the HIV/AIDS response and opportunities to advance rights-based responses to health.

References

Altman, D. (2001), *Global Sex*, University of Chicago Press, Chicago.

Barnett, T. (2006), "A Long-wave Event. HIV/AIDS, Politics, Governance and 'Security': Sundering the Intergenerational Bond?", *International Affairs*, Vol. 82 No. 1, pp. 297–313.

Barnett, T. and Prins, G. (2006), "HIV/AIDS and Security: Fact, Fiction and Evidence – a Report to UNAIDS", *International Affairs*, Vol. 82 No. 2, pp. 359–368.

Bayer, R. and Fairchild, A. (2006), "Changing the Paradigm for HIV Testing – the End of Exceptionalism", *The New England Journal of medicine*, Vol. 355 No. 7, pp. 647–649.

Behrman, G. (2004), *The Invisible People: How the U.S. has Slept through the Global AIDS Pandemic, the Greatest Humanitarian Catastrophe of Our Time*, Free Press, New York.

Bonnel, R. (2013), *Funding Mechanisms for Civil Society: The Experience of the AIDS Response*, World Bank, Washington, D.C.

Chapman, A. (2009), "Globalization, Human Rights, and the Social Determinants of Health", *Bioethics*, Vol. 23 No. 2, pp. 97–111.

Collins, C. (2013), "If We Want an AIDS-Free Generation, Why are We Cutting PEPFAR?", *Huffington Post*, 18 April, available at: http://www.huffingtonpost.com/chris-collins/pepfar-cuts-hiv-aids_b_3101250.html (accessed 9 August 2014).

El-Sadre, W., Mayer, K. and Hodder, S. (2010), "AIDS in America – Forgotten but Not Gone", *New England Journal of Medicine*, Vol. 362 No. 11, pp. 967–970.

England, R. (2007a), "Are We Spending Too Much on HIV?", *British Medical Journal*, Vol. 334, p. 344.

England, R. (2007b), "The Dangers of Disease Specific Aid Programmes", *British Medical Journal*, Vol. 335, p. 565.

England, R. (2008), "The Writing is on the Wall for UNAIDS", *British Medical Journal*, Vol. 336, p. 1072.

Epstein, H. (2007), *The Invisible Cure: Africa, the West, and the Fight against AIDS*, Penguin, London.

Fee, E. (1995), "Understanding AIDS: Historical Interpretations and the Limits of Biomedical Individualism", *American Journal of Public Health*, Vol. 83 No. 10, pp. 1477–1486.

Fidler, D. (2009), "After the Revolution: Global Health Politics in a Time of Economic Crisis and Threatening Future Trends", *Global Health Governance*, Vol. 2 No. 2, pp. 1–21.

Fineberg, H. (1989), "Education to Prevent AIDS: Prospects and Obstacles", *Science*, Vol. 239, pp. 592–596.

Forman, L. (2011), "Global AIDS Funding and the Re-emergence of AIDS 'Exceptionalism'", *Social Medicine*, Vol. 6 No. 1, pp. 45–51.

Gamson, J. (1988), "Silence, Death and the Invisible Enemy: AIDS Activism and Social Movement 'Newness'", *Social Problems*, Vol. 36, pp. 351–367.

Garrett, L. (2007), "The Challenge of Global Health", *Foreign Affairs*, January/February, pp. 14–38.

GFATM (2013), Global Fund Overview, available at: http://www.theglobalfund.org/en/overview/ (accessed 20 April 2013).

Gordenker, L., Coate, R., Johsson, C. and Soderholm, P. (1995), *International Cooperation in Response to AIDS*, St. Martin's Press, London.

Hampton, J. (1991), *Living Positively with AIDS: The AIDS Support Organization (TASO), Uganda*, Action Aid, London.

Harman, S. (2007), "The World Bank: Failing the Multi-Country AIDS Program, Failing HIV/AIDS", *Global Governance*, Vol. 13 No. 4, pp. 485–492.

Horton, R. (2012), "Offline: The Rights and Wrongs of 'an AIDS-free Generation'", *The Lancet*, Vol. 380 No. 9839, p. 324.

Ingram, A. (2009), "Biosecurity and the International Response to HIV/AIDS: Governmentality, Globalisation and Security", *Area*, Vol. 42 No. 3, pp. 293–301.

Ingram, A. (2012), "After the Exception: HIV/AIDS Beyond Salvation and Scarcity", *Antipode*, Vol. 45 No. 2, pp. 436–454.

Institute for Health Metrics and Evaluation (IHME) (2012), *Financing Global Health 2012: The End of the Golden Age?*, University of Washington, Seattle.

International AIDS Society (2013), Episode 2 – The History of the IAS, available at: http://www.iasociety.org/Default.aspx?pageId=696 (accessed 7 August 2014).

International HIV/AIDS Alliance (2012), *Don't Stop Now: How Underfunding the Global Fund to Fight Aids, Tuberculosis and Malaria Impacts on the HIV Response*, HIV/AIDS Alliance, Brighton.

IRIN News (2011), "HIV/AIDS: Global Fund Cancels Funding", 24 November, available at: http://www.irinnews.org/report/94293/hiv-aids-global-fund-cancels-funding (accessed 14 August 2014).

Knight, L. (2008), *UNAIDS: The First 10 Years, 1996–2007*, Joint United Nations Programme on HIV/AIDS, Geneva.

The Lancet (2008), "The World Bank and HIV/AIDS in Africa", *The Lancet*, Vol. 371 No. 9626, p. 1724.

Mann, J. and Tarantola, D. (1998), "Responding to HIV/AIDS: A Historical Perspective", *Health and Human Rights*, Vol. 2 No. 4, pp. 5–8.

Merson, M., O'Malley, J., Serwadda, D. and Apisuk, C. (2008), "The History and Challenge of HIV Prevention", *The Lancet*, Vol. 372 No. 9637, pp. 475–488.

Morin, J.F. (2011), "The Life-Cycle of Transnational Issues: Lessons from the Access to Medicines Controversy", *Global Society*, Vol. 25 No. 2, pp. 227–247.

Médicins Sans Frontières (MSF) (2010), *No Time to Quit: HIV/AIDS Treatment Gap Widening in Africa*, Médicins Sans Frontières, Geneva.

Nattrass, N. and Gonsalves, G. (2009), *Economics and the Backlash Against AIDS-Specific Funding: Paper for the WHO/World Bank/UNAIDS Economics Reference Group*. Washington D.C., 21 April.

Nguyen, V.-K. (2010), *The Republic of Therapy: Triage and Sovereignty in West Africa's Time of AIDS: Body, Commodity, Text*, Duke University Press, Durham, NC.

O'Manique, C. (2004), *Neoliberalism and AIDS Crisis in Sub-Saharan Africa: Globalization's Pandemic*, Palgrave Macmillan, New York.

ONE (2012), *The Beginning of the End? Tracking Global Commitments on AIDS*, ONE, Washington D.C.

Oomman, N., Bernstein, M. and Rosenzweig, S. (2007), *Following the Funding for HIV/AIDS: A Comparative Analysis of the Funding Practices of PEPFAR, the Global Fund and World Bank MAP in Mozambique, Uganda and Zambia*, Center for Global Development, Washington D.C.

Parker, R. (2011), "Grassroots Activism, Civil Society Mobilization, and the Politics of the Global HIV/ AIDS Epidemic", *Brown Journal of World Affairs*, Vol. 21 No. 2, pp. 2–37.

Pisani, E. (2008), *The Wisdom of Whores: Bureaucrats, Brothels and the Business of AIDS*, Granta, London.

Potts, H. (2008), *Participation and the Right to the Highest Attainable Standard of Health*, University of Essex, Colchester.

Rosenbrock, R., Dubois-Arber, F., Moers, M., Pinell, P., Schaeffer, D. and Setbon, M. (2000), "The Normalization of AIDS in Western European Countries", *Social Science & Medicine*, Vol. 50 No. 11, pp. 1607–1629.

Rushton, S. (2010), "Framing AIDS: Securitization, Development-ization, Rights-ization", *Global Health Governance*, Vol. 4 No. 1, pp. 1–17.

Sachs, J. and Pronyk, P. (2009), "Correspondence", *The Lancet*, Vol. 373, p. 2111.

Sandoval, C. and Cáceres, C.F. (2013), "Influence of Health Rights Discourses and Community Organizing on Equitable Access to Health: The Case of HIV, Tuberculosis and Cancer in Peru", *Globalization and Health*, Vol. 9 No. 1, p. 23.

Seckinelgin, H. (2012), "The Global Governance of Success in HIV/AIDS Policy: Emergency Action, Everyday Lives and Sen's Capabilities", *Health & Place*, Vol. 18 No. 3, pp. 453–460.

Shiffman, J., Berland, D. and Hafner, T. (2009), "Has Aid for AIDS Raised All Health Funding Boats?", *Journal of AIDS*, Vol. 52 No. 1, pp. S45–S48.

Smith, J., Ahmed, K. and Whiteside, A. (2011), "Why HIV/AIDS should be Treated as Exceptional: Arguments from Sub-Saharan Africa and Eastern Europe", *African Journal of AIDS Research*, Vol. 10 Suppl. 1, pp. 345–356.

Söderholm, P. (1997), *Global Governance of AIDS: Partnerships with Civil Society*, Lund University Press, Lund / Chartwell-Bratt, Bromley.

UNAIDS (2007), *Policy Brief: The Greater Involvement of People Living with HIV/ AIDS*, Geneva, available at: http://www.unaids.org/en/resources/presscentre/featur estories/2007/march/20070330gipapolicybrief (accessed 15 December 2015).

UNAIDS (2008), *World AIDS Report*, UNAIDS, Geneva.

UNAIDS (2013), *Global AIDS Response Progress Reporting 2013: Construction of Core Indicators for Monitoring the 2011 UN Political Declaration on HIV/AIDS*, UNAIDS, Geneva.

UN General Assembly (2001), *United Nations General Assembly Declaration on HIV/AIDS*, United Nations General Assembly, Geneva.

Whiteside, A. and Smith, J. (2009), "Exceptional Epidemics: AIDS Still Deserves a Global Response", *Globalization and Health*, Vol. 5 No. 1, p. 15.

World Bank (2008), *Integrating Gender Issues into HIV/AIDS Programs: An Operational Guide*, World Bank, Washington D.C.

3 Advocating for AIDS
CSOs and UNAIDS

In 1996 UNAIDS became the first UN agency, and GHI, to formally include civil society in its governance body – the Program Coordinating Board (PCB). The CSO movements described in the previous chapter used their expertise and access to decision-makers to demand a space within the unique joint programme. Within a context of calls for UN reform, civil society participation was justified on grounds of AIDS exceptionalism, and with arguments that CSO presence would make decision-making more responsive to affected communities, strengthen institutional legitimacy and improve downward accountability. Great expectations were set for the first global HIV/AIDS institution and its CSO allies.

UNAIDS has continued to expand its participatory governance structures, reiterating that civil society participation improves processes. Its Guidance for Partnerships with Civil Society states that:

> Among multiple other benefits, partnership with people living with HIV, key populations and broader civil society enables UNAIDS to be more grounded and stay alert to the real needs, issues and resources of individuals, communities and countries affected by HIV. Informed by that knowledge and understanding, UNAIDS is better able to support countries and communities to develop more effective responses to the epidemic, guided by lived realities and successful outcomes, responding to epidemiology and evidence, not to ideology.
>
> (UNAIDS 2012b, 12)

Similarly, a commentary written by UNAIDS staff argues that UNAIDS derives its leadership position in the HIV/AIDS response through its pioneering role in creating governance spaces open to the meaningful participation of civil society, and remains accountable to the broader HIV/AIDS movement because of this participation (Sidibe et al. 2010). These assertions are repeated by observers and academics (Horton 2012; CSO Representative 2013 #31), with only a handful of critical perspectives on such claims (Seckinelgin 2009). In particular UNAIDS argues it has set a precedent of CSO participation to be learned from and built on.

This chapter documents CSO contributions to UNAIDS governance, asking if CSO participation has lived up to expectations for a more rights-based, inclusive and responsive HIV/AIDS response. Recognizing that CSO participation in UNAIDS' regional and national initiatives is not uniform, and therefore requires case-by-case analysis, the focus is on how civil society engages with UNAIDS at the global level, though linkages to regional, national and local processes will be discussed when relevant. Furthermore, the focus is on civil society participation in the UNAIDS PCB and Secretariat, not the cosponsoring organizations. Each cosponsor has its own model of engaging with civil society (or lack thereof), and therefore analysis of these processes would require greater depth and space than is possible here.

History

In the 1980s, the UN agency best positioned to respond to the HIV/AIDS epidemic, the WHO, was slow to initiate action. Merson, the Executive Director, originally saw the disease as primarily affecting high-income countries that could respond without external assistance. Though some African countries tried to raise awareness about the epidemic, stating it was spreading "like bush fire", they got little response from the WHO (Lisk 2010, 35). Meanwhile, highly affected countries' public health systems were constricted by numerous health demands, reduced budgets under International Monetary Fund (IMF) structural adjustment policies, and political-cultural resistance to discussing issues of sexuality. With little support coming from national or international institutions, CSOs filled the void by providing home-based care, support and counselling. As these groups became connected with and got support from global advocacy networks, their concerns reached international forums. Activists began to demand a global response, lobbying the WHO to set international standards and provide assistance in developing countries (GHI Representative 2013 #3).

Finally, in 1987, the WHO General Assembly acknowledged the pandemic proportions of HIV/AIDS, and through Special Resolution 42/8, WHO's Special Program on AIDS was created, with the aim of addressing the health and other impacts of the epidemic (Lisk 2010, 40). Jonathon Mann, a physician and human rights advocate, was appointed Director. He immediately drew on the expertise of activists and NGO partners to ensure the new programme adopted the human rights approach developed by the now burgeoning global network. This level of collaboration with CSOs was unprecedented for the WHO (Merson et al. 2008, 481). The Global Program on AIDS (GPA), as the Special Program was renamed in 1988, adopted the discourse of AIDS exceptionalism to frame HIV/AIDS as a social, economic and political, as well as a health, issue.

By 1989, over 100 requests for technical assistance had been received by GPA from member states, most concerning development of national HIV/AIDS plans. Within three years it was the largest WHO programme. The USA, for

example, by the early 1990s was putting three-fifths of its extra-budgetary contributions to the WHO into the GPA (Goodlee 1995, 178). However, the GPA under Mann, while effective in getting international support for the HIV/ AIDS response, did not sit easily within the broader WHO framework. The success of the GPA created funding competition. While WHO's main budget was frozen for much of the late 1980s and early 1990s, commitments to GPA rose from US\$30.3 million in 1987 to US\$82.4 million in 1990 (Lisk 2010). Donor countries preferred to fund the extra-budgetary programme, which they had more control over, than the member state governed general budget. Furthermore, Mann challenged the biomedical approach of WHO by adopting the human rights frame pioneered by HIV/AIDS activists, and upset the state-centric approach of the organization by welcoming the participation of CSOs.

The tension between the GPA and the rest of WHO intensified with the change of Director General in 1988. Former Director General Mahler had let Mann implement the programme with little oversight, often tolerating missteps in bureaucratic process. He had also supported Mann's adoption of human rights approaches to the epidemic and his partnership approach with civil society. The new Director General, Hiroshi Nakajima, was not so tolerant, prioritized bureaucracy, and favoured biomedical state-based approaches. Davies writes that Nakajima's leadership, "can be best characterized as a return to technical initiatives, but largely based on the neoliberal model" (2010, 37). Nakajima viewed HIV/AIDS as getting too much attention, compared to the rest of WHO's mandate (Lisk 2010, 44). As he attempted to rein in the GPA, conflicts emerged between Mann and Nakajima, causing Mann to resign in 1990.

Following Mann's departure, tensions developed between the WHO and CSOs. Mann commented, "As the winds of change within WHO moved the organization back to status-quo ante thinking, the GPA and non-governmental organization relationship suffered" (Mann & Kay 1991, 227). These tensions were exacerbated by a sense of competition. CSOs were working directly with the communities most affected. This gave them credibility and a degree of control in producing knowledge around HIV/AIDS. CSOs had the further advantage of being closely connected to programmes around the world and linked together in networks. They could provide rapid information about the epidemic and what responses were and were not working (Martin 1999, 62). CSOs' active involvement in the response justified assistance for HIV/AIDS going directly to them, bypassing expensive international systems, such as the WHO. By 1990, CSOs received 17 per cent of the US\$480 million distributed for external HIV/AIDS assistance (Lee 2003, 27).

Differences in approaches created further rifts between CSOs and WHO. A WHO statement claimed: "NGOs do not possess an overall appreciation of the AIDS pandemic and all its manifestations and, moreover, usually represent a specific interest group and hence possess only a specific or limited orientation toward the dilemma as a whole" (quoted in Gordenker et al. 1995, 90). In

contrast, the GPA approach was criticized for its one size fits all implementation strategy: "These packages were all more or less the same as they were manufactured and exported from Geneva to the countries of Africa, Asia and Latin America" (Knight 2008, 34–35). Civil society presented dynamic systems for implementing programmes in contexts that were changing rapidly as new knowledge about the epidemic emerged and increasing numbers of actors became involved. WHO's cumbersome state-centred bureaucracy was much slower to adapt (Söderholm 1997, 165).

Calls for UN reform followed the end of the Cold War and WHO in particular was singled out as a problem agency. In 1993, Nakajima was re-elected amidst allegations of vote rigging, and external auditors reported serious financial mismanagement (Goodlee 1994, 1491). Söderholm writes: "WHO itself was under attack. Donors were ill at ease with how the Director-General conducted his work. This criticism spilled over into the AIDS strategy. National governments saw reasons to withdraw support from GPA, as did other UN agencies" (1997, 101). Funding for the GPA stagnated for the first time in 1990. In 1992, an external review of the GPA was published, which criticized WHO for failing to coordinate interagency responses, poor collaboration with other institutions, and interagency rivalries, which detracted from a coherent UN response.

The multisectoral response called for by activists and NGOs justified the involvement of other UN agencies in the HIV/AIDS response. In particular UNDP (which had strong relationships with CSOs) and UNICEF (which was concerned with issues related to HIV transmission from mother to child, and orphaning) began implementing interventions. However, as the UN agencies had little history of working together well, efforts to collaborate on HIV/AIDS interventions were short lived and fraught with tensions. As a result, the external review of the GPA called for a "new or alternative mechanism for ensuring effective coordination of the global efforts to combat AIDS at the country level and adequate collaboration within and beyond the UN system" (Lisk 2010, 48). In response, a General Management Committee was established to explore options. In 1992, the committee produced a report stating:

> One of the most important lessons ... has been that no single agency is capable of responding to the totality of the problems posed by AIDS; and, as never before, a cooperative effort, which is broadly based but guided by a shared sense of purpose, is essential.
>
> (quoted in Knight 2008, 20)

Global HIV/AIDS governance was to become a testing ground for a multisector, multi-actor response.

Donor countries pushed for an option outside WHO, stressing the need for greater cooperation between UN agencies and for UN reform. CSOs used these dynamics to enhance their demands for a more inclusive UN response. The GIPWA principle, which had been adopted by most donor states at the

Paris AIDS Summit in 1994, was now reasserted to demand CSO inclusion in the new global programme. CSO participation was further justified by the key role they had filled in being the first to respond to the epidemic, providing services to those affected, and advocating a global response. One early UNAIDS staff member noted civil society involvement was assured:

> Because of the [GIPWA] principle, because the AIDS response has been completely different to so many public health responses and it changed the way the global health community works. In that PWAs in the early days of the epidemic demanded to be front and centre in the response so the phrase "nothing about us without us" was key.
>
> (GHI Representative 2013 #24)

The desire for a new type of UN entity was evident from donors, combined with participation demands from CSOs to put pressure on the UN system to be more inclusive.

The resulting task force, the Interagency Advisory Group on AIDS, included 12 members: three representatives from donor countries (the Netherlands, Sweden and the USA); three from low-income countries (Bulgaria, India and Sudan); three from UN agencies (the World Bank, WHO and UNDP); and three from civil society organizations (the Netherlands-based AIDS Coordination Group, GNP+ and ENDA Tiers Monde from Senegal). The inclusion of CSOs on this task force, especially in equal number to the institutional and state actors, was unprecedented: "With the intention of facilitating the negotiation process, a radically new method was devised. ... On the task force, NGOs could provide input to the same extent that governments could, thus breaking out of sovereignty-bound practice" (Söderholm 1997, 166).

However, the role of CSOs in the new entity continued to be contentious. China and Cuba were against formal involvement of CSOs (because of their particular resistance to CSO activity in their domestic settings), as were some European countries, which argued UN entities should remain state-based. Amongst the cosponsoring organizations, the World Bank and UNDP were supportive of civil society involvement while WHO, UNICEF and UNESCO were initially against it (GHI Representative 2013 #24). After some negotiations, it was agreed that CSOs would continue to have a formal role in the new organizations, on the condition that this would not set a precedent in the UN system. The perceived need for an exceptional multisector response to the HIV/AIDS epidemic, calls for UN reform, and CSO leadership in the early response combined to justify this unique arrangement.

In July 1994, ECOSOC endorsed the creation of UNAIDS through resolution 1994/24. The memorandum of understanding for the new programme was signed by the cosponsors in October 1995, and UNAIDS was publicly launched on World AIDS Day of the same year. UNAIDS was to be governed by the PCB, which became the first UN governing body to include CSOs. Nay writes:

The ECOSOC decision to include CSOs in the governance of UNAIDS was a major step. It acknowledged the key role of these organizations in the development of the global response to the epidemic, based on the assumption that they can provide useful information and expertise because of their grass-roots activity and connection to vulnerable populations.

(2009, 10)

The role CSOs had played in providing HIV/AIDS related services, advocating a global rights-based response and challenging the WHO led to their incorporation into the only joint programme in the UN system to tackle a single health issue.

CSOs had great expectations of this new institution, as did the new staff, many of whom came from CSO backgrounds. One early staff member recalls:

We really felt that we were on the cutting edge of UN reform. We felt we had an opportunity of testing new ways of doing business, of being more efficient, being more responsive, of trying to get out of some of the traps that go with any UN bureaucracy.

(quoted in Knight 2008, 36)

It was hoped that the unique governance arrangement within UNAIDS would result in an institution that was responsive to and representative of those it claimed to serve.

However, a distinct feature of UNAIDS was that it was confined to being a coordinating agency, not an implementing one. The cosponsors were suppose to implement programmes under the auspices of UNAIDS, but were resistant to surrendering leadership. Due to continued infighting, and anxieties about the new governance format, many donor governments pledged less to UNAIDS than they had to the WHO's GPA. The limited budget (US$120– 40 million for the biennium 1996–1997) restricted the type of activity UNAIDS could engage in. Former GPA chief, Merson, recalled "UNAIDS was disabled from the start" (quoted in Knight 2008, 44). During the 1990s UNAIDS' activities largely revolved around collecting reports of all the cosponsor activities and attempting to combine them to present a coherent project (Nay 2009).

The limits of the new institution frustrated CSO expectations. UNAIDS held regional meetings to introduce the new programme to civil society, but these usually resulted in more confusion than clarity:

people attending these regional meetings were confused by what they heard about UNAIDS. If UNAIDS was being created because the epidemic was such a major problem, why was it so much smaller than GPA? And what was happening to the funding that GPA used to provide to countries?

(Knight 2008, 37)

Those CSOs that attended PCB meetings quickly discerned that the cosponsor governance format led to cautious resolutions, based on compromises,

which did not satisfy CSO expectations for the rapid advancement of a rights-based response (Nay 2009, 13). Furthermore, the consensus-based governance format depended on the agreement of conservative states resistant to both CSO involvement and rights-based responses to the epidemic. As UNAIDS did not provide funding, and remained hampered by UN protocols, the high expectations CSOs had for the organization were soon regulated to more modest hopes.

Still, the relationship between UNAIDS and CSOs was an improvement on that of the WHO: "UNAIDS was able to reach out to and work with activists in a way WHO could not" (GHI Representative 2013 #3). The new institution had recruited staff from civil society and had strong networks with CSOs around the world. Peter Piot, the first Executive Director, had worked with CSOs in the past, and now often collaborated with them to push agendas member states were resistant to (GHI Representative 2013 #24). One informant noted:

> UNAIDS was not created to support communities. On the other hand there were people involved in the creation of UNAIDS who shared an understanding and belief in the centrality of community responses. And I hoped that regardless of what happened … that UNAIDS would bring a much needed multisectoral perspective, not just multisectoral in terms of different ministries, that was needed as well, but also multisectoral in terms of public–private community.
>
> (GHI Representative 2013 #3)

While tensions persisted between UN bureaucracy and CSO's aspirations, the new organization had greater flexibility than the WHO. Despite contradictions and challenges, UNAIDS created expanded institutional space for CSOs to engage in and influence the global governance of the HIV/AIDS response.

UNAIDS' position in GHG

Throughout its 20 year history (from 1994 to 2014) UNAIDS has continued to be something of an anomaly in the UN system. It remains the only joint programme, the only single health issue entity, and the only UN institution with formal space for civil society on its board. It describes itself as "an innovative partnership that leads and inspires the world in achieving universal access to HIV prevention, treatment, care and support" (UNAIDS 2013). Interviewees particularly perceive UNAIDS as an advocacy institution, stating, "I think that was one of the big successes of UNAIDS – keeping AIDS on the agenda" (GHI Representative 2013 #6), and "I do think UNAIDS was absolutely central to the advocacy efforts that led to the dramatic increase in development assistance and world attention to HIV" (GHI Representative 2013 #3). One example of UNAIDS' advocacy role is fostering support for UN Political Commitments/Declarations on HIV/AIDS in 2001,

2006 and 2011, which have continued to position HIV/AIDS as a global public goods issue. Many actors also note the key, and not unrelated, role UNAIDS plays in gathering and disseminating information: "In no other issues do you have a global commitment and a UN agency that collects the stats at the country level, and collects global indicators for progress for global aims" (CSO Representative 2013 #1). UNAIDS has developed as an information broker in the HIV/AIDS response, and an advocate for exceptional political attention and resources.

However, since the decline of HIV/AIDS exceptionalism (described in the previous chapter), UNAIDS has had to increasingly justify its place within the UN system and broader GHG. This is largely the result of the backlash against vertical health interventions, in which UNAIDS, as the only disease-specific UN entity, is a prime target. An opinion piece in the *British Medical Journal* in 2007 called for dissolution of UNAIDS as "the biggest vertical program in history" (England 2008, 1072). The declining popularity of vertical health initiatives combined with the impacts of the economic crisis in donor countries in 2008 to cause stagnation in funding for HIV/AIDS programmes; since 2008 UNAIDS' budget has remained constant at US$485 million, which in real terms indicates a reduction in financing (UNAIDS 2015).

UNAIDS' position is further impacted by the shifting role of the UN within global governance processes in general. Nay writes, "In this new international landscape, the UN system is no longer in a position of leadership when it comes to designing and implementing international development policies" (2009, 4). In the crowded GHG arena, UN agencies compete with better-resourced entities, such as the Global Fund (discussed in the next chapter), and private foundations, such as the Bill and Melinda Gates Foundation.

Noting these developments, many informants raised questions about the continued relevance of UNAIDS. One interviewee asked, "if it [UNAIDS] went, what would the AIDS movement lose?" (CSO Representative 2013 #26). Another noted, "I wouldn't be surprised if UNAIDS was dissolved and reorganized back into the WHO" (CSO Representative 2013 #15). A state representative asked:

> UNAIDS was certainly necessary at the beginning because this was a disease that required a response that is big, quite different than others and targeted marginalized populations. But now, is it really necessary? What is the added value that WHO in a more mainstream way could not provide?
> (State Representative 2013 #14)

UNAIDS' role within the current GHG order is increasingly being questioned.

UNAIDS is aware of its precarious position and has responded by attempting to reposition itself away from being a proponent of AIDS exceptionalism, and towards being seen as an innovator within the broader GHG architecture. Recent messaging campaigns argue that the success of the HIV/AIDS response can be used to inform the SDG and other development/health agendas (Kim

et al. 2011; Sidibe et al. 2010; UNAIDS 2013). A UNAIDS representative explains:

> UNAIDS sees itself as having – based on the AIDS response and the progress of the AIDS response – having the legitimacy to say "you know this is how we have accomplished this so far" and other health and development issues can really learn from this experience ... So increasingly we are positioning ourselves as an organization that while driving advocating for the end of AIDS. We are hoping to drive progress across a lot of other different issues.
>
> (GHI Representative 2013 #31)

In particular, UNAIDS argues that as it has pioneered inclusive governance structures that engage civil society, other organizations can learn from its example (UNAIDS 2013, 5).

Influence in decision-making

CSOs engage in both the UNAIDS Secretariat and PCB in a variety of capacities, aiming to influence decision-making to better reflect a rights-based response to the epidemic. The mission of the NGO Delegation to UNAIDS' PCB is, "to ensure that their [constituent] human rights and equitable, gender sensitive access to comprehensive HIV prevention, treatment, care and support are reinforced by the policies, programmes, strategies and actions of the PCB and UNAIDS" (NGO Delegation 2013b). However, CSOs bring their own hierarchies to UNAIDS, and operate within what remain primarily state-based structures, shaped by multiple ideological and material influences (Seckinelgin 2009). This raises questions about how their participation and influence is shaped by existing structures, and how/if CSO participants are able to influence decision-making to promote alternatives.

The UNAIDS PCB, the main governance body, includes 22 member states, 11 cosponsoring organizations and five NGO delegates. According to the 1994 ECOSOC resolution on the formation of UNAIDS:

> NGOs invited [to participate in the PCB] should be those either in consultative status with the Economic and Social Council or in relationship with one of the six co-sponsoring organizations or on the roster of non-governmental organizations dealing with matters pertaining to HIV/AIDS, in accordance with the rules, procedures and well-established practice of the United Nations system.
>
> (ECOSOC 1994, 2)

Seckinelgin (2009) argues such restrictions reinforce a "durable inequality" between state members and NGOs, because only NGOs that complement the UN system are included, and only at the will of states. However, the current

process of delegate selection is somewhat different than what was likely envisioned by the authors of the 1994 resolution.

According to the ECOSOC resolution (1994/24) the five NGO seats should be filled by three delegates representing NGOs from developing countries and two delegates from developed, or in transition, countries. In practice, currently, the Delegation includes five board members and five alternates (10 in total, all of whom usually attend the meetings), representing the geographical regions of North America, Europe, Asia, South and Central America, and Africa. Though individuals are nominated to be NGO delegates, it is actually the NGOs they represent that hold the seat, in order to ensure continuity if an individual is unable to continue to meet their commitments (i.e. if one person has to abdicate, the NGO can put forward another member, who must be approved by the Delegation). In the call for nominations, which goes out to a list serve of over 3000 addresses, and is posted online, eligible NGOs are defined as local, national, regional and international organizations, networks of people living with HIV, ASOs, community-based organizations (CBOs), AIDS activist organizations, faith-based organizations (FBOs), and networks or coalitions of AIDS organizations. NGO delegates often come from regional networks, such as the Asia Pacific Network of People Living with HIV/AIDS, key population networks, such as the International Network of People Who Use Drugs, or national organizations, such as the Ghana HIV/AIDS Network.

In order to qualify, individual representatives from NGOs must meet the following criteria:

> Be actively and principally involved with HIV work in the country and/or region for which the applicant is applying; maintain a comprehensive understanding of the health, political, and social consequences and needs of the AIDS pandemic, particularly as it relates to the region; be strongly connected to and actively liaise with national and regional civil society networks; and have extensive experience in national, regional, and/or international policy making and advocacy.
>
> (NGO Delegation 2013b)

The individual delegates are not meant to particularly represent their NGO, but the broader civil society response in their region. Furthermore, though regional representation structures their participation, other affiliations to particular key populations (such as sex workers) or issue areas (such as treatment access) are also considered in the selection process. Though not explicitly stated, efforts are made to ensure equal gender representation on the Delegation, and PWA delegates are encouraged (GHI Representative 2013 #29).

Short-listed nominations are selected by the current NGO Delegation, in consultation with broader civil society, and interviewed by current delegates. The PCB approves finalists but, to date, there has not been a case of the PCB refusing a candidate put forward by the existing Delegation. The approval process is viewed more as a formality and opportunity to introduce the new

delegates to the PCB (CSO Representative 2013 #30). The Delegation's ability to essentially self-select members from civil society, according to criteria CSOs establish, indicates they have a high degree of autonomy.

However, there are also directives on who can be a delegate, restricting access to decision-making forums in less direct but influential ways. Delegates must have working knowledge of English, which means the pool of people from some regions (such as Sub-Saharan Africa) is much smaller than from others (such as Europe and North America). In practice, most delegates have university level education and professional backgrounds, which eliminates the majority of PWAs (GHI Representative 2013 #6). While there are practical rationales behind such requirements (delegates must have the language skills and knowledge of policy processes to participate in bureaucratic decision-making), it also means that access remains exclusive, especially for delegates from those regions with the majority of PWAs and key populations.

In addition to the NGO Delegation, observer NGOs can attend the PCB meetings. They must register in advance, and the Executive Director has the right to refuse permission to attend, though this has rarely been used. Observers note the UNAIDS PCB is one of the most accessible UN forums (CSO Representative 2013 #30). NGO observers may speak in plenary after all PCB members (member states, cosponsors and the Delegation) have done so at the discretion of the chair. Prior, during and after board meetings, the NGO Delegation invites NGO observers to attend briefings in order to inform participation strategies and interventions. The number of observers who attend meetings can vary greatly, depending on agenda items and current concerns in the HIV/AIDS response, but on average there have been about 60 NGO observers at meetings since 2007 (GHI Representative 2013 #28).

As observers must attend at their own cost, the majority come from Europe (due to its close proximity to Geneva headquarters) and North America (as these CSOs have greater resources). There are few observers from low- and middle-income countries. At the June 2013 PCB Meeting, only three (of approximately 60) observers were from CSOs based outside Europe and North America. The costs of observing the PCB means that well resourced and European CSOs are able to participate, while others are largely excluded.

Even for those who have access to the PCB, ability to participate is constrained by bureaucratic practices. In addition to the PCB, there are side meetings to be attended, as well as informal negotiations (GHI Representative 2013 #12). Delegates and observers note the challenges of deciphering how to gain access and influence in these less formal negotiations that shape outcomes in plenary, as they lack diplomatic know-how, coming from community back-grounds not political training (CSO Representative 2013 #23). The formal speaking process of the PCB, and the UN setting, can be overwhelming to new delegates. One representative states:

> That is one thing I find about being on the PCB. Is that you do need to have a highly level of academia to be an effective voice at times. And I

struggled. To be honest I struggled being on the PCB because it is a little bit above my level. I never worked in this kind of advocacy, policy level before. It has been a huge learning curve. ... I've struggled to the point where I sort of have anxiety attacks because I don't feel I am doing enough.

(CSO Representative 2013 #15)

As this informant has postgraduate university qualifications and is a native English speaker and is therefore likely better prepared than many others, the quote demonstrates that the learning curve for engagement is steep. It also illustrates the anxiety that results from the desire to participate effectively to represent those who do not have access, and barriers to doing so. This suggests that the delegate is committed to representing, to the best of their ability, those who do not have access to decision-making, but their capacity to do so is restricted by bureaucratic procedures.

In 2005, the NGO Delegation requested an evaluation of NGO/Civil Society involvement in the PCB. The NGO Delegation hoped this would promote governance changes, such as increased funding to support communications and coordination amongst CSOs involved in UNAIDS. Reflections by current actors on the NGO Delegation's role prior to the review, suggest that the Delegation had suffered from poor organization, and frequent internal (with each other) and external (with other board members) conflicts (GHI Representative 2013 #29). One long time observer notes, "I mean it was quite shocking in the early days. I mean there was some stunning people, some really inspiring people involved. But to be honest, it was all a bit of a mess. It was very impromptu" (CSO Representative 2013 #30). Self-recognition of these inadequacies, as well as long-standing frustrations with perceived lack of support from UNAIDS, prompted the Delegation to suggest the review.

The review was widely supported by the Delegation, partner CSOs, cosponsors and the Secretariat. It resulted in a number of notable, and generally agreed beneficial, changes. For example, a Communications Facility was established to provide support to delegates in terms of internal and external communication, organizing logistics and facilitating information exchange. Following the evaluation, more specific terms of reference were developed for delegates and an accountability mechanism was put in place in order to monitor their commitments. Furthermore, though the ECOSOC resolution does not include reference to an "NGO Delegation", instead referring to individual NGO delegates, following the 2007 review, the group made concerted efforts to act as one delegation, consolidating influence (UNAIDS 2012a; CSO Representative 2013 #30; GHI Representative 2013 #29). As a single delegation, they agreed to focus on promoting the rights of key populations and universal access.

UNAIDS Secretariat staff and external civil society observers agree that these changes have had a positive impact on the NGO Delegation's participation (GHI Representative 2013 #29; CSO Representative 2013 #30). One observer compares the current role of the Delegation to its participation prior to the review, "I think without a doubt the Delegation has really got its act

together. A lot more, a lot better. It's a hell of a lot more professional" (GHI Representative 2013 #29). The Delegation used the review process to increase its capacity to participate effectively within the decision-making bureaucracy.

Research on the NGO Delegation to the UNAIDS PCB argues that its influence is particularly limited because it does not have voting rights, which are reserved for states. The 1994 ECOSOC resolution on the formation of UNAIDS stipulated the NGOs, "would not participate in any part of the formal decision-making process, including right to vote, which is reserved for representatives of governments" (ECOSOC 1994, 3). Rittberger et al. find that "these disparities in decision-making rights means the UNAIDS only meets the minimum requirements of inclusiveness" (2008, 23). Seckinelgin notes, "While NGOs roles are recognised in relation to HIV/AIDS through their inclusion into the formal architecture of the governance, the resolution still asserts that priority be given to state members by constraining the formal procedures of participation" (2009, 219). Lack of voting rights is viewed, by these analyses, as a barrier to meaningful participation.

For the NGO Delegation, the issue of the vote has shifted over the years. An early UNAIDS staff member noted that when UNAIDS was formed the NGOs involved did not want voting rights as they felt this would compromise their independence:

> in the early days of UNAIDS, NGOs explicitly did not want to have voting right at all, because they said, then we become part of the system, we become responsible for the decisions and we want to keep our independence and our kind of watchdog function.
>
> (GHI Representative 2013 #24)

Later, around the turn of the millennium, the Delegation began campaigning for voting rights, a demand that was generally resisted by other board members and the Secretariat. The 2007 NGO/Civil Society Review suggested NGOs should be given voting rights, but this was not adopted.

It was recognized that changes to the board structure would require opening the resolution on the creation of UNAIDS, which would result in extensive bureaucratic processes and create space for numerous other competing issues to become contentious. Some actors felt that in the process the NGO Delegation might lose more than they gained, as a minority of state members have expressed displeasure over the role of NGOs in the PCB and might suggest reforms to curb their influence, as opposed to increase it (GHI Representative 2013 #29). Since 2007, the NGO Delegation has largely given up its campaign for voting rights. Voting is not seen as particularly crucial to its interests, being more of a symbolic power, as the board is consensus-based and has never actually voted, as opposed to related to direct influence over decision-making (GHI Representative 2013 #29; CSO Representative 2013 #15).

One forum where the NGO Delegation and observers are recognized as having influence is during thematic sessions. At every second UNAIDS PCB

meeting the last day is dedicated to a thematic topic, such as criminalization, gender or youth. A number of informants note that on thematic days the NGO Delegation and observers play particularly active roles, as the topics under discussion are often those issues they are most concerned with, knowledgeable about, and experienced in (related to human rights, gender equality, etc.) (GHI Representative 2013 #28; CSO Representative 2013 #15) – and therefore NGO Delegates and observers are able to apply their expertise in sharing knowledge, and exercising discursive influence and emotive force.

For example, at the 34th PCB in June 2014, the NGO Delegation prepared a background document and case studies on social drivers of the HIV/AIDS epidemic (the designated theme), taking a lead role in knowledge production. They explicitly aimed to shift the discussion away from purely legal responses to stigma and discrimination, to responses that consider the political, social and economic drivers of the epidemic. To this end they invited observers from various regions to share personal accounts of experiencing barriers to treatment, care and prevention, and community-based strategies for overcoming them. A transgender former sex worker from Asia spoke about the need for health services to reach out to marginalized populations, and a woman from Kenya shared her experience forming a barmaids' association in order to empower women at risk of HIV infections (NGO Delegation 2014). These personal accounts added emotive force to discursive arguments for a more holistic rights-based response.

However, thematic days do not result in decision points, as it is argued that this allows board members to speak freely, without being hampered by national policies and cosponsor responsibilities (GHI Representative 2013 #28). This limits the outcomes of any influence CSO representatives have during thematic days. Because of the importance of topics discussed during thematic days, the NGO Delegation first campaigned for a change in policies, so that thematic days might result in decision points. The argument, from the NGO Delegation, was that "the absence of decision points is a wasted opportunity" (NGO Delegation 2013a). While this campaign failed – due to lack of support by both other board members and the Secretariat – the Delegation successfully campaigned for follow-up to thematic days to be a standing item on the proceeding PCB agenda, at which point related decision points could be proposed. This created an opportunity for the NGO Delegation to advance its influence during thematic sessions to decision-making processes. For example, though the NGO Delegation did not feel its interventions in the thematic session on social drivers adequately shifted the discussion from legal to socio-economic rights, it was able to draft a decision point to this effect for the next PCB meeting in December 2014, in order to reiterate its argument (NGO Delegation 2014).

Many interviewees refer to the ability of the Delegation to "shift the discourse" in this way: "it is actually very clear, in particular how they changed the nuances and tone of the discussion and decision points in the PCB" (CSO Representative 2013 #30). A Secretariat staff member notes, "I think the

NGOs have huge influence at the table … and have impact on being able to say things in the right way that can perhaps move an agenda" (GHI Representative 2013 #27). The Delegation has influence over the language of decision points as it is able to go into the drafting room during board meetings (GHI Representative 2013 #28). Delegates persistently use these opportunities to make incremental changes: "And slowly, each time we get one thing more past … Having been involved in the process now I can see it. And I do see that we make a difference, we do get through" (CSO Representative 2013 #15). Similarly, the 2012 evaluation notes, "The NGO Delegation plays a vital watchdog role – monitoring, as necessary, issues and agenda items of relevance to civil society that risk slipping off the agenda" (UNAIDS 2012a).

CSO influence within the Secretariat

CSOs also engage with the UNAIDS Secretariat in multiple ways to influence decision-making. The Civil Society and Private Sector Division of the UNAIDS Secretariat collaborates with global HIV/AIDS related networks, and includes staff members who focus on specific groups, such as women's networks, key populations, religious organizations and PWAs. It also draws on the expertise of, and supports, about 60 community mobilization, gender and human rights advisors in the field (GHI Representative 2013 #28). The Secretariat works with CSOs in preparation for and during the High Level Meetings on HIV/AIDS. Prior to the 2011 meeting, for example, it provided technical and coordination support to the Civil Society Task Force, which was convened to support the President of the General Assembly and advised on civil society engagement in the global review processes. The UNAIDS Secretariat encourages member states to include civil society representatives in their delegations, and for CSOs to attend as observers (GHI Representative 2013 #28).

In particular, CSOs influence Secretariat processes through various Reference Groups. The Reference Group on HIV and Human Rights reviews the rights-based language and messaging in UNAIDS documents and policies. For example, it promoted stronger language on the decriminalization of the sex trade in UNAIDS policies, as is discussed in Chapter 5. Members of the Reference Group (all of whom come from civil society) meet with Secretariat staff working on issues related to human rights in order to share suggestions, information and advice, and comment on draft papers and policies. The Reference Group on Human Rights also has the capacity to put out its own statements and publications, which may present a different position than UNAIDS. In this way it influences discussions from both within and outside the institution through the independent production of knowledge.

Advocating rights-based legal environments

The particular manner in which civil society delegates, observers and participants in Secretariat processes influence decision-making in UNAIDS can be

illustrated through the case of mobilization around issues related to HIV/AIDS and legal rights. Briefly, the legal issues concerned revolve around: the criminalization of HIV transmission, which raises questions about shared responsibility and what constitutes informed consent; the criminalization of homosexuality, sex work and drug use, which inhibits these groups from accessing HIV/AIDS services; and stigma and discrimination perpetuated by law officials and judicial systems, which results in inadequate protection and recourse for key populations. Since 2010, these issues have become an increasing concern for CSOs involved in the HIV/AIDS response due to high profile cases of PWAs being charged over HIV transmission; new penalties in countries, such as Uganda, for homosexuality; and growing campaigns around harm reduction and the rights of sex trade workers. Due to its primarily state-based membership, within UNAIDS there has been a particular focus on improving legal environments.

In 2011, the NGO Delegation began conducting research on HIV/AIDS and legal environments. The findings of this research were then presented in the Delegation's annual NGO Report at the 29th PCB meeting in December 2011. The report drew on 27 focus groups with over 250 participants who shared direct experience and expertise about how laws around the criminalization of sex work, drug use and HIV transmission impede prevention and treatment programmes – using case studies from programme implementers to strengthen arguments. The Delegation circulated the report ahead of the PCB meeting, along with decision points that called for countries to repeal prohibitive laws, such as those around homosexuality, as well as address related issues, such as ensuring the right to safe abortion – points that were purposefully inflammatory. Then, after introducing the full report, and recognizing that once a document is rejected by the PCB it cannot be reintroduced, the Delegation withdrew these decision points, listing them as recommendations instead. A delegate explains this strategy of influencing the discourse, if not the decisions:

> So that opened the door to allow us to bring the topic back at the next board meeting. Because otherwise the report would have been discarded and not accepted. So by withdrawing, it created a big stink amongst anyone who read it and then we withdrew them. So we put our point across and I think everyone saw what we wanted. So we've been able to every board meeting go back to it. Bring it back.
>
> (CSO Representative 2013 #15)

In this case the Delegation recognized the limits of its power, especially as confined by the authority of the member states and the bureaucratic system, but was able to retain influence for further discussions.

The Delegation continued to exercise this influence by highlighting issues around HIV/AIDS and legal environments at further meetings. For example, the Delegation secured external funding to bring in an NGO observer, who spoke at the following thematic session about his experience of being

imprisoned for HIV transmission in the USA. Then, at the next PCB, during the follow-up to the thematic session on HIV/AIDS and Legal Environments, an incoming NGO delegate from Africa, an openly gay man, took the floor during a heated debate to insist that key populations exist in all contexts, regardless of state assertions to the contrary. The rest of the Delegation, and NGO observers, stood in solidarity when he spoke.

The Delegation and observers used their influence, as members of key populations and those most affected by the epidemic and punitive legal systems, to counter the negative politicization of rights issues with both personal experience of abuses and emotive force about the effects of such abuse. This resulted in relatively strong language in the decision point that followed calling for enabling legal environments, and "Increased access to justice for people living with, and affected by HIV, including their families, women, young persons, children, and key populations" (UNAIDS PCB 2012, 6.1). The reference to key populations is crucial here as it included a footnote defining key populations as including MSM, a category some states had previously resisted recognizing. It also included a call to eliminate "all forms of violence against women and girls, including harmful traditional and customary practices" (UNAIDS PCB 2012, 6.1). For UNAIDS' consensus and sovereignty-based governance format, this was unprecedentedly strong language (CSO Representative 2013 #23).

At the 31st PCB meeting, the Delegation returned to controversial issues on women's rights. During an agenda item on gender issues, the NGO Delegation ensured language on "women from key populations" and "women's rights and health organizations" was included in decision points on gender (Coulterman 2012). The strong language infuriated some countries and it looked as if the PCB might vote for the first time in its history, which would have excluded the Delegation from decision-making. However, the chair asked the Delegation if they would agree to a vote being taken, indicating a recognition of the importance of their consent and, though the delegation assented, the vote was eventually averted. This demonstrates that though the formal influence of the Delegation is limited, its compliance is still sought.

During these heated PCB meetings, the NGO Delegation was supported not only by NGO observers, but also by members of the HIV and Human Rights Reference Group who attended the meeting. The Reference Group had been engaging in its own meetings with the UNAIDS Secretariat and representatives from cosponsor organizations around enabling legal environments for the HIV/AIDS response. While the NGO Delegation and observers aimed to influence states, the Reference Group worked on the UN agencies. One influential outcome of these discussions was a joint statement by all cosponsors and the Secretariat on the closure of compulsory drug detention and rehabilitation centres – a rather impressive feat considering the previous resistance of some organizations, such as UNODC, to approaches that prioritize human rights over punitive laws around drug use (GHI Representative 2013 #6). By asserting discursive and emotive influence, the NGO Delegation and CSOs

involved in the Secretariat were able to shape policies to reflect a rights-based approach.

The case of civil society involvement around HIV/AIDS and legal environments, demonstrates the influence of CSOs in advocating the rights of key populations within the UNAIDS PCB and Secretariat. Bureaucratic processes and the dominance of state power, which prevent changes to dominate structures, restrict this influence, but civil society actors have proven astute at working within these confines to promote a rights-based response. As one informant noted:

> I think we had some really small victories, I mean they were big, but in the bigger scheme of things they were small, but they were really significant for civil society and for people directly affected by and living with HIV, because we have really been able to push the agenda quite significantly. I think some of the outcomes we had in terms of discussion at the board were really interesting I think because you wouldn't expect to get those kinds of outcomes out of a UN discussion.
>
> (CSO Representative 2013 #8)

CSOs that engage with UNAIDS have been able to apply discursive and emotive force to make incremental changes, influencing discussions, if not decisions, around human rights.

Balancing legitimacies

Both the UNAIDS PCB and Secretariat claim legitimacy based on civil society participation. An article written by Secretariat staff asks, "how has UNAIDS acquired a degree of legitimacy to espouse a vision for the future of the entire AIDS response?" (Sidibe et al. 2010, 4). The answer provided includes a list of UNAIDS lead innovations in the HIV/AIDS response, including having created, "expanded political space for affected people, communities and civil society in the governance of a health-related development challenges" (Sidibe et al. 2010, 4). However, considering the limits placed on CSO participation in UNAIDS governance and the challenges global institutions face in generating both input and output legitimacy, such claims require critical assessment.

The mission statement of the NGO Delegation is, "to bring to the PCB the perspectives and expertise of people living with, most affected by, and most at risk of, vulnerable to, marginalized by, and affected by HIV and AIDS, as well as civil society and nongovernmental entities actively involved in HIV work" (NGO Delegation 2013b). The Delegation claims input legitimacy based on representation of those most affected by the epidemic. However, the ability of the Delegation to be truly representative is restricted by regulations and practical expectations around participation in the PCB. For example, while the NGO Delegation is structured by regions, these do not necessarily

represent the contours of HIV/AIDS geography; there is no delegate for the Middle East and only one seat for Africa; though the majority of PWAs live in Africa, and some of the fastest growing epidemics are in the Middle East (GHI Representative 2013; UNAIDS 2015). Therefore, those regions most affected by the epidemic do not necessarily have corresponding representation on the delegation. This is exacerbated by the skill requirements for delegates (outlined above), which means that the pool of qualified people from some regions (particularly those that are not English speaking) and population groups (such as those with lower education levels, such as sex workers) is much smaller than from others.

One interviewee notes:

> it just really worries me that you do just see the same old people on these delegations. … Not to take anything away from those individuals, most of them are fantastic at what they do. But it does become a sort of self-filling sort of thing. You don't always get newer people in.
>
> (CSO Representative #30 2013)

Interviewees identify a revolving door from the UNAIDS NGO Delegation to the civil society delegations of other international institutions. NGO delegates also recognize that access to the PCB is restricted: "Sometimes our constituents say that 'its only certain people', but it is. You need a degree. You need a masters or a bachelors, otherwise you don't get in" (CSO Representative #15 2013). These dynamics substantiate Boedeltje and Cornips argument that in interactive governance forums "a trade-off must be made in which the principle of competence dominates at the expense of the criterion of fairness" (2004, 2). In the selection process for NGO delegates, competence in terms of education and skills trumps other possible criteria that could strengthen legitimacy, such as representation.

Recognizing it has weak representation claims, the NGO Delegation instead claims legitimacy based on membership in key population groups. As one observer noted:

> You know we have been stuck with this problem of does any one person, or two people, can they represent a movement? Can they represent the diversity of what you see in the civil society or non-governmental sector? And the probably the answer is no, but what you can do is that you can bring a unique voice to the table based on your experience.
>
> (GHI Representative 2013 #27)

When relevant issues are discussed the Delegation ensures it is represented by a member of that population group or region, or ensures that NGO observers attend who represent these groups. For example, in advocating strong policies around rights and legal environments, as discussed above, the Delegation had an openly gay African man speak about homosexuality in order to assert

membership (if not representation) of that key population group. This type of legitimacy is not based on democratic norms of representation, but membership to key population groups.

The NGO Delegation contributes to institutional output legitimacy by contributing expertise in responding to the HIV/AIDS epidemic. A UNAIDS observer notes:

> When you have civil society, when you have people living with HIV and you know representatives of MSM, and drug users and sex workers, in the room with ministers, and the government minister puts a phrase up on the screen, this is what we want to say, and the Delegation says no we want these words in here, because without that there will be repercussions at the country level. ... In those negotiations they have a very strong influence in that way.
>
> (GHI Representative 2013 #28)

Because the NGO Delegation consists of individuals with direct experience responding to the epidemic it is able to promote responsive policies. Other governance actors defer to this expertise because the Delegation is viewed as representative of those responding to the epidemic (in terms of having experience in service delivery), as opposed to representing government policies (as states do) or institutional priorities (as the Secretariat and cosponsors must).

The Delegation is also recognized as contributing to output legitimacy by shifting processes beyond diplomatic confines through sharing experiences of living with or responding to the epidemic, and appealing to moral commitments. Such interventions push the boundaries of UN bureaucracy, but are recognized as promoting responsiveness. One UNAIDS representative explains:

> In many of these board meetings, many government delegations say "I wish I could work like you guys. I wish I could say what I wanted to say, instead I have a speech from my capital and I just have to repeat it in a meeting." Whereas NGOs are a bit more flexible in approaching how to influence and how to put forward an idea that others adopted, and take on a position that the community feels will be really important to them.
>
> (GHI Representative #28 2013)

Similarly cosponsors, on the whole, appreciate that the Delegation is present because "NGOs can say things that we cannot" (GHI Representative 2013 #11). This is not to imply that cosponsors and governments all, or even mostly, agree with the NGO Delegation's interventions, but that they recognize it strengthens output legitimacy by, at times, superseding the rigidity of the UN system to ensure relevance and greater responsiveness.

One of the reasons the NGO Delegation is able to promote greater responsiveness is that it agrees to participate within established and accepted bureaucratic procedures. In order to increase its legitimacy, from the

perspective of other governance actors, the Delegation takes on diplomatic roles. These roles fulfill state and institutional expectations of effective governance, and enable communication with other governance actors (Lencucha et al. 2010). The NGO Delegation has developed its diplomatic role by adopting institutional practices of deliberation, presentation and rational argument. Such behaviour enables it to contribute to the output legitimacy of the organizations by promoting effective cooperation. One observer notes:

> They work as a team, they prepare their interventions. They work together to put forward their comments on decision points. They really have their act together ... So with that also comes more acceptances from the other stakeholders around the table of the PCB.
>
> (CSO Representative #30 2013)

The 2012 NGO/Civil Society Review notes that all but two member states, and all cosponsors, welcome the participation of the NGO Delegation because it behaves "professionally" (UNAIDS 2012a). By working within institutional processes, the delegation gains acceptance by other governance actors, while contributing to the output legitimacy of UNAIDS.

However, the diplomatic role played by the Delegation alienates civil society peers, weakening its input legitimacy. Delegates note that, when they do engage with broader civil society, their legitimacy is often questioned due to the compromises they have to make in order to work within the UN system. One civil society representative explains:

> You can't go in there [PCB meetings] as an activist because you will just be ignored. So you have to learn to play the game. ... You know we have to go back to our constituents and tell them what we are doing and often, because they are sort of more fast moving and connected they don't understand why we are taking what appears to be a softly softly approach.
>
> (CSO Representative #15 2013)

CSO peers do not recognize the delegation's diplomatic methods as representing their experiences of the epidemic and response, which (from their perspective) require urgency and action. The characteristics that make the delegation an effective (and therefore legitimate) governance actor, from the perspective of other PCB members, are the opposite to those that other CSOs recognize as representing their interests, creating a tension between input and output legitimacy.

As a result, the Delegation suffers from having to wear "multiple hats" as both an activist and a member of advocacy groups, and a participant in an institutional bureaucracy. The 2012 Review of NGO/Civil Society Participation notes, "Some respondents question if the delegation has a clear enough identity (as 'diplomat' or 'activist')" (UNAIDSa 2012, 5). The legitimacy of the delegation

itself is threatened by this lack of a valid identity. The NGO Delegation finds it has to adhere to the norms of a state-based UN bureaucracy to have influence, gain legitimacy from other PCB members, and contribute to output legitimacy. However, these means of participation weaken its input legitimacy because they do not correspond with CSO peer expectations and place restrictions on who can participate (only those with the skills to engage in bureaucratic processes).

This tension between input and output legitimacy is further complicated because successful governance in UNAIDS is indicated by consensus; meaning lack of agreement threatens output legitimacy. One civil society member noted:

> governments are corrupt, and have different priorities, they can be against homosexuality … there is nothing UNAIDS can do about that. They could kick them off the UNAIDS delegation but they never do. That is not what they want … They want to keep everyone on board because you are better being on board and accessible than being off.
>
> (CSO Representative #15 2013)

In order to maintain consensus, and therefore legitimacy, the NGO Delegation is sometimes asked to modify its demands: "They [UNAIDS Secretariat and PCB] don't like disruptions, and quite often we are asked as the NGO Delegation to temper our claims and to calm down our wording" (CSO Representative #23 2013). Toning down demands, especially during confrontations with conservative states, pits (perceived) effective governance against civil society goals to advocate a rights-based response; it requires a trade off between input and output legitimacy.

For example, at the June 2012 meeting, mentioned above, the NGO Delegation and allied member states engaged in nine hours of negotiations with Egypt and Iran over language in the decision points, with the two countries finally deciding to disassociate themselves from the particular points (UNAIDS PCB 2012). At the December 2012 meeting, consensus again broke down around the language on decision points related to gender, with Iran and Egypt again disassociating from the final point (NGO Delegation 2012a). For the NGO Delegation, the resulting decision points were successful because the issues that they felt to be important to their constituents were included. However, other actors did not feel the same:

> I think that the NGO Delegation has been blamed a little bit for it, and I think mainly, because the aim at UNAIDS level is for consensus, and if you don't reach consensus then it is almost like there has been a failure. … And while from an NGO perspective we are happy about that because it means that things are moving forward, it is not really seen, not celebrated, while we did celebrate it I guess. It is seen as quite a failure on behalf of UNAIDS and the coordinating board.
>
> (CSO Representative #15 2013)

Indeed such protracted debates caused one observer to complain that the PCB was becoming "something of a circus" (CSO Representative #30 2013). In this case, the NGO Delegation sacrificed output legitimacy (in terms of achieving consensus) of the PCB in order to insist on language reflecting civil society concerns. The constant trade-off between input and output legitimacy means that it is almost impossible for the delegation to be legitimate from both the perspective of other PCB members and external CSOs; to contribute to effective institutional governance while promoting a rights-based response in ways identifiable to other civil society actors.

Downward accountability

Much like legitimacy, the argument put forward (by UNAIDS and allied CSOs) is that CSO involvement strengthens downward accountability. One of the missions of the NGO Delegation is:

> enhancing the transparency and accountability of relevant PCB decision-making and policy-setting, helping to meet requirements for upwards accountability (towards the PCB and other delegations) and downwards accountability (towards the people, communities and constituencies affected by HIV).
>
> (NGO Delegation 2013b)

As part of its mandate to contribute to downward accountability, the delegation undertakes a number of measures to attempt to communicate UNAIDS' activities and outcomes to, and gather feedback from, civil society. Newsletters and communiqués are sent to over 3000 people on the Delegation's and UNAIDS' lists (GHI Representative 2013 #29). The NGO Delegation's website includes blogs that are posted almost immediately after PCB meetings, reports and other documentation in English, French, Arabic, Chinese, Russian and Spanish. YouTube clips from meetings and interventions are also posted online. The annual NGO Report is a consultative process including regional focus groups with civil society actors, e-surveys and online forums. The delegation holds conference calls prior to board meetings, and briefings with NGO observers throughout. They disseminate information through global and regional networks, hoping it will trickle down to local groups who will feed responses back up. They also actively pressure the UNAIDS Secretariat to share information (GHI Representative 2013, #29).

The delegation aims to expose UNAIDS' policy choices to public scrutiny, but faces particular challenges in being an effective "transmission belt" of accountability (Nanz & Steffek 2004). Though the delegation goes to extensive efforts to publicize itself, and share UNAIDS information, there is little response from external civil society. At the International AIDS Conferences in 2012, which brought together over 23,000 participants, the NGO Delegation hosted a Meet Your Representative event. However, this only attracted 20 to 30 individuals

(GHI Representative 2013 #29). Prior to the June 2013 board meeting, the NGO Delegation coordinated a conference call to go over agenda items and discussion points with civil society. An invitation to the call was sent to the over 3000 email addresses; two call times were scheduled in order to take into consideration the different time zones. However, one call was cancelled due to lack of participants and the other only attracted five non-UNAIDS associated participants. One delegate explained, "So often we find there is very little response when we do things like that … it is definitely an area we need to work on and we are trying to work on" (CSO Representative 2013 #15). Despite ongoing efforts to engage with broader civil society in HIV/AIDS, the NGO Delegation gets little response.

The cause of weak accountability relationships relates to the reputation of UNAIDS as a bureaucracy, which is not seen as relevant to those implementing programmes. UNAIDS does not provide funding, and does not have strong in-country presence, as cosponsors are responsible for implementation. Instead UNAIDS coordinates UN activities and advocates for the HIV/AIDS response in global forums. Such governance processes, characterized by having meetings and writing reports, are removed from the daily activities of most CSOs. As one interviewee noted:

> I think that it is that people still don't know about the PCB, they still don't know about the NGO Delegation. When they do know they don't especially care about it. Because it doesn't seem relevant. If they take two hours to read through some papers, they don't really see that is going to make a whole lot of difference that will affect their work on the ground.
>
> (CSO Representative 2013 #30)

Even for those who are aware of and engaged with UNAIDS, the relevance of the PCB is questioned because of the bureaucratic processes it must engage with: "The problem with these things it that you want the community representation on these kinds of panels but it takes up a great deal of people's time, a great deal of effort, it costs a lot of time. And you always ask – what is the point of all of this?" (CSO Representative 2013 #2). Reflecting similar challenges to those the NGO Delegation faces in generating input legitimacy (as discussed above) broader civil society actors generally do not recognize connections between their work and the bureaucracy of UNAIDS – a disconnect that raises questions about the role of the NGO Delegation, as one of its purposes is to provide such links, as well as about the legitimacy of UNAIDS as a whole.

Challenges to building accountable relationships also relate to difficulties communicating UNAIDS' processes and outcomes effectively to wider civil society. Board meeting papers can be over a hundred pages and are often released just days before a meeting. The turnaround time for delegates to translate these into other languages, as well as accessible English, distribute them to their networks and incorporate feedback is exceptionally tight, particularly

considering that the delegates are volunteers with other full time jobs. One delegate notes:

> We are all working full time and are busy people. Because we are all so busy, and because we can't reach out, because time is too short there is not enough connection between us and our constituents. ... And to be honest, I'm not sure how we can change that, but we are going to have to look at it.
>
> (CSO Representative 2013 #15)

Delegates' restricted time and resources limit their ability to be accountable to constituents.

A number of processes have been attempted to improve accountability relationships, but demonstrate an unwillingness or inability of UNAIDS' bureaucracy to adapt to meet CSO needs. An independent evaluation of UNAIDS' relationship with civil society noted that the Civil Society Partnership Unit remains under-resourced and marginalized within the organization (UNAIDS PCB 2009). And the 2012 review of civil society participation found:

> Civil society participation has maintained a high profile on the PCB agenda. The resulting decision points – notably at the 20th, 23rd and 25th meetings – remain valid. However, while some have been effectively implemented and led to concrete results, others have received only partial or no follow-up.
>
> (UNAIDS 2012a)

The decision points referenced above recommended, based on the 2007 NGO Review, that PCB documents be produced eight weeks ahead of meetings in order to allow the NGO Delegation time to translate, circulate and gather feedback on them. Though the PCB accepted this recommendation, it was not consistently implemented, inhibiting the ability of the Delegation to consult broader civil society in a timely manner. Similarly, following the 2007 review, member states were encouraged, and cosponsors were requested, to include representatives from civil society on their delegations, in order to increase the participation of civil society and build links with other PCB actors. However, to date, neither cosponsors nor states have acted on these decision points (GHI Representative 2013 #28). While the practical planning and financial challenges of preparing documentation in advance and increasing delegations to include civil society can be appreciated, the lack of follow through on these decision points indicates that where CSOs have tried to strengthen downward accountability, these processes have not been prioritized by other PCB members or the Secretariat.

Following the most recent evaluation of civil society participation in UNAIDS, 13 recommendations for the Secretariat and PCB were put forward on how to improve civil society participation; however these were translated into only four draft decision points for the PCB – something some observers

viewed as a watering down (GHI Representative 2013 #29; CSO Representative 2013 #30). It was further felt, by some, that these recommendations were not acted on beyond "making check lists and ticking things off" (GHI Representative 2013 #29), demonstrating weak outcomes from a key accountability process between the board, NGO Delegation and broader civil society response.

The cosponsor structure of UNAIDS creates a particularly complex accountability framework for CSOs to negotiate. Because CSOs do not participate in cosponsors' governance structures (which are all state-based), engagement is inconsistent, especially at country level, with some cosponsors readily and frequently including CSOs and others resisting CSO participation (GHI Representative 2013 #29). National and regional HIV/AIDS related initiatives are often implemented by cosponsors without communicating with the PCB NGO delegate for the region (CSO Representative 2013 #30). NGO delegates argue this impedes their ability to build strong networks with regional and national civil society groups, and makes downward accountability mechanisms overly complex. External CSOs argue that the cosponsor format makes it difficult to know which cosponsor to approach, and how to do so, depending on what HIV/AIDS interventions are being implemented where, or what policies they aim to influence.

In order to overcome the challenges of the cosponsor format, CSOs pushed for a formal UNAIDS partnership strategy to guide cosponsor and Secretariat engagement with civil society, which ultimately resulted in a Guidance Note on Civil Society Participation in UNAIDS (2011). This document was well received by civil society as it included a number of useful tools, such as checklists on civil society involvement. However, it lacks an accountability structure to ensure its implementation, and so once again does not result in meaningful outcomes. The extensive bureaucratic systems of UNAIDS PCB and Secretariat alienate CSOs, rather than creating opportunities to strengthen downward accountability relationships.

Unified budget, results and accountability framework

The NGO Delegation has also tried to gain more clarity on cosponsor involvement with civil society through participation in the revision process for the Unified Budget, Results and Accountability Framework (UBRAF) – UNAIDS' primary accountability mechanism. Revisions of this tool began in 2014 due to a number of concerns about it – mostly revolving around its extensive length (the 2013 report was over 200 pages) and lack of technical merit (indicators, outputs and outcomes demonstrate weak relationships). As one observer noted, the UBRAF is, "very vast and quite inadequate" (CSO Representative 2014 #33). Though it is not necessary to go into the details of the UBRAF here, generally the complexity and length frustrates cosponsors, the weak technical merit concerns donors, and the lack of consideration of issues related to key populations and PWA participation upsets CSOs.

The process of improving the UBRAF has been complex, due to the numerous actors involved, and inherent complications of developing a monitoring mechanism for 11 cosponsors. Throughout the process, CSO representatives have expressed frustration at what they have felt to be unnecessary delays in addressing issues of civil society participation, and lack of sufficient consultation with civil society on the part of UNAIDS and cosponsors (GHI Representative 2013 #29; NGO Delegation 2012b). Although at first not included in the revision processes, spearheaded by the Monitoring and Evaluation Reference Group (MERG), the NGO Delegation was able to demand space to participate. In this role they have focused on the need to improve accountability between CSOs and cosponsors.

The 2013 UBRAF included 11 (out of 123) indicators directly related to civil society participation. However, the NGO Delegation expressed concerns that these are "without the rigor required to effectively measure meaningful engagement and support for civil society" (NGO Delegation 2013a). In particular, the delegation argued for greater transparency about resources for civil society (i.e. how much and what type of funding cosponsors and the Secretariat provide to civil society organizations they partner with); for greater qualitative analysis of how PWAs and key populations are being engaged with, and whether that engagement is meaningful or tokenistic; and that, as opposed to highlighting only positive outcomes, reporting should also discuss challenges in order for it to be more useful to cosponsors and credible to donors. Based on these concerns, the delegation requested improved indicators that better reflect the engagement of cosponsors and the Secretariat with civil society, and put forward 12 new indicators. The Secretariat felt these were over ambitious, and reduced them to three. In return the delegation expressed concerns that these were inadequate.

In mid 2013, the UNAIDS Secretariat agreed to a proposal made by the delegation to hire a specialist to review the civil society indicators. The consultant, who was required to work within the confines of the existing indicators rather than suggesting new ones, proposed that those civil society related indicators with strong technical merit (seven of the 11) remain, and that in addition the checklist already present in the UNAIDS Partnership Guidance document be used to collect background information. The consultant also recommended that cosponsors continue the practice, pioneered at the request of the NGO Delegation in 2013, of producing an annual Civil Society Working Paper outlining their engagement with civil society on HIV/AIDS related interventions. In 2013, working papers from UNWomen, UNESCO and UNPF provided percentage estimates of their direct financial support to civil society. The consultant suggested that other cosponsors do the same, including actual amounts of support (as opposed to just percentages). In addition, it was recommended that more case studies and qualitative data, collected by objective third parties, be incorporated into monitoring processes. At the 33rd PCB, in December 2013, it was announced that, in response to the consultant's recommendations, the Secretariat and cosponsors had organized

a Cosponsors' Evaluation Working Group on Civil Society, including two members of the NGO Delegation, to shape the questionnaire and the annual working paper. At the 34th PCB, in June 2014, the first outcomes of this working group were shared, including greater financial information on cosponsors' commitments to civil society.

GARP reporting

Civil society has had some success in contributing to the downward account-ability of member states through participation in the UNAIDS Secretariat lead processes of Global AIDS Response Progress (GARP) reporting. GARP reports monitor progress towards the Declaration of Commitment (2001), and Political Declarations (2006 and 2011) on HIV/AIDS. Taylor et al. write:

> the Declaration of Commitment, with its reporting mechanism, is con-sidered among the most effective models of a non-binding instrument in global health policy. The reporting mechanism has evolved and come to have a substantial impact on domestic AIDS legal and policy environments and has significantly improved accountability at both national and global levels.
>
> (2014, 3)

Ninety-six per cent of UN member states completed UNGASS reporting in 2012.

In addition to being a widely supported accountability tool, GARP reporting demonstrates that CSO participation in UNAIDS can directly improve downward accountability. Civil society is included in all aspects of reporting, from participating on the UNAIDS MERG, which develops the indicators, to holding civil society hearings prior to, and participating in, the most recent High Level Meeting on HIV/AIDS, at which the goals were agreed to. CSO participants successfully advocate the most recent version of the GARP guidelines to include an indicator to reduce intimate partner violence, and another on the elimination of stigma and discrimination (GHI representative 2013 #33).

UNAIDS strongly encourages national governments to involve CSOs in the monitoring and reporting process as a source of information and expertise. This encouragement has proven impactful, with the majority of governments that complete reports including CSOs in consultations and data collection, and then presenting findings through validation workshops. Taylor et al. note, "In countries with little previous history of multistakeholder collaboration on AIDS, the unprecedented manner in which civil society actors were often involved in reporting may be the most immediate and tangible result of the process" (2014, 7). The National Policy Commitment documents, completed every two years by each state, include a section to be completed by govern-ment and a section to be completed by civil society. This provides a tool for CSOs to hold governments to account on promises to engage with civil

society and honour commitments to a rights-based response. CSOs are also able to use the data from the reports, widely available on the website AIDSinfo.org, to lobby governments to address neglected issues and key populations (Taylor et al. 2014, 7).

Where civil society feels excluded, that government data is inconsistent, or the indicators used are not indicative of needs and results in their particular context, CSOs can produce Shadow Reports with what they feel are more representative indicators and data. UNAIDS explains:

> Wherever possible UNAIDS encourages civil society integration into national reporting processes. … Shadow reports are intended to provide an alternative perspective where it is strongly felt that civil society was not adequately included in the national reporting process, where governments do not submit a report, or where data provided by government differs considerably from data collected by civil society monitoring government progress in service delivery.
>
> (2013, 15)

Shadow Reports are also produced by CSOs to present an alternative view on national responses. For example, in 2008, the Global Youth Coalition on HIV/AIDS produced Shadow Report for 10 countries in order to increase awareness of the unmet prevention, treatment and care needs of youth at risk of and affected by HIV/AIDS. Shadow Reports created an opportunity to draw attention to the particular human rights issues that affect youth. UNAIDS uses both shadow and state reports to compile its annual Report on the Global AIDS Response.

The number of Shadow Reports increased from 103 in 2003 to 176 in 2010 – indicating increasing involvement of civil society in GARP reporting (Sidibe et al. 2010, 3). Even more telling is that the number of Shadow Reports has dropped over the last two years, due to improved reporting by governments (often with the involvement of CSOs), and improved indicators produced by UNAIDS (Taylor et al. 2014). This demonstrates that the pressure CSOs and UNAIDS put on governments to be accountable to GARP commitments, and to report more effectively – as well as the pressure CSOs exerted on UNAIDS to develop better indicators – has had system-wide outcomes; reporting has become more reflective of rights-based goals and so the need for shadow reports has declined. The reporting on GARP targets presents an example of UNAIDS, civil society and states working together, sometimes cooperatively and sometimes through struggles, to produce innovative downward accountability mechanism and outcomes.

Chapter conclusion

The prominent role CSOs played in advocating a global response to HIV/ AIDS, combined with the failure of WHO to develop an effective

multisectoral response, led to the unprecedented inclusion of civil society actors in a UN body – UNAIDS. However, aspirations for transformation through CSO participation have been curbed by bureaucratic restrictions and state dominance. CSOs have struggled to assert influence in decision-making within the confines of governance structures that limit accessibility and resist change. However, CSOs have been able to use their unique role to shape discussions, if not decisions, around human rights. Because CSO participants have not been able to influence how governance processes are conducted, they have to continually negotiate input and output legitimacy. In order to contribute to effective governance they have to play by bureaucratic rules that alienate their constituents; when they prioritize promoting alternatives reflective of constituent interests, such as human rights issues, they are accused of threatening effectiveness. The resistance of UNAIDS to adapting to CSO participatory requirements further limits the ability of CSOs to be successful conduits for downward accountability between the institution and broader civil society response. External CSOs remain alienated by extensive bureaucratic processes, and internal CSO participants are frustrated by the inflexible bureaucracy. However, the case of CSOs, state and UNAIDS Secretariat cooperation around GARP reporting demonstrates the potential for CSO participation to strengthen accountability processes.

The limits of CSO participation in transforming UNAIDS into a responsive and representative GHI were established at its formation. Considering these restrictions CSO participants have exercised considerable influence while continuing to advocate the rights of those most affected by the epidemic. While claims that CSO participation strengthens legitimacy and accountability are overstated, the potential utility of having CSOs involved in institutional governance is demonstrated.

References

Boedeltje, M. and Cornips. J. (2004), *Input and Output Legitimacy in Interactive Governance*. Netherlands Institute for Governance, Amsterdam, available at: http://repub.eur.nl/pub/1750/ (accessed 15 December 2015).

Coulterman, A. (2012), *Report Back: 30th Meeting of the UNAIDS Programme Coordinating Board*, Geneva.

Davies, S.E. (2010), *Global Politics of Health*, Polity, Cambridge.

ECOSOC (1994), *Joint and Co-sponsored United Nations Programme on Human Immunodeficiency Virus/Acquired Immunodeficiency Syndrome (HIV/AIDS): Resolution 24/1994*. UN Economic and Social Council, Geneva, available at http://data.unaids.org/pub/externaldocument/1994/ecosoc_resolutions_establishing_unaids_en.pdf (accessed 20 July 2016).

England, R. (2008), "The Writing is on the Wall for UNAIDS", *British Medical Journal*, Vol. 336, p. 1072.

Goodlee, F. (1994), "WHO in Retreat? Is it Losing its Influence?", *British Medical Journal*, Vol. 309 p. 1491.

Goodlee, F. (1995). "WHO's Special Programs: Undermining from Above", *British Medical Journal*, Vol. 310, p. 178.

Gordenker, L., Coate, R., Johsson, C. and Soderholm, P. (1995), *International Cooperation in Response to AIDS*, St. Martin's Press, London.

Horton, R. (2012), "Offline: The Rights and Wrongs of 'an AIDS-free Generation'", *The Lancet*, Vol. 380 No. 9839, p. 324.

Kaul, I., Isabelle, G. and Stern, M. (Eds) (1999), *Global Public Goods: International Co-operation in the 21st Century*, United Nations Development Program, New York.

Kim, J., Lutz, B., Dhaliwal, M. and O'Malley, J. (2011), "AIDS and MDGs", *Third World Quarterly*, Vol. 32 No. 1, pp. 141–163.

Knight, L. (2008), *UNAIDS: The First 10 Years, 1996–2007*, Joint United Nations Programme on HIV/AIDS, UNAIDS, Geneva.

Lee, K. (Ed.) (2003), *Globalization and Health: An Introduction*, Palgrave Macmillan, New York.

Lee, K. and Zwi, A. (2003), "A Global Political Economy Approach to AIDS: Ideology, Interests and Implications", in Lee, K. (Ed.), *Globalization and Health: An Introduction*, Palgrave Macmillan, New York, pp. 13–32.

Lencucha, R., Labonté, R. and Rouse, M.J. (2010), "Beyond Idealism and Realism: Canadian NGO/Government Relations during the Negotiation of the FCTC ", *Journal of Public Health Policy*, Vol. 31 No. 1, pp. 74–87.

Lisk, F. (2010), *Global Institutions and the HIV/AIDS Epidemic: Responding to an International Crisis*, Routledge, London.

Mann, J.M. and Kay, K. (1991), "Confronting the Pandemic: The World Health Organization's Global Programme on AIDS, 1986–1989", *AIDS*, Vol. 5 Suppl. 2, pp. S221–S229.

Martin, L. (1999), "The Political Economy of International Cooperation", in Kaul, I., Isabelle, G. and Stern, M. (Eds), *Global Public Goods: International Co-operation in the 21st Century*, United Nations Development Program, New York, pp. 51–64.

Merson, M., O'Malley, J., Serwadda, D. and Apisuk, C. (2008), "The History and Challenge of HIV Prevention", *The Lancet*, Vol. 372 No. 9637, pp. 475–488.

Nanz, P. and Steffek, J. (2004), "Global Governance, Participation and the Public Sphere", *Government and Opposition*, Vol. 39 No. 2, pp. 314–335.

Nay, O. (2009), *What Drives Reforms in International Organizations? External Pressure and Bureaucratic Entrepreneurs in the UN Response to AIDS*, University of Lille, Lille.

NGO Delegation (2012a), *31st UNAIDS Programme Coordinating Board Meeting Talking Points NGO Delegate For Europe*, Geneva, available at: http://unaidsp cbngo.org/wp-content/uploads/2012/12/1.3-executive-report-ngo-delegate-europ e-ukraine.pdf (accessed 15 December 2015).

NGO Delegation (2012b), *Report Back: 30th Meeting of the UNAIDS Programme Coordinating Board*, Geneva, available at: http://unaidspcbngo.org/?P=18531 (accessed 15 December 2015).

NGO Delegation (2013a), 32nd PCB Communique, available at: http://www.unaidsp cbngo.org/2013/07/32nd-pcb-communique/ (accessed 15 December 2015).

NGO Delegation (2013b), Mandate, available at: http://unaidspcbngo.org (accessed 15 December 2015).

NGO Delegation (2014), Communiqué: The 34th Meeting of the UNAIDS Programme Coordinating Board Communique, available at: http://www.unaidspcbngo. org/pcb-meeting-archive/ (accessed 15 December 2015).

Rittberger, V., Huckel, C., Rieth, L. and Zimmer, M. (2008), "Inclusive Global Institutions for a Global Political Economy", in Rittberger, V., Nettesheim, M. and Huckel, C. (Eds), *Authority in the Global Political Economy*, Palgrave Macmillan, New York, pp. 13–54.

Seckinelgin, H. (2009), "Global Social Policy and International Organizations: Linking Social Exclusion to Durable Inequality", *Global Social Policy*, Vol. 9 No. 2, pp. 205–227.

Sidibe, M., Tanaka, S. and Buse, K. (2010), "People, Passion and Politics: Looking Back and Moving Forward in the Governance of the AIDS Response", *Global Health Governance*, Vol. 4 No. 1, pp. 1–17.

Söderholm, P. (1997), *Global Governance of AIDS: Partnerships with Civil Society*, Lund University Press, Lund.

Taylor, A., Alfven, T., Hougendobler, D., Tanaka, S. and Buse, K. (2014), "Leveraging Non-binding Instruments for Global Health Governance: Reflections from the Global AIDS Reporting Mechanism for WHO Reform", *Public Health*, Vol. 128 No. 2, pp. 151–160.

UNAIDS (2007), *Results of the Review of NGO/Civil Society Participation in the Programme Coordinating Board: Presented at Results of the Review of NGO/Civil Society Participation in the Programme Coordinating Board*, Geneva, available at: http://www.unaids.org/en/aboutunaids/unaidsprogrammecoordinatingboard/ngoci vilsocietyparticipationinpcb (accessed 15 December 2015).

UNAIDS (2012a), *Independent Review: NGO/Civil Society Participation in the UNAIDS Programme Coordinating Board*, Geneva, available at: http://www.unaids. org/en/aboutunaids/unaidsprogrammecoordinatingboard/ngocivilsocietyparticipatio ninpcb (accessed 15 December 2015).

UNAIDS (2012b), *UNAIDS Guidance for Partnerships with Civil Society, Including People Living with HIV and Key Populations*, Geneva, available at: http://www.una ids.org/en/resources/documents/2012/20120124_JC2236_guidance_partnership_civil society (accessed 15 December 2015).

UNAIDS (2013), *Global AIDs Response Progress Reporting 2013: Construction of Core Indicators for Monitoring the 2011 UN Political Declaration on HIV/AIDS*, UNAIDS, Geneva.

UNAIDS (2015), Fact Sheet 2015, available at: http://www.unaids.org/en/resources/ campaigns/HowAIDSchangedeverything/factsheet (accessed 15 December 2015).

UNAIDS PCB (2009), *25th Meeting of the UNAIDS Programme Coordinating Board: Conference Room Paper Second Independent Evaluation of UNAIDS PCB NGO Response to SIE*, UNAIDS PCB, Geneva.

UNAIDS PCB (2012), *30th Meeting of the UNAIDS Programme Coordinating Board Geneva, Switzerland*, UNAIDS PCB, Geneva.

UNAIDS PCB (2013), *Agenda Item 1.2 Report of the 31st Meeting of the Programme Coordinating Board*, UNAIDS PCB, Geneva.

4   Money plus

CSOs and the Global Fund to Fight AIDS, Tuberculosis and Malaria

The Global Fund was formed at the turn of the millennium, embodying hope that a unique multistakeholder partnership would be able to curb the epidemic through more efficient and effective aid delivery. Civil society actors were given unprecedented space within the governance of this new institution, positioned as equal and essential partners. The aspirations for inclusive and effective governance, embodied in the Global Fund, continue to be held up as an example of a uniquely participatory governance arrangement (Rittberger et al. 2008).

This chapter documents how these aspirations have been put into practice and to what effect. Structured similarly to the preceding chapter, the focus is on CSO influence in decision-making, and contributions to building institutional legitimacy and accountable relationships. Recognizing that the Global Fund is primarily a resource governance institution, the last section of the chapter analyses how CSOs attempt to influence resource distribution to promote a rights-based response.

While recognizing that the Global Fund provides funding for three diseases and so includes CSOs from various health backgrounds, the focus of this chapter is on HIV/AIDS CSOs. This is not a particularly limiting factor, as the majority of civil society actors that engage in the Fund come from HIV/AIDS CSOs (Bartsch 2007). Furthermore, in keeping with the scope of the discussion here, the analysis is of CSO participation at the global level and so regional and national processes (such as CSO participation on CCMs) are addressed only where they overlap with global level processes.

History

A number of dynamics contributed to the formation of the Global Fund in general, and the participation of CSOs in its governance in particular. These include: the growing recognition of HIV/AIDS as a global security threat, which mobilized donor states; civil society campaigns for universal access to treatment, which created demand for increased funding for HIV/AIDS; and awareness of the limits of UNAIDS in mobilizing a global response to the epidemic, which led to calls for an institution outside the UN system.

Combined, these dynamics created demand for an innovative governance structure, with increased space for CSO participation.

As Chapter 2 outlines, the concept of AIDS exceptionalism facilitated multiple framings of the epidemic, for example as a human rights issue. A further frame was the securitization of the epidemic – the argument that HIV/AIDS had to be responded to urgently because it had global security implications. The securitization of the epidemic was advanced by a number of advocates within the HIV/AIDS response such as Peter Piot, the Executive Director of UNAIDS – who saw securitization as an opportunity to gain greater international attention for the potential implications of the epidemic (Piot & Marshall 2012) – and the US Ambassador to the UN at the time, Richard Holbrock – who while on a trip in Africa visited an AIDS orphanage and was overwhelmed by the degree of suffering caused by the epidemic. Holbrock lobbied UN Secretary General Kofi Annan to raise awareness about the epidemic among member states (Barnett & Prins 2006, 360). As a result, the first UN Security Council meeting of the new millennium was also the first meeting to focus on a health issue as a security threat. At that meeting Annan stated:

> Today marks the first time, after more than 4,000 meetings stretching back more than half a century, that the Security Council will discuss a health issue as a security threat. We tend to think of a threat to security in terms of war and peace. Yet no one can doubt the havoc wreaked and the toll exacted by HIV/AIDS.
>
> (2001)

Other leaders followed Annan's lead, with the President of the World Bank stating, "Many of us used to think of AIDS as a health issue. We were wrong … We face a major development crisis, and more than that, a security crisis" (quoted in Elbe 2005, 404). The resulting resolution positioned HIV/AIDS as the cause-célèbre of shifting notions of security, which suggested that not only could viruses be used as a biological weapon, but also that the impacts of HIV/AIDS (such as widespread orphaning and deaths within the labour force) could contribute to state collapse and social breakdown, which in turn could lead to civil unrest and terrorism. Despite the lack of evidence to support such hypotheses, securitization propelled the HIV/AIDS response to the top of international agendas (Barnett & Prins 2006). This framing positioned the epidemic as a threat to both developing and developed states, generating demands for increased financing to contain the epidemic.

As states focused on the security implications of the epidemic, most CSOs continued to advocate a rights-based response. Around the turn of the millennium, much of this mobilization centred around the right to treatment access. In 1996, ART was announced at the IAS Conference in Canada, potentially transforming AIDS from a lethal disease to a chronic condition. Soon after high-income countries began public provision of treatment.

Pharmaceutical companies justified high prices on medications (over US $25,000 per patient per year in 1996) by referring to intellectual property rights, and research and development costs. It was unthinkable to states and institutions that concepts of rights and equity could interfere with intellectual property norms or trade regimes, and so it was accepted that ART was a life prolonging option only for those who could afford it (O'Manique 2004, 83). Initially, policy-makers and public health professionals in the HIV/AIDS response accepted this rationalization, believing that ART delivery was not a possibility in less developed countries due to limited technological capacity. Hein et al. write:

> [International organizations] active in the fight against HIV/AIDS in developing countries – basically the WHO and the World Bank – concentrated on strategies of prevention, as this was seen as the most cost- effective strategy. This approach took the extremely high price of ART for granted.
>
> (2007, 50)

Furthermore, health interventions in the developing world rarely addressed chronic health issues, as donors preferred short-term technical solutions, such as preventative vaccines, to long-term commitments.

However, for global networks of PWAs, and their allies, the inequality created by the high cost of ART was too obvious and devastating to ignore: some members were able to live healthy lives, while those sitting across from them at meetings were dying. Activists around the world began extensive campaigns against pharmaceutical companies and their political allies, arguing that the prices of ART needed to be reduced, and that the production and trade of generic medications should be allowed in high-prevalence low-income countries. Activists critiqued organizations, like the WHO and the newly formed UNAIDS, for not taking a radical stance on treatment. In order to advance their cause, they worked with and created organizations such as MSF, Oxfam, Consumer Project for Technology, Treatment Action Group, ACT UP, Health Global Access Project, Health Action International, Treatment Action Campaign, Kenyan Coalition for Access to Essential Medicines, and the Ugandan Coalition, among others (O'Manique 2004). These groups protested at political and business events, and implemented programmes to prove that treatment delivery could be effectively implemented in resource-poor contexts.

CSO activism and advocacy campaigns created a demand for treatment in resource-poor countries. Former UNAIDS Executive Director Piot remembers, "The donor's strategy of demand containment was slowly disintegrating" as activists staged die-ins in front of government and pharmaceutical representatives, and developing countries took the pharmaceutical companies to court (Piot & Marshall 2012, 316–317). India began manufacturing generic drugs, which activists smuggled into highly affected countries, such as South Africa.

In response to these campaigns, at the 2001 Doha Round of the WTO negotiations, it was agreed that intellectual property agreements should not prevent countries from protecting public health – enabling low- and middle-income countries to manufacture and import generic HIV/AIDS medications for public programmes. Despite success in reducing prices and increasing access to generics, it remained clear to CSOs that mid and high HIV/AIDS prevalence contexts, most of which were in low-income countries, would still not be able to afford public ART provision without donor support. CSOs began to mobilize not only for reduced prices and access to generics, but also for greater funding.

While demand for universal access to ART created contentions regarding intellectual property laws, and challenged previous global health norms around providing medications for complex chronic illnesses, it also complemented biomedical neoliberal approaches. Treatment presented a quantifiable and technical "solution" to the HIV/AIDS epidemic: "The Lazarus effect of ART, which brought life back to the dying, made spectacular and poignant human stories, and also could be relatively easily measured and quantified" (Piot & Marshall 2012, 317). ART appealed to donors, CSOs and recipient states, as it not only curbed death and suffering, but also applied market and medical approaches to address the epidemic. The effects of ART could be easily measured, and the stories of survival made for good press to galvanize fundraising. As recipient states became increasingly aware of growing death tolls, and donor states feared the global security implications of the epidemic, treatment became conceived of as a solution that could meet a variety of interests. The persistent problem, however, was how to mobilize funding to provide treatment.

UNAIDS was already in existence and was, by some, considered a possible institution through which to coordinate resources. Furthermore, as noted in the previous section, the unique structure of UNAIDS reflected an attempt by donor states to try to overcome the shortcomings of the UN system (Nay 2009, 11). But, as also already noted, UNAIDS did not live up to these ambitions, as the cosponsor format resulted in cautious compromises in the PCB and a lack of implementation capacity for the Secretariat. Dissatisfaction with the UN system prevailed, and donors remained unwilling to commit funding to a UN entity. Even when they offered resources, as DFID did, UNAIDS lacked the administrative capacity to implement projects, being dependent on UNDP and WHO for logistics (Piot & Marshall 2012, 316).

As the limits of UNAIDS' capacity became more apparent, and concern over the increasing epidemic in the developing world grew, various proposals emerged for the establishment of new multilateral funding mechanisms outside the UN system (Piot & Marshall 2012, 319). The USA, EU and Japan said they would only increase funding for HIV/AIDS if the UN was not involved – reflecting continued perceptions of inefficiency within the UN, and recognition of the limited capacity of UNAIDS. The UNAIDS Executive

Director at the time recalls, "The major donor countries and the European Commission agreed on one thing: they were on a warpath against the UN" (Piot & Marshall 2012, 320). CSOs, while still generally supportive of UNAIDS, realized that it was not the funding mechanism they and their constituents needed to access treatment, and so also advocated the formation of a new institution.

Hein et al. (2007) argue that the HIV/AIDS response went through a process of forum shifting, from the WHO, to UNAIDS and then to the Global Fund, changing institutional practices and allowing for new resources and actor coalitions in each case. In advocating an option outside the UN, donors expressed dissatisfaction with the current multilateral system. However, it is also crucial to note that the development of the Global Fund both responded to the limits of UNAIDS, and built on its precedents. As one observer noted, the creation of the Global Fund:

> probably would not have been possible without UNAIDS. The Global Fund was set up seven years after UNAIDS and so benefited from the ground that had been laid by UNAIDS. So each of these things grows of what has been laid before.
>
> (GHI Representative 2013 #3)

UNAIDS was an experiment within the UN system, the limits of which were recognized and used to conceptualize a further innovations in GHG.

At the G8 summit in Okinawa, in 2000, leaders proposed the creation of a partnership for addressing Malaria, TB and HIV/AIDS – the diseases that caused the highest number of combined deaths worldwide, and that were as a result prioritized in MDG 6. In April 2001, African heads of state met in Abuja for a special summit of the Organization of African Unity, which focused on infectious disease. They produced the Abuja Declaration calling for a "Global AIDS Fund capitalized by the donor community to the tune of US $5–10 billion accessible to all affected countries". In response, UN Secretary General Kofi Annan, also at the summit, called for a "war chest to fight AIDS" (Annan 2001). Finally, at a Special Session of the UN General Assembly on HIV/AIDS, in June 2001, member states adopted a Declaration of Commitment, pledging to "support the establishment, on an urgent basis, of a global HIV/AIDS and health fund to finance an urgent and expanded response to the epidemic." In July, the G8 committed US$1.3 billion to the fund, which had yet to be established. This resource mobilization happened relatively quickly, presenting a unique example of rapid international cooperation (Bartsch 2007, 150).

In 2001, a Transitional Working Group was created to develop the structure of the new institution. It included 40 members representing developing countries, donors, CSOs, the private sector and the UN system. Concurrently, the UK AIDS Consortium coordinated regional CSO consultations on issues related to governance, country processes and eligibility criteria. These were

communicated to CSO representatives in the working group, who made the following recommendations:

1 NGO participation must be ensured in Global Fund decision-making activities at all levels.
2 The composition of the Global Fund Board should reflect the following proportions and statuses:

   a NGO participants should have full voting status (not less than 30 per cent);
   b UN/multilateral organization participants should have observer status;
   c Donors and recipient nations should have equal representation;
   d There should be a dedicated position on the Secretariat with responsibility for NGO liaison and outreach.

3 In order to ensure maximum transparency in Global Fund activities, all proposals, interim and final reports as well as other supporting/review documentation and working documents of the Global Fund Board, Secretariat and Partnership Forum should be available publicly and for comment in a timely way.
4 In circumstances where NGOs or vulnerable groups are not recognized by national governments, mechanisms must be in place to allow them to have access to the Global Fund.
5 The key roles of the Country Coordinating Mechanisms (CCMs) should be to bring together all key stakeholders, including NGOs, civil society and representatives of people living with and affected by the three diseases covered by the Global Fund, set country priorities and monitor programmes supported by the Global Fund (GFATM 2001).

These recommendations were supported by the soon-to-be Executive Director, Richard Feachmen, and other key insiders, who had a history of working with CSOs, and recognized the powerful advocacy role they filled in creating demand for funding (Piot & Marshall 2012). They were incorporated into the new institution's governance structure, enshrining an unprecedented degree of CSO participation and promoting accountability between the institution and CSOs.

CSOs, mobilized by the promise of resources for treatment and space in Global Fund governance, used their networks to fundraise for the new initiative. They pressured governments at the Abuja meeting to commit to increasing global spending for the three diseases (GFATM 2007, 10). Piot remembers that during fundraising efforts, "Pressure from outside, by AIDS activists was intense" (Piot & Marshall 2012, 321). By applying pressure on both donor states (to give generously) and recipient states (to create demand), CSOs played a key role in mobilizing resources for the first round of Global Fund grants:

The internationally recognized role that civil society played in launching Round 1 and in participating in the conceptualization and design of the Global Fund led to a sense of ownership; the Global Fund was an initiative that they had helped to create, fund and govern.

(GFATM 2007, 10)

Similarly, key informants state, for example, "the Global Fund originated from demand coming from civil society" (GHI Representative 2013 #21). This history of ownership has continued to shape CSO participation and influence in the Fund.

The formation of the Global Fund reflects a desire by donors to do aid differently. At the G8 Genoa summit, in 2001, heads of state affirmed:

[The fund] will operate according to principles of proven scientific and medical effectiveness, rapid resource transfer, low transaction costs, and light governance with a strong focus on outcomes. We hope that the existence of the Fund will promote improved coordination among donors and provide further incentives for private sector research and development.

The aim was to overcome the politicization of aid delivery in favour of technical approaches, increasing the role of private actors and emphasis on results.

Williams and Rushton note that:

In many senses, the establishment of the Global Fund was an attempt to redress the political shortcomings of multilateral UN efforts. ... In summary, the Global Fund was an attempt to create a depoliticized and more accountable mode of global health governance.

(2011, 54)

They question this ambition, noting that:

the multisectoral and technically oriented design of the Global Fund is in fact based, in large part, on political drivers ... in other words, despite the insistence that the Global Fund is a non-political organization, the reasoning which underwrote its creation as its operating procedures reflects inherently political normative concerns.

(Williams & Rushton 2011, 58)

The Global Fund's private-partnership model and focus on results-based management reflected prioritization of technical, medical interventions – reiterating biomedical neoliberal approaches to global health – and so was only innovative within these confines.

While CSOs understood that the Fund was not created to respond to human rights demands, they saw it as a potential site to advance their fight for the rights of PWAs and affected communities in three ways. First, it

reflected a remarkable ambition to mobilize resources for health, which CSOs hoped could be channelled to meet rights goals. As one observer noted, "It was huge amounts of money for the Global Fund, as an antithesis, to the standard bilateral donors, was something we had never seen" (GHI Representative 2013 #32). Second, because it embraced a public–private multistakeholder model, the Fund was open to the participation of non-state actors, creating unprecedented space for CSO involvement. Third, because the new entity was "to be different than anything before" it was flexible, open to continued innovation. One early CSO activist recalled, "And with the Global Fund you know, we could develop a model from scratch, whereas when other models were being developed, you can only move incrementally. With the Global Fund it was developed from scratch, nothing ever existed before" (GHI Representative 2013 #27). Starting from scratch provided the chance for CSOs to advocate a dynamic institution that, even if it did not specifically aim to focus on human rights, could be more responsive to CSO influence.

Position in GHG

In addition to its inclusion of civil society, the Global Fund governance structure presents a number of unique features. It is a performance-based fund, which means grant disbursements are reduced, suspended or cancelled in cases of poor grant performance. Over the course of the grant, Principal Recipients (PRs) are responsible for regularly reporting to the Global Fund on results, expenditures and changes. As the fund is not an implementing organization, aiming instead to strengthen country capacity to respond, funding proposals and disbursement processes are managed by CCMs, consisting of representatives of government, civil society and the private sector. Proposals are judged by the Technical Review Panel (TRP), which makes recommendations to the board. The Fund "takes an unusually hands-off approach compared to most donors, leaving much of the responsibility for program design and implementation to country representatives and local groups" (Radelet 2004, 3). The CCM model of disbursement, with performance-based oversight from the Secretariat in Geneva, creates a unique model of aid delivery.

This model did not initially fit easily within existing GHG systems and relationships, especially as various actors brought pre-established interests to the Fund:

> The Global Fund assumed a win-win situation for all participating actors in the pursuit of the common goal to fight HIV/AIDS, TB and malaria and thus expected its partners to fully support all Global Fund activities. It did not consider sufficiently, however, that competing interests, different organizational cultures, a lack of mutual trust, or resource constraints could hamper an effective operation.
>
> (Bartsch 2011, 51)

For example, Piot notes it was not always easy to maintain good relations between UNAIDS and the Global Fund (Piot & Marshall 2012, 323). In order to write proposals for the fund, CCMs required the assistance of highly paid experts. This resulted in the WHO and UNAIDS investing resources in Global Fund proposal development without receiving any compensation, creating frustrations. Furthermore, the dependence on external (usually Western) experts to write the highly technical proposals raised questions about how committed to country ownership the Fund was able to be in practice (GFATM 2011a). These questions were exacerbated as tensions became apparent within the Fund's ambitions to be country driven, responsive to civil society, and accountable to donors (GHI Representative 2013 #3). Governments and civil society often disagreed over priorities, especially in relation to addressing human rights, and donors wanted more control over how the funds were used than recipient governments. Meanwhile, the fact that the USA formed PEPFAR so soon after the Global Fund demonstrated American dissatisfaction with the Fund's inclusion of civil society, and resulted in two large funding bodies in GHG, which often duplicated efforts, and created double reporting and administrative burdens for recipient countries. The five-year evaluation of the Fund, conducted in 2007, found that despite rhetorical commitment to partnerships, the Fund had not worked well with other actors in GHG, often duplicating efforts as opposed to building synergies.

Despite these challenges, due to its vast resources and ongoing, if often frustrated, support from multiple stakeholders, the Global Fund became a major player in GHG. Between 2002 and December 2006, the Global Fund approved six rounds of grants and disbursed US$3.2 billion (CGD 2012). It became one of the highest profile international aid bodies and a prominent forum for decision-making on global health. Bartsch writes, "The GF is not only an important financing mechanism in global health, it is also a major organizational interface, linking different kinds of stakeholder groups in its governing and administrative bodies" (2011, 47). Walker argues the Global Fund became increasingly involved in normative policy-making as it matured, due to the substantial influence it exercised by determining grant requirements and priorities (2011, 72). Similarly, one key informant states:

> What makes the Global Fund an amazing institution is that at the end of the day it is a global funding mechanism that has these amazing policies attached to it. Because it could have so easily become just a sort of conduit for money. But it is money plus.
>
> (CSO Representative 2013 #1)

As the Global Fund became one of the most influential actors in GHG, it shaped both donor and recipient health priorities, shifting attitudes and practices around resource mobilization, monitoring and use, and successfully mobilized other actors – including UNAIDS, WHO and various CSOs – to achieve its aims.

As a result of its growing influence and increasing funding, a certain optimism accompanied the Fund's first 10 rounds of grants. One early board member recalls:

> We were funding round after round with lots of fights and lots of debates, but still it happened. The funding was there in principle. There was more funding at the time than there was demand. ... I mean we were building the ship while sailing, which was fun too.
>
> (CSO Representative 2013 #26)

The fund rapidly scaled up programmes, often at the expense of planning and oversight (GFATM 2011a, 7). Such practices were justified by the emergency rhetoric of AIDS exceptionalism, which prioritized quick delivery over planning.

Then, in January 2011, the Associated Press published an article on several instances of fraud and corruption at the Global Fund. As the article noted, this corruption had been discovered and disclosed several months earlier by the Office of the Inspector General (OIG) and was being dealt with by the Fund. However, the article labelled the level of fraud "astonishing", with "as much as two-thirds of some grants eaten up by corruption" (Heilprin 2011). In fact, the affected funds represented 0.3 per cent of the Global Fund's total disbursements between 2002 and 2010 – an amount many observers, such a Bill Gates (2014), noted was negligible compared to many other international donors.

However, the Global Fund did not handle the bad press proactively. One staff member remembers:

> My personal opinion is that we did a very poor job of responding to that. The arrogance of the organization of the time, through all levels, was that we didn't need to do anything. The article was wrong, and everybody would see through to the truth.
>
> (GHI Representative 2013 #16)

The Fund did not responded until April with its own report, *Results with Integrity*, which reiterated the Fund's "zero-tolerance" approach to corruption.

In the meantime donors, such as Germany and Sweden, suspended aid to the Fund, and others began calling for inquiries and reforms. Civil society advocates and the Secretariat felt that donors were using the corruption accusations as an excuse to reduce funding during the economic recession (CSO Representative 2013 #1; GHI Representative 2013 #17). The corruption charges, backlash against AIDS exceptionalism, and financial crisis converged to create "the perfect storm for the Global Fund" (CSO Representative 2013 #26), which culminated in the cancellation of Round 11, due to lack of resources and because of donor demands for restructuring.

The Global Fund formed a High Level Panel to assess practices in financial oversight and implementation. The panel examined grants in 40 countries in different risk categories, drawing conclusions and making recommendations, including improving financial and board oversight, simplifying grant application processes, and putting in place a robust risk management framework. The Global Fund subsequently underwent a series of reforms. In January 2012, the board appointed Gabriel Jaramillo as General Manager to lead the Fund's restructuring for a year. Immediately thereafter, the Executive Director, Michel Kazatchkine, resigned in response to the board's decision to transfer many of his responsibilities to Jaramillo. In his resignation Kazatchkine (2012) noted:

> Today, the Global Fund stands at a crossroad. In the international political economy, power-balances are shifting and new alignments of countries and decision-making institutions are emerging or will have to be developed to achieve global goals. Within the area of global health, the emergency approaches of the past decade are giving way to concerns about how to ensure long-term sustainability, while at the same time, efficiency is becoming a dominant measure of success.

As Kazatchkine notes, changes within the Fund reflected broader shifts in GHG, beyond the mere corruption accusations. The paradigm of global health aid delivery was shifting from the emergency response characterized by rapid scale-up and a prioritization of delivery over processes, to more systematic processes focused on sustainability. In this shifting context, the efficiency and purpose of the Fund's model was called into question – generating discussions about how decisions were made, what the Fund's legitimacy rested on, and how accountable it was to both donors and recipients.

From the civil society perspective, the crisis and resultant changes created multiple concerns. Grant recipients and CSOs in implementing countries had dealt with the strict reporting procedures and accountability measures from the Fund for a decade. To have been constantly called to account and then hear there was poor management at the top made both implementing states and CSOs feel mistreated (CSO Representative 2013 #10). The cancellation of the round caused panic and damaged trust:

> When we found out the work we were doing was threatened because Round 11 was cancelled, it's alarm, alarm, alarm, what are we going to do? … And it was at the same time, where the OIG was criticizing everyone. Realistically so, but from our perspective, we felt that as much as the Global Fund now has an OIG who can name and shame everyone, it is a bit unfair of the Global Fund to do that. … And while we appreciate the Global Fund's stance, we were very angry, because we said, you know from the beginning, you should have put controls in place.
>
> (CSO Representative 2013 #8)

The conditions some donors began to demand before releasing further funding, also made CSOs feel that the principles of equality that had shaped their relationships with other governance actors previously were at risk – they were denied funding to scale up their work and told they could only access future funds on the basis of donor approval (CSO Representative 2013 #20). Furthermore, the acting Executive Director, Jaramillo, was not seen as particularly open to CSO involvement, and one of his reforms included disbanding the Civil Society Team in the Secretariat. The cancellation of the round, exposure of corruption in the Fund, restructuring and donor country reactions created tensions between the board, Secretariat and CSOs.

In 2013, Mark Dyble, former Global AIDS Coordinator at PEPFAR, was appointed the new Executive Director of the Global Fund, and a New Funding Model was announced. These changes, along with the reforms, eased donor concerns (which also relaxed with the relative recovery from the economic crisis) and renewed the hope of other partners, including CSOs. In December 2013, US$12 billion was pledged to the Global Fund, which began accepting applications under the New Funding Model.

Interviewees reflect a sense that the Fund has gone through some necessary growing pains, but has emerged stronger:

> So I think on the whole it was a rough time for the fund but I think in some cases there were self-inflicted wounds by the fund along the way. But I do think now we have come out the other side and I think Mark Dyble as the new Executive Director, will help drive some of these reforms in a positive way.
>
> (CSO Representative 2013 #26)

And:

> Now that the Global Fund has reformed, we have been very happy, we strongly lobbied for more aid effective approach. ... I think there is still an expectation that things will get better, things are getting better, last year was a bad year. But I think we will see where we move with the fallout.
>
> (State Representative 2013 #39)

Relationships between the many stakeholders within the fund appeared to be on the mend as the New Funding Model was rolled out.

As a result, the Global Fund has largely regained its prominent place in GHG. It remains the preferred method for multilateral aid disbursements for health, the focus of CSO campaigns for greater resources, and an influential policy driver. By mid-August 2012 the Global Fund had disbursed US$17.1 billion, through 1,050 grants in 150 countries. This resulted in:

- 4.2 million people receiving ART
- 9.7 million people receiving effective TB treatment

- 310 million insecticide-treated bed nets being distributed to protect families from malaria
- 250 million people being reached with HIV counselling and testing
- 4.2 billion condoms being distributed
- 1.7 million women receiving treatment for prevention of mother-to-child transmission of HIV
- 30 million services being provided to most-at-risk populations. (GFATM 2012b)

While actual attribution of what funding, by which organization, has achieved these goals, is debatable (as Global Fund grants are distributed alongside domestic resources and other funding mechanism) it is clear that the Global Fund has made a substantial contribution to scaling up the HIV/AIDS response. Walker writes, "The Global Fund has become a leader in terms of its institutional size, the magnitude of the resources it has mobilized and distributed and its authority at global and country levels" (2011, 32). The Global Fund continues to not only influence the GHG landscape, but also shape national and local responses to the three diseases. However, the recent crisis raises pertinent questions about the Fund's relationship with civil society partners, decision-making structure, legitimacy and accountability.

Influence in decision-making

The Global Fund is celebrated for its innovative structure that includes civil society in all aspects of decision-making. Its mission states:

> Under the Global Fund business model, the work is carried out by all stakeholders working together, including government, civil society, communities living with the disease, technical partners, the private sector, faith-based organizations, academics, and other multilateral and bilateral agencies. All those involved in the fight should be involved in the decision-making process.
>
> (GFATM 2013)

Interviewees agree that the Global Fund's participatory structure is remarkably inclusive stating, for example, "We call it 'The Model', the best example of how civil society can be engaged in governance at all levels" (CSO Representative 2013 #26). But what influence do CSOs actually have at the global level? And how is CSO influence shaped by governance structures, how is it applied, and to what effect? Are CSO board members and Secretariat partners able to advance the human rights agendas within Global Fund governance?

Influence within the board

At the global level, the Global Fund's governance board includes 20 voting members (donor countries with eight votes, implementing countries with

seven votes, the private sector with one vote, private foundations with one vote and civil society with three votes), and 10 non-voting members (the Chair and Vice Chair, UNAIDS, WHO, the World Bank, Stop TB Partnership, Roll Back Malaria, UNITAIDS, the Executive Director and a Swiss resident). Board members serve as representatives of their constituencies, as opposed to as individuals, or organizational or country representatives. For implementing states, constituencies are based on WHO regions; for civil society they are divided into Developing Country NGOs, Developed Country NGOs and Affected Communities; donor constituencies reflect geographic regions (such as the Scandinavian countries) or common approaches (for example Canada and Switzerland share a seat). The board is responsible for "strategy development; governance oversight; commitment of financial resources; assessment of organizational performance; risk management; [and] partner engagement, resource mobilization, and advocacy" (GFAN 2013). It meets at least twice a year, and attempts to make all decisions by consensus. When disagreements arise decisions are taken by a two-thirds majority of those present.

Each board member (apart from the Chair and Vice-Chair) is permitted to come to the board meetings with a delegation of up to 10 people, including the alternate board member, and a communications focal point, which is responsible for coordinating information sharing with the delegation and constituency. Each delegation determines how the board member, alternate, communications focal point, and members of the core delegation are selected.

The Affected Communities Delegation was originally a non-voting member, choosing to distance itself from decision-making as it felt there might be a conflict of interest if CSOs on the delegation were to benefit from Global Fund grants. However, once it became clear that the board remained at arm's length from grant decisions (because grants are essentially decided by the TRP and only approved in batches by the board), and that the vast majority of funding went to states, the Affected Communities Delegation requested to be a voting member, and has been able to vote since 2004. The ability of the Affected Communities Delegation to switch from non-voting to voting membership demonstrates not only the power of CSOs to participate in governance processes, but also their ability to shape the terms of participation.

The Affected Communities Delegation has a particular type of influence because of its status as representing those communities most affected – the main beneficiaries of the fund. This provides the delegation with a degree of expert status based on their lived experience with one of the three diseases. As one observer notes, "I think the presence of communities on the board, are actually very active, very strong, they can actually push for an issue, create a block, very easily. To the point that if you want to pass a decision you have to consult with communities" (GHI Representative 2013 #19). Another participant states, "You see the other board members and the Secretariat always look to that [Communities] delegation to see whether they approve it" (CSO Representative 2014 #34). The status of the Communities Delegations as

representatives of those most affected provides them with influence as experts for other actors to consult in decision-making.

The Developed Country NGO Delegation enjoys influence due to its access to resources and networks. Most delegates work for relatively well-funded CSOs, and participation in the Global Fund is part of their jobs. Therefore, coordinating between meetings, communicating with other actors, and lobbying the Secretariat and other board members are supported by their organizations. Delegates are well resourced and coordinated, and able to prepare extensively before board meetings. As a result of this advantage, the Developed Country NGO Delegation has substantial influence on the board. One observer noted, "I would say that it is mostly the northern NGOs that are far more dominating than the Southern NGOs, and that is a matter of capacity" (GHI Representative 2013 #24). The ability of the Developed Country NGO Delegation to dedicate time and resources to board processes allows it significant influence.

The Developed Country NGO Delegations add to this influence by building relationships with key donor states. One Global Fund staff member notes:

> there are particular donors which have the ear of the Developed Country NGOs, and so when something comes up that the Developed Country NGOs complain about, it is remarkable how quickly those particular donors come in and find out about it as well.
>
> (GHI Representative 2013 #16)

The informant goes on to note that this alliance has advantages: "I think that from a governance perspective that is not unhelpful. I think it helps the donor keep things real as well." For example, the Developed Country NGOs have collaborated with the Scandinavian block of donors to promote greater attention to LGBT rights, and with the UK to assert support for harm reduction for PWID in Eastern Europe (CSO Representative 2013 #1). The alliance between some donor states and the Developing Country NGOs converges financial and constituency interests.

It also consolidates power amongst northern-based delegations. This causes some observers to note, "The Global Fund becomes driven by [northern] NGOs and the Donors. And that is the problem" (GHI Representative 2013 #3). The aspired-for equality in decision-making between actor types and regions is subverted by the dominant influence of northern delegations. The influence of the Developed Country NGO Delegation, when combined with particular donors, consolidates power among those coming from northern contexts, raising questions about whether decision-making within the fund is as equally balanced as espoused. As in other multilateral arrangements, the well resourced have greater influence than those meant to benefit from funding (Williams & Rushton 2011, 72).

This dynamic is exacerbated by the relatively weaker role of governance actors from the implementing states. The Developing Country NGO

Delegation's influence at the board meetings is difficult to summarize as it represents a coalition of malaria-, HIV/AIDS- and TB-focused CSOs from Latin America, Africa, Eastern Europe and Central Asia and South Asia. This extremely diverse grouping creates a number of difficulties in developing a unified voice and position. Certain actors within the Developing Country NGO Delegation have greater influence than others. Delegates from Eastern Europe and Central Asia (EECA) note that they struggle to represent the interests of CSOs because of the overt focus on Africa, as the region with the highest prevalence of the three diseases (Developing Country NGO Delegation 2008). The diverse make-up of the Developing Country NGO Delegation limits its ability to have influence because of lack of consensus and competing interests within it.

When the three civil society delegations (Developing Country NGOs, Developed Country NGOs and Affected Communities) work together on the board, which they often do, they have substantial influence in that they only need one additional delegation to join their coalition in order to block a vote, and if they mobilize four allies they have a majority. Such influence is celebrated by CSOs as evidence that the Fund's structure is as inclusive of civil society voices as of other stakeholders:

> The Global Fund is a model on how civil society delegations can have equal say on a board discussion. And I think the influence is significant. The northern NGO Delegation influence is as significant as the US [government], which puts in all that money. And there isn't another institution where civil society has so much influence.
>
> (CSO Representative 2013 #1)

Governance participants argue this influence translates into decision-making power that rivals that of state board members.

An example of how the civil society delegations are able to influence not only decision-making in the Global Fund board room, but also decision-making processes and the broader HIV/AIDS response, comes from a November 2007 board meeting in China. In the lead-up to the board meeting the Communities Delegation became aware that in order to travel to China individuals had to declare their HIV status on their landing cards and could be denied entry based on a positive status (CSO Representative 2014 #34). Not only could this prevent some of the delegates from attending the meeting, it violated the principles of non-discrimination that the delegation, as representatives of the broader PWA community, honoured. Travel restrictions had been a human rights concern for PWA since the 1990 IAS Conference (discussed in Chapter 3). Following that conference, the IAS pledged not to hold a conference in any country with travel restrictions, and global networks of HIV/AIDS CSOs began campaigns against travel restrictions arguing that they were not only discriminatory and put PWAs at risk of harassment, but were also ineffective in controlling the epidemic (UNAIDS 2009).

The Affected Communities Delegation, many of whom were HIV positive, communicated their concerns about holding a Global Fund board meeting in a country with travel restrictions with the board leadership and Secretariat. About three months before the meeting, as the board and Secretariat had not acted on the delegation's concerns, the Affected Communities Delegation decided to boycott the meeting in protest against the Chinese policy on travel restrictions and the Global Fund's lack of action (CSO Representative 2014 #34). The delegation informed the Global Fund leadership of their reasons for not attending, but got little response – likely because the board could still function without the Affected Communities Delegation (despite some minor political fall-out). Then the Communities Delegation reached out to other delegations asking them, in solidarity, to also not attend. They got four other delegations to agree to boycott the meeting, which meant that the board would not have a quorum. This got the attention of the Global Fund Chair and Secretariat, who asked the delegation what it proposed.

The delegation put forward the following demands: 1) there be a clear timeline as to when the Chinese travel restrictions would be lifted prior to the board meeting; 2) the board and Global Fund leadership make a high powered statement against the travel restrictions; 3) a meeting be held between the board leadership, Global Fund leadership and government representatives in China; 4) the establishment of an international task team to address the issue of travel restrictions; 5) the Global Fund establish a policy to never again hold a board meeting in a country with travel restrictions against PWAs (Rivers 2007). Because the Communities Delegation had built a coalition that had the power to stop the meeting, causing a crisis in Global Fund governance, and embarrassment for the Chinese government, it was successful in securing all of its demands.

This demonstrates a number of dynamics about the influence of the Affected Communities Delegation particularly, and the civil society delegations in general. First, civil society was able to build a coalition to assert influence to address a human rights issue. It prevailed over institutional influence (of the Global Fund) and state influence (of the Government of China). Second, this coalition was able to affect decision-making and change institutional policies – effectively ensuring that the issue of travel restrictions would not arise again. Third, the demands made by the Communities Delegation had impacts beyond the Global Fund board. The High Level Task Team, which was formed in response to the Communities Delegation's demands, successfully lobbied for the removal of travel restrictions in key countries, including China and the USA. While these changes were likely due to a number of different political factors, such as the change in administration in the USA, the task team took a lead roll in the process, particularly advocating against travel restrictions prior to the 2008 UN High Level Meeting on HIV/AIDS. The civil society delegations not only influenced board decision-making outcomes and processes, but also the global HIV/AIDS response in order to advance the rights of PWAs.

Influence with the Secretariat

The influence of CSOs on decision-making in the Global Fund Secretariat is difficult to summarize because of varying processes across divisions, and the numerous changes that have occurred in the Secretariat over the last few years. However, both Secretariat staff and CSO representatives refer to a "continuous flow of information" between the institution and external CSOs (GHI Representative 2013 #21; CSO Representative 2013 #1). Sometimes this is through board delegates, but CSOs also contact staff directly by email and phone. Secretariat offices that work closely with civil society, for example the Community Rights and Gender (CRG) Department hold monthly telephone conferences with partners (mostly regional networks representing key populations). The invitation to join the calls is open and is distributed to a list of over 100 organizations and about 60 CSOs participate each month (GHI Representative 2013 #19; GHI Representative 2013 #21). A survey conducted in 2014 indicated that CSOs found the calls useful, with 95 per cent of respondents requesting that the calls continue. The CRG and other relevant departments also hold quarterly meetings with CSOs, and meet with both the Global Fund Advocates Network and World AIDS Campaign when needed or requested. Through these communications channels, CSOs are able to exert discursive influence within the Secretariat by providing information based on their experiences, and offering feedback on proposed policies and processes.

For example, CSOs have advocated the greater involvement of key populations on the CCMs. This campaign was partly initiated through CSO lead research. Aids Accountability, based in South Africa, held workshops with CSOs and conducted primary research on access to CCMs, finding that youth and LGBT populations are not adequately represented or consulted (Oberth et al. 2012). Concurrently, CSOs participants used Secretariat trainings on CCM procedures to lobby staff about the need for improved access of key populations to the CCMs (GHI Representative 2013 #21). In response to these demands, the Global Fund launched a pilot project in 10 countries to provide additional funding to CCMs that include key populations. A review of the pilot found it to have improved the engagement of key populations in CCMs, and recommended the approach be integrated into broader Global Fund key population strategies (ICASO 2015). This informed the development of the Community Rights and Gender Technical Assistance Program, which provides support for CSOs to engage in CCMs and related processes. In this case, CSO advocates at the global level were able to increase access to decision-making for key populations at the country level by sharing knowledge, and promoting further discussions on a rights-based response within the Secretariat.

Competing legitimacies

The involvement of CSOs in Global Fund governance aims to strengthen the institution's legitimacy by mitigating the democratic deficit multilateral

institutions are accused of through representation of those that the Global Fund claims to serve (health service providers and communities affected by the three disease). In turn, it is assumed this inclusion will result in greater institutional responsiveness and efficiencies. As Williams and Rushton note, "By including state and non-state actors from the South, the Global Fund strives at gaining legitimacy both in terms of input and output legitimacy" (2011, 154).

One of the implicit purposes of having civil society delegations on the Global Fund board is to strengthen input legitimacy (Doyle & Patel 2008, 1929). The structure of the Global Fund's board, with three civil society seats with substantial influence, has led some observers to argue such input legitimacy has been achieved: "in terms of the goal of representation or the objective of representation I think, the Global Fund probably provides the best example for how these principles of representation and inclusion have been adopted into a very large mechanism" (CSO Representative 2013 #26). However, others note the challenges the three delegations, of just 10 people each, face in representing a global and diverse movement: "There is still a lot of tokenism, and absurd tokenism. Having someone who once had malaria sitting in a room, is not representing an adequate health community voice" (GHI Representative 2013 #29). Such comments demonstrate a tension between legitimacy-related justifications for, and claims around, civil society participation, and the ability of civil society delegates to fulfill them. These tensions play out slightly differently for each of the civil society delegations to the board, as they have varying strategies of representation.

The Developing Country NGO Delegation's mission is to "represent the diverse NGO / CBO response from the global south when it comes to AIDS, TB and Malaria on the GFATM Board". It consists of approximately 23 representatives from the four "developing" regions of Latin America–Caribbean (LAC), Eastern Europe–Central Asia (EECA), Africa and Asia. Each region has a "focal point" member whose job it is to communicate with CSOs in that region. It is hard to over-emphasize the magnitude of the task of a delegation of 23 people to represent CSOs that engage in HIV/AIDS, TB and Malaria interventions in over half the world – the following discusses the challenge just one region faces.

Delegates from EECA report difficulties in connecting with CSOs in their region due to: language barriers; the self-incurred costs of communication, printing and consulting with stakeholders; and the time translation, travelling and consultation takes, when all delegates are also working in full-time jobs. In addition, delegates find that when they do consult CSOs they do not get sufficient responses because CSOs are not aware of the work of the Global Fund, and/or do not believe that their voice will be heard. These challenges are specific to the EECA context, where there is lack of public information about HIV/AIDS interventions, and states are largely resistant to civil society involvement in policy-making (Spicer et al. 2011). There is little tradition of CSOs influencing policy, and many CSOs are scared of engaging in advocacy,

or exposing corruption issues that occur during grant implementation, fearing government retribution. Most HIV/AIDS CSOs in EECA work with PWID and are at risk of government harassment. As a result of the challenges of engaging with regional and national CSOs, delegates find it hard to claim representation of CSOs in their region (Developing Country NGO Delegation 2008).

However, its the Developed Country NGO Delegation that faces the greatest legitimacy challenges, though this at first seems contradictory considering its relative advantages in terms of resources and communications networks. The delegation consists of representatives from North America, Western Europe, Australia and Japan. The core delegation of 10, who attend board meetings, engage with a larger contact group of about 60 people, which it keeps informed about and consults with on processes and decision-making (CSO Representative 2014 #34). These individuals are members of other CSO networks, such as the Interagency Coalition on AIDS and Development (ICAD) and GNP+, who in turn share information with their members. The Developed Country NGO Delegation does not struggle with communications challenges as there is a consolidated, relatively small group of NGOs that engaged in resource mobilization for the three diseases, most of which have access to communication services and organizational support. Therefore, being a valid representative of its direct constituents is relatively unproblematic for the Developed Country NGO Delegation.

However, the legitimacy of the Developed Country NGO Delegation is questioned when it claims representation beyond this constituency. Many members of the Developed Country NGO Delegation have been involved in the HIV/AIDS response for decades as pioneers of the rights-based response, and were directly involved in the formation of the Global Fund. Based on this experience they assume a global leadership role, which is reasserted by their substantial influence on the board. They speak of "mentoring" CSOs from other regions, and claim "ownership" of the Fund (CSO Representative 2013 #1). However, this leadership role is not recognized by other board members. As one observer notes, "there has been resentment at times, where for instance certain members of the North [Developed Country] NGO Delegation speak as if they just know what is right, not just for civil society, but for the implementing world" (CSO Representative 2013 #30). Because the Delegates come from relatively well-resourced CSOs, largely based in the global north and connected to donors, their claims of broader leadership are questioned by board members from implementing states and CSOs.

The Developed Country NGO Delegation's role as funding recipients generates further legitimacy concerns related to conflicts of interest. Some Developing Country NGO delegates work for CSOs that receive resources from the Fund to implement grants, from which the CSOs necessarily take an administrative cut. For example, the International HIV/AIDS Alliance has always had a staff member on the Developed Country NGO Delegation, and is also the largest CSO recipient of Global Fund grants. Though there is little evidence

of the Developed Country NGO Delegation using their influence to advance their own positions, legitimacy is based on perceptions as much as (or perhaps more than) evidence (Doyle & Patel 2008). Therefore, perceived conflicts of interests, as both decision-maker and recipient, cause other governance participants to describe members of the Developing Country NGO Delegation as "paid lobbyists, that are there to get what they need from the fund because that is how that person has made their living for 10 years" (GHI Representative 2013 #16). Because being on the board is part of their job in an organization receiving financing from the Fund, some delegates are seen as promoting their own careers, as opposed to the interests of those affected by the three diseases (as does the Communities Delegation) or the interests of those implementing programmes (as does the Developing Country NGO Delegation). One Secretariat staff member notes:

> At least the implementing [Developing] Country NGOs are doing the work. The communities, are the people living with the diseases, and other people are here to serve. But the Developed NGOs are sometimes there because they've all got very good Western salaries. ... they are rights-based people, and they are there to hold the Global Fund accountable to the human rights and all those kinds of things, but there is a tension, where people say what is your skin in the game? What do you bring to the table?
> (GHI Representative 2013 #16)

These questions about both the validity and utility of the Developed Country NGO Delegation's influence, demonstrate that including CSOs in institutional governance can raise new legitimacy questions, particularly where CSOs are filling dual roles as decision-makers and receivers of grants.

The Affected Communities Delegation's purpose is "to ensure the voices and issues of people living with and affected by HIV, TB and malaria influence the deliberations and decisions on investments and programs of the Global Fund to achieve greater and sustained impact for communities." In practice the majority of members of this delegation are people affected by HIV/AIDS (Hein et al. 2007). Neither the TB nor the Malaria response has an organized global network to the same extent as HIV/AIDS. While some observers note that the PWA dominance in the Affected Communities Delegation limits its ability to be representative, these limitations are well understood by most governance actors, and do not seem to detract from its legitimacy (GHI Representative 2013 #21; CSO Representative 2014 #34). There is an unspoken acceptance that "affected communities" refers to PWAs and key populations, with minimal representation from TB and Malaria constituencies.

The Communities Delegation makes concerted efforts to be a valid representative of those affected by HIV/AIDS and the other diseases. Each member of the support delegation (20–40 people) aims to have 10 further contacts they communicate with, who then have another 10 contacts each, increasing the network exponentially by degrees of separation. The feasibility

of creating this web of connections is largely based on personal commitments, abilities and resources (capital, human and social) of the individuals involved (CSO Representative 2014 #34). While this effort to create representation through network building is highly variable and difficult to monitor, it appears to have achieved a sort of web of representation, as opposed to linear structure, which is perhaps more realistic considering the impossible task of establishing relationships with such a diverse and vast constituency base. In addition, the delegation signs memorandums of understanding on partnership agreements with organizations that have their own networks, such as Roll Back Malaria, Stop TB and GNP+. This intentional networking allows the Affected Communities Delegation to contribute a degree of input legitimacy, as it is recognized that it makes a concerted effort to communicate with constituents within recognized limitations.

The Affected Communities Delegation attempts to build further legitimacy through open and transparent processes. Board members for the Communities Delegation are drawn from a core and support delegation. The core delegation consists of 10 CSO representatives who attend board meetings and provide advisory and communications support to the board delegates (main, alternate and communications focal point). Core delegates are recruited from the support delegation of 20–40 members, who participate in governance processes from remote locations. The board and alternate board member serve for 18 months, and the board member can only serve one term. The board member must be a PWA and must come from the global south – the alternative usually comes from a different geographical region. Efforts are made to ensure key populations are represented on the delegation, and that it reflects gender balance (most often the board and alternate board member are of different genders). This process constructs validity based on transparent processes, established regulations and population presence, combining input and output legitimacy.

In the decision-making section above, it is noted that the Communities Delegation has a specific type of influence on the board, based on its role as representing those most affected – with other board members "looking to it" when making decisions. In other words, it has a "normative validity" (Bartsch 2007, 5). The legacy of the GIPWA principle continues to provide moral legitimacy to the Communities Delegation as it reinforces "a generalized perception or assumption that the actions of an entity are desirable, proper, or appropriate within some socially constructed system of norms, values, beliefs, and definitions" (Suchman 1995, 574). Other governance actors view the Communities Delegation as representing those most affected by the three diseases, which strengthens the delegation's and institution's legitimacy.

Though it first appears input based, this legitimacy is largely output orientated as it reflects assumptions that having representation of affected communities promotes effectiveness; that the presence of a PWA on the board will enable the Global Fund to better meet the needs of PWAs. While this assumption is largely untested, it does generate significant legitimacy. Because of the

established GIPWA norm in the HIV/AIDS response – that the representation of those most affected is essential and effective – the Communities Delegation is viewed as legitimate, and as adding legitimacy to the institution, despite its variable ability to actually represent constituents. While there are few direct links between constituents and the delegation, legitimacy is partly generated by the delegation's efforts to create networks of communication and transparent processes of representation, and is then reasserted by normative claims.

Some donor states and Secretariat staff members express concern that the substantial influence the civil society delegations have in decision-making (as described above) negatively impacts the output legitimacy of the institution. They argue the civil society delegations have "too much power" (State Representative 2013 #38), and "They have much more influence than we would hope for" (State Representative 2013 # 39). While not taking issue with the rights-based agenda of the CSO delegations, they argue that the way the delegations exercise influence threatens output legitimacy. For example, one member of the donor block remarked that during a particularly crucial board meeting, in which the new Executive Director was appointed and the New Founding Model proposed, the civil society coalition blocked a vote over a seemingly small detail:

> It was really important, the board said, we need to come out of this meeting with a new Executive Director, with a new funding model, and the message needs to be clear. And then they [the civil society delegations] blocked the vote, after it was discussed. These people were sitting on the committee that looked at every word [of the proposed decision-point], and over something where they thought could be a misinterpretation; they voted the whole thing down ... so they did that because they thought "we can renegotiate that". So of course it worked out, but nobody understood what the fuss was all about. ... If you have a fundamental problem you deal with it beforehand and do not do these games, and that is really bad governance I would say.
>
> (State Representative #38 2013)

The donor's concern was not with the proposed change the civil society coalition pushed through, but how they engaged in the governance process. Similarly, a member of the Global Fund staff noted that the civil society delegations often appear to be "writing decisions in bathroom stalls" and lobbying as activists, as opposed to acting cooperatively in governance processes (GHI Representative 2013 #16).

In contrast, other observers note that, "they [civil society delegations] are probably by far the most organized, even if you compare them to the governments. Even if, in terms of consultation, in terms of issues, they have discussed them and they have a position" (GHI Representative 2013 #21). Similarly, the report of the General Manager notes that, "The civil-society groups on the Board have maintained a much more stable and disciplined

membership over the years" (GFATM 2012b, 27). CSO policies related to rotations of delegates, terms served, and communication strategies tend to be more transparent and credible, than the other delegations. A Global Fund Staff member notes, "I also think that some of that tension [between civil society and other actors] can be good and healthy. It keeps us on our toes" (GHI Representative 2013 #16). From these perspectives, the civil society delegations contribute positively to board governance by being well prepared, presenting a strong position, and challenging the Global Fund to remain responsive.

Because the civil society delegations have substantial influence in the board, and can shape how decisions are made, as well as what decisions are made, they do not have to behave by the rules of bureaucratic multilateral governance – they are not dependent on the approval of other governance actors. Therefore, though civil society delegations often resist bureaucratic processes, this may not necessarily result in inefficiencies – especially for an organization that aims to avoid doing business as usual. The five-year evaluation of the Fund notes that, "Civil society stakeholders continue to remind the Global Fund that it is an evolving institution with a unique model" (MACRO 2009, 10). Quick acting on the part of the delegation (by, for example, drafting new decision-points in bathroom stalls) may make the board more responsive to changing circumstances and new ideas, strengthening its output legitimacy.

Walker argues that "Rather than a source of input-oriented legitimacy which provides some form of global deliberative equality, the Global Fund's board can better be understood as a source of output-oriented legitimacy" (2011, 7). She argues that this is because the balance of power on the board favours donors. While donor influence is dominant, the influence of the civil society delegations is also, as noted in the above section, significant. However, Walker's argument stands up in relation to the civil society delegations as well. The civil society delegations cannot claim to represent the diverse HIV/ AIDS organizations and individuals affected by the three diseases. The Communities Delegation makes the most successful attempt at this, but their legitimacy is derived more from normative output functions, than representative input legitimacy. The Developing Countries Delegation has the impossible task of representing varied movements across half the globe, which it admittedly struggles with. The Developed Country NGO Delegation lacks a valid leadership role, and raises new legitimacy challenges around conflicts of interest.

Despite the limited input legitimacy they bring to the fund, the substantial influence of the civil society delegations enables them to contribute to governance processes in a way that makes some observers feel they threaten output legitimacy with their advocacy tactics, while others feel they strengthen it by forcing responsiveness. The civil society delegations do not need to depend on legitimacy from constituents, or develop it by following pre-established processes. Instead they demand it by asserting their influence in the Fund, building on output related assumptions that CSO participation breeds greater responsiveness, if not representation.

Downward accountability

The Global Fund argues that the inclusion of CSOs in its governance improves its ability to be accountable to those most affected by the three diseases. It states that civil society actors that engage in board and Secretariat processes serve as "an important channel for influencing policy decisions for all civil society stakeholders" (GFATM 2012a, 4). However, considering that, as demonstrated above, civil society board members struggle to represent constituents, suffering from weak input legitimacy, their ability to act as downward accountability conduits is compromised.

There is a sense that the Global Fund "is run by a section of good old friends" or "a small family, a group" (State Representative 2013 #38). While CSOs draw on networks of influence, as described in the previous sections, these tend to be based on established relationships and relatively select connections. Indeed, the five year evaluation of the Fund stated, "The Global Fund's approach during its first five years more accurately reflects a 'friendship model' than a genuine 'partnership model'" (MACRO 2009, 34). While the challenge of reaching out beyond existing contacts to the massive and diverse global movements – and organizations with different aims and processes – is immense, even civil society participants note that more could be done to diversify input: "It worries me at the end of the day. There is still this critique of global advocates doing the rounds, and they are fantastic people, but I just don't know that we have really sussed that communication and consultation thing" (CSO Representative 2013 #30). Lack of networks beyond a select group of CSOs impacts downward accountability as access to the Global Fund is viewed as a closed group.

A further restriction on downward accountability is the type of function board members fill. Civil society board members influence decisions about Global Fund policy and governance, but these are not always, or even most often, the aspects of the Fund that are most crucial to those implementing programmes or affected by the three diseases. For example, Walker argues that the Global Fund has a "double accountability gap" in that it is not accountable to those whose lives it affects (2011, 34). Using the case of Malawi's unsuccessful proposal to the TRP, and challenges with ART provisions, she argues that the Malawians who were impacted by the TRP's negative decisions and delayed grant disbursements, did not have a process of recourse – they cannot hold the Global Fund to account when access to ART is threatened because of Global Fund decisions.

The role of civil society delegates on the board does not fill this gap as they are rarely connected to country health providers and local patient groups. Furthermore, the board approves the TRP's recommendations in batches (not by particular country), and to date has always accepted the TRP's recommendations in full. Civil society delegates do not have influence over the specifics of funding decisions, or what factors are taken into consideration when they are made. CSOs that engage in the Secretariat at the global level

also do not fill this gap, as the majority of them collaborate on global advocacy goals, not operational challenges. In other words, the structures that civil society actors engage in, through the board and Secretariat, do not provide accountability links between those affected by funding decisions and the people that make the decisions at the global level. Williams and Rushton find that "the stakeholder group with perhaps the least opportunity to demand such accountability is those people affected by the three diseases" (2011, 69). The civil society actors who engage with the Global Fund board and Secretariat do not fulfill a role that connects them with those affected by funding decisions.

Arguably, connections could be made by the Secretariat's Fund Portfolio Managers (FPMs) who are, among their many roles, responsible for communicating with local civil society actors and service providers, and for informing the Secretariat of realities on the ground. However, the 2007 review found that at the country level many civil society groups are "unaware of whom it should speak to within the Secretariat to voice concerns or challenges regarding Global Fund processes and, therefore, may not invite an FPM visiting the country to address those concerns" (MACRO 2009, 26). Similarly, many CSOs view the FPMs as inaccessible, and complain that they only communicate with CCM heads and Secretariats, as opposed to CSOs that are not represented on the CCMs (Kageni 2012). Such Secretariat structures do not provide adequate accountability relationships beyond the CCMs.

Partnership forum

In an attempt to promote accountability to those civil society actors beyond the board delegation and key partners of the Fund, the Global Fund holds Partnership Forums every 24 to 36 months. Partnership Forums aim to allow a wide range of stakeholders "to express their views on the Global Fund's policies and strategies" by serving as a "visible platform for debate, advocacy, continued fund raising, and inclusion of new partners" (GFATM 2015b). The core functions of the Partnership Forum are to:

a Review progress based on reports from the board and provide advice to the Global Fund on general policies;
b Provide an important and visible platform for debate, advocacy, continued fundraising and inclusion of new partners;
c Mobilize and sustain high-level coordination, political commitment and momentum to achieve the Global Fund's objectives; and
d Provide a communication channel for those stakeholders who are not formally represented elsewhere in the governance structure.

Though there are decision-making and resource mobilization functions related to the Partnership Forum, its primary purpose is to build communication networks with stakeholders to strengthen downward accountability.

Up until 2015, the Partnership Forum included e-forums, regional consultations and global meetings of 200–500 participants from affected communities, NGOs and FBOs, donors, multilateral development cooperation agencies, technical and research agencies, foundations and the private sector. The largest group of participants was always from civil society (29 per cent of participants at the 2011 forum) (Fremont Center 2011). At the forums CSOs, states and other partners make presentations on a range of topics in order to share experiences and lessons learned. Partnership Forums were held in Bangkok, Thailand, in 2004; in Durban, South Africa, in July 2006; in Dakar, Senegal, in December 2008; and in São Paulo, Brazil, in June 2011. In 2015 three regional partnership forums were conducted (Addis Ababa, Ethiopia; Bangkok, Thailand; Buenos Aires, Argentina), as well as an online consultation process.

The forums result in recommendations that go to the Strategy Investment and Impact Committee, in order to be presented to the board for consideration. This provides a sense of accountability – that decision-makers will hear topics of concern. One participants describes his impressions after participating in the forum:

> I think that it was an amazing, amazing meeting ... where you have a person who uses drugs sitting next to an African minister, sitting next to a donor or whatever. So it was phenomenal conversations, it really went to the heart of the issues of the fund. And at the time you know that the recommendations are going to go somewhere.
>
> (CSO Representative 2013 #26)

The aim is to ensure that civil society groups and other partners have an opportunity to speak directly (via the committee) to the board and Secretariat.

However, the accountability relationship generated by the Partnership Forum is one-dimensional. Participants can access information and share concerns, but the board is not required to be responsive, and participants have no recourse to follow up on suggestions that result from the Partnership Forum. This weakens the ability of the Partnership Forum to hold decision-makers accountable. For example, the 2008 Partnership Forum produced the following recommendation, which led to the development of the Global Fund's Gender Strategy:

> That the Board instruct the Secretariat to ensure that the implementation plan for the gender equality strategy is produced in consultation with women's organizations and other groups working on gender equality, and that it has specific, measurable goals and objectives with indicators to track progress by the fund and countries against defined benchmarks and within defined time frames. This implementation plan should reflect progress at the country level, in particular, linking disbursements with outcomes for girls and women.
>
> (GFATM 2008)

This recommendation was taken to the committee responsible for developing the Gender Strategy. However, as will be discussed in the next chapter, the resulting strategy was not adequately resourced or communicated. Furthermore, it did not include the monitoring structure recommended by the Partnership Forum, and it has had only minimal impact on Global Fund processes (Fleischman 2008).

In this case, the Partnership Forum provided an opportunity for CSOs to promote human rights concerns – particularly related to gender – but had no recourse to follow up on how these recommendations were implemented. In the absence of an internal accountability mechanism for the strategy, CSOs have tried to hold the Global Fund to account by producing external evaluations of the Gender Strategy, which highlight weak implementation. The Partnership Forum, while allowing broader civil society to communicate with the board and Secretariat, does not provide mechanisms to hold decision-makers to account.

The limits on creating downward accountability through the Partnership Forum are highlighted by the evaluation of the 2011 forum (Fremont Center 2011), which included an e-survey, an e-forum, and a main conference in São Paulo, Brazil from 28 to 30 June. Two hundred and eighty-nine people attended the São Paulo meeting, representing 107 countries. As the Partnership Forum occurred during the development of the Global Fund's 2012–2016 strategy, it provided CSOs with the opportunity to influence planning. Consultations were organized around the following themes: 1) maximizing impact; 2) delivering on a human rights approach for the three diseases; 3) using the money wisely; 4) Implementing for increased impact.

The evaluation found that "the consultations did not result in bold, new thinking" (Fremont Center 2011, 18). The Partnership Forum resulted in more of a reassertion of pre-existing ideas, than a challenging of current practice. While lack of critique does not necessarily imply weak accountability – accountability processes can be affirming as well as critical – to some this was a concern:

> participants indicated some value in the Partnership Forum serving as an echo chamber, a sounding board, or a way to gain buy-in to proposed directions and calls to action. But others criticized the facilitation for not pushing dialogue into new territory.
>
> (Fremont Center 2011, 18)

Creating buy-in and mobilizing action is not the same as generating accountability; it could instead be view as a process of co-option.

The lack of new thinking at the forum suggests a gathering of the usual suspects; and therefore the usual debates. At the 2011 forum, two-thirds of participants reported (through a survey) already being engaged in Global Fund processes (Fremont Center 2011). The process of selecting who participates in the Partnership Forum raises further accountability questions as it has not been particularly transparent. In 2011, the Civil Society Team at the

Secretariat reached out to its networks with CSOs asking them to nominate three names for consideration. These were then evaluated based on regional and key population balance to develop a list, which was shared with relevant staff for finalization. Individuals on the final list were sent invitations. Participants and other stakeholders express confusion over how this process is actually carried out, with some arguing the civil society delegations to the board should be consulted, and others arguing their influence would be in a conflict of interest as they might select CSOs that reflect their shared views (Fremont Center 2011). All respondents noted that the selection process should be more transparent. The system of bringing together those already involved in the Fund raises questions about what added value the partnership forum has (if one of its goals is to bring together actors who do not usually engage in the fund) and perhaps explains the lack of "bold new thinking".

Interestingly, the one consultation at the 2011 forum where new ideas were put forward was the Human Rights Break Out Group. In this case, the group was able to demand that the Global Fund honour its commitment to human rights by promoting stronger language in the strategy document. Due to CSO consultations, language was changed in the first draft of the 2011–2016 strategy, prior to the Partnership Forum, from "Stimulate greater programmatic attention and investment to overcome stigma and discrimination" to "Increase investments in programs that address human rights-related barriers to access" (GFATM 2011c; GFATM 2011b; emphasis added). Similarly, wording was strengthen from, "Take steps to ensure the Global Fund is not supporting programs that violate human rights" to "Ensure that the Global Fund does not support programs that infringe human rights" (GFATM 2011c; GFATM 2011b; emphasis added). These much more direct commitments to human rights are attributed to the input of CSOs during the Partnership Forum (GHI Representative 2013 #16).

However, while the forum provided an opportunity for CSOs to hold the Global Fund to account on rights commitments, the way decision-makers interpret and implement this language remains at their own discretion. While the Partnership Forum provides an opportunity for civil society actors to come together to build connections, support the Global Fund, and provide input into policies and strategies, it does not fulfill its accountability mandate because the relationship between participants and decision-makers is one directional.

As a result both CSOs and Global Fund representatives question the purpose and utility of the Partnership Forum. One observer notes:

> I think you always have to question the cost effectiveness of a meeting of 500 people and you know I haven't a clue how to evaluate value for money, cost effectiveness of something like that. And I think that is going to be a really difficult decision for the Fund in the future ... I mean from a governance point of view, I think it was an interesting sort of experience and sort of experiment. But the extent to which it is sustainable as a

model and the extent to which it is cost effective as a model I really don't know.

(CSO Representative 2013 #30)

Due to the weak accountability outcomes of the Partnership Forum it is not surprising that both external CSOs, and Global Fund staff and board members have questioned its utility, especially in light of the substantial costs (the Fund spent more than $1.5 million on the 2011 Partnership Forum) (Fremont Center 2011).

In a letter in August 2013 board leadership stated it was discussing "an evolving Partnership Forum model" that took into consideration recommendations and critiques from past forums. What emerged was a new model that included three regional forums and an online consultation. While an assessment of this new process is yet to be published, so it is not possible to determine whether it has resulted in an improved accountability processes, two outcomes are apparent. First, reports from the three regional forums and online consultation demonstrate that the majority of participants continue to be CSOs, and they continue to advocate more human rights-based responses (GFATM 2015b). CSOs particularly stressed the need for improved accountability mechanisms to improve rights-based monitoring – for example developing key performance indicators to measure equitable gender outcomes for women and girls. Second, the Global Fund remains adaptive and willing to change accountability practices based on CSO and others' concerns. This demonstrates potential to enhance CSO ability to act as conduits for downward accountability.

CSOs as watchdogs

Strong downward accountability relationships require accessible information, something CSOs that work with the Global Fund continually advocate. The 2007 evaluation of the Fund found that:

> Civil society stakeholders continue to report the difficulty they have in accessing up-to-date and easily-digestible information on the Global Fund and its processes, in particular feedback from Global Fund Board meetings on key decisions taken, information on the functioning of CCMs and the roles and responsibilities of its members and information on how to become involved in the different levels of the Global Fund architecture.
>
> (MACRO 2009, 46)

Global Fund documents are famously long and complex. For example, prior to one board meeting over 900 pages of documentation and PowerPoint presentations were distributed to board members (MACRO 2009, 51). Furthermore, because the Fund prides itself on its dynamism, it can change

policies and procedures rapidly, causing CSOs to feel like they are constantly playing a game of catch-up. Research in Latin America found that, for example, many women's groups felt unable to engage with Global Fund processes because of the high level of education required to understand rapidly changing policies (CSO Representative 2013 #13; ICW Global 2012). CSOs continue to complain of the difficulty in accessing up-to-date and easily digestible information on Global Fund procedures, particularly on how civil society is represented in the Global Fund – knowledge essential to building downward accountability relationships (GFATM 2012a, 5).

Noting these challenges, some CSOs (such as the International HIV/AIDS Alliance, the Open Society Institute, Aids Accountability and ICASO) have taken on the role of synthesizing and distributing Global Fund information in more accessible formats by publishing bulletins and updates. In Latin America, a group of CSOs established El Observatorio Latino, which reports on Global Fund disbursements in the region, aiming to increase the accountability of recipients of Global Fund grants, identify technical support for CSOs, and promote more involvement of CSOs in Global Fund processes (GFATM 2012a, 17). By producing and sharing information, CSO coalitions make it possible for other organizations to communicate with the Global Fund from an informed position. This in turn forces the Global Fund to be more responsive to affected communities. The evaluation notes, "This watchdog role has in many places forced the Global Fund to adapt its policies and countries to re-evaluate their targets to ensure the needs of people living with and affected by the three diseases are sufficiently met" (MACRO 2009). By sharing information in accessible formats, CSOs create opportunities for accountability relationships between the fund and those it aims to serve.

One of the most active accountability-focused CSOs is Aidspan, which was set up soon after the creation of the Global Fund to:

> reinforce the effectiveness of the Fund through its watchdog role and to act as an independent source of information for stakeholders both involved and not involved in Global Fund processes, including people and organizations in all sectors within developing countries who are applying for and implementing Global Fund grants, stakeholders who wish the organization to be more successful and members of the Global Fund Board delegations.
>
> (Aidspan 2013)

Aidspan offers two particular services. First, it publishes a Guide to the Global Fund, which simplifies processes so that they are easily understandable. Not only does this increase the ability of CSOs to hold the Global Fund to account, it also has the spin-off effect of challenging the Global Fund Secretariat to make its information more clear (Civil Society Representative 2013 #15). Second, Aidspan publishes the Global Fund Observer (GFO), a monthly e-newsletter that reports on happenings at the Global Fund Secretariat, in

CCMs and at the board. It is distributed to over 10,000 subscribers, in over 170 countries, and published on the Aidspan website. The GFO includes factual articles, as well as some commentary. Participants note that even the factual reports serve a watchdog function: "To some extent, just by reporting the facts we are facilitating the accountability process, even if it is not us wagging our fingers. Other people can wag their fingers based on what we are reporting" (CSO Representative 2013 #5). By making Global Fund information accessible Aidspan enables other CSOs to engage in accountability relationships.

Civil society representatives on the board, and who engage with the Secretariat, do not have the relationships with constituents, or role in governance, to provide those affected by Global Fund decisions with recourse; they can question lack of adherence to policy and procedure, and reiterated rights claims, but have little influence over how decisions are implemented. Despite their substantial influence in decision-making, they do not fulfill ambitions to make the Global Fund accountable to constituents. The Partnership Forum, which explicitly aims to link the Global Fund with the broader response to the three diseases, also has not resulted in a reciprocal accountability process that allows CSOs to hold the Fund to account on human rights, or other, commitments. Many of the CSOs that participate in these processes, and others, are a select group of friends – the result is a network of horizontal accountability, as opposed to downward. Aidspan, and other information sharing focused CSOs, however do strengthen downward accountability by disseminating information in accessible formats, which provides opportunities for others to act as watchdogs.

Resource governance

When asked how civil society partners contribute to the Global Fund, one staff member stated, "One, to help us with governance, two to hold us accountable, and three advocacy for resource mobilization" (GHI Representative 2013 #19). As outlined above, CSOs played a key role in arguing for the initial resources for the creation of the fund, and they have since continued to advocate a continued increase in those resources. CSOs play a crucial role during replenishment campaigns. CSOs in donor countries lobby their governments to make sizeable commitments through direct advocacy and fundraising events. Prior to the 2013 funding round, CSOs based in Europe collaborated with the Global Fund to coordinate a replenishment meeting at the European Commission in Brussels. CSO representatives from all over the world attended the event, using it as an opportunity to voice their particular needs for funding from their regions. The replenishment meeting was then followed with a demonstration in front of the European institutions, calling for full funding for the Global Fund. Similar activities occurred in the USA and UK, at international HIV/AIDS conferences, and at other major events.

The Global Fund Advocates Network (GFAN) was specifically formed, in 2008, by a coalition of CSOs to support such events and lobby for continued and increased resources for the Global Fund. The network, based in the

Netherlands, supports fundraising and advocacy, aiming to build a social movement in support of the Fund. In 2013, it held a Global Resource Mobilization Meeting to brief civil society groups about the changes in the fund and to develop joint fundraising strategies. About 70 CSO representatives attended, as well as representatives from the Global Fund board and Secretariat, including the Executive Director. The delegates contributed suggestions to inform the Global Fund's fundraising strategies. In particular, CSO participants took issue with the Global Fund's plan to propose three funding scenarios to donors, pointing out that in such cases donors generally chose the lowest option (GFAN 2013, 15). Instead, CSO representatives suggested a single ask be put forth, and suggested the figure of US$15 billion, which was adopted by the Global Fund. This was followed up with a call for action petition, which was signed by 2000 individuals asking donor and implementing countries to: recommit to the goals of increased strategic investments and scaling-up of treatment, prevention, care and support programmes for people living with and affected by HIV/AIDS, tuberculosis and malaria; fully fund the Global Fund by collectively committing at least US$15 billion in new contributions for 2014–16; recommit to increased domestic investment targets for health. The call to action petition was distributed prior to the major replenishment meeting in the USA in 2013 (GFAN 2013). CSOs not only influenced resource mobilization by advocating greater donor resources, but also provided input into Global Fund resource mobilization strategies.

CSO representatives in recipient countries contribute to replenishment efforts by participating in events, and increasing awareness of the needs for greater resources in their regions. The Africa Regional Civil Society Platform on Health and Universal Access campaigned for the Global Fund replenishment by promoting greater domestic commitments to health, which they argue demonstrates the willingness of recipient countries to partner with the Global Fund towards achieving universal access (ARCSP 2013). The Platform also coordinated advocacy efforts at the BRICS summit held in South Africa in 2013.

Other organizations, such as the AIDS and Rights Alliance of Southern Africa (ARASA), set up meetings with various stakeholders from both implementing and donor states. They lobbied the four African countries that agreed to contribute to the fund to do so. ARASA also held a major campaign in Kenya, aimed at exposing gaps in the current health budget and the need for additional resources, holding street demonstrations and making presentations to parliament (Civil Society Representative 2013 #20). Such activities expose the need for greater resources in low-income countries, promote domestic investments in health, and agitate for the involvement of middle-income countries in resource mobilization.

Members from implementing country CSOs also participated in the Here I Am Campaign, writing and producing video blogs about living with HIV/AIDS, TB and Malaria. These were distributed widely via social media and the online news site the *Huffington Post*. The title of the campaign, "Here I Am",

confronted perceptions in donor countries that the HIV/AIDS epidemic was somehow less severe than previously feared by purposefully demonstrating what it is like to live with the virus and be reliant on international support for life prolonging treatment and care (GFAN 2013). This campaign was officially developed by ICSS, but received much mentoring, marketing and technical support from the Global Fund Secretariat. As with many CSO resource mobilization activities, there was a high level of crossover and sharing of resources, expertise and connections between CSOs and the Global Fund Secretariat.

In December 2013, donors committed to US$12 billion over three years for the Global Fund – US$3 billion short of the civil society ask. It is not possible to conclude how much of this funding is because of CSO advocacy, compared to other factors, but anecdotal evidence suggests that CSOs played a key role in the fundraising. Staff members within the Global Fund noted that they would not have been able to carry out fundraising efforts on the current scale without CSO support (GHI Representative 2013 #3). These views were reiterated in public statements by Global Fund leadership. The Executive Director noted that, "Civil society and communities are key for advocacy around the Fund, including as we seek new resources" (GFAN 2013). Observers suggest that the reason other organizations, such as UNITAID and The Vaccine Alliance (GAVI), followed the Global Fund's example of including civil society in their governance structures is that they realize the key role these groups played in mobilizing resources (CSO Representative 2013 #1), suggesting that CSOs' potential for generating institutional resources is substantial.

Activist and other groups that advocated the creation of the Global Fund had hoped that it would provide funding to CSOs in order to support interventions aimed at addressing the rights of key populations. However, the majority of financing continues to be distributed to government ministries for both pragmatic and ideological reasons. On the practical side, the size of the grants distributed requires bureaucracies that can absorb and manage the funds, which most CSOs cannot. The decision to provide such large grants is based on the desire to keep the Global Fund Secretariat small, and not require numerous country offices; providing many smaller grants to CSOs would require greater supervision and therefore overhead costs at the Secretariat (CSO Representative 2013 #1). Ideologically, this preference for states as PRs reflects a desire for Global Fund resources to be distributed in line with government policies, which ideally means they will reflect national needs. In practice this only occurs where and if the government is responsive to the communities and populations most affected.

While the Fund aims to support "country ownership", promoting a national multisectoral response, Walker (2011) notes that the dominant approach reflects more of a policy of "state ownership", in which CSOs have little power compared to governmental actors. Though the CCMs, which nominate the PRs of Global Fund grants, consist of both state and non-state actors, these are often dominated by state interests, and CSOs that are friendly to them, with a notable lack of participation of key populations (Oberth 2012).

Though the majority of funding continues to be directed to government ministries, in the minority of situations CSOs act as PRs. CSOs take on PR responsibilities where governments are unable or unwilling to do so, or where CSOs have specific expertise that provides a particular advantage. For example, the International HIV/AIDS Alliance (the CSO that receives the largest amount of Global Fund grants) is a PR in the Ukraine, due to its expertise in, and government opposition to, harm reduction (CSO Representative 2013 #1). The Alliance is recognized as able to provide a rights-based approach, which the government is unwilling to do.

CSOs appear to be particularly effective in implementing grants. The Global Fund's evaluation system rates grants along one of five categories: A1 (exceeding expectations), A2 (meeting expectations), B1 (adequate), B2 (inadequate but potential demonstrated), and C (unacceptable). These ratings guide decisions on disbursement amounts, and whether or not to renew a grant. Grants with a C rating will usually not receive subsequent disbursements. CSO PRs receive the majority of top ratings for performance, with over 50 per cent of CSO PR grants ranking in "A" categories between 2008 and 2010 (comparable to government PR grants, of which just over 30 per cent ranked in A categories) (GFATM 2011a, 3). Informants argue that CSOs' higher performance in grant implementation relates to their ability to develop strong networks with affected communities, and their historical commitment to advancing rights-based approaches (CSO Representative 2013 #2). However, no sustained analysis has been done on why CSOs perform better than other PRs. The high ranking of CSO PRs demonstrates that where CSOs have the opportunity they contribute to more effective resource use (according to the Global Fund's standards).

Pointing out the demonstrated success of CSO PRs in reaching key populations and implementing grants effectively, CSO representatives on the Global Fund board and committees have advocated Dual Track Financing (DTF). DTF encourages proposals to the Global Fund to include both government and non-government PRs. A number of interviewees note the adoption of DTF was the direct result of the efforts by the communities and NGO delegations on the Global Fund board, and their continued campaigns for a greater role of CSOs in grant implementation (GHI Representative 2013 #3; GHI Representative 2013 #21). At the 15th Board Meeting, in 2007, under the heading of "Strengthening the Role of Civil Society and the Private Sector in the Global Fund's Work" the board approved the recommendation for routine use of DTF (GFATM 2007). The Secretariat then, in consultations with CSOs, produced guidelines that encouraged CCMs to nominate at least one government and one non-government PR to lead programme implementation. The guidelines did not require proposals to include DTF, but included the following caveat: "If a proposal does not include both government and non-government PRs, it should contain an explanation of the reason for this" (GFATM & International HIV/AIDS Alliance 2008, 7).

However, DTF has not become a dominant approach within Global Fund grant disbursements. In 2009, 70 DTF proposals were received (out of 159 proposals in total) and 35 were approved (out of a total of 85 approved proposals) (TRP 2009). In 2010, 52 DTF proposals were received (out of 150 proposals in total), and 27 approved (out of an approved total of 79) (TRP 2010). Despite strong language within the board resolution and guidance documents, the majority of proposals, successful and unsuccessful, did not include DTF. Furthermore, the number of DTF proposals decreased between funding rounds, demonstrating declining commitment to DTF. One reason provided by the TRP for CCM's not submitting DTF proposals was that current PRs felt they were performing well, and so the need to add an additional PR was not recognized (TRP 2008). Such rationales indicate that, despite advocacy by CSOs and directives from the Global Fund, the majority of CCMs do not recognize the benefits of increasing the role of CSOs as PRs.

Where governments do include CSOs, they often do so because they believe it will increase the chances of submitting a successful proposal, as opposed to out of recognition of the benefits of partnering with CSOs: "Government-dominated CCMs may have less understanding of the role of CSOs and often make the decision to nominate a CSO as a PR because the Global Fund recommends doing so, rather than because they recognise civil society as a key partner" (ICASO 2012a, 11). This superficial sense of partnership results in poor cooperation between government and CSO PRs. For example, though the India HIV/AIDS Alliance, a local CSO, has a record of successfully implementing grants as a PR under DTF, it does not have a strong relationship with the government PR. Furthermore, because it was a PR, the Alliance could not participate in the CCM, and was frustrated to see CSO seats on the CCM remain empty because of government apathy to CSO involvement. A report found:

> The result is a situation where civil society is poorly represented and implementing organizations such as the Alliance cannot contribute. This situation, coupled with many government agencies' critical view of the capacities and governance of civil society organizations in general, has had a negative impact on the ability of civil society to be considered equal and/or significant players to date for the Global Fund.
>
> (ICASO 2012a, 17)

DTF, while having marginally increased access to resources and influence over distribution for CSOs, has not transformed the approach of those governments who remain resistant to sharing power and funding.

Directing resources to communities and key populations

CSOs have continually advocated funding streams that aim to provide resources more directly to communities through local CSOs, faith-based groups and

other actors. One avenue they have pursued is the promotion of funding specifically for Community Systems Strengthening (CSS). The Global Fund defines CSS as "the provision of financial, technical and other kinds of support to organizations and agencies that work directly with and in communities" (GFATM 2014). The key principles of CSS are:

> Significant and equitable role in all aspects of program planning, design, implementation and monitoring for community-based organizations and key affected populations and communities, in collaboration with other actors; programming based on human rights; programming informed by evidence and responsive to community experience and knowledge; commitment to increasing accessibility, uptake and effective use of services to improve the health and well-being of communities, and accountability to communities.
>
> (GFATM 2014, 9)

This formalized approach to increasing the involvement of affected communities and key populations in Global Fund resource governance represents an effort to systematically strengthen community responses, and support human rights interventions, providing a corrective to the usual distribution channels, which neglect these aspects of the response (as outlined in section one of this chapter).

Much like DTF, key informants note the prominent influence of CSOs in advocating the creation of CSS. Civil society board members continually pushed for funding structures that direct resources to local CSOs, arguing that funding that flows through governments and international organizations rarely reaches community-based organizations (CBOs) and key populations (CSO Representative 2013 #1). Pressure also came from CSO representatives on CCMs, who argued that in order for local CSOs to participate in Global Fund processes they required greater support and capacity building (ICASO 2012b). In response to this pressure, the Global Fund began referring to the need for CSS in communications with CCMs and partners in 2006. That year it produced, in partnership with the International HIV/AIDS Alliance, case studies of successful CSO participation in implementing Global Fund grants as CCM members, PRs and sub-recipients, labelling these activities CSS. The report read:

> These interventions, known as community systems strengthening (CSS), are increasingly becoming a core part of the Global Fund's preferred strategy across its programs. More and more civil society groups are receiving not only financial support but also crucial technical support in areas including accounting and monitoring and evaluation.
>
> (GFATM & International HIV/AIDS Alliance 2008, 5)

The following year the Global Fund issued information notes advising applicants on how to include CSS in proposals. Under pressure from CSO delegates, in 2008, the board recommended "the routine inclusion, in proposals

for Global Fund financing, of requests for funding of relevant measures to strengthen community systems necessary for the effective implementation of Global Fund grants" (GFATM and International HIV/AIDS Alliance 2008, 6). Applicants were specifically encouraged to include CSS activities in proposals, and indicate how resources would reach local-level groups and key populations.

However, the opportunity to include greater focus on CSS was infrequently and inconsistently adopted by applicants. During the following funding round the TRP reported:

> As in round seven, the TRP was disappointed to see that the majority of proposals submitted to the Global Fund for support (and HIV proposals especially) failed to include any real discussion on whether particular groups are under-represented in accessing and/or receiving prevention, treatment, and/or care and support services relevant to the particular country context.
>
> (2008, 23)

Round 9 saw only a slight increase in proposals including CSS. Furthermore, many of the activities labelled as CSS more closely resembled health systems strengthening: "activities included microscopes and training for microscope operators in community health centres; renovation of local, regional, and national health facilities; capacity building for local government units in HIV planning; and training of health care professionals" (GFMSM 2013, 5). These inputs were not the sort of community support, such as funding for peer support groups and advocacy activities, that CSO proponents had envisioned. Despite CSO advocacy and Global Fund Secretariat promotion of CSS, the majority of applicants did not seize the opportunity to include requests for rights-based interventions.

CSOs attribute the weak adoption of CSS to the challenges of communicating CSS results within the Global Funds performance-based management framework (ICASO 2012a). Local CSOs often have limited time and capacity to engage in extensive monitoring and reporting procedures, making them risky sub-recipients of grants. Furthermore, support activities, such as peer counselling, and advocacy efforts, such as promoting legal rights of key populations, did not deliver easily measurable results. The Global Fund found that:

> it has been difficult for community actors to clearly explain the connections between health outcomes and community activities that have potential impacts on health but are not directly related to health service delivery, for example advocacy, social protection and welfare services, home-based care or legal services.
>
> (GFATM 2014, 8)

Because CSS outcomes were not easily measured, they were viewed as detracting from the strength of proposals, despite Global Fund calls for a greater focus

on CSS. While CSS was adopted and promoted in principle by the Global Fund, it did not fit into pre-established systems and governance processes, which restricted implementation.

In response to these challenges, and under continued pressure from CSO representatives on the board to improve its capacity to support CSS, in 2010, the Global Fund released an extensive framework to encourage greater focus on CSS in Round 10. This framework was developed in collaboration with a range of CSOs, such as the Coalition of Asia Pacific Regional Networks on HIV/AIDS, and other organizations, such as UNAIDS and the World Bank. A draft was consulted on through interviews, meetings, workshops and an online questionnaire with CSOs around the world, giving CSOs multiple opportunities to influence the final draft (GFATM 2014, iv–v). The resulting framework was well received by CSOs who saw it "as an opportunity to frame and strengthen their efforts in the response to AIDS, tuberculosis, and malaria and to redress the balance of programming toward the most neglected groups" (GFMSM 2013, 3).

Following the development of the framework, in Round 10, CSS interventions were included in 65 of the 150 eligible disease proposals (43 per cent), and in six of the 28 crosscutting health system strengthening requests (21 per cent) (Rivers 2010). However, the majority of requests continued to be for community service delivery interventions, which the GFMSM notes "is significant because service delivery does not reflect the more traditional notions of community system strengthening like advocacy, capacity building and leadership development" (2013, 9). In some cases, the Global Fund encouraged CSOs to include greater service delivery components at the expense of advocacy activities. During Round 10, a regional network of sex worker organizations in Latin America and the Caribbean applied for CSS funding with a proposal aimed at reducing stigma towards sex workers in health care settings. Initially, the network did not include direct service delivery in the proposal because it did not want to overlap with national efforts. However, Global Fund Secretariat staff pressured the proposal developers to include high-level impact indicators related to service delivery, because these were better reflected in the monitoring framework (GFMSM 2013, 13). Even with the new CSS framework, the disconnect between the ideal of CSS, as promoting enabling environments at the local level, and the confines of Global Fund reporting priorities, shifted resources away from advocacy and support, to technical interventions.

During the same round, over half of CSS funding went to government recipients, not CSOs, raising concerns that resources would continue to be spent at the national, not local level, and on government sanctioned interventions, as opposed to advocacy and rights projects for marginalized groups. The GFMSM noted:

> The fact that such a high proportion of CSS funding is used by the governmental sector indicates that a smaller proportion of CSS funding is

being used for activities that the government neglects or that are most effectively carried out by civil society organizations. This is particularly true for interventions targeting key populations.

(2013, 9)

While CSS had been conceived of as a corrective to provide resources to communities, populations and organizations neglected by dominant resource distribution patterns, the majority of funding was still provided to governments for generalized programmes. In contexts where governments denied existence of key populations, for example MSM populations, directing CSS funds through a Ministry of Health was unlikely to reach those most in need. The GFMSM found, "efforts to use CSS for key populations have faced the same challenges that key population programming has faced since the creation of the Global Fund" (2013, 14). In other words, the status quo was maintained.

Any further potential of the new framework was stemmed by the cancellation of Round 11, in November 2011, and the resulting period of upheaval within the Global Fund. One key informant sums up the process of promoting CSS:

The role of the community representatives involved in the board, as well as those who are working within the Secretariat, pushed hard for the creation of the CSS framework. That got developed, but it really hasn't been implemented. Many of the recommendations that have been made repeatedly to the Global Fund about how it could improve its CSS approaches, how it can better utilize funding structures for key affected populations, those ideas have not really been adapted and adopted to the extent that they could or should be.

(CSO Representative 2013 #2)

Despite successfully advocating a CSS Framework, which espoused ideals of community participation and human rights, the overarching structures of the Global Fund, the dominant role of states as PRs, and performance-based management limited its potential to providing a corrective to current distribution priorities.

In addition to promoting CSS, CSOs on the Global Fund board, and through groups such as the GFAN, continued to advocate greater resources for interventions focused on key populations. Between 2002 and 2010, only about 10 per cent of the Global Fund's cumulative approved funding for HIV prevention was allocated to interventions targeting the key populations of sex workers, people who inject drugs and men who have sex with men (Avdeeva et al. 2011, 8). Recognizing this gap, in 2010, the board approved the creation of a dedicated reserve of funding for most at risk populations (MARPs). The MARP Reserve, created only for Round 10, set aside a maximum of US$75 million over two years to fund proposals from applicants who focused interventions towards key populations affected by HIV/AIDS. Applicants

who wished to address the needs of MARPs could either submit a regular HIV/AIDS proposal focusing partly, predominantly or only on MARPs through the general process, or submit an HIV proposal focusing on MARPs through the reserve (GFATM 2010).

This reserve aimed to particularly provide funding to support interventions targeting key populations in upper middle- and lower middle-income countries. In this way it was different from CSS, which was largely directed towards supporting community interventions in low-income countries. Instead the MARP Reserve recognized that in contexts of low prevalence, but concentrated epidemics, there was a need for specific funding for key populations, especially considering that concentrated epidemics were characteristic of middle-income countries, which were not prioritized in grant distribution. Through this new route, proposals from middle-income countries focusing on key populations did not have to compete with proposals responding to generalized epidemics.

In 2010, 25 MARP proposals were received, and 12 were approved (with total funding of US$46.9 million) (TRP 2010). This was a somewhat higher success rate than for general proposals (48 compared to 41 per cent), leading the TRP to conclude, "Overall, the quality of focus on these populations was greatly enhanced in the proposals submitted under this funding reserve in Round 10, suggesting that this mechanism provided an appropriate incentive for applicants to focus on these groups" (TRP 2010, 4). Approved MARP proposals contained 11 per cent more activities related to prevention, care and support, and to addressing stigma targeting key populations than general HIV proposals – a modest increase of rights-based interventions. Furthermore, the TRP found that proposals to the general category of funding also included greater focus on MARPs in Round 10, noting:

> This could suggest that all Round 10 applicants, regardless of their choice of HIV proposal type, were appropriately made more aware by the board's message and Secretariat information notes on this topic. This initiative most likely resulted in a better prioritization of interventions focused on those that are most at-risk of being infected.
>
> (TRP 2010, 12–13)

The TRP recommended that the MARP Reserve be continued. However, like the CSS process, the development of the MARP Reserve was stalled by the cancellation of Round 11 and subsequent upheaval in the Fund.

Despite efforts to promote CSO participation in resource distribution through CSS and the MARP Reserve only a minority of Global Fund resources were dedicated to addressing the human rights issues of key populations and affected communities. The TRP consistently reported, in its reviews following funding rounds, disappointment in the relatively low prioritization of programmes for key populations, and to address human rights and gender inequality in funding proposals (TRP 2010). Despite CSO efforts to develop distribution channels so that resources would better reach affected communities and key

populations, funding has not reflected these rights goals. The creation of the MARP Reserve reflected recognition that demand was outpacing supply for the Global Fund. By advocating the Reserve, CSOs tried to protect funding for key populations in middle-income countries, a struggle that would continue with the introduction of the New Funding Model.

The New Funding Model

Following the cancellation of Round 11, the Global Fund went through a period of substantial restructuring. Throughout the process, CSOs continually advocated greater resources being directed towards community responses and key populations, often struggling with the competing interests and priorities of other governance actors. As consultations about the NFM unfolded, CSOs fought to hold on to the modest gains they had made in terms of funding for CSOs, CSS and the MARP Reserve.

This process occurred following accusations of corruption in the Fund, cancellation of Round 11, and subsequent restructuring, which in turn occurred within the broader context of economic recession in donor countries and the backlash against AIDS exceptionalism (discussed in Chapter 2). These external dynamics, though not focused on in this analysis, were influential factors, particularly making the Secretariat and Board sensitive to donors' interests, due to fear of lack of resources.

The development of the NFM aimed to be participatory and inclusive. CSOs engaged in conference calls, and meetings with board and committee members of the Global Fund, as well as the Secretariat. However, a number of respondents found it frustrating to work with a leadership team that was not necessarily familiar with human rights approaches, or used to working with CSOs. The interim Executive Director during much of this process, Gabriel Jaramillo, had a background in banking, as opposed to global health, and was viewed by a number of informants as not particularly open to CSO input (CSO Representative 2013 #1; CSO Representative 2013 #30). Furthermore, CSOs expressed irritation that the numerous consultants involved in the process often usurped their expertise. One key informant reflects on the processes, "So you could say, yeah we've been involved but the question is whether we have been effective" (Civil Society Representative 2013 #26). Others complain of having participated in "hundreds of useless consultations" (CSO Representative 2013 #30).

Of the various networks involved, GFAN worked particularly closely with civil society members to gather input to inform the content of the NFM. Early in the process it began advocating a pledging opportunity in 2012. However, this did not materialize as the Secretariat and Board felt it was imperative to focus on reforms before asking donors to give. GFAN then consulted with its members to develop a common CSO position on the NFM. Key components of the resulting position paper were: the rejection of pre-set country funding allocations/ envelopes as these would prevent full expressions of country demand; a suggestion that, if funding is insufficient, high quality

asks be prioritized if further funding became available; and an ask for a more flexible resource mobilization strategy that would provide predictable and sufficient funding opportunities (GFAN 2013).

The GFAN had limited success in ensuring that the NFM reflected these priorities. In terms of country allocations, the NFM is structured so that countries can access three types of funding: indicative funds, based on the allocation they have been awarded; incentive funds, which represent an opportunity for further financing based on achieving performance targets; and unfunded quality demand, for innovative and ambitious projects that, if there are cost savings or additional resources available, will be funded on a case-by-case basis (Garmaise 2014). Though CSOs managed to influence the model to avoid completely restrictive caps on funding by successfully advocating the creation of the unfunded quality demand, indicative funding (the majority of resources to be distributed) is capped by country allocations, something CSOs opposed. Furthermore, while the incentive funding reflects CSO calls for the prioritization of high quality asks, the fact that this is presented as an extra resource pool, to be distributed only if additional funding is available, means it does not provide predictable financing. Instead it is to be distributed on a case-by-case basis, and therefore more evidence of its use is needed in order to analyse whether it will be implemented in a way that provides funding to rights-based interventions, and mitigates the negative effects of restrictive country allocations.

Early in the process of developing the NFM, donors voiced opposition to funding responses in middle-income countries, arguing governments in middle-income countries had the ability to cover the costs themselves. A number of countries that received grants from the Global Fund had recently made the transition from low- to middle-income country status. This raised questions about their dependence on international aid to fund their HIV/AIDS response, with donors arguing that, in a context of resource scarcity, due to the global recession, funding should be dedicated to where it could have the largest impact, or the "greatest return on investment", which was in low-income, high HIV/AIDS prevalence states (State Representative #14; Garmaise 2012).

Debates over the provision of international aid to countries that have shifted to middle-income status, is by no means unique to the HIV/AIDS response or Global Fund resource governance. What makes resource considerations particularly tense in this case is that many middle-income countries have concentrated epidemics amongst key populations, such as PWIDs and MSM, who remain marginalized and often criminalized by their governments (for example homosexuality is illegal in Nigeria, impeding programmes targeted at MSM). Domestic resources are sufficient to cover the majority of the costs of HIV/AIDS interventions, justifying Global Fund withdrawal, but states are unlikely to fill the resource gap because of lack of concern for, and sometimes outright opposition to, key populations. As one key informant noted, "It is not a financing challenge, it is a political challenge" (State Representative 2013 #14). The role of the Global Fund becomes tenuous in these contexts, as the

withdrawal of funding threatens to exacerbate the epidemic and human rights violations, but its continued provision enables governments to neglect the HIV/AIDS response and key populations.

For many CSOs, donor driven decisions to reduce funding to middle-income countries represented a retreat from the idea of a global response, indicating instead the more common development assistance approach of transfers from the north to the south. At the 2012 International AIDS Conference, CSOs protested with signs that read "keep the Global Fund global". CSOs also viewed the decline of support for funding to middle-income countries as a reversal on commitments to universal access, noting that treatment coverage in Eastern European countries was lower than in Sub-Saharan Africa (Civil Society Representative 2013 #2). For CSOs operating in middle-income countries, the potential decline of Global Fund resources threatened their survival, as they relied on international funding and did not benefit from domestic support. They also expressed fear that the shift from international to national funding would result in a retreat on rights-based programmes, as many middle-income governments have restrictive approaches to drug use and sexual rights.

CSO representatives on the Global Fund board and committees continually voiced opposition to reducing funding in middle-income countries with concentrated epidemics. In May 2012, the Developed Country NGO Delegation to the board submitted a paper arguing:

> Many countries are transitioning from low to middle income, but poverty in middle-income countries remains high. … Middle-income countries have higher burdens of HIV and TB than low-income countries. … The capacity of middle-income countries to pay for health and their disease responses varies. … The Global Fund will only achieve its targets if investment is proportionate to disease burden.
>
> (Garmaise 2012)

External CSOs used forums, such as the GFAN meetings, to express concerns over plans to decrease funding to middle-income countries (GFAN 2013). They produced research demonstrating the potential negative impact of cuts to HIV/AIDS resources and lobbied both donor governments and the Global Fund Secretariat (International HIV/AIDS Alliance 2012; Raminta et al. 2013). In a commentary in the Global Fund Observer, CSO representatives wrote that though one of the five strategic objectives outlined in the strategy for transitioning to the NFM was to protect and promote human rights, such "noble aspirations are to some extent undermined by the absence of any concrete effort to ensure that populations specifically affected are not left behind. Focus is again constrained to those countries where the greatest gains can be made" (Kapilashrami & Hanefeld 2014).

The debate over funding for middle-income countries (between CSOs and donor states) revolves around differing understandings of greatest need. For

donors, who are concerned about dependence on their resources, the withdrawal from middle-income countries is based on economic rationales that consider supply and demand, and returns on investments (there is more demand in Sub-Saharan Africa and implementing interventions is cheaper). From the rights-based perspective of most CSOs, greatest need is not only indicated by poverty, but also unequal access to resources. For example, CSOs from Latin America argue that many middle-income countries also have high degrees of inequality, which prevents the majority of the population from enjoying the benefits of economic development (CSO Representative 2013 #13). They further note that such gross inequality generates marginalization and discrimination, which increases vulnerability to HIV. As one CSO representative summarizes:

> much of the discussion around driving funding for middle-income countries has been very much focused on the economics of it, that middle-income countries have money, they should take responsibility for paying for their own, and that makes all the sense in the world until you start talking about gay men in Nigeria, drug users in Russia, sex workers anywhere.
>
> (CSO Representative 2013 #2)

CSOs repeatedly point out – in board meetings, consultations and publications – the numerous flaws in the World Bank classification of country incomes, noting such classifications do not take into account inequalities within countries, human rights concerns or the willingness of states to respond to the HIV/AIDS epidemic and needs of key populations.

The development of the NFM was dominated by the economic rationale of donor states concerned with investment impacts. Whereas previous frames around HIV/AIDS exceptionalism had created space for CSO arguments for the need for a truly global response, in the context of economic recession and restructuring of the Global Fund, donors were able to assert their preferences, which tended towards more traditional resource transfers from the global north to south. One advocate notes, "CSO concerns to be honest were kind of ignored because the Global Fund was going through its own internal crisis" (CSO Representative 2013 #20). The funding crisis in the Fund made it more sensitive to donor interests, which justified funding priorities on the basis of perceived resource scarcity.

As a result, those countries that were identified as having had receiving more than their fair share of Global Fund resources were told to expect funding decreases. In a letter received by the Ukraine CCM, the Global Fund Secretariat said:

> The allocation formula used in the new funding model indicates that Ukraine's HIV and TB components are receiving more funding than the country's fair share of Global Fund resources. ... Given the need to balance limited resources across the entire Global Fund portfolio, with focus on

the highest disease burden and lowest income level countries, this allocation will need to be gradually reduced.

(Quoted in Gelfand 2014)

In response, the PR for the Ukraine, the International HIV/AIDS Alliance, reported:

> The Ukrainian situation is a quite evident example of how the country AIDS response can suffer from the NFM math. Common sense says to me that the existing grant pipeline should be realistic, up-to-date. As we see it, this not the case, assuming this funding level for 2014, the funding for the next year will dramatically decrease. Legally the Global Fund might have stronger arguments, but programmatically – not! And with the Global Fund we are not battling a legal case in a court, we are jointly fighting the epidemic, and disarming us makes fighting the epidemic in Ukraine weaker.

(Quoted in Gelfand 2014)

While the impacts of decreasing allocations to middle-income countries have yet to play out, CSOs continue to argue against the logic promoted by donors and adopted by the Secretariat, suggesting (as the quote above demonstrates) that reducing funding for middle-income countries threatens a global compact to fight the epidemic. At the 2015 Partnership Forums CSOs suggested using different criteria than World Bank country classifications to determine country eligibility, and creating funding streams to continue support for rights-based programmes in countries that transition from Global Fund to domestic resources (GFATM 2015b). However, CSOs have not been able to shift resource governance principles to reflect earlier aspirations for exceptional global solidarity.

The lack of funding for key populations in middle-income countries is exacerbated by the lack of continuation of the MARP Reserve. The MARP Reserve is not incorporated into the NFM, as funding for key populations is expected to be included in both indicative and incentive funds. However, based on the first round of Concept Notes received by the TRP, the increased focus on the rights of key populations noted in Round 10 has not been maintained (TRP 2014). Instead, the TRP found that Concept Notes lacked reliable and appropriate size estimates for key populations, and that there were only two proposals (out of five) in which human rights policy changes were cited as critical enabling factors, and these were only related to minimal requests for investments. The short-term success of the MARP Reserve in Round 10 has not been carried over to the NFM. CSO gains in promoting this special fund for key populations are stalled and possibly reversed.

Furthermore, the separation of indicative and incentive funding, and unfunded quality demand, may have further marginalized programmes focused on human rights. The TRP found that proposals regulated such interventions to

the above indicative funding requests; meaning rights-based interventions would only be funded in the case of surplus resources or exceptional performance. The TRP concluded that "these cases suggest that the Global Fund has missed opportunities to leverage its considerable influence to advance policy issues that are critical for program success and sustainability" (quoted in Garmaise 2012). It went on to recommend that the Secretariat develop a strategy to work with partners to promote greater focus on the rights of key populations. Similarly, a gender review of 20 Concept Notes in 2014 found that most only included programming to address gender-related barriers to services in "above allocation" requests, as opposed to core allocation (GFATM 2015a).

CSOs particularly fought to ensure the continuation of CSS in the NFM, bringing up the importance of CSS in consultations with Global Fund staff, in board meetings, and through consortium meetings. Organizations such as the GFMSM (2013) published analysis of the limitations of the previous CSS framework and recommendations for how to better incorporate CSS in the NFM to support the rights of key populations and affected communities. In early 2013, the Secretariat released information that CSS would be combined with health systems strengthening. This was opposed by CSOs, who noted that health systems strengthening efforts tend to focus on infrastructure, personnel and technical inputs, and so rarely address less formal care work and efforts to address the social and economic determinants of health (GFMSM 2013, 8). Based on these arguments, the decision to combine the two was reversed (GFAN 2013, 12; GHI Representative 2013 #21).

Instead, the Secretariat worked with institutional partners, such as UNAIDS and UNDP, as well as regional CSOs, such as the Coalition of the Asia Pacific Regional Networks on HIV/AIDS, to develop a guidance document on how CSS fits within the NFM. The draft was circulated through an international consultation with civil society, using an online questionnaire, interviews and a two-day meeting with key informants (GFATM 2014, v).

Within this framework, the scope of CSS and the range of community sector activities remain relatively unchanged (GFATM 2014, iii). However, the CSS can no longer include community-led programme implementation or service delivery. This change responds to concerns expressed by CSOs that CSS service delivery interventions had caused confusion and duplication of efforts with health system strengthening in the past (GFMSM 2013). Instead, service delivery components must be included in core programming within other modules. Where applicants decide that these services should be carried out by community organizations, they are to include strengthening interventions from the CSS framework to ensure the organizations can fulfill these roles (GFATM 2014, 27). The continuation of CSS, consultations with CSOs on its revisions, and clear delineation from service delivery funding, demonstrate that CSOs have been able to ensure this funding stream continues to adapt towards a rights-based response. However, the TRP has continued to note a general lack of CSS activities within Concept Notes. As with gender and key population programming, CSS programming is most often only included in

above-allocation requests, demonstrating that CSS is not prioritized by most PRs (GFATM 2015a, 16).

Under the NFM system, instead of CCMs producing a proposal to then be reviewed by the TRP during established funding rounds, CCMs are to produce a Concept Note, which can be developed in conjunction with their other health and related planning schedules, such as national strategic plans, and which then initiates a dialogue with the Global Fund in order to develop a full proposal. Within this processes there is the potential for both greater and more restricted CSO participation and influence. Kapilashrami and Hanefeld write:

> Provided that such dialogue is a process and not a one-off meeting, drawing both national and sub-national engagement in an open and transparent and inclusive series of consultations that are not restricted to pre-existing Global Fund networks of civil society, there is an opportunity for civil society to better prepare for grant management and implementation. … How this model will allow for community-level engagement in decision-making, particularly among vulnerable populations and groups who have hitherto remained invisible or marginalized in the decision-making and grant application processes, remains to be seen. Here again is the challenge of tremendous opportunity pitted against a historical legacy of coming up short.
>
> (2014)

CSOs are hopeful the new system will result in inclusivity and responsiveness, but fear prevalent practices of government control and bureaucratic requirements will limit opportunities for change.

CSOs in Zimbabwe found that the impetus to develop a Concept Note that reflects a country's national strategic plan (a key pillar of the new process) meant that, because their government denies some key populations (such as MSM) exist, opportunities to include CSOs and interventions that target key populations are restricted. Indeed, the TRP feedback on the Zimbabwean Concept Note found it suffered from programming gaps for key populations, such as MSM and PWID (Zimbabwe CCM 2013, 17). Furthermore, CSOs felt that during the Concept Note development process, Global Fund staff and other CCM participants pressured them to direct their efforts primarily to the health system strengthening component, which focuses on service delivery and the health workforce, not towards the needs of key populations, community infrastructure and enabling environments (Zimbabwe CCM 2013, 28). Similar concerns were reiterated at the 2015 Partnership Forums where it was noted that the need to integrate Concept Notes with strategic plans meant the rights-based responses were excluded, because countries failed to prioritize key populations in their domestic policies (GFATM 2015a). An analysis by the Access to Funding Department in 2015 found that just 59 per cent of the 111 Concept Notes submitted in 2014 clearly documented efforts to engage key population groups (GFATM 2015a, 20).

The ability of CSOs to participate in the Country Dialogue process is restricted by continued confusion over the NFM and demands for highly technical proposals. CSOs that gathered for a GFAN meeting expressed concerns and confusion over how civil society participation in country dialogues will be structured (GFAN 2013, 11). Following a workshop on the NFM, attended by 60 representatives from government and CSOs in Cote d'Ivoire, participants expressed dismay at the complexities of the process, and the need for a high level of technical expertise to develop a Concept Note through the country dialogue process. One CCM member was quoted as reflecting "The methodology is extremely demanding. ... We don't have all the necessary skills; we need a team that is better-equipped" (quoted in Fontaine 2014). Experience in Zimbabwe found the Concept Note process no less time demanding or complicated than the previous proposal development process, and recommended that it be simplified and the length of the Concept Note be shortened (Zimbabwe CCM 2013). Partnership Forum members also stressed the need for a simplified and adaptable Concept Note and funding disbursement system.

In response to these trends, civil society delegations to the Global Fund board and partners of the Secretariat pressured the fund to provide more strategic support so that CSOs meaningfully engaged in Concept Note development. In April 2014, the board approved the Community Rights and Gender Technical Assistance Program – a US$15 million project to provide technical assistance to civil society organizations for participation in country dialogue and Concept Note development, and to support the long-term capacity development of civil society networks. Local and national CSOs can apply to be qualified as technical assistance providers, and then receive funding to assist CCMs in developing Concept Notes. The positioning of CSOs as experts within this programme demonstrates their considerable influence and credibility with the Secretariat and board, and provides resources for closer partnerships with state. The intention is that this increased CSO expert presence will not only simplify the Concept Note process but also result in greater consideration of key populations in final proposals (GFATM 2015a, 17). In addition to advocating the technical assistance programme, the Developing Countries NGO Delegation successfully proposed a review of the Global Fund's progress towards its strategic objective on human rights. The Delegation requested that the report:

> outline key activities and budgetary allocations, activities undertaken with partners to realize the strategic objective, an analysis of relevant approved grants, and an update on the status of enforcement of the Technical Review Panel's ("TRP") recommendations on human rights, gender and key populations.

The review, completed in March 2015, identified the limits of funding for human rights interventions within the NFM, which the Global Fund committed to addressing.

Chapter conclusion

The creation of the Global Fund was prompted by aspirations to create an institution to facilitate treatment access and address global security concerns, which was not confined by UN bureaucracy. Calls for innovation created opportunities for CSOs to demand space for participation to advance rights agendas, which they gained by demonstrating the productive role they filled as fundraising advocates. Despite the changes of 2011–12, the Fund remains one of the most influential GHIs, but questions about its partnership model, structure, legitimacy and accountability have become increasingly pertinent.

Within the dynamic structure of the fund, the influence CSOs generate as those most affected, as advocates, and through networks, provides opportunities for CSOs to influence not only decision-making, but also governance processes. While influence is uneven, disproportionately exercised by northern actors, there are examples of CSOs from all regions advancing the Fund's capacity to address human rights issues.

The civil society delegations to the Global Fund board are unable to be representative of their large and diverse constituencies. The Developed Country NGO Delegation in particular exacerbates, as opposed to mitigating, input legitimacy challenges. Instead, the civil society delegations generate output legitimacy: for the Affected Communities Delegation this is tied to the normative validity of the GIPWA principle; for the others it reflects their (often contentious) demands that the board remain responsive and dynamic. Due to weak input legitimacy, the civil society delegations are unable to strengthen downward accountability to those most affected by the epidemic, or to hold the Fund to account. Similarly, the Partnership Forum and Secretariat processes reflect more of a horizontal accountability, than downward, structure. However, efforts by external CSOs to make information from and about the Global Fund accessible have enabled external CSOs to act as watchdogs. Though civil society participants in the governance of the Global Fund have substantial influence, which they often use to promote human rights, claims that they are representative of and accountability to a broader movement are overstated.

Since advocating the creation of the Global Fund, CSOs have consistently tried to direct greater resources to non-state actors, affected communities and key populations. In these efforts they have achieved some progress in terms of promoting policies such as DTF, CSS and the MARP Reserve. However, implementation of these policies has continually faced barriers related to the demand for performance-based results, the dominant position of states as PRs, and the restrictions created by the changing political economy of global health. What modest gains were initially achieved were then stalled by the cancellation of Round 11, and subsequent upheaval in the Fund. CSOs have tried to protect funding for key populations and CSS, through participation in the development and implementation of the NFM, but have switched from an offensive position of advocating greater resources for rights-based responses, to defending what gains they have previously achieved.

References

Aidspan (2013), About Us, available at: http://www.aidspan.org/page/what-we-are (accessed 10 August 2014).

Annan, K. (2001), Secretary-General Proposes Global Fund for Fight Against HIV/ AIDS and Other Infectious Diseases at African Leaders Summit, available at: http:// www.un.org/press/en/2001/SGSM7779R1.doc.htm (accessed 15 December 2015).

ARCSP (2013), *Advocacy Strategy*, Africa Regional Civil Society Platform, Kigali.

Avdeeva, O., Lazarus, J.V., Aziz, M. and Atun, R. (2011), "The Global Fund's Resource Allocation Decisions for HIV Programmes: Addressing those in Need", *Journal of the International AIDS Society*, Vol. 14 No. 1, p. 51.

Barnett, T. and Prins, G. (2006), "HIV/AIDS and Security: Fact, Fiction and Evidence – a Report to UNAIDS", *International Affairs*, Vol. 82 No. 2, pp. 359–368.

Bartsch, S. (2007), "The Global Fund to Fight AIDS, Tuberculosis and Malaria", in Hein, W., Bartsch, S. and Kohlmorgen, L. (Eds), *Global Health Governance and the Fight against HIV/AIDS*, Palgrave Macmillan, New York, pp. 146–171.

Bartsch, S. (2011), "A Critical Appraisal of Global Health Partnerships", in Williams, O.D. and Rushton, S. (Eds), *Partnerships and Foundations in Global Health Governance*, Palgrave Macmillan, New York, pp. 32–52.

CGD (2012), *The Global Fund to Fight AIDS, Tuberculosis, and Malaria: Background Paper Prepared for the Working Group on Value for Money: An Agenda for Global Health Funding Agencies*, Center for Global Development, Washington D.C.

Developing Country NGO Delegation (2008), *Developing Countries NGO Delegation in the Global Fund Board*, Geneva.

Doyle, C. and Patel, P. (2008), "Civil Society Organisations and Global Health Initiatives: Problems of Legitimacy", *Social Science & Medicine*, Vol. 66 No. 9, pp. 1928–1938.

Elbe, S. (2005), "AIDS, Security, Biopolitics", *International Relations*, Vol. 19 No. 4, pp. 403–419.

Fontaine, A. (2014), "Hope and Unease Accompany Inaugural Training on New Funding Model in Côte d'Ivoire". *Global Fund Observer*, 2 April, available at: www. aidspan.org/gfo_article/hope-and-unease-accompany-inaugural-training-new-fun ding-model-c%c3%b4te-divoire (accessed 15 December 2015).

Fleischman, H. (2008), *An Analysis of the Gender Policies of the Three Major AIDS Financing Institutions: The Global Fund to Fight AIDS, Tuberculosis and Malaria, the World Bank and the President's Emergency Plan for AIDS Relief*, UNAIDS, Geneva.

Fremont Center (2011), *2011 Global Fund Partnership Forum: An Independent Evaluation*, Fremont Center, New York.

Garmaise, D. (2012), "TRP Observations and Lessons Learned on First Wave of Concept Notes", *Global Fund Observer*, 14 June, available at: http://www.aidspan. org/gfo_article/trp-observations-and-lessons-learned-first-wave-concept-notes (accessed 7 August 2014).

Garmaise, D. (2014), "Transition to the NFM Marred by Unanticipated Consequences", *Global Fund Observer*, 28 May, available at: http://www.aidspan.org/ gfo_article/transition-nfm-marred-unanticipated-consequences (accessed 7 August 2014).

Gates, B. (2014), Bill Gates Q&A: Fighting Corruption, the Future of Aid, available at: https://www.weforum.org/agenda/2014/02/bill-gates-qa-fighting-corruption-future-aid/ (accessed 7 August 2014).

Gelfand, L. (2014), "Global Fund Announces Country Allocations under NFM", *Global Fund Observer*, 19 March, available at: http://www.aidspan.org/gfo_article/global-fund-announces-country-allocations-under-nfm (accessed 12 August 2014).

GFAN (2013), *Strategy Meeting on Resource Mobilization for the Global Fund to Fight AIDS, Tuberculosis and Malaria*, Global Fund Advocates Network, Amsterdam.

GFATM (2001), *Key Recommendations From the NGO Consultation Meeting*, GFATM, Brussels.

GFATM (2007), *Decision Points: Fifteenth Board Meeting*, Geneva, available at: http://www.theglobalfund.org/en/board/decisions/ (accessed 12 August 2014).

GFATM (2008), *Recommendations From the Global Fund Partnership Forum*, GFATM, Dakar.

GFATM (2010), *Creation of a Dedicated Reserve for Most at Risk Populations for HIV/AIDS for Round 10*, Geneva, available at: http://www.theglobalfund.org/Knowledge/Decisions/GF/B21/DP18/ (accessed 12 August 2014).

GFATM (2011a), *Report of the High Level Independent Review Panel on Fiduciary Controls and Oversight Mechanisms*, Geneva, available at: www.theglobalfund.org/.../oig/reports/OIG_GF-OIG-15-009_Report_en/ (accessed 12 August 2014).

GFATM (2011b), *The Global Fund Strategy 2012–2016: Investing for Impact*, Geneva, available at: http://www.theglobalfund.org/en/strategy/ (accessed 12 August 2014).

GFATM (2011c), *A Strategy Framework for the Global Fund 2012–2016: Draft Revision 1.2*, GFATM, Geneva.

GFATM (2012a), *An Evolving Partnership: The Global Fund and Civil Society in the Fight Against AIDS, Tuberculosis and Malaria*, Geneva, available at: http://www.infocenter.nercha.org.sz/node/847 (accessed 12 August 2014).

GFATM (2012b), *Report Of The General Manager: Twenty-Seventh Board Meeting*, Geneva, available at: http://www.theglobalfund.org/en/board/meetings/27/ (accessed 12 August 2014).

GFATM (2014), *Community Systems Strengthening Framework*, Geneva, available at: www.theglobalfund.org/.../core/framework/Core_CSS_Framework_en (accessed 10 December 2014).

GFATM (2015a), *Community Rights and Gender Report*, Geneva, available at: http://www.theglobalfund.org/en/fundingmodel/technicalcooperation/communityrightsgender/ (accessed 15 December 2015).

GFATM (2015b), *Partnership Forum*, Geneva, available at: http://www.theglobalfund.org/en/partnershipforum/ (accessed 15 December 2015).

GFATM and International HIV/AIDS Alliance (2008), *Civil Society Success on the Ground. Community Systems Strengthening and Dual-track Financing: Nine Illustrative Case Studies*, GFATM, Geneva / HIV/AIDS Alliance, Brighton.

GFMSM (2013), *Community Systems Strengthening and Key Populations*, Global Fund for Men who have Sex with Men, Oakland, CA.

Heilprin, J. (2011), "Fraud Plagues Celebrity-Backed Global Health Fund", *Associated Press*, 23 January, available at: http://www.huffingtonpost.com/2011/01/23/global-health-fund-fraud_n_812801.html (accessed 10 August 2014).

Hein, W., Bartsch, S. and Kohlmorgen, L. (Eds) (2007), *Global Health Governance and the Fight against HIV/AIDS*, Palgrave Macmillan, New York.

ICASO (2012a), *Lessons Learned from Efforts to Strengthen CCMs*, Toronto, available at: http://unaidspcbngo.org/?tag=communique, (accessed 15 December 2015).

ICASO (2012b), *Technical Support Needs of Indigenous Civil Society Principal Recipients of Global Fund Grants*, Toronto, available at: http://www.icaso.org/files/technical-supp

ort-needs-of-indigenous-civil-society-principal-recipients-of-global-fund-grants (accessed 15 December 2015).

ICASO (2015), *Country Coordinating Mechanism: Key Affected Populations and People*, Toronto, available at: http://www.icaso.org/media/files/23993-CCMKAPPilo tEvaluationReportShortVersionFINAL.pdf (accessed 15 December 2015).

ICW Global (2012), *Governance Manual*, International Community of Women with HIV/AIDS, Buenos Aires.

International HIV/AIDS Alliance (2012), *Don't Stop Now: How Underfunding the Global Fund To Fight Aids, Tuberculosis and Malaria Impacts on the HIV Response*, International HIV/AIDS Alliance, Brighton.

Kageni, A. (2012), "New Structure at Global Fund Will Reduce Influence of Civil Society", *Global Fund Observer*, 10 May, available at: http://www.aidspan.org/gfo_a rticle/new-structure-global-fund-will-reduce-influence-civil-society (accessed 10 August 2014).

Kapilashrami, A. and HanefeldJ. (2014), "Meaningful Change or More of the Same Rhetoric? The Global Fund's New Funding Model and the Politics of HIV Scale-up", *Global Fund Observer*, 18 March, available at: http://www.aidspan.org/gfo_arti cle/meaningful-change-or-more-same-rhetoric-global-fund%E2%80%99s-new-funding-model-and-politics-hiv (accessed 12 March 2014).

Kazatchkine, M. (2012), *A Message to Staff, Partners and Friends from the Executive Director*, GFATM, Geneva.

MACRO (2009), *The Five-Year Evaluation of the Global Fund to Fight AIDS, Tuberculosis, and Malaria: Synthesis of Study Areas 1, 2 and 3*, GFATM, Geneva.

Nay, O. (2009), *What Drives Reforms in International Organizations? External Pressure and Bureaucratic Entrepreneurs in the UN Response to AIDS*, University of Lille, Lille.

Oberth, G. (2012), *Who is Really Affecting the Global Fund Decision Making Processes?*, Aids Accountability, Cape Town.

O'Manique, C. (2004), *Neoliberalism and AIDS Crisis in Sub-Saharan Africa: Globalization's Pandemic*, Palgrave Macmillan, New York.

Piot, P. and Marshall, R. (2012), *No Time to Lose: A Life in Pursuit of Deadly Viruses*, W.W. Norton & Co, New York.

Radelet, S. (2004), *The Global Fund to Fight AIDS, Tuberculosis and Malaria: Progress, Potential, and Challenges for the Future*, Center for Global Development, Washington D.C.

Raminta, S., Sergey, V. and Pinkham, S. (2013), *Quitting While Not Ahead: The Global Fund's Retrenchment and the Looming Crisis for Harm Reduction in Eastern Europe and Central Asia, EHRN, 2013*, Eurasian Harm Reduction Network, Vilnius.

Rittberger, V., Huckel, C., Rieth, L. and Zimmer, M. (2008), "Inclusive Global Institutions for a Global Political Economy", in Rittberger, V., Nettesheim, M. and Huckel, C. (Eds), *Authority in the Global Political Economy*, Palgrave Macmillan, New York.

Rivers, B. (2007), "Main Decisions Made at November Board Meeting", *Global Fund Observer*, 14 November, available at: http://www.aidspan.org/sites/default/files/gfo/ 80/English/GFO-Issue-80.pdf (accessed 10 August 2014).

Rivers, B. (2010), "Global Fund Board Approves Round 10 Proposals", *Global Fund Observer*, 16 December, available at: http://www.aidspan.org/gfo_article/globa l-fund-board-approves-round-10-proposals (accessed 12 August 2014).

Spicer, N., Harmer, A., Aleshkina, J., Bogdan, D., Chkhatarashvili, K., Murzalieva, G., Rukhadze, N., Samiev, A. and Walt, G. (2011), "Circus Monkeys or Change

Agents? Civil Society Advocacy for HIV/AIDS in Adverse Policy Environments", *Social Science & Medicine*, Vol. 73 No. 12, pp. 1748–1755.

Suchman, M. (1995), "Managing Legitimacy: Strategic and Institutional Approaches", *The Academy of Management Review*, Vol. 20 No. 3, pp. 571–610.

TRP (2008), *Report of The Technical Review Panel and the Secretariat on Round 8 Proposals*, GFATM, Geneva.

TRP (2009), *Report of the Technical Review Panel and the Secretariat on Round 9 Proposals*, GFATM, Geneva.

TRP (2010), *Report of the Technical Review Panel and the Secretariat on Round 10 Proposals*, GFATM, Geneva.

TRP (2014), *Report of the Technical Review Panel on the First Wave of Early Applicants in the Transition to the New Funding Model*, GFATM, Geneva.

UNAIDS (2009), *Denying Entry, Stay and Residence due to HIV Status*, UNAIDS, Geneva.

Walker, L. (2011), *Healing Power: The Global Fund, Disrupted Multilateralism and Mediated Country Ownership*, University of Warwick, Warwick.

Williams, O.D. and Rushton, S. (Eds) (2011), *Partnerships and Foundations in Global Health Governance*, Palgrave Macmillan, New York.

Zimbabwe CCM (2013), *The Experience of Zimbabwe with the Global Fund's New Funding Model*, Ministry of Health of Zimbabwe, Harare.

5 CSO participation in the shifting context of global health governance

The creation of UNAIDS and the Global Fund, as set out in the previous chapters, coincided with a period of increasing political attention to global health issues and corresponding resources. As is also set out in Chapters 1 and 2, since approximately 2008 global health resources have stagnated and the priorities of GHIs and donors have been called into question, particularly around HIV/AIDS. This context has demanded a repositioning of the HIV/AIDS response, and CSOs' positions within it, in the broader context of GHG.

This chapter outlines how changes in the broader political economy of health resulted in a reassertion of biomedical and neoliberal approaches. In this shifting context HIV/AIDS CSOs have struggled to maintain their privileged position and ability to advance a rights-based response to health. While they have attempted to transfer their expertise and rights-based frames to sectors beyond the HIV/AIDS response, they are restricted by the legacy of AIDS exceptionalism. This is illustrated by the inability of HIV/AIDS CSOs to ensure strong right-to-health language in the SDG agenda. However, CSOs have been more successful in continuing to champion rights-based responses through the key populations frame. Examples of how this frame has been used to advance the rights of specific key populations at the global, regional and national levels demonstrate both the opportunities and limits HIV/AIDS CSOs continue to engage with.

CSO survival and the end of AIDS (exceptionalism)

Following the 2012 IAS conference *The Lancet* reported:

> The most commonly used phrase at the XIX International AIDS Conference, held in Washington, DC, this week was "an AIDS-free generation". The frequently expressed view of almost all leaders of the HIV community was that an AIDS-free generation was a rapidly approaching reality.
>
> (Horton 2012, 324)

Key leaders, epistemic communities and institutions argue it is possible to "End AIDS" or achieve an "AIDS Free Generation" by stopping new infections

and providing treatment to those who are HIV positive. As one interviewee noted, "Well the biggest, probably the biggest change [in the HIV/AIDS response] is that people dare to speak about ending AIDS" (CSO Representative 2013 #26). Hillary Clinton, then US Secretary of State, reiterated PEPFAR's call for an AIDS Free Generation; UNAIDS Executive Director, Michele Sidibe insisted, "We can end AIDS" (quoted in Horton 2012, 324). The end of AIDS framing is an attempt to re-galvanize support in the context of perceived scarcity. Horton notes that, "these words [AIDS free generation] rallied a faltering AIDS movement" (2012, 324). Arguments that HIV/AIDS could be ended were reiterated in order to advocate a "final" new injection of resources in the HIV/AIDS response.

The rationale that HIV/AIDS can be ended was based on scientific and technical arguments. Das and Horton noted, "Scientific advances have to some extent prompted a renewal in efforts towards achieving an AIDS-Free Generation" (2012, 309). End of AIDS messaging celebrated technological developments related to treatment and prevention as enabling a final push to end the epidemic. For example, UNAIDS insiders argued that "the science exists to make an AIDS-free generation a reality" (Buse et al. 2012, 42). At the 2014 IAS conference this rhetoric continued with reference to "the last mile" of the HIV/AIDS response. UNAIDS introduced the slogan "90, 90, 90" (90 per cent of people living with HIV will know their status, 90 per cent of those with diagnosed infection will be receiving sustained antiretroviral therapy, and 90 per cent of those will have durable viral suppression), which was framed within the broader concept of ending AIDS. UNAIDS stated "a final set of targets is needed to drive progress towards the concluding chapter of the AIDS epidemic, promote accountability and unite diverse stakeholders in a common effort" (UNAIDS 2014, 2).

CSOs have been more cautious of adopting and applying the end of AIDS frame. The CSO ONE has instead promoted the phrase, "the beginning of the end", arguing that predicting the end of AIDS is unrealistic (2012). A minority of HIV/AIDS CSOs hope that the end of AIDS frame can be used to advocate greater human rights, suggesting that by recognizing that technical solutions exist, the remaining barriers, which they identify as human rights related, become more crucial to overcome:

> The most significant scientific hurdles have been addressed. We have very effective, relatively low cost, relatively safe, sustainable treatment that people can be on for a long time and now, we know that we have, a variety, and there are very effective prevention interventions. ... So that kind of ratchets up the human rights challenges, because we have the tools now. So the human rights impediments become the major obstacle
>
> (CSO Representative 2013 #2)

From this perspective, it is hoped that policy-makers and leaders will recognize that the missing piece of the puzzle to ending HIV/AIDS lies in a rights-based response.

However, the majority of CSOs see the end of AIDS frame as obscuring crucial rights arguments. Prominent South African activist Mark Heywood argued, at the 2013 International Conference on AIDS and STIs in Africa, that the end to AIDS frame is "misleading, potentially demobilizing, and irresponsible, and does not fully consider the realities on ground". Pointing out the need to address persistent inequalities and human rights violations he went on to state:

> Let's dispose of the notion of an end to AIDS. While we acknowledge that we have made progress, we are in a more difficult space in 2013 than we were a decade ago. The end of AIDS is nowhere in sight and we need to tackle the social inequalities that continue to impact on the AIDS response.
>
> (Quoted in Cullinan 2013)

Similarly, Das and Horton write:

> The science of HIV can mislead us into thinking there are technical solutions to the epidemic. If we could only roll out more antiretrovirals in the developing world, develop the right regimen for treatment as prevention, or develop an effective vaccine or the right micro biocide all will be well. But, in truth, the underlying challenge of HIV is only partly technical. A more important barrier is cultural: stigma and alienation apply not only to the HIV epidemic among men who have sex with men but also among heterosexuals.
>
> (2012, 309)

These CSO leaders recognize the contradiction within claims that an epidemic spread largely through social discrimination and marginalization, can be ended with technological solutions.

Within UNAIDS, the NGO Delegation has pointed out that the end of AIDS framing is not explicitly rights-based:

> In this regard we are also concerned with the lack of specifics around the language proposed on the "end of AIDS", which unlike the robust 3 zero's [UNAIDS' strategy], does not have an explicit and pronounced focus on human rights, stigma reduction and people-centeredness.
>
> (NGO Delegation 2013)

The 32nd PCB meeting included extensive discussion of the limits and drawbacks of the end of AIDS frame, making it clear that HIV/AIDS CSOs find little space to advance human rights arguments within it.

As opposed to being a new frame, the focus on technical "solutions" in the end of AIDS frame is reminiscent of the early HIV/AIDS response, when government officials argued that once the virus was discovered the epidemic would be curbed. The US congress insisted then that, "yet another terrible

disease is about to yield to patience, persistence and outright genius" (quoted in Nolen 2009, 199). Since the 1980s, the introduction of successful prevention methods, such as condoms, and of treatment, such as ART, generated predictions that the epidemic would soon be over. The messaging now is that because there is increasingly accessible treatment and combination prevention, the epidemic will be defeated. However, these technologies are not particularly new (for example, treatment has been available since 1998, it has just not been widely available), and implementation faces both old (lack of funding) and new (drug resistance) limitations. In this sense it is unclear what advantage the current political and economic context has, with decreased prioritization, in ending HIV/AIDS. The end of AIDS frame represents a recycling of biomedical neoliberal narratives of technical solutions, within which there is restricted space for human rights arguments.

Rather than presenting an opportunity for HIV/AIDS CSOs to propose alternatives, the end of AIDS frame represents a resurgence of biomedical neo-liberalism in the post AIDS exceptionalism context (discussed in Chapter 2). Within this political economy both the rights-based frame and the role of HIV/AIDS CSOs have become precarious. Members of epistemic communities and institutions note that HIV/AIDS focused CSOs are lagging behind the shift away from AIDS exceptionalism (CSO Representative #36 2013). Harman writes, "A fundamental problem within this has been the uneasy relationship between the state and civil society. ... Civil society campaigns have maintained exceptionalism" (2012, 108). CSOs forged their identity, and solidified their right to participate in GHG, within the space provided by exceptionalism and so struggle to adapt to the shifting political economy of GHG. One GHI staff member asks:

> Can civil society get out of the AIDS incubators and get into health dialogue? The AIDS movement is not ready or equipped to engage in fancy discussions on global health, it is totally in contradiction to the way the AIDS movement has been geared. Because the AIDS movement has always been geared on, we are dying, we have to do something. This is our issue. ... It is not the nature of these organizations. If they were they wouldn't be the organizations that they are. They would lose their status.
>
> (GHI Representative 2013 #12)

Engaging in broad global health processes is difficult for HIV/AIDS CSOs because their influence is justified on exceptionalist grounds that typical public health approaches are insufficient to address the unique characteristics and threats of the epidemic. Now these characteristics and threats are becoming normalized the relationship between HIV/AIDS CSOs and the broader public health community is in flux. For example, where treatment is available HIV/AIDS is changing from a death sentence to a chronic disease, and HIV/AIDS CSOs have no unique claim for chronic care resources above and beyond that of CSOs representing other long-term illnesses.

This transition is further influenced by the decline in urgency around the HIV/AIDS response, which changes the role of CSO advocacy and activism. One activist notes, "So I think activism won't be as important as it was in the beginning. Where at that time it was really necessary to get press attention, to make big statements, to act violently" (CSO Representative 2013 #18). Dramatic demonstrations, such as sit- and die-ins, and other activist HIV/AIDS CSO techniques are becoming less common. Instead HIV/AIDS CSOs note that they have to "be smarter" and "more sophisticated" and "find a balance" in order to influence current governance practices (GHI Representative 2013 #29; CSO Representative 2013 #23). For example, treatment activists engage in lengthy legal negotiations over intellectual property rights, instead of throwing blood on politicians. Though crucial, these processes are much more difficult to explain to constituencies, citizens and donors, and almost impossible to get media coverage for (CSO Representative 2013 #9). Morin (2011) documents how media attention to universal access to ART campaigns declined exponentially as the issue moved from high profile court cases and protests, to negotiations and legal proceedings with pharmaceutical companies and governments. Furthermore, as HIV/AIDS-specific campaigns expanded to include broader access to medication issues the media attention and public awareness plummeted.

Despite these challenges, HIV/AIDS CSOs argue that other health CSOs can further learn from their example:

> I think that other communities look to the AIDS community to say, you guys have been so successful in terms of raising money, raising the profile of the issue, driving real scale-up of services, so I think there are a lot of lessons to be learned from the AIDS community that other disease are trying to tap into as well.
>
> (CSO Representative 2013 #7)

The relative success HIV/AIDS CSOs have achieved in influencing the framing of the HIV/AIDS response to reflect human rights concerns is perceived as something to be expanded in order to influence other health sectors (GHI Representative 2013 #12).

However, the assertion that HIV/AIDS CSOs have something to teach other CSOs demonstrates a degree of hubris. The legacy of AIDS exceptionalism created a division between HIV/AIDS CSOs and other health and rights groups. Many CSOs involved in other health priorities resented the prioritization of AIDS during the period of exceptionalism. A CSO representative states: "There has always been some conflict between NGOs that mobilize around a vertical response to HIV and those that said it should be health system strengthening, it should be money going to budget support" (Civil Society Representative 2013 #1). The vertical nature of AIDS exceptionalism directed great resources and attention to HIV/AIDS CSOs at the perceived detriment of other health issues (England 2008). Now that AIDS exceptionalism has declined CSOs continue to pit HIV/AIDS against other health issues.

Referring to a meeting about a Gates Foundation funded health project one observer notes:

> At the start there were quite a lot of anti-HIV political messages: AIDS gets too much money, if a fraction of what went to HIV went to diarrhoea or maternal health then it would make a huge impact. And you saw people making presentations that showed how much money HIV got compared to other causes.
>
> (CSO Representative 2013 #1)

In such contexts it is difficult for HIV/AIDS CSOs to collaborate with other health CSOs, never mind lead or provide an example to them. The unique involvement of HIV/AIDS CSOs in GHG often alienated, as opposed to inspired, other health movements.

Framing the Sustainable Development Goals

The challenges HIV/AIDS CSOs face in maintaining influence in the post exceptionalism context is evident in their attempts to influence the post-MDG agenda around health. The MDGs have guided development interventions since 2000. Goal six specifically refers to HIV/AIDS (combat HIV/AIDS, malaria, and other diseases), and includes the following targets: have halted by 2015 and begun to reverse the spread of HIV/AIDS; and have achieved, by 2010, universal access to treatment for HIV/AIDS for all those who need it. The inclusion of HIV/AIDS in the MDGs was a coup for a then still emerging HIV/AIDS response. It was the result of extensive lobbying by UNAIDS, personal commitment to the issue by then UN Secretary General Kofi Annan, and advocacy efforts by HIV/AIDS CSOs (Piot & Marshall 2012). The inclusion of HIV/AIDS in the MDGs spurred the exceptional HIV/AIDS response that unfolded over the next decade.

However, while global progress towards MDG 6 has been noted, in that HIV infections declined by 24 per cent between 2001 and 2011, infections also more than doubled in certain regions, such as the Caucasus and Central Asia, meaning that the goal to halt and reverse the spread of HIV will not be met (Action for Global Health 2009). Meanwhile goals towards universal access to ART are still mere ambitions, as approximately 59 per cent of PWAs still do not have access to treatment (UNAIDS 2015). Due to this uneven progress, HIV/AIDS remains an unfinished MDG.

Around 2012, as evidence of progress, or lack thereof, towards the MDGs began to be consolidated, global institutions, states and CSOs began to articulate the next version of a global development agenda. HIV/AIDS CSOs were the first actors to express concerns that the post-MDG process was not prioritizing HIV/AIDS, and to take action in response, demonstrating their sole continued allegiance to AIDS exceptionalism. The International HIV/AIDS Alliance, in the UK, presented evidence supporting the continued prioritization

of HIV/AIDS to DFID as early as October 2012 (CSO Representative 2013 #1). At the annual Freespace meeting of the International Civil Society Support (ICSS), in January 2013, partners noted that there was no organized mobilization from the HIV/AIDS response in the post-MDG processes, and asked ICSS to follow up. ICSS found that HIV/AIDS was not present on most health agendas, and began facilitating consultations among CSOs (CSO Representative 2013 #26).

HIV/AIDS CSOs, such as ICASO, led and participated in an e-discussion on HIV, Health and Post-2015 Agenda, sponsored by UNAIDS. Six representatives from civil society monitored forums on the following themes: the unfinished HIV agenda; AIDS, health and development; decision-making and accountability. The over 200 contributions to these discussions were overwhelmingly from CSOs, who constantly reaffirmed the need for a rights-based response led by those most affected by the epidemic. One participant noted: "A key success of the AIDS response is that it has come, first and foremost, from the advocacy efforts of many affected communities and groups, without which the global response may never have taken off" (UNAIDS 2013). The synthesis report from the e-consultation was distributed to various actors involved in the post-MDG process, including participants of the High Level Thematic Meeting on Health.

Despite these concerted efforts, HIV/AIDS was not prioritized in SDG planning. In a letter to UN Secretary General, the NGO Delegation to UNAIDS wrote:

> However, despite the unrelenting efforts, HIV currently has limited visibility in all the key Post 2015 documents, including the 11 thematic outcomes, in the High Level Panel report – and is alarmingly omitted in the recent report from the Open Working Group meeting on Health that was held last May.
>
> (NGO Delegation 2013)

When HIV/AIDS CSOs engaged with the NGO platform that was mobilizing around the SDG agenda – Beyond 2015 the World We Want – they found a distinct absence of HIV/AIDS in health and related position papers and statements (CSO Representative 2013 #9). Lack of attention to HIV/AIDS demonstrated that not only was AIDS exceptionalism over, but also that HIV/AIDS CSOs did not have the same influence, and perhaps allies, as they did during the original MDG framing.

This is particularly noteworthy because overall the SDG process is perceived as including greater CSO involvement than previous processes. HIV/AIDS CSOs and other actors see this greater participation as evidence that the HIV/AIDS response has contributed transformation in GHG towards more inclusive global governance (CSO Representative 2013 #1); a belief that is supported by continued reference to the role of HIV/AIDS CSOs in previous processes. One report on a civil society consultation notes:

> During the Town Hall meeting it was acknowledged that the HIV response has catalyzed a new form of activism around health, comprising the centrality and leadership of the people most affected by the epidemic; the non-negotiability of gender equality and human rights as essential to successful health outcomes; and the value of multi-sectorial partnerships and governance models.
>
> (World We Want 2015)

The precedent HIV/AIDS CSOs set in influencing GHG is being expanded on in the SDG process. However, the reference noted above is also the only mention of HIV/AIDS in the consultation briefing, demonstrating that despite a desire to build on the history of activism around HIV/AIDS, it is also being relegated to the sidelines of current global health agendas.

Somewhat ironically, the high level of CSO participation in the SDG process means HIV/AIDS CSOs have a difficult time getting their voice heard over that of other issue areas, especially due to perceptions that HIV/AIDS has already had more than its fair share of attention and resources. The legacy of jealousy and division from the exceptionalism period continues to play out through CSO competitions to influence the SDG processes. One representative from an advocacy organization notes HIV/AIDS CSOs have to fight for space to participate in broader health CSO consultations, "whereas before we would have been part of the mainstream NGO asks" (CSO Representative 2013 #1). Nilo (2013) refers to the advocacy context around the MDGs as one of "fierce competition", noting that getting HIV/AIDS on to the agenda is a "huge challenge posed to AIDS activists". In the crowded environment of CSO mobilization around the MDGs, the HIV/AIDS voice is just one of many, and one that is viewed as having already had its turn.

Recognizing their limited power as a single-issue lobby, HIV/AIDS CSOs tried to work with other health related CSOs to promote continued focus on HIV/AIDS within broader health goals, and to ensure reference to human rights approaches to health in the final health goal. As one participant in SDG processes noted, "AIDS exceptionality is over. We have to use universal health coverage to promote rights" (CSO Representative 2013 #10). E-consultations reflected opinions from CSOs that approaches to universal health coverage could be complementary to human rights approaches by improving health systems for the under-served and promoting integration between HIV/AIDS, sexual and reproductive health rights movements. Interview informants further argued that integration could reduce the stigma associated with HIV/AIDS by normalizing it (CSO Representative 2013 #18). HIV/AIDS CSOs have identified opportunities, for both the HIV/AIDS response and broader health goals, to advance the rights frame within broader health goals.

However, HIV/AIDS CSOs note that throughout discussions the idea of a universal health goal was predominantly framed within a biomedical paradigm, with limited space for human rights frames. They worried that a broad health goal would become "selective primary health care … a watered down

Alma Ata", and that it would be used to reduce prioritization for not only HIV/AIDS, but the universal right to health in general to purely biomedical approaches (CSO Representative 2013 #10). Such an approach would prioritize service delivery CSOs over advocacy-based organizations that do not contribute to technical targets. One representative commented:

> The question for us is how helpful is it [universal health coverage] in relation to HIV. I think the question is not a question any more. We see it as unhelpful. It may be a good goal in promoting health systems, but less helpful in terms of promoting the work that is more complex than just health systems, which AIDS is. HIV has to do with key populations, with human rights, with all these other issues, that are not just health system related, but are you know cultural, social, legal.
>
> (CSO Representative 2013 #26)

HIV/AIDS CSOs wrote to the Secretary General to stress the need to "go beyond a biomedical focus" with a universal health goal, and include "pro-nounced focus on human rights, stigma reduction and people-centeredness" (NGO Delegation 2013). They continued to advocate greater attention to both HIV/AIDS and the right to health within the SDG agenda in international forums. At the July 2014 UNAIDS PCB an observer intervened to note that:

> We remain concerned, that in the last report of the Open Working Group, HIV has not received the necessary attention and that sexual rights, sexu-ality education, gender identity risk to disappear from the agenda. ... The need for a stronger human rights based post-2015 Framework, with specific attention to marginalized, excluded and stigmatized populations, in par-ticular under the health and the equality goals.
>
> (NGO Delegation 2014)

CSOs fears about a universal health goal were well founded. The SDGs, finalized in 2015, include the health goal "Ensure healthy lives and promote well-being for all at all ages". Under unfinished MDGs, a HIV/AIDS sub-goal is listed as, "by 2030 end HIV/AIDS, tuberculosis, malaria, and neglected tropi-cal diseases". However, while commitment to human rights is asserted in the preamble to the SDGs, there is no specific reference to a rights-based approach to health within the language of SDG Three. HIV/AIDS CSOs continue to assert the need to include more explicit language on the right to health, but are restricted by their lack of influence within a crowded CSO environment, and the post-exceptionalism context of reasserted biomedical neoliberalism.

From human rights to key populations

HIV/AIDS CSOs have responded to shifts away from a rights-based response to global health, and structures that restrict their participation and influence,

by adopting the key populations frame. "Key populations" refers to those groups at higher risk of HIV infection and of being more greatly affected by the epidemic (UNAIDS 2011b). The term usually refers to PWAs and their partners, MSM, PWID, sex workers and their clients. The key population approach seeks to overcome the contradiction of normalizing an epidemic that remains exceptional for those groups that have higher prevalence and risk of HIV infection. Arguments within this frame counter the post-exceptionalist context, with its shift away from HIV/AIDS and human rights, by arguing that for certain groups HIV/AIDS remains a prevalent threat, and that because key populations are neglected by public health programmes and marginalized by society, reaching them with prevention and treatment services requires rights-based interventions, usually led by CSOs.

For example, the International HIV/AIDS Alliance's "What's Preventing Prevention" campaign argued that prevention efforts would only be effective when interventions focused on the rights of key populations. The campaign countered post-exceptionalist arguments that HIV/AIDS prevention programmes were often based on poor evidence (Epstein 2007), by arguing that an evidence-based approach identified key populations as a target group. The campaign further emphasized, through extensive reviews and subsequent publications that, so far, the HIV/AIDS response failed to prioritize key populations, a gap that was presented as the missing piece of the prevention puzzle. The Alliance's campaign both addressed critiques of exceptionalist approaches (that they were not based on sound evidence), and asserted that the human rights frame was essential to the HIV/AIDS response.

The key populations frame also fitted into the end of AIDS discourse, outlined above, by suggesting that recently improved knowledge about who is most at risk of HIV creates new opportunities for high impact, targeted interventions. For example, one research institute writes:

> In spite of an aggregate decline in HIV incidence worldwide, a growing body of epidemiological evidence shows that key populations continue to bear a disproportionately high burden of HIV infection in both low- and high-prevalence countries. With HIV/AIDS concentrated among these populations, efforts to achieve an AIDS-free generation will not succeed unless much greater attention and adequate resources are directed to address their HIV-related needs.
>
> (amfAR 2013)

Similarly, Whiteside and Smith (2009) argued AIDS remains exceptional in Eastern Europe because of high prevalence amongst key populations, such as PWID. The confluence of exceptionalism arguments and end of AIDS terminology within such policy discussions demonstrates how the concept of key populations is adaptable to multiple frames.

In addition to CSOs, GHIs and donors promote the key populations frame through biomedical and economic rationales, as well as human rights

arguments. A study by the World Bank, UNPF and John Hopkins School of Public Health (World Bank 2012) notes that technical interventions, such as condom provision and needle exchanges, which target key populations are cost effective, as "resources need to target the most effective interventions, based on sound evidence." The World Bank report goes on to note:

> This means focusing on some of the hardest-to-reach and most stigmatized populations, including sex workers, people who inject drugs, and men who have sex with men. The public health urgency to address these key populations is consistent with the human rights imperative to include those most in need of HIV prevention, treatment, and care.
>
> (2012)

Similarly, a key informant from the Global Fund notes that the economic recession helped spur the focus on key populations, as such approaches were seen as more efficient: "This is a positive result of austerity. ... In countries where there is not enough resources, people want to know is there a way to identify three populations who represents 80 per cent of the epidemic" (GHI Representative 2013 #21). Economic and rights frames become mutually supportive within arguments that it is most effective to address the epidemic by focusing on key populations.

The term "key populations" is appealing to donors and GHIs as it is politically palatable, suggesting a neutral and more technical approach than human rights, with its highly political connotations. It can also obscure just who these populations are, turning heroin addicts and gay men, for example, into sanitized acronyms (PWID and MSM) that require technical interventions, such as clean needles and condoms to address vulnerability. Through the language of key populations, it is argued that ensuring the rights of those most vulnerable to HIV/AIDS is both cost effective and efficient – representing a (perhaps uneasy) marriage of human rights and biomedical neoliberal rationales.

Due to its broad appeal, the term has gained policy traction with institutions, policy-makers and HIV/AIDS CSOs. One representative from the Global Fund states: "I think key population is becoming a buzzword, it is super sexy, and if you work in key populations you are cool guy ... And now everybody is talking about key populations" (GHI Representative 2013 #21). Reflecting this prioritization, PEPFAR, the WHO and UNAIDS developed a comprehensive package of services for key populations to guide national HIV/AIDS plans, funding requests and donor policies (USAID 2014). Article 29 of the 2011 UN General Assembly Political Declaration on HIV and AIDS specifically refers, for the first time, to the need to address key populations, noting "that many national HIV-prevention strategies inadequately focus on populations that epidemiological evidence shows are at higher risk, specifically men who have sex with men, people who inject drugs and sex workers". The concept of key populations in the response to HIV/AIDS has gained widespread use and popularity.

HIV/AIDS CSOs use the key populations frame to justify their continued participation in GHG through the argument that in order to provide effective services to key populations, participation of representatives from these groups, and CSOs that work with them, is required. Since most states and institutions rarely have positive relationships with such groups, the role of CSOs in global HIV/AIDS governance processes remains necessary. Furthermore, though states may adopt the language of key populations in declarations and national plans and resolutions, they also often continue to criminalize, marginalize and/or neglect these groups, necessitating CSO involvement. The Global Fund states, "In particular, civil society organizations have a key role to play in reaching out to those key affected populations not usually reached by government services" (GFATM 2014, 2). HIV/AIDS CSOs have found continued space to engage in GHG and advocate human rights approaches by applying the key populations frame. The sections that follow explore how CSOs have attempted to utilize this frame to advance struggles for human rights globally, and how these link to regional, national and local struggles.

People who inject drugs (PWID)

An editorial in the *International Journal of Drug Policy* argues that drug issues rarely enter into discussions on international human rights obligations, creating a vacuum in which "human rights abuses flourish with little public comment" (Lines & Elliot 2007, 454). These human rights violations, such as lack of access to health services and police harassment, increase the vulnerability of PWID to HIV infection and prevent them from accessing treatment when they are infected. In almost all regions of the world, "those who inject drugs are among the most marginalized people in society and unnecessarily put at increased risk of preventable [HIV] infections" (Persson et al. 2011, 469). As a result, PWID are one of the population groups with a growing epidemic, making up 5–10 per cent of PWAs globally (UNAIDS 2013).

Harm reduction programmes, such as opiate substitutes and needle exchanges, have been proven to be an effective approach to preventing HIV infections and in helping PWID access rehabilitation services, and HIV/AIDS treatment and care (UNAIDS 2013). However, in countries with concentrated HIV/AIDS epidemics among PWID – such as those in Eastern Europe – harm reduction approaches are often resisted as contradicting condemnation of drug use, and PWID are stigmatized and criminalized. Even in most countries where harm reduction is available, PWID are still viewed as "bad citizens" and resources are inadequate (CSO Representative 2013 #18). PWID and allied CSOs have increasingly tried to argue that increasing access to harm reduction both prevents further spread of the epidemic among PWID, and is consistent with a rights-based response to the epidemic – arguments that are supported by extensive research on methadone clinics, needle exchanges and supervised injection sites (IHRA 2009). However, harm reduction advocates face numerous barriers, sometimes (in contexts such as Russia and China) as

severe as harassment and imprisonment for advocacy efforts (IHRA 2009). As a result, "while significant progress has been made in other areas of the HIV response, the vast majority of people who use drugs – a marginalized and largely criminalized population – have been the last to benefit from HIV prevention, treatment and care services" (IHRA 2009, 5).

The key populations frame provides an opportunity to move PWID from the margins to the centre of the HIV/AIDS response. CSOs that advocate the rights of PWID have used the key populations frame to gain access to, and influence over, global governance forums in order to promote harm reduction as a human right. An example of this comes from efforts by the International Network of People Who Use Drugs (INPUD) – a global organization aimed to defend the rights and promote the health of PWID. The group initiated global lobbying efforts at the 2009 High Level Meeting on the Commission of Narcotic Drugs, chaired by UNODC, but reported, "people who use drugs were made to feel extremely unwelcome and Executive Director Costa went out of his way to question the value of our participation" (Southwall 2012). INPUD representatives also joined the UK delegation to the UNODC, but once again found their participation was sidelined by the UN agency, which has a reputation for being unfriendly to civil society and for interpreting its commitments to CSO participation "in the most narrow terms" (IHRA 2009).

As a strategic move, INPUD then decided to influence UNODC through UNAIDS, where there was already an established practice of CSO involvement, and where the participation of key populations groups was encouraged (CSO Representative 2013 #23). INPUD used this opportunity to call for a unified response to injection drug use within the UN system, pointing out the vast differences between UNODC arguments against harm reduction and UNAIDS support for it, as well as varying levels of engagement with civil society. Over the next few years, INPUD, and other CSOs engaged in the rights of PWID, attended PCB meetings, sometimes sharing personal accounts of discrimination and living with both addiction and HIV/AIDS, and sometimes presenting efficiency arguments for better prevention and treatment services for PWID (CSO Representative 2013 #23).

Meanwhile, organizations of PWID engaged with both UNAIDS and the WHO around policies related to drug use, and participated in forums with other stakeholders, such as UNAIDS led dialogues with faith-based groups and key populations. At the December 2012 UNAIDS PCB meeting, the NGO delegate from INPUD outlined the success of these processes in advancing policies around the meaningful participation and rights of PWID, particularly in relation to harm reduction. However, he also noted:

> Sadly our experience with UNODC, our lead cosponsor, could not have been more different. In three years we have had only three opportunities for meaningful participation and the absence of any systematic form of engagement means that civil society has very limited knowledge of

> UNODC's plans, activities and results. This inhibits meaningful participation and the community watchdog function.
>
> (Southwall 2012)

He went on to critique the Executive Director of UNODC for failing to mention harm reduction during his speech on World AIDS Day. This intervention by the NGO delegate pushed the limits of what was acceptable criticism in the UNAIDS PCB, and would likely not have been tolerated in most other UN bodies (CSO Representative 2013 #23). It was made possible by the acceptance of key population representation in HIV/AIDS governance, which created space for a PWID to challenge current UN practice.

In many ways this was a successful engagement. Staff members of UNODC were impressed with civil society participation in the PCB, and advocated that UNODC develop a similar model:

> So the effectiveness of civil society in raising that issue [harm reduction] and pushing it basically lead to UNODC following this meeting, becoming really engaged saying, "we want to become, the inclusiveness of civil society in the PCB, we want to achieve that in UNODC".
>
> (CSO Representative 2013 #1)

The UNODC's Global Coordinator for HIV/AIDS invited international and regional organizations to a high-level meeting at the UNODC headquarters in Vienna, with CSOs reporting that, "the meeting was very positive" (CSO Representative 2013 #23). It was also agreed that the group of NGOs would meet with the UNODC every six months, a meeting that was informally referred to as a "mini PCB", as it mimicked UNAIDS' inclusive format (CSO Representative 2013 #23). While such developments may have partially resulted from leadership transitions within UNODC, and shifting ideas around harm reduction in general, the space created by the HIV/AIDS response for key population involvement contributed to a spill-over effect that allowed for greater CSO participation in global drug policy in order to further promote the rights of PWID and harm reduction policies.

Such opportunities to engage in global HIV/AIDS governance processes enable PWID to challenge national denial about the existence of PWID populations. Some countries, for example Rwanda and Eritrea, claim that since there are no reported incidents of injection drug use there is no need to report on it or develop programmes to address it (Persson 2011, 470). Such claims are supported by the fact that PWID in such contexts hide from authorities, out of fear of prosecution, and only access health services in the most extreme circumstances – greatly impeding HIV/AIDS prevention and treatment activities. In order to overcome state denial about PWID populations, and therefore improve access to services, CSOs use global HIV/AIDS governance spaces to speak out within the safety provided to key population representatives. The NGO Delegation to UNAIDS brought a PWID from Afghanistan to a PCB

meeting in order to "stop people from saying these things don't exist" (GHI Representative 2013 #29). Spicer et al. quote a PWID advocate explaining, "I started the advocacy on the international stage because I felt safe there" (2011, 1752). Acceptance, and even encouragement, of key population participation in global HIV/AIDS forums can counter national repression of, and failure to recognize, PWID as a key population.

CSO representatives of PWID use the acceptance of key populations in global governance forums to influence national policies. In the Ukraine, the International HIV/AIDS Alliance and the GNP+, the two Global Fund grant principal recipients, successfully advocated the introduction of methadone as drug substitution therapy despite initial state resistance to harm reduction (Spicer et al. 2011). Though at one point the Ukrainian government tried to impose customs (of about US$2000–3000) on needles the HIV/AIDS Alliance was importing for its harm reduction programmes, the Alliance was able to use its influence with donor governments and GHIs to pressure the Ukrainian government to remove the tax (CSO Representative 2013 #1). Such cases demonstrate the power of global networks, with a shared frame, in influencing national policies and practices towards a rights-based approach.

However, a disconnect persists between the empowerment opportunities in global forums, and the continued repression of local CSOs implementing harm reduction programmes. Spicer et al. find that in three Eastern European countries the difference between international CSOs and local CSOs is distinct: "smaller CSOs in all three countries with limited resources, fewer skills and less knowledge and experience continued to have limited influence, although some interviewees reported that they were starting to gain knowledge and advocacy experience" (2011, 1752). Though local CSOs that are members of global networks, and/or closely connected to international CSOs, benefit from increased access to resources and mentoring around advocacy, most continue to focus on service delivery programmes as they fear government reprisals if they engage in advocacy (Spicer et al. 2011, 1753).

CSOs have used the space available due to the acceptance of the key population frame in global HIV/AIDS governance, to promote the participation of PWID in global drug governance and advance acceptance of harm reduction policies, often subverting repressive state influences. However, the top down approach of HIV/AIDS CSOs and allies has yet to overcome the gap between the inclusiveness of global forums and restrictive national/local contexts.

Men who have sex with men (MSM)

HIV/AIDS research has demonstrated that the denial of sexual and legal rights, and homophobia, increases the risk of HIV infection for MSM, and prevents them from accessing treatment and care (Das & Horton 2012). However, the majority of hyper-endemic countries (such as those in Southern Africa) and countries with growing HIV epidemics (such as those in Eastern Europe and the Middle East) continue to criminalize same-sex acts. Some HIV/AIDS

CSOs also engage in the denial of sexual rights (Seckinelgin 2012a). Examination of the origins and power politics imbedded in this homophobia is complex and beyond the scope of this book. What is crucial here is how those HIV/AIDS CSOs that invoke a rights-based approach have engaged in struggles, using the key population frame, to promote the rights of MSM – and to what effect.

Advocates for the rights of MSM have been well represented in global HIV/AIDS governance, and therefore do not have to fight for space as PWID did (as described above). Because the early HIV/AIDS movement in North America and Western Europe grew largely out of the gay rights movement, this component of the HIV/AIDS response has had extensive influence on global HIV/AIDS governance (which remains located in North America and Western Europe and dominated by interests from these regions). This is not to deny homophobia in these contexts, but to simply note that HIV/AIDS CSOs representing MSM have not had to use the key populations frame to demand space in GHG, as this space had already been established. Instead the dominance of Western interests in advocating the rights of MSM has influenced how the key populations frame has developed globally, and been transmitted to national and local contexts.

Since the early activism of the 1980s, HIV/AIDS interventions have promoted global identities based on sexual behaviours, which have been overwhelmingly dominated by Western concepts of sexuality. For example, the confessional technologies of coming out as HIV positive are derived from the Western gay rights experience (Nguyen 2010). Altman notes that the terminology used in HIV/AIDS sexual rights frames comes from a Western context: "Ironically the term 'men who have sex with men' was coined to reach men who rejected any sense of identity based upon their sexual practices, but fairly quickly became used in ways which just repeated the old confusions between behaviour and identity" (2001, 74). The prominent role gay rights movements played in the early response resulted in Western terms and practices being promoted through globalized networks to other regions.

However, attempts to create solidarity from a distance through terms such as MSM, and practices such as coming out, are complicated by cultural and personal understandings and experiences of sexuality. As Seckinelgin notes, "sex is always about crossing multiple boundaries and sexuality follows from this and at its base it is about a crossing between the public and the private spheres" (2012a, 2). Similarly, Altman notes that:

> Speaking openly of homosexuality and transvestism, which is often the consequence of Western influence, can unsettle what is accepted but not acknowledged. Indeed there is some evidence in a number of societies that those who proclaim themselves "gay" or lesbian, that is seek a public identification based on their sexuality, encounter a hostility which may not have been previously apparent.
>
> (2001, 92)

He goes on to note that "modern (i.e. Western) ways of being homosexual threaten not only the custodians of 'traditional' morality, they also threaten the position of 'traditional' forms of homosexuality, those which are centered around gender nonconformity and transvestism" (2001, 88). Western approaches to MSM rights can exacerbate tensions and discrimination in other contexts by upsetting cultural norms, such as around privacy. This makes the construction of a global rights frame for MSM highly complicated as it interacts with cultural identities and personal experiences.

These complications are apparent in the attempts of Western-based HIV/AIDS CSOs to use the key populations frame to advocate legal reforms in non-Western countries that punish homosexual acts. In 2010, CSOs, academics, and legal and medical professionals formed the Commonwealth HIV/AIDS Action Group. Together with the Commonwealth Foundation and Secretariat it launched a project that aimed to increase understanding of how legal frameworks that discriminate against key populations restrict the HIV/AIDS response. The project, which collaborated with the UNAIDS Reference Group on Human Rights, lobbied the Commonwealth of Nations to promote law reform, with a particular focus on addressing anti-homosexuality laws in Commonwealth countries though online petitions, letters to Commonwealth Ministers of Foreign Affairs (18,000 were sent), CSO–government dialogues and media campaigns. The extensive briefing papers and reports produced by the programme and its partners repeatedly point out that ensuring MSM rights is essential for an effective HIV/AIDS response focused on key populations (International HIV/AIDS Alliance 2010).

Following this campaign, Foreign Ministers from Commonwealth countries agreed to recommendations that prioritized law reform for a more effective response to HIV/AIDS, though what actual laws would be changed and how was not specified. Furthermore, while HIV/AIDS CSOs celebrated the Commonwealth agreement as a success (International HIV/AIDS Alliance 2012), there have been no known positive changes in anti-homosexuality laws in Commonwealth countries since. In fact, in January 2014, Nigeria passed legislations that will punish anyone who promotes gay rights with a 10-year prison sentence – the opposite type of law to that it agreed to at the 2012 Commonwealth meeting. In this case, the identification of MSM rights with key populations approaches to the epidemic failed to move beyond global rhetoric.

Two factors limit the transformative potential of the Commonwealth campaign for MSM rights. First, the focus on legal reforms reflects a predominately liberal understanding of rights that neglects social, cultural and economic contexts. As Essa points out, "The fact is, protective laws themselves will not change the lived experience of gays in most of these countries, not in their current state, at least" (2014). High HIV/AIDS prevalence countries with legal rights for sexual minorities, such as South Africa, still suffer from extreme repression of these groups, restricting the effectiveness of HIV/AIDS interventions. Furthermore, legal protection only assists those who are "out" about their sexuality, as opposed to those who wish to keep it private. In addition to legal

prosecution, MSM who disclose their orientation in Sub-Saharan African countries report family rejection, public humiliation, harassment by authorities, and ridicule by health-care workers, challenges that require a more holistic, and culturally appropriate, rights-based response. While changing legal environments may be a step in addressing the rights of key populations, it presents a technical solution to a social problem.

Second, promoting legal change at the global level represents an attempt to interfere in governance realms (legislature and judiciary) protected by national sovereignty. As a result, in contexts where homosexuality is conceived of as a Western or neo-colonial import into African cultures, pressure to change laws can be framed as a threat to national sovereignty. Despite extensive evidence of same-sex acts and relationships in all contexts and cultures, the high levels of participation of MSM from Western contexts in the HIV/AIDS responses supports the impression that the focus on key populations rights is a Western led campaign, and resistant governments use Western dominance as an excuse to discredit rights claims (Essa 2014; Altman 2001). Such accusations are facilitated when Western leaders – such as British Prime Minister David Cameron, and US President Barack Obama – speak out about the rights of MSM, and when other donor states, such as Netherlands and Denmark, prioritize funding for HIV/AIDS programmes that promote the rights of MSM in Sub-Saharan Africa. These advocacy and funding efforts create the impression that the HIV/AIDS response is a conduit for spreading Western cultural norms to other regions, and for interfering with state sovereignty. Such interference results in a backlash, with accusations of cultural imperialism coming from both governments and some national CSOs (GHI Representative 2013 #11). While the key populations frame has drawn attention to MSM rights globally, the Western dominance of this particular aspect of the HIV/AIDS response limits its applicability in other contexts.

However, where global actors are willing to let local organizations lead, the key populations frame can be linked with local conceptions of rights to protect key populations. Recognizing the limits on global engagement around MSM rights in national contexts, a representative from the Global Fund (who has a long history of working with national and regional CSOs in Southern Africa) noted that when news emerged that an HIV/AIDS activist who had spoken about the rights of MSM on Zambian television had been arrested she cautioned the institution and other colleagues to not speak until a national response was organized:

> So I rang everyone. I alerted them and said "this is what is happening in Zambia, but no action until the Zambians tell us what to do. Because we do not want to make noise and this noise is not useful. … Your noise can be made useful, but in some instances your noise is not useful."
>
> (GHI Representative 2013 #19)

The need for national CSO leadership on this issue was respected as not only appropriate, but more effective than external involvement.

Regional HIV/AIDS CSOs, and other rights groups, took the lead in condemning the arrest of the activist. The HIV/AIDS Rights Alliance of Southern Africa (ARASA) responded by linking the denial of MSM rights with the HIV/AIDS key populations frame, with the Executive Director stating:

> Apart from being a gross violation of his right to freedom of expression, Kasonkomona's arrest and charge are particularly concerning because he was on a commercial television station, defending the rights of marginalized populations, who are not being reached by HIV services due to the criminalized nature of their sexual orientation and/or gender identity.
>
> (Clayton quoted in ARASA 2013)

ARASA used the key populations frame to legitimize its condemnation of the arrest, by linking the denial of sexual rights with the need for an effective HIV/AIDS response.

In February 2014, Kasonkomona was acquitted of the charges against him. The court ruled that he had the right to speak his opinion, even when contradicting Zambian law and cultural norms. The ruling demonstrates that by linking sexual rights with another already accepted right (of freedom of speech) Kasonkomona's release was allowed without violating cultural codes. This suggests that there maybe be further opportunities for HIV/AIDS activists to assert a rights-based response by connecting local conceptions of rights with global key populations frames.

ARASA has witnessed a shift in how its members, CSOs in Southern Africa, view sexual rights issues. Up until a few years ago ARASA partners were resistant to working on sexual rights, not only because of personal prejudices, but also out of fear of legal reprisals. However, a few years ago ARASA began dialogues with partners on sexual rights. This coincided with increased funding from donors for interventions that target key populations, and the high profile cases against HIV/AIDS activists in member countries (such as the one noted above), which members clearly identified as violating other human rights, such as freedom of speech (CSO Representative 2013 #8). One member representative explains, "All of a sudden our partners were being threatened for working on this issue and as a regional partnership, we needed to form a strong voice that stood behind these partners and said, wherever it exists, human right violations are wrong" (CSO Representative 2013 #8).

As a result, ARASA members voted for sexual rights to be their advocacy priority during 2013. They promoted this agenda in international forums, such as at the WHO and UNAIDS/UNDP Human Rights Reference group; at the regional level, through advocacy targeting the South African Development Community, and at the national level by lobbying governments, and locally by challenging homophobic attitudes. They produced reports, and engaged in advocacy activities, particularly exploring interactions between sexual rights, African cultures and Christian values. While the outcomes of these initiatives are hard to measure, the ability of ARASA to foster ongoing discussions

about key populations' rights suggests that where global solidarity around sexual identity is limited, regional and national mobilization presents possibilities when such rights are linked to domestic understandings of justice. Furthermore, it may be that the global campaigns, while creating a backlash against MSM rights, have also provided resources to build local struggles around sexual rights, fostering further potential for change.

Sex workers

HIV/AIDS CSOs have used the key populations frame to shift policy discussions around sex work. Sex workers are 14 times more likely to be infected with HIV than their peers and so are identified as a key population in the response to HIV/AIDS (UNAIDS 2013). The identification of sex workers as a key population has directed resources towards sex worker rights initiatives. Currently, HIV/AIDS programmes provide the majority of global funding for sex worker support interventions, providing crucial resources for programmes that are chronically underfunded (OSI 2006). The key populations frame has also generated government and donor attention towards sex work. Representatives from sex worker organizations in India state, "The country woke up to issues of sex workers, only when HIV became a threat. Till then, about a million female sex workers in this country were a silent minority; preferably forgotten" (Pragati 2012). The key populations frame has increased attention and resources to addressing the vulnerability of sex workers to HIV infection.

However, recognition of sex workers as a key population does not always have positive effects. Brijnath notes that the correlation between HIV and sex work "has seen an additional layer of discrimination levelled at urban women who in addition to having to endure the stigma of whore, are also characterized as repositories of infection and disease" (2007, 378). Similarly, Scambler and Paoli (2008) note that the emergence of HIV/AIDS resurrected the association of sex work with sexually transmitted infections (STIs). Such stigma is exacerbated by a continuing focus on sex workers as "the problem" with little attention paid to their clients (O'Manique 2004, 28). Negative attitudes towards sex work mean that the key populations frame within the HIV/AIDS response can be either repressive or transformative – and in practice has played out as a mix of both.

The identification of sex workers as a key population brought the HIV/AIDS response into complex struggles over conceptions of rights. Some women's organizations, as well as a number of Christian-based CSOs, argue that sex work is universally degrading and must be criminalized. These abolitionist approaches to sex work focus on enforcing legal punishments for buying and selling sex, and on providing economic alternatives for sex workers. While this approach is more acceptable within biomedical neoliberalism – because of the focus on legalities, and integration into the formal economy – and is supported by a number of religious organizations, it is generally opposed by people who do, or have, worked in the sex trade as stigmatizing, responsible for driving

sex work underground where it is more dangerous, and failing to promote the rights of sex workers who do not want to, or cannot, leave the trade (Ahmed 2011).

In contrast, advocates of a "sex-positive" approach argue that sex work should be decriminalized to ensure workers have access to public health, state protection and legal services, and that empowerment interventions should respect the rights of sex workers whether they leave the trade or not (Ahmed 2011). Sex-positive activists have used the key populations frame of the HIV/AIDS response to counter abolitionist approaches to sex work.

In 2007, when UNAIDS statements shifted from sex-positive to abolitionist approaches (probably due to American influence), NGO delegates at the UNAIDS PCB lobbied on behalf of sex worker rights. The NGO meeting report noted:

> Following the UNAIDS Guidance Note on HIV and Sex Work was released in April 2007, there has been extensive criticism from networks of sex workers and sex work projects from across the world due to the undermining of a human rights-based approach and the promotion of repressive approaches to sex work and HIV, which are known to have an adverse impact on working conditions, and increasing stigma surrounding sex work.
>
> (Quoted in Ahmed 2011, 240)

CSOs used HIV/AIDS governance forums to argue that an abolitionist approach to sex work was ineffective and repressive.

In response UNAIDS formed an advisory group with the Global Network of Sex Trade Projects. Based on the advice of this group, and continued emphasis on creating enabling legal environments for key populations, UNAIDS shifted its policies back towards decriminalization. In addition, the UNDP-led Global Commission on HIV and the Law, made up of UN and civil society actors, took up the cause of sex workers, explicitly advocating decriminalization. These actions culminated in 2013, with the WHO publishing a guide for implementing health projects with sex workers, which openly called for decriminalization and a rights-based response. By arguing that a sex-positive approach to sex work was essential to an effective global HIV/AIDS response, HIV/AIDS and sex-worker rights CSOs were able to influence the policies and statements of GHIs.

HIV/AIDS CSOs then aimed to use global forums and principles to influence national policies. As Ahmed writes, "sex-positive feminists are attempting to use top-down global governance structures to constrain the power of national authorities at the state and local level" (2011, 240). For example, following the Human Rights Reference Group's campaigns and UNAIDS' shift in policy to promote decriminalization of sex work, CSOs were able to convince Vietnam to stop putting sex workers in rehabilitation centres (GHI representative 2013 #32). Global HIV/AIDS governance forums have become a site of struggle

where the key populations frame draws attention to sex worker rights, and creates opportunities to influence national policies.

However, the influence of these global processes is less notable in high-income countries. In February 2014, the European Parliament voted in favour of a resolution to adopt the Nordic model towards sex work throughout the region, putting pressure on member states to revise their stance on sex work in line with this policy. The Nordic model – so named because it is implemented in Sweden, Norway and Iceland – criminalizes buying and benefiting from the profits of sex work, but does not criminalize selling sex. This approach is supported by some radical feminists, who argue any subjugation of a woman's body is violence against all women, and by religious groups who view it as punishing the purchasers of sex, not those selling sex, who they argue are victims (Ahmed 2011). Supporters of the Nordic model argue prostitution is inherently wrong and that all sex workers are victims, forced into the trade by others or circumstances; while sex workers should not be punished themselves, prostitution ought to be eliminated by decreasing demand through criminalizing buying sex.

The Nordic model contradicts both WHO and UNAIDS policy, and is generally condemned by sex worker organizations and HIV/AIDS CSOs as inhibiting, not supporting, a rights-based approach to sex work and HIV/AIDS. Because the Nordic model prohibits buying sex, workers are isolated to obscure locations where their clients are not at risk of getting caught. In such places sex workers are less able to screen potentially dangerous clients, such as those who do not want to use condoms or who are violent. Clients are also unlikely to report abuse they may witness in brothels for fear of prosecution. Because the Nordic model prohibits benefiting from the income of sex workers, workers cannot employ bodyguards to protect themselves from unprotected and violent sex (Ka Hon Chu & Glass 2013). According to key informants, the Nordic model increases risk of HIV infection and prohibits sex workers from accessing health services: "We have seen so much evidence that the control sex workers have over their working conditions, including protecting themselves from HIV, has a huge impact in driving this wedge between sex workers and health care" (CSO Representative 2014 #37).

A coalition of 450 civil society organizations and 45 researchers protested against the European Parliament's acceptance of the Nordic model (ICRSE 2014). Some member states, such as Germany, have also publicly expressed resistance to the Nordic model. However, the European Parliament's adoption of this approach demonstrates the limits of global guidelines – such as those promoted by UNAIDS and WHO – to influence regional processes.

The concept of the Nordic model has spread across the Atlantic, where struggles for rights-based approaches to sex work gain little traction from international process. For example, the Canadian HIV/AIDS Legal Network played a key role on the UNAIDS Human Rights Reference Group and Global Commission on HIV/AIDS and the law, promoting decriminalization of sex work as best HIV/AIDS practice. It also played a key role in efforts to

reform sex-work conditions in Canada. However the Legal Network has not had the same influence with its own government as with the GHIs.

In 2007, the HIV/AIDS Legal Network combined forces with other CSOs to take the Canadian government to court over existing sex work-related legislation, which it argued violated the country's Charter of Rights and Freedoms, by forcing sex workers to work in unsafe locations and prohibiting them from taking measures to protect themselves (both working out of a brothel and hiring a bodyguard were prohibited under the legislation, forcing workers on to the streets without any security). In December 2013, the Supreme Court ruled in favour of the plaintiff, and gave the Canadian government one year to develop new legislation that ensured sex workers could exercise their constitutional rights (Bennett 2013). This decision was heralded by HIV/AIDS and sex worker CSOs as an opportunity to decriminalize sex work, in line with the global standards set by the WHO and UNAIDS.

The new legislation, introduced in May 2014 and deemed "a Canadian Model" by the government, reflects many aspects of the Nordic Model, while also criminalizing further activities related to sex work, such as communicating for the purposes of selling sex in certain locations and prohibiting the advertising of sexual services. Both Canadian and global HIV/AIDS and sex worker rights CSOs argue these provisions contradict a rights-based approach to HIV prevention and sex work (Smith 2014). During the 2015 federal election the Liberal Party promised to revisit the legislation but, having won the election, has yet to do so. Meanwhile, CSOs are bringing another constitutional challenge against the legislation. This is expected to take between three and five years, and as one representative of a CSO preparing for this eventuality notes:

> The sad reality is that in the meantime circumstances on the ground for sex workers are not going to change. These laws go further than the previous laws did in terms of creating an environment where sex workers are far more vulnerable to exploitation and violence.
>
> (CSO Representative 2014, #37)

Debates over approaches to sex work within HIV/AIDS responses have been most contentious within the US government's global HIV/AIDS programme, PEPFAR, where CSOs have taken opposing stances. When PEPFAR was formed under the Bush administration in 2003 it brought together a diverse group of allies – ranging from gay rights groups to evangelical Christian CSOs. In particular Evangelical groups had "significant impact" in determining how then President George W. Bush understood the epidemic and appropriate responses to it (Diven 2009, 253; Dietrich 2007). A large portion of the Christian-based CSOs that influenced the formation and delivery of PEPFAR had a history of engaging in anti-trafficking initiatives, and argued that all sex workers were essentially trafficked victims. During the development of the Leadership Act to form PEPFAR, with prompting from such CSOs, Republican Congressman Christopher Smith proposed an amendment which became known as the

Anti-Prostitution Pledge. The pledge mandated that organizations receiving PEPFAR funding explicitly oppose prostitution and sex trafficking, and banned PEPFAR recipients from promoting or advocating decriminalization of sex work. This language was nearly identical to the Trafficking Victims Protection Act drafted in 2000 by evangelical Christian CSOs. The amendment was included, and Christian CSOs ensured it was implemented. In 2005, the Christian Medical Association, Alabama Physicians for Life, World Religion and the Traditional Values Coalition sent a letter to President Bush, urging him to resist any efforts to remove the Anti-Prostitution Pledge (Ahmed 2011, 245).

For HIV/AIDS CSOs the pledge restricted a rights-based approach to HIV/AIDS programming, denying services to a key population affected by the epidemic. HIV/AIDS and women's rights organizations (such as the International Women's Health Coalition) submitted letters to Health and Human Services expressing concern about the Anti-Prostitution Pledge, and seeking clarification on what the pledge meant by opposing prostitution. Organizations asked if this extended to conducting research on sex workers' vulnerability to HIV, and on providing support to sex work collectives to better protect themselves and access health services, but did not receive clear answers. In 2007, 170 individuals and organizations, including the Global Network of Sex Work Projects, submitted another letter seeking further clarification. The response was again vague and maintained language that conflated sex work with trafficking, and opposed any form of support for decriminalization (Ahmed 2011).

A coalition of rights-based CSOs (including the Alliance for Open Society International, the Open Society Institute, Pathfinder International, the Global Health Council, and Interaction) then filed a lawsuit against PEPFAR, arguing that the prostitution pledge violated the First Amendment because it compelled recipients to adopt the government's viewpoint and restricted freedom of speech (Ahmed 2011). In May 2013, after 10 years, the US Supreme Court ruled that the prostitution oath did violate the First Amendment. While HIV/AIDS, sex worker and women's rights CSOs celebrated this apparent victory, their success was immediately squashed by a narrow interpretation of the ruling, which determined that the pledge could not be required of US based organizations, but could still apply to foreign and affiliate organizations. Therefore, for example, CARE US did not have to sign the pledge, but Care Botswana did. As a result, the pledge was essentially still in effect; still included in PEPFAR contracts, and still being signed by recipients of PEPFAR funding. HIV/AIDS CSO representatives involved were "mystified" by the interpretation of the ruling, and unable to comprehend the political reasoning behind it. One informant reflects:

> It is a great example of how agonizingly slow advocacy is. And how even when you get a big high profile win, like the supreme court of finding the clause unconstitutional as applied, you still have to keep fighting for forever. You never really get to pop Champagne.
>
> (CSO Representative 2013 #31)

However, in January 2015, after further campaigns and legal battles by CSOs InterAction and Pathfinder International, the Supreme Court ruled that the "first amendment doesn't stop at the US boarder" (Krueger 2015). In other words, PEPFAR could not force overseas affiliates of American organizations to sign the pledge (though it could still force foreign organizations). This was finally heralded as a success in increasing access to HIV/AIDS resources for sex workers, and in fighting stigma and discrimination towards them. The long campaign to remove the prostitution pledge demonstrates how campaigns for key population rights at the global level can have only limited impact on national policies (even where they relate to and impact global health), which have to be fought through local processes.

The other population – women

The experiences of HIV/AIDS CSOs in advocating the rights of sex workers as a key population demonstrates the limits of applying global frames to regional and national struggles. A further limitation relates to those human rights issues that do not fit within the key population paradigm – such as women's rights. Women, though the majority of PWAs (making up 60 per cent of PWA worldwide), are not a "key population" in their own right, but are only so in specific circumstances (particularly when they are giving birth or breastfeeding). Despite concerted efforts by HIV/AIDS CSOs, women's rights have remained a neglected priority within the rights-based response, a marginalization that the key populations frame continues, as opposed to overcoming.

As the early HIV/AIDS response focused on the plight of gay men in Western countries, attention to the initial impact of the epidemic on women was delayed (O'Manique 2004, 22). However, as data from Sub-Saharan Africa improved, and evidence emerged that, in the context of a generalized epidemic, women were most vulnerable, calls for specific attention to the biological and social factors that put women at risk developed. HIV/AIDS CSOs, especially in Sub-Saharan Africa, began linking arguments for women's rights with the rights frame of the HIV/AIDS response. This frame convergence occurred at an opportune time: the rise of HIV/AIDS on international agendas coincided with increased attention to women's rights; the international women's rights movement achieved status in global governance forums with the Beijing Declaration in 1995, the same year UNAIDS was formed. Braun and Dreiling write, "With support from transnational networks and international agencies, the re-framing of women's grievances into a human rights language occurred as the HIV/AIDS crisis peaked" (2010, 468).

Women's rights activists recognized that in order to achieve long-standing goals around women's sexual and reproductive rights they needed to cooperate with other organizations, international institutions and social movements, and found allies in the HIV/AIDS response (Tallis 2012). The creation of organizations such as UNAIDS and the Global Fund provided opportunities for women's rights focused CSOs to participate in global forums, "bringing

together women's rights claims with health" (Braun & Dreiling 2010, 469). CSOs concerned with women's rights dedicated time and resources to engaging in these processes by serving on boards and advisory bodies, and participating in organizations such as the Global Commission on Women and HIV/AIDS. The relative openness of HIV/AIDS institutions to civil society participation, and adoption of human rights frames, suggested that the global HIV/AIDS response could provide an opportunity to advance women's rights. However, the ability of CSOs to use HIV/AIDS governance institutions as an entry point to transform women's rights was restricted by the dominance of state power. Describing early efforts within WHO, Booth (1998) argues that "femocrats" were caught in a contradiction of promoting a global vision of social and political change, and pressure to conform to organizational norms that prioritized state sovereignty. Within these norms there were few opportunities to challenge state policies to advance women's health-related rights.

While it might be argued that a more multi-actor approach has developed since Booth's analysis in 1998, women's rights advocates engaged with current GHIs continue to struggle to promote women's rights. A review of the primary institutions in the global governance of the HIV/AIDS response (UNAIDS, PEPFAR, World Bank, WHO and Global Fund), suggests efforts to advance women's rights have had limited impacts in a context that is dominated by state priorities (Fleischman 2008, 5). For example, Fleischman notes that:

> World Bank officials stress that the institution is demand driven i.e. directed by the expressed needs of their clients – national governments – and that its assistance is developed largely in consultation with these governments, with some civil society participation, and in collaboration with other development partners and donors. Accordingly, the issues of both gender and AIDS have to be prioritized by the country itself, which is not often the case.
>
> (2008, 7)

Similarly, a CSO representative who advocates greater attention to women's rights in the UNAIDS PCB notes that:

> it is pretty difficult to tell a country want to do – Egypt and Iran and some of the other countries. … And one of the things, especially Egypt keeps popping up, [and saying] well that's interfering with sovereignty, you are telling us how to run our country.
>
> (CSO Representative 2013 #15)

Advocates of women's rights have been unable to overcome the rigidity of state-based systems that respond to the interests of governments before women affected by HIV/AIDS (whose interests are rarely represented by government). As a result, as one advocate notes:

I don't know that the AIDS response has made any huge, significant changes [in relation to women's rights], but I think what it has done is brought to the surface more for the discussion. It has raised awareness around it more and they are certainly pushing it more in their policies, it is just getting countries to do anything about it.

(CSO Representative 2013 #15)

HIV/AIDS institutions have not proven to be a fruitful site for struggles towards greater gender equality.

The Global Fund, with its public–private partnership model, suggests an opportunity to challenge state dominance. However, an NGO observer to the Global Fund also notes that "they use country ownership as an excuse for not addressing women's rights" (CSO Representative 2013 #25). At the 2011 Partnership Forum, CSOs attempted to overcome this resistance by recommending that the Fund develop a gender strategy, which it did. It then hired one person (in a Secretariat of over 200) to implement this strategy, did not provide a budget for implementation, and did not communicate the strategy to staff, fund recipients, donors or other partners (ATHENA 2013). Therefore, it is not surprising that three subsequent external evaluations of the gender strategy were damning. The most recent review, led by the ATHENA Network of southern based CSOs involved in HIV/AIDS and gender interventions, said that the strategy was "commendably progressive on paper", but that it had not been adequately budgeted, that its implementation had been limited, and that no adequate communications strategy had been launched to explain or promote it (2013, 1). As a result, "many people remain unaware of the existence of the GES and the importance assigned to addressing gender equality through the Global Fund" (ATHENA 2013, 2). This lack of follow-through on commitments to promoting gender equality demonstrates the persistent neglect of women's rights in the largest donor organization of the HIV/AIDS response.

The increased focus on key populations threatens to exacerbate this marginalization of women's rights agendas within the global governance of the HIV/AIDS response, and to divert attention and resources. While women and girls are occasionally mentioned in definitions of key populations (most notably in Global Fund documents), most often they are not. For example, both the WHO's and USAID's definitions of key populations do not include women (WHO 2014; USAID 2015).

In a context of perceived resources scarcity, the key populations frame diverts HIV/AIDS resources and attention away from struggles for women's rights. For example, CSOs from Southern Africa report that they are having to shift resources away from programmes that focus on women to those that focus on key population groups: "Because the LGTB advocacy and the advocacy around key populations is really strong, some of the money is shifting that way ... funding for home-based care and women is decreasing" (CSO Representative 2013 #8). This shift exacerbates burdens on caregivers,

the vast majority of whom are predominantly women. A Kaiser Foundation survey found that over two-thirds of primary caregivers for PWAs were women (Peacock & Weston 2008, 2); a South African national evaluation of home-based care found 91 per cent of caregivers were women (Chella 2006, 8).

In many high prevalence countries in Sub-Saharan Africa, these women provide the majority of HIV/AIDS care work, as public health systems are generally unable to meet health care needs. In Zimbabwe, an evaluation of community responses found that unpaid volunteers provided 69 per cent of human resources for local CSOs (Katietek 2012). Another study found that volunteers made up more than half of the staff in locally based HIV/AIDS CSOs (International HIV/AIDS Alliance 2010). Most care workers receive little to no support from GHIs or states. They might receive stipends but these are often insufficient and inconsistent. Similarly care programmes report struggling to access basic supplies. Furthermore, Esplen (2009) notes that most HIV/AIDS programmes do not address the gendered nature of care work. In 2010 only 12 per cent of the global HIV/AIDS resources directed to treatment and care interventions went to supporting home-based care programmes (UNAIDS 2011a).

As a result of the lack of meaningful support for care work, caregivers sacrifice their own resources, time and opportunities to care for the sick, exacerbating their own poverty and vulnerability to HIV infection. Rau notes that, "while governments and international institutions have argued for more money to support HIV/AIDS programs and bureaucracies, civil society (individuals, families and local organizations) have remained the largest funders of HIV/AIDS activities" (2006, 293). Household expenditures include the cost of clean water, food, primary health care and transportation to health care. These costs differ based on geography and available social services, and so cannot be generalized, but are essential in all cases of HIV/AIDS care. In the absence of proper equipment, such as gloves, caregivers are exposed to HIV infection when performing care tasks (Akintola 2004, 3). Caregivers may also experience increased risk of rape due to having to travel alone in insecure environments to care for the ill (Akintola 2006, 242). With little donor recognition of, or provision for, community-based care, and continued reliance on volunteers who receive little more than training and basic supplies, those who provide the majority of HIV/AIDS care services – impoverished women – are not seen as a key population, and continue to be neglected in the global distribution of HIV/AIDS resources.

Within current global HIV/AIDS policy, women are only identified as "key" to the HIV/AIDS response as mothers who might pass on the virus to their children. Booth (1998) argues that the HIV/AIDS response frames women as either "mothers or whores", and in either case as a source of infection. In other words, women's issues are only considered if they are sex workers (within the confines discussed above) or mothers, but the general experience of women living with and affected by HIV is neglected.

Global programmes reflect this perception, placing a particular emphasis on preventing vertical transmission (from mother to child), obscuring principles of women's right to health for its own sake. For example, UNAIDS and PEPFAR

implemented a "Global Plan Towards the Elimination of New Infections Among Children by 2015 and Keeping Their Mothers Alive". In response to a plan report, the President of CSO Family Care International expressed frustration that it "almost completely ignores the second target [keeping mother's alive]", and goes on to note that the 15 page report only includes one "glancing" reference to the fact that women have the right to ART for their own sake (Starrs 2013). Her commentary represents a continued frustration by women's rights advocates around the failure of HIV/AIDS interventions and policies to recognize women's rights as essential to the response, beyond their role as mothers. The identification of women as key to the HIV/AIDS response only when they are pregnant or breastfeeding fails to transform ideas about women's right to health – and neglects HIV positive women who are not mothers.

The recent rollout of Option B+ demonstrates the continued lack of consideration of women's rights and focus on vertical transmission. Option B+ is the method of starting HIV positive pregnant women on treatment even when their CD4 count is above 350 (the usual threshold for starting treatment), and keeping them on treatment for the duration of their life. This differs from Option A and Option B, under which women stop treatment after having given birth or stopped breast feeding respectively, and then return to treatment when their CD4 count falls below 350 (UNICEF 2013). The rationale is that this introduces treatment when women are in health facilities, access they may not normally enjoy, and is highly effective in preventing vertical transmission. It also includes a simplified ART regime of one pill, as opposed to the combination methods provided to pregnant women in better-resourced contexts. Option B+ is deemed cost-effective: "potentially saving more than 250,000 maternal life years, compared to other practices of preventing vertical transmission, and yields incremental cost effectiveness ratios of US$ 455 per life year gained over current practices" (Fasawe et al. 2013, e57778). A further benefit is that PWAs on ART are less likely to pass on HIV to sexual partners – therefore Option B+ has prevention impacts. As a result, Option B+ is celebrated by UNAIDS, UNICEF and WHO as a powerful new tool for preventing vertical infection. A UNICEF document reads:

> this new approach called "Option B+" has already begun to show impressive results in "real world", resource-constrained settings, dramatically increasing the numbers of pregnant women enrolling on ART. The tide is turning – now is the time to move with the momentum and embrace a bold public health approach to effectively eliminate new paediatric HIV infections.
>
> (2013, 2)

To date, Option B+ has been implemented in Malawi, since 2011, and in Uganda, since 2012.

While not opposed to Option B+, HIV/AIDS and women's rights CSOs point out a number of contradictions within approaches to rolling it out and are attempting to influence delivery to include a greater rights focus.

A primary concern is that Option B+ lacks adequate consideration of the implications of starting ART earlier than necessary on women's long-term wellbeing. The chances of PWAs developing drug resistance and side effects increase the longer they are on ART. In the general PWA population about 20 per cent of people on ART develop drug resistance, requiring more expensive (and therefore less available) second line medications. Research from Malawi indicates that women who start treatment as Option B+ are more likely to be lost to follow up than women who start on Option A or B, and therefore are at greater risk of drug resistance (and therefore AIDS related death) (Landes et al. 2012). This suggests that Option B+, while having immediate benefits for infants, may have negative long-term outcomes in terms of drug resistance for mothers.

In order to influence policy discussions around Option B+, ICW and GNP+ conducted research in Uganda and Malawi with pregnant women. Evidence from these focus groups notes that women understand Option B+ to be primarily about protecting the baby from infection, not the wellbeing of the mother, which "caused concern among some participants" (ICW & GNP+ 2013, 2). Such findings expose the assumption that women will ultimately sacrifice their own wellbeing for that of the child, an assumption that Option B+ proponents capitalize on. The research further demonstrates that Option B+ is implemented in a way that denies pregnant women an informed choice. As one CSO representative stated, "These women wouldn't generally have a choice. You don't get asked if you would like to be on medication. You can get forced into it" (CSO Representative 2013 #15). The research report notes that:

> Despite being called an "option", Option B+ is being offered as the only available method in Malawi to prevent vertical transmission. Pregnant women were generally expected to start treatment as soon as they tested HIV positive, either the same day or within a week, but often did not receive enough information to understand the choices involved. Women reported little or no support to make decisions about their treatment.
>
> (GNP+ & ICW 2013, 3)

Many women feel ill-informed about Option B+, what it entails and what it means for their and their children's health. This contradicts the rights-based principles of the HIV/AIDS response, as promoted by CSOs, of patient empowerment and participation in decision-making.

CSO research also illuminated broader community equity issues inherent in the Option B+ approach, which are largely ignored by state and institutional proponents. Focus group participants expressed concern over increased risk of gender-based violence, due to unequal treatment access – making explicit the consequences of providing treatment for mothers but not for fathers (GNP+ & ICW 2013). As there is no global goal to prevent paternal HIV related deaths (to keep fathers alive), men are not prioritized for treatment, which

can create resentment and violence within families. The failure to provide treatment for fathers also illustrates rigid conceptions of gender roles, which prioritize women as child carriers and caregivers, failing to consider that fathers are also essential family members who contribute to the wellbeing of mothers and infants. Furthermore, as Coutsoudis et al. (2013) note, prioritizing pregnant women over non-pregnant women and men who may have higher viral loads, raises ethical issues and may contribute to community conflicts and impact behaviours (for example, encouraging HIV positive women to get pregnant, in order to access treatment). While the argument can be made that in contexts of resource scarcity certain lives have to be prioritized, the Option B+ triage approach to ART delivery produces multiple consequences, some including rights violations that are not acknowledged or mitigated within the current rollout programme.

Women's rights advocates are concerned that the WHO and national health programmes are primarily promoting Option B+ because it is cost effective and has immediate efficiency gains:

> From a public health perspective it is easier to just put a person on a pill, rather than monitoring ok, this person has a CD4 of 600, let's put them on medications until after the baby, then they come off the medications. That's all too complicated so let's put them all on meds.
>
> (CSO Representative 2013 #15)

Advocates note the contradiction of claiming cost efficiency and lives saved, when the effects on women starting treatment early, and on infants breast-feeding while their mothers are on treatment, remain largely unknown: "The business case, which supports use of Option B+ in resource-limited settings, does not fully address four critical considerations: ethics, medical safety and benefits, program feasibility, and economic concerns" (Coutsoudis et al. 2013, 269). CSO representatives argue that Option B+ is based on untested assumptions that low recruitment costs will balance out the costs of prolonged medical care and increased risk of drug resistance, with little concern for the long-term wellbeing of the women involved.

The rollout of Option B+ raises questions around who claims success and how, highlighting the "disjuncture between the assumed ideal governance of the disease and people's needs to obtain healthy lives" (Seckinelgin 2012b, 453). In the case of Option B+, preventing vertical transmission is deemed successful even if it has long-term negative impacts on mother and infant wellbeing. For example, a UNICEF and WHO document reports:

> Malawi envisioned that Option B+ would be easier to implement due to its simple "one size fits all" approach which would enable women to access ART at high levels even in settings with poor access to CD4 testing. The early experience with Option B+ in Malawi has borne this out, being extraordinarily successful, with a more than fivefold increase in the

numbers of pregnant women being enrolled on ART in only the first quarter of full nationwide implementation.

(2013, 3)

Success in this statement is based on increased numbers of women on ART without considering how many of these women actually required ART for their own health, will have to deal with side effects and adverse impacts on their wellbeing because of ART, and are at risk of drug resistance. Having more mothers on ART demonstrates progress to achieving international goals, but not necessarily improved wellbeing for mother and infant.

Questioning such claims, CSOs continue to voice concerns that Option B+ interventions need to include a stronger and more holistic women's health and rights focus. A global women's rights advocate summarizes:

> It's just like, [the organizations say] we just need to fix this right now ... and the voice of positive people is just bring everyone back and said "have you thought of this, and have you thought of that?" And you need to think of this and you need to think of that. And also bringing it back to human rights.
>
> (CSO Representative 2013 #15)

It is unclear if women's rights advocates will be able to bring the response "back to human rights" but they continue to try. While it is too early to determine the outcomes of CSO efforts to impact Option B+ rollout, efforts are underway to scale up Option B+ in Sub-Saharan Africa.

As Tallis (2012) writes:

> Without an understanding of power inequalities, especially in intimate relationships which essentially provide the framing for sexual and reproductive issues, mainstreaming sexual and reproductive health and rights can only improve the health of the women they reach and will do little to shift the status quo.

The lack of critical consideration of power inequalities is apparent in institutional approaches to women's rights, and through the predominately biomedical endeavours that focus on vertical prevention, as opposed to women's rights and wellbeing. The key populations frame does little to challenge persistent gender inequality, at best considering women "key" only when they are pregnant and within the biomedical confines of reproductive health. Through continued CSO advocacy these contradictions are exposed.

Chapter conclusion

From 2012 on, the concept of ending AIDS began to be used within the global HIV/AIDS response. This frame attempted to re-galvanize support within the

post-exceptionalism context but raised difficult questions about the role of HIV/ AIDS CSOs in "post-AIDS" GHG, as their participation had been justified based on exceptionalism. As biomedical and technical approaches were heralded as the solution to ending the epidemic, CSOs found space for social and political projects shrinking. As the case of the development of the SDGs demonstrates, in the post-AIDS exceptionalism context of reasserted biomedical neoliberalism, both the human rights frame and the role of HIV/AIDS CSOs have become vulnerable.

In response to this shifting context, HIV/AIDS CSOs, in collaboration with institutions and donor states, promote the frame of key populations. The key populations frame enables an uneasy marriage between human rights and biomedical neoliberalism, and justifies continued CSO participation in global HIV/AIDS governance. HIV/AIDS CSOs have used this opportunity to advance the rights of key populations in global forums, advocating acceptance of harm reduction for PWID, campaigning for the end of repressive laws against MSM, and challenging abolitionist approaches to sex work. These governance struggles interact with regional, national and local rights struggles with varying outcomes. For PWID, global mobilization around harm reduction has increased opportunities for engagement in governance processes and greater access to harm reduction services, but local CSOs still struggle within repressive environments. For MSM, top down approaches have resulted in a backlash against Western led HIV/AIDS responses, raising questions about the appropriateness and utility of global frames in addressing rights related to personal experiences and cultural understandings. However, there is evidence of local CSOs linking sexual rights with local rights frames more successfully. The increased attention to sex work has advanced rights-based policies at the global level, but these have had little influence on regional and national policy contexts, illustrating the greater opportunities CSOs find in promoting change in global institutions as opposed to states. The recent changes in PEPFAR demonstrate the continued potential for transformation through CSO activism.

While the key populations frame has created continued space for rights claims in global HIV/AIDS governance, how these global struggles interact with the lived realities of those affected by HIV/AIDS is by no means straightfor ward, or necessarily transformative. This is most clear in relation to those groups whose rights do not fit within this paradigm – the most obvious example being women. Despite the fact that women make up the majority of PWAs, provide the majority of HIV/AIDS related care work, and are most at risk of infection, women's rights have been and continue to be neglected by the HIV/AIDS response, except for where they relate to biological maternal functions. While HIV/AIDS CSOs have attempted to promote a more holistic approach to women's rights, so far – as is demonstrated by the rollout of Option B+ – they have had little success beyond exposing current contradictions.

References

Action for Global Health (2009), Achieving the Health MDGs by 2015: What the EU Needs to Do! available at: http://www.actionforglobalhealth.eu/our-work/health-m dgs.html (accessed 15 December 2015).

Ahmed, A. (2011), "Feminism, Power, and Sex Work in the Context of HIV/AIDS: Consequences for Women's Health", *Harvard Journal of Law & Gender*, Vol. 34, pp. 225–258.

Akintola, O. (2004), *A Gendered Analysis of the Burden of Care on Family and Volunteer Caregivers in Uganda and South Africa*, Health Economics and HIV/AIDS Research Division, Durban.

Akintola, O. (2006), "Gendered Home-based Care in South Africa: More Trouble for the Troubled", *African Journal of AIDS Research*, Vol. 5 No. 3, pp. 237–247.

Altman, D. (2001), *Global Sex*, University of Chicago Press, Chicago.

amfAR (2013), *Tackling HIV/AIDS Among Key Populations: Essential to Achieving an AIDS-Free Generation*, amfAR Public Policy Office, Washington D.C.

ARASA (2013), *Press Statement: African Civil Society Groups Condemn Limitation of Freedom of Expression in Zambia*, Windhoek, Namibia, available at: http://www.ara sa.info/news/press-statement/ (accessed 15 December 2015).

ATHENA (2013), Strengthening Women's Engagement with the Global Fund to Champion Gender Equality through the New Funding Model and Beyond, available at: http://asapltd.com/wp-content/uploads/2013/08/GF-Gender-Outcomes_Document_FINAL_26July.pdf (accessed 15 December 2015).

Bennett, D. (2013), *Canada v. Bedford – The Decision in 705 Words*, Vancouver, available at: http://www.pivotlegal.org/canada_v_bedford_a_synopsis_of_the_sup reme_court_of_canada_ruling (accessed 15 December 2015).

Booth, K. (1998), "National Mother, Global Whore, and Transnational Femocrats: The Politics of AIDS and the Construction of Women at the World Health Organization", *Feminist Studies*, Vol. 24 No. 1, pp. 115–139.

Braun, Y. and Dreiling, M. (2010), "From Developmentalism to the HIV/AIDS Crisis", *International Feminist Journal of Politics*, Vol. 12 No. 3, pp. 464–483.

Brijnath, B. (2007), "It's about TIME. Engendering AIDS in Africa", *Culture, Health & Sexuality*, Vol. 9 No. 4, pp. 371–386.

Buse, K., Blackshaw, R. and Ndayisaba, M.G. (2012), "Zeroing in on AIDS and Global Health Post-2015", *Globalization and Health*, Vol. 8 No. 1, p. 42.

Chella, A. (2006), *Reducing the Burden of HIV and AIDS Care on Women and Girls*, Volunteer Services Overseas, London.

Coutsoudis, A., Goga, A., Desmond, C., Barron, P., Black, V. and Coovadia, H. (2013), "Is Option B+ the Best Choice?", *The Lancet*, Vol. 381 No. 9863, pp. 269–271.

Cullinan, K. (2013), "Very Far from the End of AIDS", *Health-E News*, 10 December, available at: http://www.health-e.org.za/2013/12/10/far-end-aids/ (accessed 15 December 2015).

Das, P. and Horton, R. (2012), "The Cultural Challenge of HIV/AIDS", *The Lancet*, Vol. 380 No. 9839, pp. 309–310.

Dietrich, J.W. (2007), "The Politics of PEPFAR: The President's Emergency Plan for AIDS Relief", *Ethics & International Affairs*, Vol. 21 No. 3, pp. 277–292.

Diven, P. (2009), *The Hyperpluralism of US Development Policy: Managing the Multiple Objectives of PEPFAR*, Aids Accountability, Cape Town.

England, R. (2008), "The Writing is on the Wall for UNAIDS", *British Medical Journal*, Vol. 336, p. 1072.

Epstein, H. (2007), *The Invisible Cure: Africa, the West, and the Fight against AIDS*, Penguin, London.

Esplen, E. (2009), *Gender and Care Overview Report*, Institute for Development Studies, Brighton.

Essa, A. (2014), "Homophobia: Africa's New Apartheid. Both African and Western Governments are Using Gay Rights as a Political Tool", *Al Jazeera*, 1 February, available at: http://www.aljazeera.com/indepth/opinion/2014/02/homophobia-africa -new-apartheid-20142194711993773.html (accessed 7 August 2014).

Fasawe, O., Avila, C., Shaffer, N., Schouten, E., Chimbwandira, F., Hoos, D., Nakakeeto, O., de Lay, P. and Braitstein, P. (2013), "Cost-Effectiveness Analysis of Option B+ for HIV Prevention and Treatment of Mothers and Children in Malawi", *PLoS ONE*, Vol. 8 No. 3, p. e57778.

Fee, E. (1995), "Understanding AIDS: Historical Interpretations and the Limits of Biomedical Individualism", *American Journal of Public Health*, Vol. 83 No. 10, pp. 1477–1486.

Fleischman, H. (2008), *An Analysis of the Gender Policies of the Three Major AIDS Financing Institutions: The Global Fund to Fight AIDS, Tuberculosis and Malaria, the World Bank and the President's Emergency Plan for AIDS Relief*, UNAIDS, Geneva.

GFATM (2014), *Community Systems Strengthening Framework*, Geneva, available at: www.theglobalfund.org/.../core/framework/Core_CSS_Framework_en (accessed 15 December 2015)

Harman, S. (2012), *Global Health Governance*, Routledge, New York.

Horton, R. (2012), "Offline: The Rights and Wrongs of 'an AIDS-free Generation'", *The Lancet*, Vol. 380 No. 9839, p. 324.

ICRSE (2014), *560 NGOs and 94 Researchers Demand Members of European Parliament To Reject Ms Honeyball Report*, Brussels, available at: http://www.sexworkeurop e.org/news/general-news/560-ngos-and-94-researchers-demand-members-european-pa rliament-reject-ms-honeyball (accessed 15 December 2015)

ICW and GNP+ (2013), *Understanding the Perspectives and/or Experiences of Women Living with HIV Regarding Option B+ in Uganda and Malawi*, Global Network of People Living with HIV/AIDS, Amsterdam.

IHRA (2009), *Harm Reduction and Human Rights: The Global Response to Drug-Related HIV Epidemics*, International Harm Reduction Association, London.

International HIV/AIDS Alliance (2010), *Mapping of Funding Mechanisms and Main Sources of Funding for the Community Response to HIV and AIDS*, International HIV/AIDS Alliance, Brighton.

International HIV/AIDS Alliance (2012), *Success! Commonwealth Agreement*, International HIV/AIDS Alliance, Brighton.

Ka Hon Chu, S. and Glass, R. (2013), "Sex Work Law Reform in Canada: Considering Problems with the Nordic Model", *Alberta Law Review*, Vol. 51 No. 1, pp. 101–124.

Katietek, J. (2012), *Flow of Funds in Community-based Organizations in Kenya, Nigeria and Zimbabwe*, World Bank, Washington D.C.

Krueger, S. (2015), A Striking Defeat for U.S. Government's Anti-Prostitution Pledge, available at: https://www.opensocietyfoundations.org/voices/striking-defeat-us-go vernment-s-anti-prostitution-pledge (accessed 15 December 2015).

Landes, M., van Lettow, M., Bedell, R., Mayuni, I., Chan, A.K., Tenthani, L., Schouten, E. and Wools-Kaloustian, K.K. (2012), "Mortality and Health Outcomes

in HIV-Infected and HIV-Uninfected Mothers at 18–20 Months Postpartum in Zomba District, Malawi", *PLoS ONE*, Vol. 7 No. 9, p. e44396.

Lines, R. and Elliot, R. (2007), "Injecting Drugs into Human Rights Advocacy", *International Journal of Drug Policy*, Vol. 18, pp. 453–457.

Morin, J.F. (2011), "The Life-Cycle of Transnational Issues: Lessons from the Access to Medicines Controversy", *Global Society*, Vol. 25 No. 2, pp. 227–247.

NGO Delegation (2013), *32nd PCB Communique*, Geneva, available at: http://www.unaidspcbngo.org/category/communiques/ (accessed 15 December 2015).

NGO Delegation (2014), *The 34th Meeting of the UNAIDS Programme Coordinating Board Communique*, Geneva, http://www.unaidspcbngo.org/category/communiques/ (accessed 15 December 2015).

Nguyen, V.K. (2010), *The Republic of Therapy: Triage and Sovereignty in West Africa's Time of AIDS, Body, Commodity, Text*, Duke University Press, Durham, NC.

Nilo, A. (2013), *The Post 2015 Agenda – Keep Both of Your Eyes On It!*, NGO Delegation to UNAIDS, Geneva, available at: http://www.icad-cisd.com/pdf/Announcements/NGO-PCB-Newsletter-November.pdf (accessed 15 December 2015).

Nolen, S. (2009), *28: Stories of AIDS in Africa*, Vintage Canada, Toronto.

O'Manique, C. (2004), *Neoliberalism and AIDS Crisis in Sub-Saharan Africa: Globalization's Pandemic*, Palgrave Macmillan, New York.

ONE (2012), *The Beginning of the End? Tracking Global Commitments on AIDS*, ONE, Washington D.C.

OSI (2006). *Sex Worker Health and Rights: Where is the Funding?* Open Society and Rights Project, New York.

Peacock, D. and Weston, M. (2008), *Men and Care in the Context of HIV and AIDS: Structure, Political Will and Greater Male Involvement*, Division for the Advancement of Women, New York.

Persson, A., Ellard, J., Newman, C., Holt, M. and de Wit, J. (2011), "Human Rights and Universal Access for Men Who Have Sex with Men and People Who Inject Drugs: A Qualitative Analysis of the 2010 UNGASS Narrative Country Progress Reports", *Social Science & Medicine*, Vol. 73 No. 3, pp. 467–474.

Piot, P. and Marshall, R. (2012), *No Time to Lose: A Life in Pursuit of Deadly Viruses*, W.W. Norton & Co, New York.

Pragati (2012), *Sex Work and HIV/AIDS in India*, Bangalore, available at: http://www.swasti.org/pragati (accessed 15 December 2015).

Rau, B. (2006), "The Politics of Civil Society in Confronting HIV/AIDS", *International Affairs*, Vol. 82, pp. 285–295.

Scambler, G. and Paoli, F. (2008), "Health Work, Female Sex Workers and HIV/AIDS: Global and Local Dimensions of Stigma and Deviance as Barriers to Effective Interventions", *Social Science & Medicine*, Vol. 66 No. 8, pp. 1848–1862.

Seckinelgin, H. (2012a), "Global Civil Society as Shepherd: Global Sexualities and the Limits of Solidarity from a Distance", *Critical Social Policy*, Vol. 32 No. 4, pp. 536–555.

Seckinelgin, H. (2012b), "The Global Governance of Success in HIV/AIDS Policy: Emergency Action, Everyday Lives and Sen's Capabilities", *Health & Place*, Vol. 18 No. 3, pp. 453–460.

Smith, J. (2014), "To Help or to Hinder? Sex Work Legislation and HIV Prevention", *Rabble*, 21 March, available at: http://rabble.ca/news/2014/03/to-help-or-to-hinder-sex-work-legislation-and-hiv-prevention (accessed 8 August 2014).

Southwall, M. (2012), *31st UNAIDS Programme Coordinating Board Meeting Talking Points NGO Delegate for Europe*, UNAIDS, Geneva.

Spicer, N., Harmer, A., Aleshkina, J., Bogdan, D., Chkhatarashvili, K., Murzalieva, G., Rukhadze, N., Samiev, A. and Walt, G. (2011), "Circus Monkeys or Change Agents? Civil Society Advocacy for HIV/AIDS in Adverse Policy Environments", *Social Science & Medicine*, Vol. 73 No. 12, pp. 1748–1755.

Starrs, A. (2013), "Forgotten Women: UNAIDS, PEPFAR, and 'Keeping Mothers Alive'", *RH Reality Check*, 27 June, available at: http://rhrealitycheck.org/article/2013/06/27/forgotten-women-unaids-pepfar-and-keeping-mothers-alive/ (accessed 8 August 2014).

Tallis, V. (2012), *Feminisms, HIV, and AIDS: Subverting Power, Reducing Vulnerability*, Palgrave Macmillan, New York.

UN General Assembly (2011), *Political Declaration on HIV and AIDS: Intensifying Our Efforts to Eliminate HIV and AIDS*, UN, New York.

UNAIDS (2011a), *State of the AIDS Response*, Geneva, available at: http://www.who.int/hiv/pub/progress_report2011/en/ (accessed 15 December 2015).

UNAIDS (2011b), *Terminology Guidelines*, Geneva, http://www.unaids.org/sites/default/files/media_asset/JC2118_terminology-guidelines_en_0.pdf (accessed 15 December 2015).

UNAIDS (2013), *Global Aids Response Progress Reporting 2013: Construction of Core Indicators for Monitoring the 2011 UN Political Declaration on HIV/AIDS*, Geneva, available at: http://www.unaids.org/sites/default/files/media_asset/GARPR_2013_guidelines_en_0.pdf (accessed 15 December 2015).

UNAIDS (2014), *Ambitous Treatment Targets: Writing the Final Chapter of the AIDS Epidemic*, Geneva, available at: http://www.unaids.org/sites/default/files/media_asset/JC2670_UNAIDS_Treatment_Targets_en.pdf (accessed 15 December 2015).

UNAIDS (2015), *Fact Sheet 2015*, Geneva, available at: http://www.unaids.org/en/resources/campaigns/HowAIDSchangedeverything/factsheet (accessed 15 December 2015).

UNICEF (2013), *Evaluation Report: IAS-ILF/UNICEF Satellite Session Beyond Option B+*, UNICEF and IAS, Kuala Lampur.

USAID (2014), *What We Do*, Washington D.C., available at: https://www.usaid.gov/what-we-do/, (accessed 15 December 2015).

USAID (2015), *Key Populations: Targeted Approaches Toward An Aids-Free Generation*, Washington D.C., available at: https://www.usaid.gov/what-we-do/global-health/hiv-and-aids/technical-areas/key-populations-targeted-approaches-toward (accessed 15 December 2015).

Whiteside, A. and Smith, J. (2009), "Exceptional Epidemics: AIDS Still Deserves a Global Response", *Globalization and Health*, Vol. 5 No. 1, p. 15.

WHO (2014), *Consolidated Guidelines on HIV Prevention, Diagnosis, Treatment and Care for Key Populations*, Geneva, available at: http://www.who.int/hiv/pub/guidelines/keypopulations/en/ (accessed 15 December 2015).

World Bank (2012), *Increased Targeting of Key Populations Can Accelerate End of Global HIV Epidemic*, Washington D.C., available at: http://www.worldbank.org/en/news/press-release/2012/11/28/increased-targeting-key-populations-can-accelerate-end-global-hiv-epidemic (accessed 15 December 2015).

World We Want (2015), *NGO Perspectives on the Post-2015 Agenda for Health*, available at: http://www.beyond2015.org/world-we-want-2015-web-platform (accessed 15 December 2015).

6 Conclusion

This book has sketched, in broad strokes, the complicated history of the global response to HIV/AIDS, and the role of CSOs within it. Broad strokes were necessary because global processes respond to and interact with uncountable local and national processes. This is a history of conflicting processes, cooperation and compromises that occurred over three decades, in varying spaces, among an ever-shifting combination of actors.

This is a narrative about change. It illustrates the challenge an unknown and lethal epidemic posed to traditional biomedical health responses, and the opportunity this created for a new type of response. It describes how a unique sense of global solidarity formed, for a moment at least, around the concept of AIDS exceptionalism, setting a precedent for addressing a global health issue. It outlines how human rights frames became increasingly interlinked with biomedical neoliberalism, and shifted into discussions around key populations with both new opportunities and limitations for transformation. It presents the uneven progress of these frames – such as around harm reduction – from local to global forums, and back to national and local contexts. It explains how the failure of biomedical state-based systems, and the use of AIDS exceptionalism, allowed new, more inclusive if not transformative, institutional forms to be created, and unprecedented levels of resources to be applied.

This narrative also illustrates what has not changed – the dominance of biomedical neoliberal approaches to GHG. This has limited rights-based outcomes: PWID still receive inadequate support and are stigmatized; the rhetoric of commitment to gender equality by HIV/AIDS institutions and leaders is not translated into policy action or resources; community and rights-based groups still struggle to access resources. As the HIV/AIDS response moves from being an exception within GHG to being normalized, opportunities for change constrict, as demonstrated by the lack of explicit human rights language within the SDG health goal and reduction of funding for key populations within middle-income countries.

The overarching narrative is one of resistance within a dominant neoliberal context, and the struggles that ensued. Within these processes, CSOs have been positioned as central agents. This is just one take on a much broader story

about GHG, the role of CSOs in global processes, and struggles for human rights. It is an important one because it demonstrates that community groups, activists and INGOs are actors to be reckoned with in global forums; and that they have promoted change, even within the confines of a political economy of biomedical neoliberalism and dominant donor state power.

Throughout this history of CSO participation, contradictions (such as between the rhetoric of supporting CCS in the Global Fund's NFM and continued restrictions created by performance-based management) and opportunities (such as the creation of the Community Rights and Gender Technical Assistance Program) have been made explicit, contributing to a more nuanced understanding of the role and influence of CSOs within GHG.

Evaluating assumptions

This book began by repeating assertions about the transformative role CSOs have played within the global AIDS response and the need to learn from these examples. There are a number of assumptions within these assertions that can be evaluated in light of the evidence presented in the preceding chapters. First, is the assumption that CSOs represent those most affected by the epidemic. The HIV/AIDS response was initiated by PWAs and their allies who formed support groups, service delivery organizations and global networks. In this sense, the origins of CSO involvement in the HIV/AIDS response are bottom up. However, within the context of AIDS exceptionalism, these grassroots forces became increasingly entwined with the interests of states, institutions and other actors. Analysis of those CSOs that engage in global institutions and resources governance demonstrates a certain elitism: CSO board members at the Global Fund are a group of "good old friends"; CSO representatives without the right (i.e. Western) skill set and resources struggle to participate effectively in UNAIDS' PCB.

At the same time these "elite" CSOs have consistently advocated increased space for other CSOs – such as by promoting greater inclusion of key populations in the Country Dialogue process of the Global Fund's NFM. The ethos of promoting the participation of those most affected remains, despite structures (such as institutional bureaucracies and northern consolidations of power) that restrict local and national access to global governance forums and processes. Marginalized populations, such as PWIDs, have been able to use the human rights and key populations framing of the response to access global governance processes and spaces.

CSOs have also continued to advocate a rights-based response to the epidemic, suggesting that even if the majority of organizations that engage in global governance processes do not directly represent marginalized and affected constituencies, they do aim to represent their interests. CSOs have pushed for global policies that create enabling legal environments; have worked with the Global Fund to direct resources towards key populations; and have fought

PEPFAR policies that deny HIV/AIDS resources to sex workers. While CSO participation in the global governance of the HIV/AIDS response does not inherently, or consistently, represent those most affected, CSO participants continue to create and seize opportunities to advance the rights-based response that community groups initiated.

The subsequent question is then, has this participation (which aims to represent, if not be representative of a broader constituency) substantially changed GHG? The argument here is that CSO participation has promoted potential alternatives within the dominant order, and maintained space for further transformations. The most apparent example of change is the CSO promoted human rights framing of the epidemic and response, and the adoption of this frame (in conjunction and competition with other frames) by global institutions and donors. This frame expanded conceptions of ill health and appropriate responses to include social, economic and political causes and correctives. Peer support and equal access to health care became key principles of the response. While Western understandings of this rights-frame remain dominant, HIV/AIDS CSOs in other parts of the world have integrated it with, and adapted it to, indigenous approaches – for example, by linking global frames around sexuality with local conceptions of rights.

While the rights-based frame emerged in conflict with biomedical neoliberal understandings, it has become increasingly entwined with these, particularly during the period of HIV/AIDS exceptionalism, raising questions such as: does this indicate a co-option of rights alternatives or a sophisticated subversion of hegemonic ideas? The evidence of how CSOs have continued to advance rights goals within the current key populations frame suggests that the linking of biomedical and rights approaches has continued to create space for CSO participants to advance claims – by linking a rights-based approach with efficiency language – but also restricted possibilities for transformation – for example, by failing to move beyond a narrow understanding of women's rights. In the current political economy of restricted opportunities, continued struggles, such as around funding for key populations in middle-income countries, demonstrate that CSO actors are well aware of the compromises and contradictions within the conflation of rights and biomedical frames, and are attempting to use the space available to advance alternatives that will better meet the needs of those most affected by the epidemic.

Widespread acceptance of rights framing, and the linked argument for CSO participation, generated global institutional forms that were more inclusive than previous arrangements (Rittberger et al. 2008). Both UNAIDS and the Global Fund have involved people from marginalized constituencies – including gay men from countries were same-sex relations are illegal, PWIDs, sex workers and women from impoverished communities. Do these individuals represent broader constituencies? They aim to represent their interests by promoting rights-based responses within the institutions. Therefore, while the institutions themselves may not be representative, they have incorporated members of marginalized constituencies to promote these interests. However,

there is also need for a nuanced analysis that illuminates the barriers CSO participants face working within rigid institutional structures.

A degree of agency has also been demonstrated, with CSOs exercising a particular type of influence – tied to their role as members (as opposed to representatives) of affected populations – and expert status based on lived experience, both of which generate discursive and emotive influence. CSOs have used this influence, as well as that derived from their global networks, to continue to advocate rights agendas, having some more clearly identifiable successes – such as ensuring indicators in global HIV/AIDS reporting that measure rights-based outcomes – than others. So while CSOs might not have transformed institutional governance, they have promoted shifts towards a more equitable order in and through institutions.

CSO efforts are complicated by the multiple agendas within a loose coalition. Not only are health related CSOs competing for resources, as demonstrated by conflicts over the framing of the SDGs, the influence of evangelical CSOs in determining PEPFAR's Anti-Prostitution Pledge demonstrates competing notions of rights-based responses. Consequently, the identification of sex workers as a key population has had both transformative and repressive impacts. This is a crucial reminder to advocates of greater CSO participation in GHG that CSO influence can take many different forms and have oppressive, as well as empowering, outcomes.

Possibilities for transformation in the HIV/AIDS response have become increasingly restricted by trends within the political economy of global health, as evidenced by the limited opportunities to continue to advance funding for key populations in middle-income countries through the Global Fund's NFM. CSOs need to ask themselves challenging questions about their participation in resource mobilization. Is it possible that they could use their role as advocates for greater funding to have more significant power over resource distribution? Currently, CSOs mobilize funds they have little control over, raising questions about whose interests their advocacy efforts serve. The continued dominance of donor states and institutions in deciding how resources are used, presents perhaps the most crucial struggle for CSOs in the HIV/AIDS response.

Yet, even when considering conservative spending directives, the narrow priorities of donors and conflicts among health and rights-based CSOs, the exceptional amount of resources dedicated to the HIV/AIDS response has not, despite some analysis, done harm. It has in fact achieved clearly identifiable "good" – 15.8 million PWAs are on treatment and new infections have decline by 35 per cent globally since 2000 (UNAIDS 2015). What has been raised, through CSO advocacy, state initiatives and donor support, should not be negated.

CSOs have contributed transformational elements to global HIV/AIDS governance by promoting an alternative human rights frame and demanding space to represent the interests of those most affected in governance forums. This transformation began among those most affected by the epidemic who

demanded a global response that was inclusive and rights-based. While governance outcomes have been limited by shifts in the broader political economy, rigid institutional forms, and a continued lack of CSO power to determine resource distribution, CSOs remain active participants. The have advanced a rights-based response in global HIV/AIDS governance, despite these limits and many changes in the response over the past 30 years, fostering continued transformative potential.

Understanding CSO functions and influence within GHG

Murphy (2000), among others, has noted that critical IR theorists have not done a good job of documenting how community groups and movements promote alternatives and influence global governance. This book aims to contribute to filling this gap by presenting a historical case of how grassroots mobilization aimed to influence a global response towards a more equitable order. This demonstrates that analysis of such processes is not only possible, but can also contribute critical perspectives on how and why change in global governance occurs. In this case, the role of CSOs is positioned as instrumental in advancing alternatives within the HIV/AIDS response, contributing to discussions on why the response has been exceptional, and on current changes within it. Such analysis adds deeper understandings of global governance processes and non-state actors within them.

This analysis is rooted in historical experience, as opposed to theoretical confines. Instead of forcing governance processes into predetermined categories, such as agenda setting, this more flexible framework starts with history, looking at how the global HIV/AIDS response has changed, why and to what effect. This ensures that the analysis is not just of stated intentions, but also of the outcomes of these intentions. CSO participation is not accepted as promoting a rights-based response because CSOs say they are rights-based, but because they created and defined a rights-based frame, and their participation has resulted in identifiable rights-based changes – such as removal of HIV/AIDS travel bans in China and the USA.

This historical account is situated within the context of the political economy of global health, demonstrating that where and why CSOs have influenced change, and where they have not, relates as much to external forces, and interests of other actors within them, as to the characteristics, motivations and agency of the CSOs. For example, CSOs were incorporated into UNAIDS' governance structure because of their successful promotion of the GWIPA principles, as well as the desire by many states to experiment with creating more responsive UN systems. Therefore, Lencucha et al.'s (2010) argument for context specific analysis of the role of and opportunities for CSOs in global governance is strengthened.

Analysis of CSO governance contributions to the Global Fund and UNAIDS suggest concepts such as legitimacy and accountability have to be adaptable to the unique global governance arrangements that are emerging. Both

institutional cases suggest that CSO participation has few positive legitimacy outcomes. CSO insistence on certain issues (such as funding for their own organizations) and methods (such as activist tactics) can detract from the legitimacy of GHIs. CSOs only contribute to both input and output legitimacy where they not only have influence over decision-making, but also can shape processes. Where CSOs' preferred engagement strategies, such as activism, are not tolerated (such as within UNAIDS) they face challenges to their input legitimacy because of the need to adapt to hegemonic interests' preferred processes, which in turn alienates their constituents. Institutions that aim to effectively include civil society must consider how to be flexible to CSOs' preferred processes.

Weak legitimacy, combined with rigid bureaucracies, necessarily affects the ability of CSO participants within institutions to generate downward accountability. In both institutional cases analysed here CSO delegations do not generate strong downward accountability relations – at best representing networks of horizontal accountability with allied CSOs. The Global Fund's Partnership Forum presents an example of a complex, but one-way accountability mechanism, the value of which is questionable. Due to weak downward accountability relationships, CSOs can contribute to, as opposed to mitigate, dominant power relations and bureaucratic processes that alienate constituents. This supports Bartsch's (2007) assertion that CSO participation can create new, as well as address old, accountability challenges.

However, there are also previously under-discussed positive outcomes of CSO participation, for example, the ability, and utility of external CSOs to strengthen accountability. External CSOs that aim to share and comment on institutional processes make greater contributions to downward accountability. For example, CSOs that produce and disseminate information about the Global Fund have forced it to be more transparent and accessible; CSOs that work with the UNAIDS Secretariat to produce the GARP reports strengthen global accountability processes. CSOs external to GHIs have influence as watchdogs, sharing information to motivate change and forcing institutions to increasingly consult civil society and improve the accessibility of their information. These cases suggest downward accountability is best generated from outside the institution, as opposed to within it.

Implicit in the analysis presented here are the questions – what types of power do CSOs have in global governance processes, where and why? While findings here are specific to the HIV/AIDS response, they may provide indications for further analysis of CSO influence in global governance. The first type of power CSOs exert is the power of an alternative. When biomedical responses failed to develop an initial response to the epidemic, CSOs were well positioned to assert a different type of response. The central role CSOs played in the early response provided them with space and credibility, on their own terms, to mitigate the risk of co-option by powerful interests.

CSO representatives have power as members of key populations. Their lived experiences of stigma and discrimination, of living with the virus, and

being on the receiving end of the response generates justification for their participation in global institutions, and also demands that other actors listen to them. This normative validity of lived experience that CSO representatives bring to governance forums presents a corrective to processes that are often accused of being dominated by technical experts and distanced from realities on the ground. Within the institutional governance arrangements discussed here, CSOs have translated key population status into discursive and emotive influence.

Within debates over the role of global governance, there are those who suggest CSOs have little influence in global governance processes, acting only as conduits of more powerful interests (Bebbington et al. 2008). Within the HIV/AIDS response there are ample examples of CSOs struggling against powerful actors, such when the NGO Delegation to UNAIDS PCB challenged Iran and Egypt with strong decision point language on human rigths. Though CSOs have frequently cooperated with other governance actors, this has most often been in order to advance their own goals within the confines of dominant biomedical neoliberalism. For example, by cooperating with like-minded members of the UNAIDS PCB, the NGO Delegation was enable to ensure its proposed decision points stood.

CSOs generate influence through their extensive networks. Despite differences, conflicts and competition between CSOs, their ability to converge around specific issues, such as the need for greater resources, provides a cumulative influence. The Communities Delegation to the Global Fund was able to convince other delegations to support its demand that China lift travel restrictions on PWAs, and together these allies worked with other organizations, such as UNAIDS, to fight travel restrictions around the world. It is these moments of cooperation that have generated the greatest CSO-initiated change in the global governance of the HIV/AIDS response.

While the outcomes of CSO struggles rarely fully achieve their goals (as the continued challenges to effectively implement a response that empowers women indicate), the struggles themselves depict resistance to co-option. Within the global HIV/AIDS response, CSOs are considered actors that should not be antagonized, but must be brought into cooperative arrangements (often through certain rights concessions in declarations, decisions and funding structures). Just as the hegemonic approach of biomedical neoliberalism within GHG cannot be ignored, neither can the rights-based agenda of CSO coalitions.

Findings support Benner et al.'s (2004) assertion that neither full-blown optimism nor pessimism is helpful in conceptualizing the role of CSOs in global governance. The role of CSOs in the HIV/AIDS response has promoted alternatives to hegemonic approaches, strengthening rights considerations, but has had limited governance outputs related to improving legitimacy and accountability, or directing resources to community groups. The outcomes of CSO participation are much more complex than previously presented, and are not all positive.

A primary limitation to this research is that the focus on global governance processes directs analysis to one level of engagement. Because the focus is on

global-level processes, the discussion of specific rights campaigns such as for PWID, MSM and sex workers are discussed in less detail than a more focused analysis might allow. There is an opportunity to expand on many of the themes in this book – such as the use of global forums to create acceptance of harm reduction and how this impacts national and local struggles – through further research. Such research would be a valuable contribution as lack of recognition of rights struggles can result in neglect, with donors and policy-makers ignoring such rights claims. By drawing attention to the struggles of CSOs to promote rights other than access to treatment, this book provides examples of resistance that are often ignored in academic literature and policy discussions about the HIV/AIDS response. There is a need for much further research on CSO campaigns for human rights through global governance forums and processes.

This book has woven feminist analysis into a broader discussion of CSOs and HIV/AIDS response, arguing that the gendered nature of the epidemic necessitates consideration of the gendered structure of the response. Feminist analysis demands the constant linking of global processes to outcomes, and subsequent re-evaluation of claims to support rights. The question behind such analysis is – but what does this mean for women and other marginalized populations? For example, the success of Option B+ is evaluated not against global targets, but the impact of the programme on the wellbeing and relationships of women affected. In particular, feminist analysis has exposed the failure of all aspects of the HIV/AIDS response to prioritize the needs of the group most affected by the epidemic (impoverished women living in Sub-Saharan Africa). Women's rights have been neglected by institutions, such as the Global Fund, under the justification of country ownership, and the key populations frame continues this neglect. In the meantime the burden of HIV/AIDS care work continues to fall on those with the least resources. Explicitly outlining these continued patterns facilitates analyses of why change does not happen, as well as why it does; questions crucial to understanding future opportunities for CSOs. Feminist analysis has demonstrated the limits of transformation, making explicit the continued dominance of biomedical neo-liberalism and its patriarchal nature. There is a need for much greater feminist critique of GHG, including of the role of CSOs within it, in order to expose continued androcentric approaches and patriarchal power structures.

CSOs and the rebuilding of GHG

Considering ongoing calls to reform and rebuild GHG, a final question that emerges is – if it is accepted that CSO participation is beneficial within GHG, or even just an established reality how can governance arrangements be crafted to make it more effective and responsive? As the quote at the beginning of the introduction demonstrates, the HIV/AIDS response is not a case of dominant global governance actors deciding to include CSOs; it is a case of CSOs creating a movement, demanding a global response and then

ensuring their own place within this response. Acceptance by states and institutions was required, but it can be argued that these other actors had little choice, considering the prominent role CSOs played in initiating the global HIV/AIDS response. Therefore, this implies that CSO participation must be self-generated, not brought in after the fact. Policies that aim to promote greater and more effective CSO participation might do well to look at existing CSO mobilization, and support CSOs in these endeavours, as opposed to trying to create social movements or networks from the top down.

Having demonstrated that CSOs have contributed to potential transformation in the global HIV/AIDS governance, a further follow-up question is – have these changes had ripple effects beyond the HIV/AIDS field to other aspects of GHG, and global governance in general? Key informants note that they had hoped the example of CSO involvement in the HIV/AIDS response would set a precedent for governance processes around other issue areas. Some express frustration that this has not been achieved, noting that many institutions, such as the WHO, still do not incorporate CSOs in a meaningful way. Others argue that now the precedent of CSO involvement in global HIV/AIDS governance has been set it would be hard for GHIs to go back to primarily state-based systems. These commentators cite the example of CSO participation in setting the SDG agenda as evidence of acceptance of CSO involvement. The history presented here suggests that CSO participation in the HIV/AIDS response has set a new precedent, or a higher bar of inclusivity – whether current and future governance arrangements will rise to meet the challenge, and perhaps advance it, remains to be seen.

What does this history indicate for the future of the HIV/AIDS response and the role of CSOs within it? CSOs are facing one of the most restrictive funding environments of the past 30 years, which is forcing questions about priorities and threatening to divide coalitions in a time where cooperation is essential. The broad goal of SDG3 demonstrates the influence of various health movements, but achieving the wide-ranging targets will require cooperation not only among these movements but beyond the health sector with environmental, trade and other activists. Despite the progress of the HIV/AIDS response over past 30 years, the challenges facing CSOs that envision a GHG that reflects the right to health are perhaps more daunting then ever. Reflecting on these challenges, Parker writes:

> In the now 30 year history of the civil society response to the epidemic, grassroots activists have managed to transform their movement into a transnational coalition capable of overcoming the resistance of some of the most powerful private interests in the world and creating an unprecedented level of mobilization of public institutions at both the national and intergovernmental level in ways that are unheard of in relation to any other global health issue. While the economic and policy challenges are significant, the persistence of the AIDS activist movement in seeking to

transform the world's response to the epidemic should give us at least some reason for hope about the future.

(2011, 35)

The sum of the findings presented here support Parker's suggestion that there is reason to hope for the future. CSOs engaged in GHIs are proving increasingly apt at working within existing systems to advance human rights discussions despite a restrictive political economy. The NFM of the Global Fund, while representing continued restrictions on CSO influence over resource use, also creates opportunities for CSOs to demand funding for rights-based interventions, and history suggests they will continue to do so with fervour. Despite repressive policies around the rights of sexual minorities in many countries, increasing global mobilization deems these unacceptable, and local actors are adapting struggles for sexual rights to the local HIV/AIDS response and society in general. CSOs continue to demand critical conversations be held around new developments in the response, such as Option B+; not opposing them, but asserting the need for a rights-based ethos to their rollout, ensuring such endeavours do more good than harm. Without CSOs, it is unlikely such conversations would occur. It is these ongoing struggles that justify Parker's "hope about the future".

This hope is not based on false promises about the End of AIDS, generated in Geneva, or an AIDS Free Generation, generated in Washington D.C. It is based on the committed individuals and organizations around the world who have struggled to promote more inclusive and responsive global governance arrangements in response to one of the most defining health threats of the past half century.

References

Bartsch, S. (2007), "The Global Fund to Fight AIDS, Tuberculosis and Malaria", in Hein, W., Bartsch, S. and Kohlmorgen, L. (Eds), *Global Health Governance and the Fight against HIV/AIDS*, Palgrave Macmillan, New York, pp. 146–171.

Bebbington, A., Hickey, S. and Mitlin, D. (Eds) (2008), *Can NGOs Make a Difference?: The Challenge of Development Alternatives*, Zed Books, London.

Benner, T., Reinicke, W.H. and Witte, J.M. (2004), "Multisectoral Networks in Global Governance: Towards a Pluralistic System of Accountability", *Government and Opposition*, Vol. 39 No. 2, pp. 191–210.

Lencucha, R., Labonté, R. and Rouse, M.J. (2010), "Beyond Idealism and Realism: Canadian NGO/Government Relations During the Negotiation of the FCTC", *Journal of Public Health Policy*, Vol. 31 No. 1, pp. 74–87.

Murphy, C. (2000), "Global Governance: Poorly Done and Poorly Understood", *International Affairs*, Vol. 76 No. 4, pp. 189–803.

Parker, R. (2011), "Grassroots Activism, Civil Society Mobilization, and the Politics of the Global HIV/AIDS Epidemic", *Brown Journal of World Affairs*, Vol. 21 No. 2, pp. 2–37.

Rittberger, V., Huckel, C., Rieth, L. and Zimmer, M. (2008), "Inclusive Global Institutions for a Global Political Economy", in Rittberger, V., Nettesheim, M. and

Huckel, C. (Eds), *Authority in the Global Political Economy*, Palgrave Macmillan, New York.

UNAIDS (2015), *Fact Sheet 2015*, Geneva, available at: http://www.unaids.org/en/resources/campaigns/HowAIDSchangedeverything/factsheet (accessed 15 December 2015).

Appendix: Key informants

Classification	Number of informants
Civil Society Representatives	20
GHI Representatives	17
State Representatives	2

Location of informants by WHO regions	
Africa	7
Americas	8
South East Asia	1
Europe	21
Eastern Mediterranean	1
Western Pacific	1

Sex	
Male	20
Female	19

Organizations represented

A number of informants were affiliated with more than one organization. All affiliations are listed here:

1 Aids Accountability International
2 Aids Coalition to Unleash Power (ActUP)
3 AIDS Rights Alliance of Southern Africa
4 Aidspan
5 Asia Pacific Network of People Living with HIV/AIDS
6 ATHENA Network

7   Canadian HIV/AIDS Legal Network
8   Center for Health and Gender Equality
9   European Treatment Action Group
10   Fermont Center
11   Global Fund to Fight AIDS, Tuberculosis and Malaria
12   Global Network for and by People Living with HIV/AIDS
13   Harm Reduction International
14   Health Economics and HIV/AIDS Research Division
15   International Coalition of AIDS Support Organizations
16   International Community of Women with HIV/AIDS
17   International HIV/AIDS Alliance
18   International Network of People Who Use Drugs
19   Médicins Sans Frontières
20   ONE
21   Pivot Legal Society
22   Positive Women's Network
23   Stop HIV/AIDS Alliance
24   Treatment Action Coalition
25   UNAIDS
26   UNDP
27   UNICEF
28   WomenArise
29   World AIDS Campaign

Index

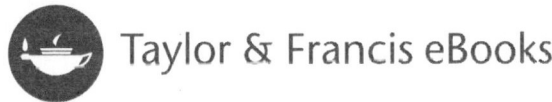
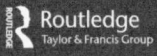